CANCER PREVENTION
AND EARLY DIAGNOSIS
IN WOMEN

CANCER PREVENTION AND EARLY DIAGNOSIS IN WOMEN

ALBERTO MANETTA, MD
Professor, Department of Obstetrics and Gynecology
Department of Internal Medicine, Division of Epidemiology
Senior Associate Dean of Education Affairs
University of California, Irvine
Orange, California

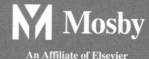 Mosby

An Affiliate of Elsevier

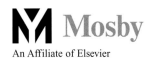

An Affiliate of Elsevier

The Curtis Center
Independence Square West
Philadelphia, Pennsylvania 19106

CANCER PREVENTION AND EARLY DIAGNOSIS IN WOMEN   ISBN 0-323-01347-3
Copyright © 2004, Elsevier Science (USA). All rights reserved.

NOTICE

Medicine is an ever-changing field. Standard safety precautions must be followed, but as new research
and clinical experience broaden our knowledge, changes in treatment and drug therapy may become
necessary or appropriate. Licensed health care providers are advised to check the most current product
information provided by the manufacturer of each drug to be administered to verify the
recommended dose, the method and duration of administration, and contraindications. It is the
responsibility of the licensed prescriber, relying on experience and knowledge of the patient, to determine dosages and the best treatment for each individual patient. Neither the publisher nor the editor
assumes any liability for any injury and/or damage to persons or property arising from this
publication.

International Standard Book Number 0-323-01347-3
Library of Congress Cataloging-in-Publication Data

Cancer prevention and early diagnosis in women / [edited by] Alberto Manetta. – 1st ed.
      p. ; cm.
   Includes bibliographical references and index.
   ISBN 0-323-01347-3
   1. Cancer in women–Prevention. 2. Cancer in women–Diagnosis. 3. Medical screening.
   I. Manetta, Alberto.
   [DNLM: 1. Neoplasms–prevention & control. 2. Neoplams–diagnosis. 3. Women's
Health. QZ 200 C2153637 2004]
   RC281. W65C365 2004
   616.99′4052′082-dc21

                                                                          2003044208

Acquisitions Editor: Stephanie Donley
Developmental Editor: Kim J. Davis
Publishing Services Manager: Patricia Tannian
Project Manager: Sharon Corell
Book Design Manager: Gail Morey Hudson
Cover Design: Liz Rohne Rudder

Printed in China

Last digit is the print number: 9   8   7   5   4   3   2   1

I wish to dedicate this book
to my family
my children **Kathryn** *and* **Edward**
and Edward's wife **Jennifer**
for their encouragement, patience, and devotion
and my wife **Nancy**
whose unwavering love and support
have made this book and indeed my career possible.

AM

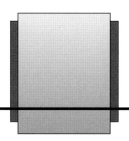

Contributors

MICHELE A. CARTER, PhD
Associate Professor of Ethics and Philosophy
Institute for the Medical Humanities
Director, Institutional Ethics Program
University of Texas Medical Branch
Galveston, Texas

HELENA R. CHANG, MD, PhD
Professor, Department of Surgery
David Geffen School of Medicine
University of California, Los Angeles;
Director, Revlon UCLA Breast Center
Los Angeles, California

ROBERT CLARK, MD, MBA
Professor and Chairman
Department of Radiology
University of South Florida College of
    Medicine;
Chief of Radiology
H. Lee Moffitt Cancer Center and Research
    Institute
Tampa, Florida

VIVIAN DICKERSON, MD
Associate Clinical Professor
Samueli Center for Complementary and
    Alternative Medicine
Department of Obstetrics and Gynecology
University of California, Irvine
Orange, California

MERRILL EISENBERG, PhD
Assistant Professor
Mel and Enid Zuckerman Arizona College of
    Public Health, The University of Arizona
Tucson, Arizona

LINDA L. GARLAND, MD
Assistant Professor of Medicine
Lung Cancer Program, Arizona Cancer Center
University of Arizona Health Sciences Center
Tucson, Arizona

HOWARD D. HOMESLEY, MD
Clinical Professor
Vanderbilt University Medical School
Gynecologic Oncology and General Surgery of
    Middle Tennessee
Nashville, Tennessee

JAMES JAKOWATZ, MD
Assistant Professor in Residence
Department of Surgery Oncology
University of California, Irvine Medical
    Center
Orange, California

KAREN TODD LANE, MD
Assistant Professor in Residence
Department of Surgery
University of California, San Francisco
San Francisco, California

SHIRAZ I. MISHRA, MD, PhD
Associate Professor
Samueli Center for Complementary and
    Alternative Medicine
Department of Medicine, University of
    California, Irvine
Irvine, California

WADIE I. NAJIM, MD
Associate Clinical Professor
Department of Family Medicine and Geriatrics
University of California, Irvine
University of California, Irvine Medical Center
Orange, California

VANDANA S. NANDA, MD
Associate Professor of Dermatology
University of California, Irvine
University of California, Irvine Medical Center
Orange, California

PAMELA J. POWERS, MS
Program Director
Network for Information and Counseling
College of Public Health
University of Arizona
Tucson, Arizona

MARK S. SHAHIN, MD
Clinical Assistant Professor
Department of Obstetrics and Gynecology
Temple University School of Medicine
Philadelphia, Pennsylvania;
Gynecologic Oncologist
Rosenfeld Cancer Center
Abington Memorial Hospital
Abington, Pennsylvania

JOEL I. SOROSKY, MD
Professor of Obstetrics and Gynecology
Director, Division of Gynecologic Oncology
The University of Iowa Hospitals and Clinics
Iowa City, Iowa

KRISHNANSU SUJATA TEWARI, MD
Assistant Clinical Professor
The Division of Gynecologic Oncology
Department of Obstetrics and Gynecology
University of California, Irvine Medical Center;
The Southern California
    Permanente Medical Group;
Kaiser Foundation
Hospitals of Bellflower,
    Baldwin Park, and
    Harbor City, California

CHARLES P. THEUER, MD, PhD
Assistant Clinical Professor
Department of Medicine and Surgery
University of California, Irvine
Irvine, California;
University of California, Irvine Medical Center
Department of Medicine and Surgery
Orange, California

Preface

Women's health care is being defined as a new discipline that transcends and blends the boundaries of traditional clinical disciplines. The interlocking specialties primarily involved in women's health include obstetrics and gynecology, internal medicine, family medicine, geriatrics, and pediatrics. There is a need for health care providers to have the knowledge to properly understand the predisposition to cancer. They also must be able to assess cancer risk, provide contemporary advice on prevention, and prescribe appropriate screening tests for early diagnosis.

The intention of this book is to address the assessment of risk, prevention, and early diagnosis of cancer in women. It is not an encyclopedic volume addressing every known cancer. It is limited to cancers that occur most frequently and are responsible for the greatest mortality in the United States, with special emphasis on gynecologic cancers. This is not a simple how-to book. It addresses the subject of cancer comprehensively, providing the most appropriate scientifically based information available. The book is divided into 12 chapters and includes the principles of cancer screening, the most common cancer sites, ethical and legal implications of genetic testing, and an evidence-based analysis of complementary therapies in cancer prevention.

Cancer screening is an important step in the prevention and early diagnosis of cancer. Many general principles of cancer screening are common to the various cancers and screening strategies. Chapter 1 outlines these principles as well as the common terms, benefits, and risks of cancer screening. Assessment of screening programs, the potential for bias and error in evaluation, and systematic methods for evaluation are also discussed in this chapter.

There are nine chapters covering specific cancers: breast, cervical, colorectal, lung, ovarian, skin, uterine corpus, vaginal, and vulvar. These chapters investigate incidence and mortality, assess associated risk factors, and explore the methods of prevention, early detection, and diagnosis available for these cancers. Age-related incidence, geographic distribution, genetic and familial risk factors, and various social and ethnic group effects are also addressed.

Chapter 11 explores the ethical and legal dimensions of genetic testing used to prevent hereditary disease. The three sections of this chapter describe issues related to the use and limitations of genetic testing for cancer susceptibility, address the emerging ethical, legal and social concerns associated with genetic testing, and provide an ethical framework for addressing these concerns.

The last chapter in this book presents an evidence-based analysis of complementary therapies in cancer prevention. The first two sections define complementary and alternative medicine (CAM) and explore literature review methodology. The potential anticarcinogenic action of several CAM therapies is presented in the next section, followed by an in-depth examination of CAM therapies associated with specific types of cancer.

Considering the redefinition and interlocking of specialties in women's health care today, it is vital for health care providers and trainees to acquire specialized knowledge that enables them to properly assess cancer risk. The dissemination of comprehensive, scientifically based, practical information focused on the prevention of women's cancer is an essential step in decreasing the devastating impact of this disease. *Cancer Prevention and Early Diagnosis in Women* is presented to furnish health care providers with the information needed for the assessment of risk, prevention, and early diagnosis of cancer in women.

Alberto Manetta, MD

Contents

1 Principles of Cancer Screening, 1
Robert Clark

2 Cancer of the Lung, 12
Linda L. Garland, Merrill Eisenberg, and Pamela J. Powers

3 Breast Cancer Risk Factors and Prevention, 48
Karen Todd Lane and Helena R. Chang

4 Colorectal Cancer, 69
Charles P. Theuer

5 Skin Cancer, 122
Vandana S. Nanda and James Jakowatz

6 Cervical Cancer, 148
Alberto Manetta

7 Cancer of the Vagina, 190
Alberto Manetta

8 Cancer of the Vulva, 197
Krishnansu Sujata Tewari

9 Prevention and Early Diagnosis of Ovarian Cancer, 249
Mark S. Shahin and Joel I. Sorosky

10 Cancer of the Uterine Corpus, 267
Howard D. Homesley and Alberto Manetta

11 Ethical and Legal Implications of Genetic Testing in
Preventive Health, 289
Michele A. Carter

12 Complementary Therapies in Cancer Prevention, 306
Shiraz I. Mishra, Wadie I. Najim, and Vivian Dickerson

CHAPTER 1

Principles of Cancer Screening

Robert Clark

INTRODUCTION

Cancer screening seems intuitively beneficial. The concept of detecting a cancer early, when the tumor is manageable and has not spread from its primary site, rather than late, when it has metastasized to other vital organs, seems reasonable. Yet, despite being intuitive, cancer screening remains controversial and often confusing. Why not screen everyone in order to detect all cancers early? Should screening always be recommended for the most common or most lethal cancers? Conversely, how can cancer screening be considered useful when most screened individuals never get the disease yet incur the costs of screening and the risk of a false-positive test?

Although the answers to these questions often are different for specific cancers, many general principles of cancer screening are common to the various cancers and screening strategies. The purposes of this chapter are to outline the principles of cancer screening, define terms common to all types of screening, articulate the expected benefits and potential risks of screening, offer criteria for assessment of proposed screening programs, delineate the potential sources of bias and error in evaluation, and propose systematic methods for evaluation of cancer screening.

Cancer screening principles should be considered ideals; few, if any, cancer screening strategies will fulfill all the degrees of proof. However, these principles should be used as a framework when reading the scientific literature and evaluating the rationale for new screening tests or proposed strategies. The farther the rationale for a new screening strategy wanders from these principles, the less justification there is for its adoption.

CANCER SCREENING

Screening is the application of a test to detect a potential cancer where no signs or symptoms of the cancer are present.[1-4] Testing for cancer screening involves both the traditional cancer detection tests and newer molecular or genetic tests for increased risk. The traditional type test ideally detects cancer before it is clinically apparent; early in its natural history; before it has become systemic; or when treatment may be more effective, less expensive, or both. An abnormal screening test in this situation leads to further diagnostic evaluation to determine whether cancer is present and if cancer is detected, leads to subsequent treatment. The second type of screening, which may become more prevalent in the future, involves screening for genetic or molecular markers that designate a high risk for developing cancer. It is not always clear what an abnormal screening test in this situation means or what recommendations should follow.[5,6]

Cancer screening is a secondary form of cancer prevention, as distinguished from primary prevention, such as avoidance of cigarette smoking to prevent lung cancer. The term "cancer screening" is synonymous with other terms, such as "detection" or "early detection,"[1-3] and has been modified by some authors as "mass," "routine," "regular," or "selective" cancer screening. However, these modifiers have no universally accepted definitions. Every cancer screening strategy must identify its target population, the proposed screening test, and the frequency of the screening test. Knowledge of these parameters for any screening strategy makes other modifier terms moot.

Cancer Screening Test

The cancer screening test is the method used to detect a specific target cancer[1-3] and may consist of a single modality or a combination of tests. Laboratory tests of blood or body fluids, physical examinations, invasive procedures, and imaging tests are examples of screening tests.

Asymptomatic

The goal of cancer screening is to detect cancer before it is clinically apparent. Therefore "asymptomatic" is defined in the perspective of the individual who has no known signs or symptoms of cancer before the screening test. For example, as a result of a digital rectal examination, a physician detects a prostate nodule on the gland of a man with no previously known signs or symptoms. The patient then has a sign of cancer detected by the physician and the screening test; nevertheless, the man was asymptomatic before the screening and the cancer was detected by screening. This example of asymptomatic status is appropriate even if the man had symptoms related to another condition, such as benign prostate hypertrophy.

Screened Individual

Screened individuals are often inappropriately called "patients." Screening involves the testing of asymptomatic people. A screened individual does not become a "patient" until the screening test is abnormal. New concerns, anxieties, costs, and discomforts begin when the individual becomes a "patient." Ideally, screened individuals should be identified as "people" or "subjects," rather than patients.

Target Population

The target population of a proposed screening strategy defines the characteristics of an individual who would be appropriate to receive the screening test. Certain characteristics identify an individual as a candidate for cancer screening. For example, because prostate cancer is rare in teenage boys, screening is inappropriate in this age group of males. Typical defining characteristics of a target population include sex, family history, specific known risk factors, geographic region of birth or residence, race or ethnicity, and age.

Screening Practitioner

The screening practitioner is the health care professional who performs the cancer screening test,[1-3] including primary care physicians, specialist physicians, nurses, physician assistants, and technicians.

Diagnosis

Screening is not diagnosis.[1,2,7] The cancer screening test identifies asymptomatic individuals with a high likelihood of having cancer. Screened individuals then are separated by the screening test into two subsequent groups: those with normal test results (high likelihood of not having cancer) and those with abnormal results (high likelihood of having cancer). In some individuals with normal results from a screening test, cancer may be subsequently detected with diagnostic tests such as biopsy (a false-negative screening test). All individuals with abnormal screening test results require some diagnostic evaluation. Some of those with abnormal results and further diagnostic evaluation will not have cancer (a false-positive screening test). Diagnosis is the clinical problem-solving process applied to symptomatic individuals or asymptomatic individuals with abnormal screening tests.

Symptomatic individuals require diagnostic evaluation to determine the cause of symptoms. A screening test applied to a symptomatic person should not be considered a screening event because diagnostic evaluation is required regardless of the results of the screening test. Moreover, the value of a screening strategy cannot be assessed if symptomatic individuals are included in the target population because these people may already have advanced disease that needs diagnostic evaluation.

Screening Strategy or Protocol

A cancer screening strategy or protocol defines the operational parameters of a cancer screening program: who, how, what, where, and when. The screening strategy or protocol defines the population to be screened (the target population) and the screening test to be used as well as when and how often the screening test should be applied. The screening strategy also may define who should perform the screening test, the conditions under which it should be applied, and the criteria for an abnormal test. A screening strategy or protocol is useful in designing clinical trials and interpreting scientific data about screening. Another function of screening strategies or protocols is to make recommendations to individuals or groups about cancer screening.[1-3]

The screening protocol design must be clearly understood when interpreting scientific evidence about cancer screening. The protocol of a screening clinical trial often is limited. Therefore the results obtained by the trial are valid only for the conditions of that protocol. For example, a cancer screening protocol that studies a target population of white European women ages 50 to 69 years, applies a screening test every 2 years for 10 years, and finds 40% fewer cancer deaths in screened women than in unscreened women suggests strong evidence of the effectiveness of cancer screening. However, it may not be applicable to women older than 69 years of age, to women younger than 50 years, or to Japanese women, and the results of this protocol may not be enough evidence alone to justify recommending cancer screening annually for all Black women older than 40 years of age. Alternatively, a cancer screening test applied to men between ages 65 and 75 years that shows no benefit to the screened group when compared with unscreened men does not signify a lack of potential benefit to screening men younger than age 65 years. The results simply show that no information about screening younger men is available from the screening test.

The scientific literature focusing on cancer screening is replete with clinical trials that have different screening strategies and protocols for the same target cancer. It is difficult to compare or combine the data from these trials to answer scientific questions that were not posed before the design of the clinical trial. However, cancer screening strategies in clinical practice are not limited to those studied by clinical trials; they may be recommended by individual practitioners, professional medical societies, public health agencies, and health maintenance organizations. Their recommendations are based on their best assessment of the available scientific evidence, as well as their best estimate of applicability to individuals or target populations not included in the original scientific protocols, which varies among groups, practitioners, and policy-makers. Therefore it is not surprising that "guidelines" for cancer screening may vary among various organizations and among practitioners.

Outcomes

The scientific evidence of the value of screening requires that outcomes of a screening protocol be measured. Outcomes are the health and economic results that are related to screening.[1,8,9] Outcomes include the benefits, harms, and costs of screening as well as its incurred diagnostic evaluations. Outcomes are measured by tracking the detailed clinical results of screened individuals (Box 1-1).

Effectiveness

The effectiveness of cancer screening is determined by comparing outcomes to ascertain if the benefits outweigh the harms and whether the health outcomes (benefits and harms) justify the costs.[1,8,9] Moreover, the outcomes and effectiveness measures of the screened population must be compared with those of a similar unscreened group. For example, for a screening program to be judged effective, the stage distribution of detected cancers in screened individuals should be lower than cancers detected in unscreened people. However, although lower stage distribution is a necessary condition of effectiveness, it is not sufficient. In addition, the case-fatality rate and, more important, the site-specific mortality rate for a screened group should be significantly less than that of an unscreened group.

Cost-effectiveness

Ideally, the total cost of the screening program (the total of screening costs, diagnostic evaluations, treatment costs of detected cancers, and value of years of life lost to cancer deaths) should be less than the total cost for the unscreened group (the total of diagnostic evaluations, treatment costs of detected cancers, and value of years of life lost to cancer deaths). Relevant costs to be considered in this evaluation are listed in Box 1-2. However, cost savings that result from screening programs have been difficult to determine.[8] Hence, other cost measures, such as cost-determination, cost-minimization, cost-effectiveness, cost-benefit, and cost-utility analyses, are often analyzed.[1,9-14]

 BOX 1-1   Outcome Measures in a Cancer Screening Program

Short-term Measures
Number of individuals in the target population who were offered screening
Number and proportion of individuals in the target population who received screening
Number and proportion of target population who were examined by multiple screens
Number or prevalence of preclinical cancers detected
Proportion of abnormal screened individuals brought to definitive diagnosis or follow-up
Monetary cost per cancer detected
Sensitivity and specificity of the screening test
Positive and negative predictive values of the screening test
Long-term Measures
Stage distribution of detected cancers
Case-fatality rate of screened individuals
Site-specific cancer mortality rate of screened target population
Total monetary costs

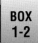

BOX 1-2   **Relevant Costs of a Cancer Screening Program**

Costs of Screening Tests
- Direct costs or charges
- Indirect costs (time, anxiety)

Costs Incurred by Abnormal Screening Test
- Direct costs or charges of diagnostic evaluation or biopsy
- Indirect costs of complications, morbidity, anxiety, time, loss of work

Costs Related to False-positive Screening Tests
- Direct costs or charges of diagnostic evaluation or biopsy
- Indirect costs of complications, morbidity, anxiety, time, loss of work

Costs Related to False-negative Screening Tests
- False sense of security
- Delay in diagnosis due to disregard of clinical symptoms

Costs Related to Treatment and Rehabilitation
- Direct costs or charges of treatment and rehabilitation
- Indirect costs of complications, morbidity, anxiety, time, loss of work

Costs Related to Death
- Direct costs or charges related to death
- Indirect costs of years of life lost

EPIDEMIOLOGIC MEASUREMENTS
Prevalence and Incidence Rates

The prevalence rate of cancer denotes the number of cancers that exist in a defined population *at* a specific time, whereas the incidence rate denotes the number of new cancers that develop in a defined population *during* a specific *period* of time.[1-3] Both are commonly expressed as the number of cancers per 100,000 individuals in the defined population. The ideal screening test would detect all the prevalent cases of cancer in the first screen of a previously unscreened population. Subsequent screening examinations would detect incidence cases developing in the population since the prior screen.

The incidence rate for a given cancer is usually lower than the prevalence rate. Theoretically, in a defined population of individuals who received three cancer screenings at yearly intervals, the first screen would detect all prevalence cases (developing for several years before the first screening). The second and third screenings would detect incidence cases (i.e., only those cases that developed since the first screening).

Positive and Negative Tests

A *true-positive* screening test is an abnormal test for cancer in an individual who subsequently is found to have cancer within a defined period of time after the test. A *true-negative* screening test is a normal test for cancer in an individual who subsequently is found not to have cancer within a defined period of time after the test.[2,15,16] A *false-positive* screening test is an abnormal test for cancer in an individual who subsequently is found not to have cancer within a defined period of time after the test. A *false-negative* screening test is a normal test for cancer in an individual who subsequently is found to have cancer within a defined period of time after the test.[2,16,17]

Sensitivity

The sensitivity of a screening test represents its ability to detect those individuals with cancer in the defined population[2,16,17] and is derived from the true-positive ratio (i.e., the proportion of positive tests in all individuals with disease). Sensitivity is defined as the number of true-positive (TP) cases divided by the total number of true-positive (TP) and false-negative (FN) cases.

$$\text{Sensitivity} = \frac{TP}{TP+FN}$$

Specificity

The specificity of a test represents its ability to identify those free of cancer in the population[2,16,17] and is derived from the true-negative ratio (i.e., the proportion of negative tests in all individuals without disease). Specificity is defined as the number of true-negative (TN) cases divided by the total number of true-negative and false-positive (FP) cases.

$$\text{Specificity} = \frac{TN}{TN+FP}$$

Positive Predictive Value

The positive predictive value is the measure of the validity of a positive test (i.e., the proportion of positive tests that are true-positive cases (Table 1-1).

$$\text{Positive Predictive Value} = \frac{TP}{TP+FP}$$

The predictive value of a test depends on the disease prevalence (Table 1-2). As the prevalence of cancer increases in the population, the positive predictive value of the screening test increases, even though its sensitivity and specificity remain unchanged.[18-20] Therefore for maximum efficiency and cost-effectiveness, screening should be focused on the populations with highest prevalence of the disease.

Negative Predictive Value

The negative predictive value is the measure of the validity of a negative test (i.e., the proportion of negative tests that are true-negative cases).

$$\text{Negative Predictive Value} = \frac{TN}{TN+FN}$$

 Table 1-1
Hypothetical Example of Validity Measures of a Screening Test

Results of Screening Test	TRUE CHARACTERISTICS IN THE POPULATION		
	Have the Disease	Do Not Have the Disease	Total
Positive test	80	100	180
Negative test	20	800	820
Total	100	900	1000

True-positive tests = 80; sensitivity = 80/(80 + 20) = 0.80.
True-negative tests = 800; specificity = 800/(800 + 100) = 0.89.
False-positive tests = 100; positive predictive value = 80/(80 + 100) = 0.44.
False-negative tests = 20; negative predictive value = 800/(800 + 20) = 0.98.

Table 1-2
Relationship of Positive Predictive Value of the Screening Test to the Prevalence of Cancer in the Population

Two Hypothetical Scenarios: Prevalence Rates of 1% and 5%

Prevalence of Cancer = 1%

Test Results	Have Disease	Do Not Have Disease	Totals	Positive Predictive Value
Positive	99	495	594	99/(495+99) = 0.17
Negative	1	9405	9406	
Total	100	9900	10,000	

Prevalence of Cancer = 5%

Test Results	Have Disease	Do Not Have Disease	Totals	Positive Predictive Value
Positive	495	475	970	495/(495+475) = 0.51
Negative	5	9025	9030	
Total	500	9500	10,000	

Sensitivity of screening test = 0.99; specificity of screening test = 0.95.
1% prevalence of cancer: TP = 99, TN = 9405, sensitivity = 99/(99 + 1) = 0.99; FP = 495, FN = 1, specificity = 9405/(9405 + 495) = 0.95.
5% prevalence of cancer: TP = 495, TN = 9025, sensitivity = 495/(495 + 5) = 0.99; FP = 475, FN = 5, specificity = 9025/(9025 + 475) = 0.95.

GOVERNING PRINCIPLES OF CANCER SCREENING

The governing principles of cancer screening are those that make a screening program worthwhile. These principles define the characteristics of the disease considered for screening, the screening test, and the outcomes (Table 1-3).[1-3,20]

The disease considered for screening should have high prevalence and incidence rates and should have serious clinical consequences measured in mortality, morbidity, and costs. The biology and natural history of the disease should be known. Ideally, the cancer should exist for a long time in a preclinical phase amenable to screening, and this preclinical phase should have a high prevalence rate in the screened population. The disease should have an effective treatment at an early stage, and this treatment should be more effective than treatment at late stage. When a disease has no effective treatment or when treatment in its early stage is no more effective than in its advanced stage, screening is problematic unless counseling is shown to be useful.

Table 1-3
Governing Principles of a Worthwhile Cancer Screening Program

Characteristics of the Disease	Characteristics of the Screening Test
High morbidity, mortality, costs	Able to detect disease in preclinical phase
High prevalence and incidence	Effective (i.e., sensitive and specific)
Known natural history and biology	Safe
Preclinical phase with high prevalence	Simple, inexpensive
Effective treatment of early stage disease	Acceptable to individuals

An effective screening test should have the ability to detect cancer in its preclinical phase with acceptable sensitivity, specificity, and predictive values. The test should be safe; screened individuals are asymptomatic and should not suffer complications of a screening examination. To be applied efficiently in large populations, the screening test should be simple, inexpensive, and accessible. Moreover, if compliance with repeated screens is expected, the test must be acceptable to the screened individuals.

The most important outcome measure of the effectiveness of a screening strategy is the demonstration that the mortality rate from the disease is significantly lower in the total screened population when compared with the cancer mortality rate in an equivalent population of unscreened people, preferably demonstrated by a randomized, controlled, defined population clinical trial.

Expected Benefits and Potential Harms

The expected benefits of screening are a lower mortality rate from the target cancer, a reduction in morbidity from the disease, and lower health care costs.

Additional benefits may include improved length and quality of life, as well as less pain, anxiety, and disability. Expected benefits of screening are derived from the true-positive results of a screening test. Although not a benefit that makes a screening program effective, a true-negative screening test result may provide reassurance that cancer has not developed.

The potential harms of screening are related to the test itself or to its results. Those related to the test are costs, inconvenience, anxiety, and discomfort. Additional potential risks (complications) may be related to invasive screening tests. The potential harms related to the results are those associated with false-positive and false-negative tests. The potential benefits of screening must outweigh the potential risks because any harm to an asymptomatic person is not to be considered lightly. A false-positive test result causes anxiety and incurs a diagnostic evaluation, with its attendant costs, potential risks, and side effects. A false-negative test result can lead to a false sense of security. Subsequent clinical signs or symptoms of cancer may be dismissed because of a prior negative screening test, thus resulting in further delay in detection.

Evaluation of a Proposed Screening Strategy

A systematic approach to cancer control research that provides a framework for the evaluation of a proposed screening strategy has been developed (Box 1-3).[21-23] The evaluation begins with knowledge about the basic biology and epidemiology of the cancer and incorporates information about characteristics of the populations at high risk, cancer prevalence and incidence rates, tumor growth rates, mortality rates, and costs of care and disability. The next step, hypothesis development, synthesizes the available scientific information and

---

BOX 1-3	**Cancer Control Phases: A Systematic Evaluation Process for Proposed Screening Strategies**

- Basic research and epidemiology
- Hypothesis development
- Methods development
- Controlled intervention trials
- Defined population studies
- Demonstration and implementation projects
- Nationwide dissemination programs

proposes possible interventions to be applied to the cancer problem. Cancer screening may not always be the appropriate intervention; primary prevention, if possible, is the optimal prevention. The proposed intervention strategy should be expressed as a testable hypothesis that can be evaluated in an objective, scientific fashion.

Next, methodologic research is necessary to characterize the variables to be controlled or monitored in subsequent clinical trials. This phase might include pilot studies to identify target populations or compliance rates of screened individuals, to evaluate application or acceptability of screening tests, or to estimate the efficacy of the screening test. Methods that have been tested adequately and proved may be incorporated into clinical intervention trials. Initial trials may be uncontrolled but, ideally, these interventions should be controlled. Cohort studies or case control trials may be used to estimate benefits from a screening intervention; however, randomized, controlled trials are likely to provide the most convincing results.

Measures of the quantitative impact of a screening intervention that uses a defined population study would identify not only barriers to widespread adoption of the intervention but also methods for overcoming these barriers. The defined population must include a large number of people to show a significan intervention benefit. The screening strategy is beneficial if the defined population study demonstrates a significant reduction in disease-specific mortality rate when compared with the unscreened group.

When screening is shown to be beneficial in defined population studies, demonstration and implementation programs are appropriate. The purpose of these programs is to apply the proven intervention in a community at large with measurement of the public health impact. A surveillance system should be in place to ensure that the application, accuracy, and effectiveness of screening in the community are equal to that demonstrated in clinical trials. Quality control processes and assessment of the adequacy of diagnostic evaluation and treatment in the community may be developed during this phase.

Finally, when demonstration and implementation programs ensure that community dissemination can be achieved, nationwide screening programs and policy recommendations may be developed.

POTENTIAL HARMS AND BIASES IN EVALUATION

All the steps in the evaluation process described above are not always completed with a new screening strategy. Pressures to circumvent the process include immediate clinical acceptance and dissemination of a new screening test, the expense of defined population studies, and preliminary recommendations for screening from professional organizations. However, without the assurance of this process, an incompletely evaluated screening strategy may deliver more harms and costs than benefits. Moreover, without the demonstrated benefit of a screening intervention in a defined population trial, the potential benefit of a screening strategy may be overestimated and invalid.

Almost invariably, individuals with cancer identified by screening will have longer survival times than those diagnosed with usual clinical detection. However, these apparent increased survival times are not always equivalent to reduction in mortality from cancer. Three biases that contribute to this spurious survival increase and potentially mask the lack of screening benefit are lead-time bias, length bias, and overdiagnosis bias. Randomized, controlled clinical trials can control for these biases and can identify and quantify more accurately the benefits of a screening strategy.

Lead-time Bias

Lead-time bias refers to clinical outcome observations that are not adjusted for the timing of the diagnosis. The length of time by which screening advances the diagnosis of cancer compared with the usual clinical detection is the lead-time. In an uncontrolled clinical trial, this lead-time appears to *increase* survival time because survival time is measured from the time of diagnosis to the time of death. However, despite the apparent increase in survival time, the natural history of the disease and the time of death remain unchanged. This apparent increase in survival time without reduction in mortality is termed lead-time bias.[1,2,20]

A beneficial screening strategy detects cancer before its systemic spread, alters the natural history of the disease, and defers the time of death. This alteration of the natural history of the disease, with prolongation of life, cannot be recognized without a randomized, controlled trial that adjusts for lead-time bias.

Length Bias

Length bias refers to clinical outcome observations that are not adjusted for the rate of progression of disease.[1,2,20] The probability that a cancer will be detected by screening is directly proportional to the length of its detectable preclinical phase, which is inversely related to its rate of progression. Individuals with rapidly progressive cancers (i.e., those with brief preclinical phases) are more likely to die of their disease and are less likely to be identified by screening. Alternatively, individuals with slowly progressive cancers (i.e., those with long preclinical phases) are less likely to die of their disease and are more likely to be identified by screening. Therefore screening tends to detect cancer subsets with long preclinical phases, less aggressive progression, and perhaps better inherent prognosis.

A barnyard analogy may help clarify the concept. Assume we are standing around a corral in a barnyard. The animals in the corral represent cancers and the quickness of each animal represents the rapidity of growth of the cancer. In the corral there are four types of animals: turtles, chickens, horses, and pigs. You, dear reader, represent the screening test. I ask you to enter the corral three times and capture an animal each time. Each of the times you enter the corral represents a screening event. Although it is possible that you will bring chickens, horses, or pigs from the corral, it is more likely that you will capture the slowest animal, the turtles. Similarly, screening tends to detect cancer subsets with slower growth rates and perhaps better inherent prognoses.

If the outcomes of individuals with screening-detected cancers in an uncontrolled clinical screening trial are compared with a general population of clinically detected cancers, the screened group may demonstrate an artificially higher survival rate because of the length bias sampling effect. A randomized, controlled trial obviates this bias.

Overdiagnosis Bias

Length bias effect may be magnified as the screening test threshold is lowered and the least aggressive tumors are detected. Among this group of neoplasms may be cases that would regress, remain stable, or progress too slowly to ever have become clinically apparent during the individual's lifetime. This effect has been termed *overdiagnosis* bias, or *pseudodisease*.[1,2,20,24]

Overdiagnosis bias is compounded by the difficulty in defining pathologically the distinct lines between benign hyperplasia, atypical hyperplasia, dysplasia, and carcinoma. As a screening strategy detects less aggressive tumors at earlier stages in the progression of disease, some cases of benign conditions will be classified as cancers, artificially elevating the apparent survival benefit. Randomized, controlled trials, with standardized pathologic review, offset the effects of this error by controlling for this bias.

CONCLUSIONS

Although screening for cancer has enormous intuitive appeal, the true benefits, harms, and costs of this cancer control approach can only be determined from appropriate clinical trials that measure the relevant parameters. Although there is evidence of benefit in some programs, such as screening for breast, colon, and cervical cancers, evidence of benefit is inconclusive or lacking for many common cancers.

REFERENCES

1. Clark RA: Principles of cancer screening. *Cancer Control* 1995;2:485-492.
2. Clark RA, Reintgen DS: Principles of cancer screening. In Reintgen DS, Clark RA, editors: *Cancer screening*, St. Louis, Mosby, 1996.
3. Eddy DM, editor: *Common screening tests,* Philadelphia, American College of Physicians, 1991, 1-21.
4. Hulka BS: Cancer screening: degrees of proof and practical application. *Cancer* 1988;62:1776-1780.
5. Hoskins KF, Stopfer JE, Calzone KA, et al: Assessment and counseling for women with a family history of breast cancer: a guide for clinicians. *JAMA* 1995;273:577-585.
6. Shattuck-Eidens D, McClure M, Simard J, et al: A collaborative survey of 80 mutations in the BRCA1 breast and ovarian cancer susceptibility gene: implications for presymptomatic testing and screening. *JAMA* 1995;273:535-541.
7. Moskowitz M: Screening is not diagnosis. *Radiology* 1979;133:265-268.
8. Ellwood PM: Shattuck lecture. Outcomes management: a technology of patient experience. *N Engl J Med* 1988;318:1549-1556.
9. Wennberg JE: Outcomes research, cost containment, and the fear of health care rationing. *N Engl J Med* 1990;323:1202-1204.
10. Fries JF, Koop CE, Beadle CE, et al: Reducing health care costs by reducing the need and demand for medical services. The Health Project Consortium. *N Engl J Med* 1993;329:321-325.
11. Doubilet P, Weinstein MC, McNeil BJ. Use and misuse of the term "cost effective" in medicine. *N Engl J Med* 1986;314:253-256.
12. Doubilet PM: "Cost-effective": a trendy, often misused term. *AJR Am J Roentgenol* 1987;148:827-828.
13. Eisenberg JM: Clinical economics: a guide to the economic analysis of clinical practices. *JAMA* 1989;262:2879-2886.
14. Detsky AS, Naglie IG: A clinician's guide to cost-effectiveness analysis. *Ann Intern Med* 1990;113: 147-154.
15. Goodwin PJ: Economic evaluations of cancer care incorporating quality-of-life issues. In Osoba D, editor: *Effect of cancer on quality of life*, Boca Raton, FL, CRC Press, 1991.
16. McNeil BJ, Keeler E, Adelstein SJ: Primer on certain elements of medical decision making. *N Engl J Med* 1975;293:211-215.
17. McNeil BJ, Adelstein SJ: Determining the value of diagnostic and screening tests. *J Nucl Med* 1976;17:439-448.
18. Moskowitz M: Impact of a priori medical decisions on screening for breast cancer. *Radiology* 1989; 171:605-608.
19. Moskowitz M: Predictive value, sensitivity, and specificity in breast cancer screening. *Radiology* 1988;167:576-578.
20. Black WC, Welch HG: Advances in diagnostic imaging and overestimations of disease prevalence and the benefits of therapy. *N Engl J Med* 1993;328: 1237-1243.
21. Cadman D, Chambers L, Feldman W, et al: Assessing the effectiveness of community screening programs. *JAMA* 1984;251:1580-1585.
22. Greenwald P, Cullen JW: The new emphasis in cancer control. *J Natl Cancer Inst* 1985;74:543-551.
23. Greenwald P, Cullen JW, McKenna JW: Cancer prevention and control: from research through applications. *J Natl Cancer Inst* 1987;79:389-400.
24. Black WC: Overdiagnosis: an under-recognized cause of confusion and harm in cancer screening. *J Natl Cancer Inst* 2000;92:1280-1282.

CHAPTER 2

Cancer of the Lung

Linda L. Garland
Merrill Eisenberg
Pamela J. Powers

INTRODUCTION

At the beginning of the 21st century, women face a health crisis of epidemic proportion related to the adverse effects of exposure to tobacco products, especially cigarette smoke. Although fewer women than men are currently smoking, the effects of a dramatic increase in smoking by women over the second half of the 20th century are now being manifested. Lung cancer has outdistanced breast cancer as the deadliest cancer in women, accounting for 25% of all cancer deaths in women today.

Although lung cancer is a major consequence of tobacco use in women, the adverse effects of tobacco products on women's health include an increase in the risk of other cancers, including esophageal, head and neck, pancreatic, cervical, renal, and bladder cancers. Tobacco exposure by women during the perinatal period has been associated with multiple adverse reproductive health outcomes. This chapter focuses on the impact of the dramatic rise in tobacco use during the 20th century on women's health.

LUNG CANCER INCIDENCE AND MORTALITY
General Trends in Lung Cancer Incidence and Mortality

Lung cancer continues to have an impact of epidemic proportion on the health of Americans and people worldwide. An estimated 169,500 new lung cancers were diagnosed in the United States in the year 2001, with somewhat fewer lung cancers diagnosed in women than men—approximately 78,800 versus 90,700, respectively. Lung cancer–related deaths represented more than one quarter of the estimated 553,400 cancer deaths in America in the year 2001. Although more American women and men were diagnosed that year with breast cancer or prostate cancer, respectively, lung cancer still remained the leading cause of cancer death for both genders.[1]

Trends in Lung Cancer Incidence and Mortality in Women
Women—Image and Smoking Prevalence

The current epidemic of lung cancer in women has its roots in the social, economic, and political trends that evolved over the course of the 20th century. At the beginning of that century, tobacco use by women was extremely rare, with smoking prevalence for women estimated at 6% in 1924.[2] Recognizing that women would be a fertile target for mass marketing of tobacco products, the tobacco industry first began its targeting of women as early as the 1920s, using the concept of "image advertising." "Reach for a Lucky instead of a sweet" was one of the first advertising campaigns that associated cigarette use with staying slim, a theme with specific appeal for women.[3] This strategic link of Lucky Strikes and other cigarette brands with weight control led to a 300% increase in sales for this brand of cigarettes in the first year of this ad campaign. Cigarettes designed specifically for women were first market-ed in the 1920s, featuring, for instance, lipstick-colored tips. Although national statistics for cigarette prevalence were not available early in the century, there were data that showed a significant upward trend in cigarette use by women. In the space of 5 years, from 1924 to 1929, smoking prevalence in women was estimated to have increased to 19%.[2] Several sur-veys undertaken in the mid-1930s reported smoking prevalences of 26% among women younger than 40[4] and 20% for women of all ages.[5]

There was a significant increase in the numbers of women as well as men who took up the habit of smoking cigarettes during World War II. Image advertising capitalized on the war effort to promote smoking in women. Chesterfields cigarette advertisements featuring glam-orous photographs of fashion models or movie stars marketed glamour and thinness to women on the home front. Women contributing directly to the war effort—WAFS, for exam-ple—were pictured engaged in cigarette smoking. Over the period of 1930 and 1945, approximately 20% of women smoked.[6] A Gallup Poll of tobacco use by women in 1944 reported that more than one third all of women used cigarettes during that year.[7]

The Narrowing of the Gender Gap

Although smoking rates for American women climbed over the first half of the 20th century, they nonetheless remained significantly lower than rates for American men, with the exis-tence of a wide gender gap in smoking prevalence. In 1955, a survey representing national smoking prevalence reported 32% of women as ever-smokers and 24% as current smokers. It was during this time period, through epidemiologic studies conducted in the 1950s and 1960s, that a causal association between tobacco smoke and lung cancer was first reported.[8,9] Nonetheless, tobacco use by women and men continued to rise during the 1950s and 1960s. The mid-1960s was the launching period of image advertising campaigns that linked ciga-rette smoking to women's freedom of choice and their burgeoning social, economic, and political opportunities, best typified by the Virginia Slims campaign featuring the slogan, "You've Come a Long Way, Baby." By 1965, one year after the groundbreaking report of the Advisory Committee to the Surgeon General that cited evidence of the adverse health effects of tobacco use was published,[10] 33.9% of women smoked cigarettes. Men's use of tobacco had continued to rise and remained greater than that of women, with 51.9% of U.S. men smoking cigarettes in 1965.

The gender gap in smoking prevalence further declined between 1965 and 1979, due mainly to a large decline in men smokers, from 51.9% to 33.9%, rather than a dramatic decline in women smokers; over this period, smoking prevalence for women declined from 33.9% to 29.9%.[11] Since the mid-1980s, the gender gap has remained around 5%, with 22% of U.S. women aged 18 or older smoking cigarettes at the end of the 20th century, in comparison to 26.4% of U.S. men.

Lung Cancer Incidence and Mortality in Women

Since the 1950s, there has been a dramatic 600% increase in lung cancer deaths in women. This rapid rise in lung cancer deaths in women has paralleled the dramatic increase in smok-ing prevalence by women that had begun earlier in the century. This trend was identified in the first U.S. Surgeon General's report devoted to women and smoking, published in 1980, which noted that smoking-related disease in women was now appearing in epidemic pro-portion.[2] Following this report, in the mid-1980s, a grim landmark in the history of women's health was recorded as lung cancer overcame breast cancer as the leading cause of cancer-related death in women (Fig. 2-1). In men, a decline in the incidence of lung cancer began in the 1980s and continued through the end of the 1990s at a rate of decrease of 3.2% per year from 1992 through 1997. For women overall, lung cancer incidence stabilized over the 1990s, although for women age 40 to 59, rates have started to decline.[12] Globally, since 1985, there has been an estimated 21% increase in the number of lung cancer cases in women, compared with 4% in men.[1]

Incidence and Ethnicity

Smoking prevalence for women varies significantly by ethnic group. Prevalence studies on women's tobacco use by ethnic group reflects a constellation of factors that includes cultural norms for tobacco use in general and by gender, socioeconomic factors, levels of education, and possibly genetic polymorphisms that may influence tobacco addiction. Studies on women and smoking, especially early studies, have been limited in their reporting by ethnic group. For much of the 1900s, large surveys on smoking prevalence for women did not include data for ethnic groups such as Hispanics and Native Americans. Smoking prevalence by ethnicity was first reported in several large studies: the National Health Interview Survey, conducted during the years 1965 to 1998, which reported on the prevalence of ever-smoking among women aged 18 or older, and the National Household Survey on Drug Abuse, United States, 1997-1998.[13,14] Prevalence data for the ethnic groups were defined as White, non-Hispanic; Black, non-Hispanic; Hispanic; American Indian or Alaska Native; and Asian or Pacific Islander. Ever-smoking was highest for women self-described as White, non-Hispanic, ranging from 42.3% to 44.8% from 1965 to 1998. Following closely in prevalence, Black, non-Hispanic women were ever-smokers at a rate of 39.4% to 32.6% during the same period. Rates for Hispanics and Asian or Pacific Islander were significantly lower in comparison; for the years 1979–1998, ever-smoking ranged from 35.4% to 25.6% and 24.3% to 16.8%, respectively. For American Indian or Alaska Native women, ever-smoking rates were significantly higher and did not fall, ranging from 56.6% in 1979 to 57.7% in 1998.

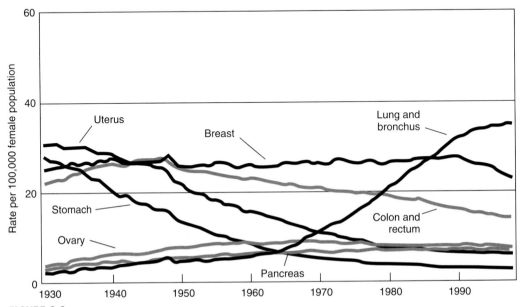

FIGURE 2-1
Lung cancer–related deaths surpasses breast cancer in the 1980s. (From Landis SH, Murray T, Bolden S, Wingo PA: Cancer statistics, 1999. *CA Cancer J Clin* 1999; 49:8-31.)

RISK FACTORS FOR LUNG CANCER IN WOMEN

Cancer develops through a multistage process that involves complex interactions between host susceptibility factors and carcinogen exposure. Host factors that determine susceptibility to carcinogens, such as those contained in tobacco smoke, include both inherited and acquired genetic factors that modulate carcinogen activation, carcinogen metabolism, and susceptibility to carcinogen exposure at the level of the target tissue(s). Attention to gender-specific aspects of cancer risk has yielded some data suggesting that women are at increased risk for the carcinogenic effects of tobacco, although more research is needed to support firm conclusions in this area.

Family History and Lung Cancer

Studies have reported an excess of cancers in family members of persons with lung cancer, suggesting a role for an inherited susceptibility for the development of cancer in these families. A case-control study of never-smokers and former smokers who developed lung cancer showed a greater probability of having a paternal history of any cancer and aerodigestive cancer, a maternal history of breast cancer, and a history of any cancer in siblings. There was a near-significant excess of lung cancer, aerodigestive cancer, and breast cancer in sisters.[15] In general, lung cancer in women is unlike breast cancer, for which distinct germline mutations of the BRCA gene confer extremely high lifetime risks for the development of breast and pelvic cancers, independent of environmental risk factors.

Genetic Factors

Genetic Factors in Carcinogen Metabolism

Genetic polymorphisms in tobacco carcinogen that activate and metabolize enzymes are thought to play significant roles in determining individual susceptibility to carcinogens. Among the most important of these polymorphisms are those that involve the genes encoding products that activate carcinogens through the cytochrome P450–activating enzymes, and the NAT2 and glutathione-S-transferase (GST)–detoxifying enzymes. Polymorphisms for the CYP1A1 and the GSTM1 genes have been associated with an increased risk of lung cancer.[16,17] Gender differences in the risk of cancer conferred by genetic polymorphisms in metabolism-related genes have been proposed. Women who have a CYP1A1 mutant genotype had a greater risk of lung cancer than men with the same genotype (odds ratio 4.98 vs. 1.37, respectively).[18] The role of CYP1A2 in combination with NAT2, a second enzyme with a key role in the metabolic activation of heterocyclic amines, has been examined in a population of Chinese women who have a relatively high rate of lung cancer despite a low smoking prevalence.[19] Those women with slow NAT2/rapid CYP1A2 activity were at the highest risk for the development of lung cancer, particularly adenocarcinomas; this phenotype suggests that procarcinogens would be activated in an enhanced fashion by CYP1A2 in combination with a reduced rate of detoxification by NAT2.

Genetics and Smoking Behavior

Genetic factors that may impact on smoking initiation and the maintenance of smoking behavior have been identified. Nicotine is the main psychoactive component in cigarette smoke that is believed to underlie tobacco addiction and dependence. The dopaminergic system of neurotransmission, which is considered a primary "reward" pathway, appears to have an important role in smoking behavior. In general, tobacco smoke enhances dopamine neurotransmission in the brain, with an enhancing effect on serotonin neurotransmission as well. Enhancement of dopamine transmission is involved in the reinforcing effects of nicotine in animal models.[20] Nicotine can stimulate the release of dopamine and can inhibit dopamine reuptake.[21,22] Variations in dopamine receptor genes may influence an individual's susceptibility to nicotine addiction. In a cohort of lung cancer patients, those with a genetic polymorphism at the D2 dopamine receptor locus initiated smoking at an earlier age and smoked more heavily than those patients who lacked the polymorphism.[23] A second study showed a relationship between the dopamine transporter gene, SLC 6A3-9, and smoking initiation at an age younger than 16.[24] An effect of gender on the expression of dopamine and serotonin transporters has been reported, which may be related to their upregulation by the sex steroids estradiol and progesterone.[25-27] An increased understanding of the individual genetics of smoking behavior, in combination with the individual's inherited metabolic risk profile, can potentially help identify individuals at high risk for lung cancer.

Cigarette Smoking

The strongest risk factor for the development of lung cancer in both women and men is active tobacco smoking, also called exposure to "mainstream smoke," which accounts for 85% to 90% of all lung cancers. Tobacco smoke contains more than 3000 chemicals, of which 40 to 50 are putative carcinogens. The polycyclic aromatic hydrocarbons (PAHs) and nitrosamines have been identified as the most important classes of tobacco carcinogens. A clear association between increased risk of lung cancer–related death and exposure by women to tobacco smoke has been shown in six prospective studies conducted worldwide that have provided data on more than one million women in four countries.[28-30] Relative risks of death from lung cancer in these studies have ranged from 2.0 to 11.9 for current smokers. Furthermore, these studies have demonstrated a clear dose-response relationship between quantity of tobacco used daily by women and their risk of death from lung cancer.

Whether women are at higher risk than men for the development of lung cancer, given the same exposure to tobacco, is currently not known. Some case-control studies have shown equal or higher smoking-related relative risks for lung cancer among women than among men.[31,32] However, differences between men and women in both patterns of smoking and tobacco use reporting are possible confounders in this type of study. The actual exposure to tobacco carcinogen a woman receives may differ from men's for the same number of cigarettes smoked because of differences in puff volume, puff frequency, and depth of inhalation. Women may underreport daily cigarette use. However, it is possible that women do have an increased susceptibility profile based on genetic and cellular mechanisms that affect tobacco smoke carcinogens, as described previously.

Gender and the Biology of Lung Cancer

There do appear to be gender-related differences in the biology of lung cancer. The anatomic distribution of lung cancers within the lung itself differs by gender; women develop more peripheral than central lesions. Women have a higher incidence of adenocarcinoma and a lower incidence of squamous cell and small cell carcinomas when compared with men. It has been proposed that greater use of filtered cigarettes by women may underlie this trend. The use of cigarette filters has been associated with altered patterns of smoke inhalation. Longstanding smokers of filtered cigarettes take larger puffs and retain smoke longer to compensate for the lower nicotine content of filtered cigarettes; thus smoke particles may be deposited in more peripheral zones of the lung where adenocarcinomas preferentially arise.[33] There is a high incidence of adenocarcinomas in non–tobacco-exposed women in

China, possibly related to the metabolism of heterocyclic amines found during the cooking of meat at high temperatures.[19]

Environmental Tobacco Smoke Exposure

Environmental tobacco smoke (ETS) is a risk factor for the development of lung cancer in never-smokers. The major component of ETS is "sidestream smoke," which contains the same carcinogens as "mainstream smoke," although at a lower concentration because of dilution with ambient air. Persons are exposed to ETS in both household and occupational settings. In the United States, the estimated risk for lung cancer has been reported to be increased 1.6-fold by ETS.[34] For women in particular, spousal smoking is an important source of ETS. A European study confirmed an elevated, albeit small, increase in risk of lung cancer caused by ETS.[35] Support for the association between ETS and the development of lung cancer in nonsmoking women includes the finding of urinary metabolites of the tobacco-specific lung carcinogen nitrosamine 4-(methylnitrosamino)-1-(3-pyridyl)-1-butanon (NNK) in non-smoking women exposed to ETS through spousal tobacco use.[36] Women never-smokers who develop lung cancer through ETS may be particularly susceptible to tobacco carcinogens because of an "at risk" genotype.[37] The role of occupational exposure to ETS has been the subject of controversy. A recent metaanalysis of five studies reported an odds ratio for lung cancer of 1.39, supporting a role for occupational ETS in the etiology of lung cancer,[38] whereas earlier metaanalyses did not show significant odds ratios ETS in lung cancer

Other Risk Factors for Lung Cancer in Women
Occupational Risks

Occupational exposures for women and men have been estimated to account for 5% and 15% to 20% of all lung cancers, respectively.[39,40] Chemical and physical agents that have been identified as lung carcinogens in the workplace include arsenic, asbestos, ethers, chromium, cadmium, nickel, PAHs, radon, and vinyl chloride. The role of workplace exposures in relation to the development of lung and other cancers in women has not been extensively investigated. Furthermore, smoking, among other exposures, is a confounder in some occupational exposure studies. Although most studies on occupational lung carcinogens have focused on agents found in male-dominated occupations, an increase in lung cancer incidence has been reported for women involved in the manufacturing of metals, clay, computers, and rubber-plastics,[41] and for laundry workers and dry cleaners.[42] For African-American women, nonsignificant risks have been reported for occupational exposure to paint and gas fumes; in farming settings and in building maintenance, African-American women had an elevated, albeit insignificant, risk for lung cancer.[43] Further study into the role of occupational exposure to lung carcinogens for women is especially relevant as women assimilate into occupations formerly occupied predominantly by men.

Nonoccupational Risks

Worldwide, there are populations of women who have not been exposed to tobacco carcinogens but who have an elevated risk of lung cancer. A risk factor for lung cancer in Chinese women, who traditionally have a low smoking prevalence, is internal air pollution from combustion products of coal burning, nonvented oil cooking fumes, or fumes generated from the cooking of meats.[19,44,45] Cooking oils are usually heated to high temperatures, a process that causes the release of large amounts of fumes that can contain volatile, mutagenic substances. Oils that have been identified with an increased risk of lung cancer include rapeseed oil, linseed oil, or the combination of both; additionally, lung cancer risk has been shown to increase with the number of years spent cooking.[46,47]

TOBACCO USE
Understanding Smokers

Smokers vary greatly in their patterns of use, levels of addiction, and willingness to quit. Many variables—age, ethnicity, gender, education, socioeconomic status, work environment, home environment, quitting history, and smoking history—come into play when assessing a person's addiction and likelihood to quit smoking. Three quarters of U.S. women who smoke want to quit smoking completely, but only 46.6% report having tried to quit during the previous year.[14]

In multiple studies, poverty and education are strong predictors of smoking status and continued smoking. Women living below the poverty level also are more likely to smoke then women whose income is at or above the poverty level; 29.6% of poor women smoke, whereas 21.6% of women at or above the poverty level smoke.[14] In addition, the unemployed are more likely to be current or ever-smokers and are less likely to have quit, compared with employed people or those not in the workforce.[48]

Education as a predictor of smoking status cuts across racial lines; 33% of adult White women with no high school diploma or General Educational Development test (GED) reported current smoking in 1998, compared with 32.8% of adult African-American women with the same education level. Among White women with a bachelor's degree or higher, 11.4% reported current smoking in the same time period, compared with 9% of African-American women with the same education level.[49] It was previously thought that smoking rates were high for groups with less than a high school education. Data analysis of the National Health Interview Survey (1983–91) showed that people with 9 to 11 years of education are most likely to be current, ever-, and heavy smokers.[48] Smoking rates and smoking cessation rates for those with zero to 8 years of education are similar to that of people with 12 or more years of education.[48] It has been theorized that those with 8 of fewer years of education may be so impoverished that they cannot afford to buy cigarettes. After 11 years of education the likelihood of smoking decreases, and the likelihood of cessation increases with each year of education.[48] Smoking among U.S. women with 9 to 11 years of education is three times that of women with 16 or more years of education (32.9% vs. 11.2%).[14]

Tobacco use is just one of many poor health behaviors in which smokers often engage.[50-53] Ever-smokers consider themselves to be less healthy[54]—and probably are. When compared with nonsmokers, smokers are more likely to be obese, lead sedentary lifestyles, have poor diets, and abuse alcohol and other drugs, and less likely to use preventive health services.[50-53] Smokers report less physical activity, more bodily pain, and less vitality than never-smokers; their reported health perceptions and bodily pain are often equivalent to never-smokers who are several years older.[54]

Smoking and abuse of alcohol and other substances often go hand in hand.[50,51,53] Women who smoke may be nearly five times as likely to abuse alcohol than women who were never smokers.[51] Metaanalyses of the literature linking smoking and alcohol show more than 90% of alcoholics are cigarette smokers.[53] Lifetime prevalence of alcohol, cannabis, cocaine, and other drugs is significantly higher among people with mild to moderate nicotine dependence when compared with never-smokers.[50] There also are significant associations between several psychiatric disorders and cigarette smoking.[51] Smoking prevalence is higher among people with major depression,[50,55-57] anxiety,[50,55,58] and schizophrenia.[55,59] The likelihood of any anxiety disorder in people who are moderately nicotine-dependent is four times higher than that in nonsmokers.[50] The risk of major depression is tenfold among smokers who also abuse other substances compared with nonsmokers with no substance dependence; this rate is twice that of smokers who use no other drugs compared with non-smokers with no substance dependence.[50] Negative affect—particularly depression—is often associated with failed cessation attempts.[14,60]

As is evident in the literature, many smokers are caught in a cycle of poverty, low education, poor health behaviors, abuse of multiple substances, and decreased use of preventive health care. Healthy behaviors and use of preventive services show a trend toward self-protection. Physicians have fewer opportunities to conduct interventions related to smoking or other lifestyle choices with people who do not demonstrate self-protective behaviors. When compared with never-smokers, female smokers are less likely to come to a physician's office for well-woman screening tests,[52] and they are less likely to bring their children in for preventive care.[61] Health care delivery systems that foster long-term physician-patient relationships may increase cancer screening rates among women.[62] Women who were older, never married, poorly educated, or rural residents, or who had larger families, were less likely to have received health care services in the past year and were more likely to have received services more than 5 years ago or never.[62] When tobacco-dependent patients do present themselves in a health care setting, health professionals at all levels should be prepared to offer a brief cessation intervention.

Nicotine Addiction

Nicotine is a powerfully addictive substance.[63] Although there are any number of reasons why people become tobacco users, continued use—without regard for the health risks to themselves or others—often indicates nicotine addiction.

Usage patterns suggest that smokers unconsciously attempt to control blood nicotine levels throughout the day by self-administering nicotine at regular intervals of 30 to 60 minutes (15–30 cigarettes per day).[63] Because nicotine is metabolized quickly,[64] smokers are driven to replenish nicotine levels by regularly lighting up. Regular smoking throughout the day also can be used to enhance cognitive performance[65] or cope with stress,[58,66] or it may be a reaction to smoking-related trigger situations.[63,67]

Many social variables are predictive of smoking behavior, but the number of cigarettes smoked per day strongly indicates an individual's level of nicotine dependence[14] and the likelihood that he or she will be able to quit tobacco.[68] More than 75% of women who smoke report one or more indicators of nicotine dependence, and close to 75% report feeling dependent upon cigarettes.[14]

At opposite ends of the smoking continuum are occasional smokers and hard-core smokers. For health care providers and others who may intervene with smokers, it is important to know how smoking patterns impact a person's level of addiction and likelihood to consider quitting.

Researchers estimate that 15% to 20% of current smokers are low-rate, irregular smokers, or chippers.[69] Many occasional smokers (79%) smoke as few as one to five cigarettes per day on the days they smoke—approximately 30 cigarettes per month.[69] In contrast, daily smokers often smoke 600 cigarettes per month.[69]

Although the classical theory of dependence suggests that continued exposure to an addictive substance will eventually lead to addiction, chippers may smoke for years and never show evidence of dependence.[63] Chippers may be biologically anomalous and, therefore, less susceptible to nicotine addiction.[63] Some occasional smokers may increase or decrease their cigarette consumption, but approximately 40% have never been moderate or heavy smokers.[69]

Smoking rates for occasional smokers may be influenced by knowledge and social norms.[67,69] They appear to be psychologically different from dependent smokers in that they are less stressed and better adapted to stress.[63] Given this theory, their need to smoke in order to cope with stress may be less than that of dependent smokers.[63] Women who are very light smokers often smoke in social situations and link smoking with pleasurable relaxation.[67]

Occasional smoking is often a temporary or transitional state.[69] Some occasional smokers may run the risk of becoming daily smokers, whereas others may consider quitting. Change in marital status—from being married to being divorced or widowed—and workplace boredom and job repetitiveness were predictors of occasional smokers becoming daily smokers.[69] This supports the theory that people use smoking to blunt stresses that are not mitigated by other coping mechanisms.[58] Characteristics that predicted occasional smokers becoming abstinent were age and education. Younger smokers and those with more education were more likely to quit.[69] Occasional smokers may benefit from cessation programs because they have a stronger intention to quit and are more likely to quit.[69] Whereas 48% of occasional smokers strongly intend to quit, only 25% of daily smokers strongly intend to quit.[69] In a large cohort study, 82% of the women who quit were light smokers (1–24 cigarettes per day).[68]

Although many studies site the government statistic that at least 70% of current smokers want to quit,[70] there is a group of smokers—dubbed hard-core smokers—who will most likely never quit.[71] Low-probability quitters are characterized by high addiction (≥15 cigarettes per day), no recent 24-hour quit attempt in the past year, and no intention of quitting in the coming 6 months.[72] This group has a 3% probability of quitting smoking 2 years in the future.[72] Hard-core smokers have been defined as a subgroup of the low-probability quitters; they are characterized by high addiction (≥15 cigarettes per day), no 24-hour quit attempt in the past year, and no intention of quitting ever.[71]

Analysis of California longitudinal data has revealed that approximately 5.2% of adult smokers can be classified as hard-core. The typical hard-core smoker is a White, non-Hispanic man older than 44 years of age who lives alone; who has 12 or fewer years of education; whose income is below $50,000; and who is retired, unemployed, or unemployable.[71] Conversely, people who report very light smoking have an educational level similar to that of nonsmokers.[67]

Hard-core smokers started smoking at an earlier age, are more addicted, and smoke more cigarettes. Only 14% of hard-core smokers have ever seriously considered quitting, compared with 50.5% of all non–hard-core smokers.[71]

Although hard-core smokers are more likely to report their health as poor, they appear to be in denial about the health dangers of cigarette smoking to themselves or to others. Only 31.7% of hard-core smokers believe that inhaling secondhand smoke causes lung cancer in nonsmokers, compared with 70.2% of non–hard-core smokers.[71] Sixty-one percent of hard-core smokers believe that smoking is harming their health, compared with 79.5% of non–hard-core smokers.[71]

Nicotine and the Brain

Tobacco use is not just a nasty habit; long-term use leads to nicotine dependence. When use is discontinued for even a short period of time, the smoker often experiences nicotine withdrawal. Nicotine dependence and withdrawal are both categorized as mental disorders in the

American Psychiatric Association's *Diagnostic and Statistical Manual of Mental Disorders* (DSM-IV). Use of all forms of tobacco—cigarettes, chewing tobacco, snuff, pipes, and cigars—and prescription medications containing nicotine—patches and gum—can lead to nicotine dependence and withdrawal.[73] The degree of dependence is related to how rapidly the nicotine is absorbed by the body and the nicotine content of the product.[73] Nicotine dependence has similarities to other substance dependencies. In general, substance dependence is characterized by continued use of the substance, despite significant problems related to that use. The pattern of repeated self-administration results in tolerance for the ever-increasing doses of the substance, withdrawal when the substance is withheld, and compulsive drug-taking behavior.[73] Dependence is defined as the existence of three or more of the following symptoms occurring at any time in the same 12-month period.

1. **Tolerance:** Dependent smokers must continuously increase the dose of nicotine to obtain the same effect. Long-term smokers often consume more than 20 cigarettes per day. This amount of smoking would have produced nausea, dizziness, and other symptoms of toxicity had they consumed this level when they began to smoke.[73]

2. **Withdrawal:** Withdrawal symptoms appear when blood or tissue concentrations of the addictive substance decline.[73] Nicotine withdrawal syndrome can characterized by the existence of any four of the following symptoms: dysphoric or depressed mood; insomnia; irritability, frustration, or anger; anxiety; difficulty concentrating; restlessness or impatience; decreased heart rate; and increased appetite or weight gain.[73] These symptoms can cause significant distress or impairment in the individual's social, occupational, or general functioning.[73] Craving for nicotine is an important part of withdrawal and may contribute significantly to relapse. After as much as 6 months of abstinence, 50% of ex-smokers report having had the desire for a cigarette in the previous 24 hours.[73]

3. **Patterns of compulsive use:** Patterns of compulsive use include smoking more or smoking over a longer period of time than was originally intended; expressing a desire to quit or cut down but being unable to; spending a significant amount of time and effort obtaining tobacco or ensuring a steady supply; planning daily activities around smoking; giving up social or recreational activities that are not conducive to smoking, and even withdrawing from friends or family to smoke; continuing to smoke, despite the realization that it is contributing to psychological or physical problems.[73]

The most common signs of nicotine dependence are tobacco odor, cough, evidence of chronic obstructive pulmonary disease, and excessive skin wrinkling.[73] Nicotine dependence is more common among people with mental disorders. Depending upon the condition, smoking prevalence can range from 55% to 90%,[73] whereas the adult smoking rate in the U.S. population is 23.3%.[70] Smoking increases the metabolism of some psychiatric drugs, and consequently smoking cessation can increase blood levels of these drugs, sometimes to a clinically significant degree.[73]

Nicotine withdrawal is associated with dry or productive cough, decreased heart rate, decreases in catecholamine and cortisol levels, changes in rapid eye movement (REM), impairment on neuropsychological testing, and decreased metabolic rate.[73] People who suffer from major depression or any anxiety disorder reported more severe nicotine withdrawal than people who do not have these conditions.[74]

Several characteristics of nicotine dependence may predict the likelihood of smoking cessation relapse: smoking soon after waking, smoking when ill, difficulty refraining from smoking, reporting that the first cigarette of the day would be the most difficult to give up, and smoking more in the morning than in the afternoon.[73] Other factors that play a role in cessation are the number of cigarettes smoked per day, the nicotine yield of the cigarettes, and the number of pack-years a person has smoked.[73] The more nicotine a person has ingested over a longer period of time, the higher his or her level of addiction and the harder it will be to quit. Lifetime prevalence of nicotine dependence in the United States is 20% among the general population and 50% to 80% among current tobacco users. Lifetime prevalence of nicotine withdrawal among current tobacco users is 50%. Furthermore, it is estimated that 50% of people who quit on their own and 75% of those who use smoking treatment programs experience withdrawal when they stop using tobacco.[73]

In the United States, approximately 45% of people who have ever smoked eventually stop smoking, but most people try and fail at least three or four times before they successfully quit.[73]

There are an infinite number of reasons why people start using tobacco, why they continue to use it, and why they may try to quit. As is evidenced above, level of addiction coupled with social and behavioral factors influences a person's lifestyle choices.

SMOKING CESSATION AS A PREVENTIVE MEASURE

Although the *primary* prevention of tobacco use may be the ideal way to address the problem of tobacco control in women, it is clear that significant numbers of American women are current smokers and that each day, girls and women initiate tobacco use. Thus smoking cessation techniques must continue to be developed such that durable cessation for large percentages of smokers, both women and men, becomes possible. Long-term smoking cessation rates have historically been extremely low; 1-year abstinence has been reported at 4.3%.[75] The Centers for Disease Control and Prevention reported overall annual cessation rates of 4.7%.[70] As a result of initiatives promoted by the 1980 Surgeon General's report, *The Health Consequences of Smoking for Women* (U.S. Department of Health and Human Services[2]), gender-specific differences in outcomes of smoking cessation have been investigated. Biopsychosocial factors that have possible gender-specific effects on smoking cessation include the influence of potential weight gain associated with cessation, general commitment to health, and social support during cessation. Other avenues of gender-specific cessation research include influence of the hormonal milieu and depression in women on cessation success, socioeconomic status and cessation, and subgroup analysis (i.e., women heavy smokers, minority women).

In general, both women and men cite "health reasons" as the overriding motivation for smoking cessation.[76] No significant gender difference in the frequency of this factor has been reported.[77] However, women have more concerns with the health effects of their smoking on others than men.[78] This includes an increased concern about the health effects of smoking on their children and other family members; this concern for the effect of a mother's smoking on her children has been used successfully to motivate smoking mothers to seek aid in smoking cessation.[79]

Weight gain after smoking cessation is an important concern for both women and men, and concern with weight gain may act as a barrier to cessation initiation and continued cessation. However, this issue may be more important in influencing cessation attempts for women than men. More women than men reported weight gain during cessation attempts than men (33% versus 21%), and concern about weight gain was cited as one reason for relapse by 33% of women compared with 21% of men.[80]

Strategies for smoking cessation encompass a wide variety of approaches that range from unaided smoking cessation to assisted techniques that include self-help, cessation counseling, and nicotine replacement therapy (NRT), and to combinations of these techniques. Unaided cessation had been the preferred technique until the 1990s, when nicotine replacement therapies came into popular use.[81] In a metaanalysis of 10 prospective studies of unaided quitters, there were no significant differences in 6-month and 12-month abstinence rates between women and men.[75]

Cessation interventions appear to improve cessation rates. In guidelines developed through a metaanalysis of randomized controlled trials of smoking cessation interventions, those smoking cessation interventions that used counseling or other psychosocial interventions led to increased cessation rates; additionally, increased intensity of health care provider contact, with increased amount of person-to-person contact time, were identified as positively influencing smoking cessation rates.[82] It appears that training in the use of self-help materials, combined with recruitment by a health professional into a treatment group and supplemented by a physician's advice, can boost abstinence rates to 13% at 6 months and up to 3.9% at 1 year.[83] Several studies have reported that, in general, women use more cessation assistance than men.[81,84]

Tobacco dependence has many of the characteristics of a chronic disease.[60] Few tobacco users reach permanent abstinence the first time they try to quit; most cycle through multiple periods of tobacco use and abstinence from tobacco use. There are a number of research-based strategies that can be employed by physicians who are attempting to motivate patients to quit using tobacco. To successfully intervene with patients, clinicians must understand the chronic nature of tobacco dependence and social and behavioral contexts of smoking.

Tobacco use cessation interventions can improve quit rates when compared with unaided cessation.[60] In 2000, the Agency for Healthcare Research and Quality (AHRQ) and the U.S. Public Health Service published the *Treating Tobacco Use and Dependence Clinical Practice Guideline*, a compilation of metaanalyses of thousands of tobacco use cessation randomized trials. The guidelines recommend behavioral strategies and pharmacologic treatment for nicotine dependence as both efficacious and cost-effective. In addition, the guidelines advocate for brief cessation interventions by physicians and health care systems changes that would institutionalize nicotine dependence treatment.

The AHRQ guidelines strongly support multisession telephone-based cessation counseling, group counseling, or individual counseling; strategies that incorporate social support outside of treatment; and seven different cessation medications (Table 2-1).

There is a strong dose-response relationship between successful tobacco use cessation, the length of a person-to-person intervention, and the number of contacts (Table 2-2).[60] Although brief cessation interventions lasting as little as 3 minutes can increase abstinence rates, intense sessions, lasting more than 10 minutes, increase the likelihood of cessation.[60] Multiple cessation counseling sessions—four or more—further increase cessation rates.[60]

Practical counseling that includes problem solving is particularly effective (odds ratio [OR] = 1.5). In addition, intra-treatment (OR = 1.3) and extra-treatment (OR = 1.5) social support significantly increase abstinence rates (Table 2-3).[60]

Pharmacologic Therapies for Cessation

By prescribing effective pharmacotherapies to their smoking patients, physicians may double or triple their patients' chances of abstinence.[60] Unfortunately, some physicians may be reluctant to prescribe medications because of commonly held beliefs. Prevailing myths associated with prescribing medications for smoking treatment include: (1) smoking is a lifestyle choice and not a true dependence disorder; (2) medications should be reserved

Table 2-1
Efficacy of and Estimated Abstinence Rates for Various Types of Formats (n=58 studies)

Format	Estimated Odds Ratio (95% C.I.)	Estimated Abstinence Rate (95% C.I.)
No format	1.0	10.8
Self-help	1.2 (1.02, 1.3)	12.3 (10.9, 13.6)
Proactive telephone counseling	1.2 (1.1, 1.4)	13.1 (11.4, 14.8)
Group counseling	1.3 (1.1, 1.6)	13.9 (11.6, 16.1)
Individual counseling	1.7 (1.4, 2.0)	16.8 (14.7, 19.1)

Source: Fiore MC, Bailey WC, Cohen SJ, et al: *Treating tobacco use and dependence.* Clinical Practice Guideline, Rockville, MD, US Department of Health and Human Services, Public Health Service, June 2000.[60]

for heavy smokers; (3) medications should be used only with behavioral treatment; (4) and smokers should try to quit on their own first. Clinical and epidemiologic data discount these myths.[60]

Five first-line cessation medications have been found effective at increasing cessation and have been approved by the Food and Drug Administration (FDA): bupropion SR (sustained release), nicotine gum, nicotine inhaler, nicotine nasal spray, and nicotine patch (Table 2-4). Additionally, two second-line medications (clonidine and nortriptyline) are available but have not yet been approved by the FDA.

In addition to the studies listed in Tables 2-1, 2-2, 2-3, and 2-4, research has been conducted to test the effectiveness of combining different types of medications and of combining medication and behavioral support. Although nicotine patch and gum have been found to be more effective when used together, this strategy may lead to nicotine overdose and should be used only with patients who are unable to quit using one medication.[60] Specific pharmacotherapy recommendations for subpopulations are not currently available through the FDA, but several studies have shown that care should be taken when prescribing some medications to pregnant smokers or patients with cardiovascular diseases.[60] Pregnant smokers should be advised to forego NRT—if at all possible—and seek behavioral support that includes postpartum intervention.[60] Some researchers believe that the safety of NRT during

Table 2-2
Efficacy of and Estimated Abstinence Rates for Various Intensity Levels of Person-to-Person Contact (n=43 studies)

Level of Contact	Estimated Odds Ratio (95% C.I.)	Estimated Abstinence Rate (95% C.I.)
No contact	1.0	10.9
Minimal counseling (< 3 minutes)	1.3 (1.01, 1.6)	13.4 (10.9, 16.1)
Low-intensity counseling (3-10 minutes)	1.6 (1.2, 2.0)	16.0 (12.8, 19.2)
Higher-intensity counseling (> 10 minutes)	2.3 (2.0, 2.7)	22.1 (19.4, 24.7)

Source: Fiore MC, Bailey WC, Cohen SJ, et al: *Treating tobacco use and dependence.* Clinical Practice Guideline, Rockville, MD, US Department of Health and Human Services, Public Health Service, June 2000.[59]

Table 2-3
Efficacy of and Estimated Abstinence Rates for Number of Person-to-Person Treatment Sessions (n=45 studies)

Level of Contact	Estimated Odds Ratio (95% C.I.)	Estimated Abstinence Rate (95% C.I.)
0-1 session	1.0	12.4
2-3 sessions	1.4 (1.1, 1.7)	16.3 (13.7, 19.0)
4-8 sessions	1.9 (1.6, 2.2)	20.9 (18.1, 23.6)
> 8 sessions	2.3 (2.1, 3.0)	24.7 (21.0, 28.4)

Source: Fiore MC, Bailey WC, Cohen SJ, et al: *Treating tobacco use and dependence*. Clinical Practice Guideline, Rockville, MD, US Department of Health and Human Services, Public Health Service, June 2000.[59]

pregnancy cannot be guaranteed and that it cannot be definitively said that NRT is safer than smoking during pregnancy.[8]

Brief Cessation Interventions By Physicians

Physicians often do not assess and intervene with their smoking patients—despite the prevalence of smoking, the lethality of nicotine addiction, and the existence of effective smoking cessation treatments.[60] Discouraging statistics about long-term quit rates leave many physicians feeling ineffective at intervening with smoking patients.[60] In reality, even minimal physician advice to quit can be a powerful motivator for smokers.

Table 2-4
Efficacy of and Estimated Abstinence Rates for Pharmacotherapies

Pharmacotherapy	Estimated Odds Ratio (95% C.I.)	Estimated Abstinence Rate (95% C.I.)
Bupropion SR, prescription (n=2 studies)	2.1 (1.5, 3.0)	30.5 (23.2, 37.8)
Nicotine gum, over-the-counter (n=13 studies)	1.5 (1.3, 1.8)	17.1 (20.6, 26.7)
Nicotine inhaler, prescription (n=4 studies)	2.5 (1.7, 3.6)	22.8 (16.4, 29.2)
Nicotine nasal spray, prescription (n=3 studies)	2.7 (1.8, 4.1)	30.5 (21.8, 39.2)
Nicotine patch over-the-counter or prescription (n=27 studies)	1.9 (1.7, 2.2)	17.7 (16.0, 19.5)
Clonidine, prescription (n=5 studies)	2.1 (1.4, 3.2)	25.6 (17.7, 33.6)
Nortriptyline, prescription (n=2 studies)	3.2 (1.8, 5.7)	30.1 (18.1, 41.6)

Source: Fiore MC, Bailey WC, Cohen SJ, et al: *Treating tobacco use and dependence*. Clinical Practice Guideline, Rockville, MD, US Department of Health and Human Services, Public Health Service, June 2000.[59]

Perpetuating the myths that there is one "magic bullet" treatment for smoking treat-ment and that cessation success should be defined only as total abstinence mask the true chronic nature of nicotine addiction.[60] Smokers often cycle through stages of quitting.[85] Numerous researchers have tested Prochaska and DiClemente's Transtheoretical Model of Staged Change since it was first proposed in the 1980s. The theory postulates that there are five stages through which a smoker cycles when he or she is trying to quit and that at any stage the smoker can move forward toward a quit attempt or backward to a previous stage or relapse.

1. **Precontemplation:** The smoker is not thinking about quitting and doesn't feel that smoking is a problem.
2. **Contemplation:** The smoker begins to think about quitting.
3. **Preparation:** The smoker plans a quit attempt.
4. **Action:** The smoker quits.
5. **Maintenance:** The smoker tries to maintain the quit attempt.

Physicians should keep the stages of change in mind when intervening with smoking patients. Patients who are in the precontemplation stage may be less receptive to physician intervention than those in the later stages. The "5 A's" have been suggested as an outline to guide clinical interventions.[60] These strategies have been designed to be brief, requiring 3 minutes or less of the physician's time.

1. **Ask** every patient at every visit if he or she uses tobacco and document status in the patient's chart.
2. **Advise** the patient to quit in a clear, strong, personalized manner.
3. **Assess** the patient's willingness to quit.
4. **Assist** the patient in making a quit attempt if he or she is ready. This could include offering cessation counseling, making a referral to services, and prescribing med-ication. Several studies have reported women use more cessation assistance than men.[81,84]
5. **Arrange** for follow-up, preferably within the first week after the quit attempt.

Brief interventions are particularly effective when incorporated into overall clinical systems changes. These changes could include cessation training for staff, recording nico-tine dependence diagnostic codes on billing forms, identification of and interventions with tobacco users at each visit, intervention follow-up protocols, and chart stickers to track patient interventions and quit attempts. Brief cessation interventions can be con-ducted by other clinic workers, including nurses and office staff—in addition to the physi-cian. The more cessation messages a smoker receives, the more likely he or she is to make a quit attempt.

Physicians can enhance the patient's motivation to quit by personalizing the interven-tion message to the smoker using the "5 R's."[60]

1. **Relevance:** Why is quitting important to the patient? Physician advice is more effective if it is tailored to the patient's personal situation, family history, or other risk factors. In general, both women and men cite "health reasons" as the overrid-ing motivation for smoking cessation.[76,86] No significant gender difference in the frequency of this factor has been reported.[77] Other top reasons for quitting includ-ed expense (60.7%), concern regarding the effects of secondhand smoke on oth-ers (55.8%), and setting a good example (55.1%).[86] Women may have more con-cerns with the health effects of their smoking on others than men.[78] This includes an increased concern about the health effects of smoking on their children and other family members; this concern for the effect of a mother's smoking on her

children has been successfully used to motivate smoking mothers to seek aid in smoking cessation.[79]

2. **Risks:** What are the patient's health risks if he or she continues to smoke? Ask the patient to identify potential negative consequences of tobacco use.

3. **Rewards:** There are many positive outcomes of smoking cessation. Ask the patient to identify personal benefits for quitting, such as improved health, feeling better about one's self, saving money, or setting a good example for children.

4. **Roadblocks:** Smoking is an addiction that generally progresses over many years. Ask the patient what barriers may prevent him or her from successfully quitting smoking, such as fear of withdrawal, weight gain, depression, or lack of support.

5. **Repetition:** Physicians should repeat the motivational intervention each time a smoking patient visits. Smokers who have tried to quit and failed should be told that most people try several times before they quit successfully.

When intervening with patients, emphasize that there are five key strategies for quitting tobacco.[87]

1. **Get ready:** Patients should be advised to plan their quit attempt by setting a quit date; changing their environment (i.e., discarding cigarettes and ashtrays, establishing a smoke-free home); reviewing what went right or wrong with past quit attempts; and planning for trigger situations that might result in relapse.

2. **Get support and encouragement:** Social support from friends, family, or trained counselors can improve an individual's chances of quitting tobacco. Many U.S. states have smoking cessation telephone quitlines or community-based classes that offer professional behavioral support.

3. **Learn new skills and behaviors:** Patients should be advised to distract themselves from urges to smoke. Strategies could include keeping busy, going for a walk, changing their daily routines (particularly those associated with smoking), drinking water, and planning something enjoyable and stress-free everyday.

4. **Get medication and use it correctly:** There are five medications that have been approved for smoking cessation treatment by the FDA: Bupropion SR, nicotine gum, nicotine patch, nicotine inhaler, and nicotine nasal spray. Using NRT or buproprion SR, a nonnicotine cessation drug, can significantly increase smoking cessation success. Nicotine gum and some patches are available over-the-counter medications, but the other medications are prescription only. Research studies have shown that many people use over-the-counter cessation medications incorrectly; this impairs their effectiveness. Physicians' advice to quit, help in choosing the right medication, and instructions in proper usage can significantly increase their patients' chances of successfully quitting smoking.

5. **Be prepared for relapse or difficult situations:** Most people relapse within the first 3 months after quitting smoking. Frequent reasons for relapse include drinking alcohol, being around others who are smoking, weight gain, and depressed mood.

Predictors of Success

Some studies have identified a number of variables that are associated with successful cessation. These include smoking fewer cigarettes per day, longer time before the first cigarette of the day, more than one previous quit attempt, a strong desire to stop smoking, the absence of other smokers in the household, higher socioeconomic status, and older age.[85,88]

Overall, variables associated with higher abstinence rates include:
1. **High motivation:** Tobacco user reports that they are motivated to quit.
2. **Ready to change:** Tobacco user reports readiness to quit within 1 month.
3. **Moderate to high self-efficacy:** Tobacco user is confident that he or she will be able to quit.
4. **Supportive social network:** Tobacco user works and lives in a smoke-free environment and has friends who do not smoke around him or her.[60]

Reasons for Relapse

Some research studies have shown that women have a harder time quitting and avoiding relapse when compared with men, whereas others have suggested that they have similar cessation success rates.[60,89] Withdrawal symptoms may play a larger role in relapse for women than men.[89] Pregnancy, fear of weight gain, depression, and the need for social support appear to be associated with smoking maintenance, cessation, or relapse in women.[14] Although women and men benefit equally from smoking cessation interventions, women face different stressors and barriers to quitting.[60]

Regardless of smoking status, depression and anxiety are major women's health problems. Clinicians should be alert to signs of postcessation depression, which often leads to relapse. Addressing withdrawal symptoms with behavioral counseling, pharmacologic treatments such as antidepressants, or both, may be especially helpful to women.[85] When compared with successful quitters, women who continued smoking reported higher consumption of alcohol and heavier smoking.[68]

Overall, variables associated with cessation relapse include the following:
1. **High nicotine dependence:** Tobacco user has experienced severe withdrawal during previous quit attempts, smokes more than 20 cigarettes per day, and has first cigarette of the day within 30 minutes of waking.
2. **History of psychiatric comorbidity:** Tobacco user has a history of depression, schizophrenia, alcoholism, or other chemical dependency.
3. **High stress level:** Tobacco user has experienced stressful life events or recent major life changes (i.e., divorce, marriage, loss of income), or both.[60]

Weight gain after smoking cessation is an important concern for both women and men, and concern with weight gain may act as a barrier to cessation initiation and continued cessation. However, this issue may be more important in influencing cessation attempts for women. More women than men reported weight gain during cessation attempts than men (33% versus 21%), and concern about weight gain was cited as one reason for relapse by 33% of women, compared with 21% of men.[80] Others have reported that actual weight gain during cessation does not predict relapse to smoking.[14] Smoking cessation is followed by early weight gain that may make most former smokers comparable in weight, after 2 years, to never-smokers of the same sex, same age, and same education level.[90]

Whereas smoking may have a short-term effect on weight that disappears within 2 years after cessation,[90] education and socioeconomic status are strong long-term predictors of body weight and variation in body weight over time.[88,90] The relationship between education and weight-related aspects of lifestyle such as diet and physical activity may be a major predictor of long-term weight history.[90] Women who gain the most weight after smoking cessation were those who do not increase their physical activity.[68] It has been suggested that moderate increases in physical activity can minimize postcessation weight gain in women[68] and that smoking cessation programs should include education components on diet and physical activity.[90]

PREGNANCY AND SMOKING

Prevalence of Smoking During Pregnancy

Women's exposure to tobacco smoke is associated with numerous adverse outcomes of pregnancy for both mother and infant. Many women smoke during their pregnancies—despite increasing public health awareness of the health risks of tobacco use during pregnancy. Prevalence estimates of smoking during pregnancy compiled from a number of studies surveying women with live births showed a downward trend in prevalence, from 19.5% in 1989 to 12.9% in 1998.[14] Other studies have reported higher prevalence rates; for instance, the 1995 National Survey of Family Growth reported a prevalence rate of 17.8% for women smoking during and after pregnancy.[91] Discrepancies in prevalence of smoking during pregnancy may be due in part to concealment of tobacco use from their clinicians by some pregnant women, leading to underreporting.[92,93]

Rates of smoking during pregnancy vary by age, education, race, ethnicity, and socioeconomic status. Black women used tobacco during pregnancy at a rate of 27% in 1988, slightly lower than that for American Indian women (35%) and White women (27%).[94] Other surveys have reported similar prevalence rankings by ethnicity, with White mothers having a higher prevalence than Blacks as well as Hispanics.[95] There appears to be an effect of place of birth on smoking prevalence in women of certain ethnicities; for Mexican mothers, those born in the United States had a prevalence rate of 6% as compared with 2% for Mexican mothers born outside the United States.[96] A similar trend has been noted for Asian or Pacific Islander women, who have an extremely low prevalence (3%) of smoking during pregnancy if born outside of the United States.

As with overall smoking prevalence, an inverse relationship has been reported between level of education and prevalence of smoking during pregnancy. In 1998, there was nearly a twelvefold difference in smoking prevalence during pregnancy when comparing women with 9 to 11 years of education (25.5%) to women with 16 or more years of education (2.2%). Tobacco use during pregnancy also varies by age of the mother; in 1998, young women aged 18 to 24 years were more likely to smoke during pregnancy than women aged 25 to 49 (15.1% versus 10.5%, respectively).[14]

Effects of Smoking on Reproductive Outcomes

There are multiple adverse effects on reproductive outcomes that have been directly or indirectly related to maternal tobacco exposure. It has been estimated that 5% of all perinatal mortality is attributable to smoking during pregnancy.[97] Maternal tobacco exposure has been associated with alterations in the physiology of fertility, placental functioning, and intrauterine fetal growth and development. Additionally, an increase in prevalence of some health conditions, including respiratory illnesses and sudden infant death syndrome, has been reported in children born to smoking mothers.

The adverse effects of chemicals contained in tobacco smoke, especially nicotine and its major metabolite, cotinine, have been described for many aspects of reproductive physiology. Nicotine crosses the placenta, with levels detectable in the fetal circulation and the amniotic fluid.[98] Nicotine, PAHs, and cigarette smoke have been shown to affect gonadotropin release and estradiol production, ovulation, gamete and ovary function, fallopian tube physiology, and ovum implantation.[99-101] Nicotine, a known vasoconstrictor, has been shown to cause decrease in uterine artery blood flow and attendant alterations in fetal oxygenation and acid-base status.[102] Nicotine affects transport function of the placenta and has been shown to inhibit placental amino acid uptake.[103] Carbon monoxide, which is present in blood in increased amounts in chronic smokers, crosses the placenta; consequences of increased carbon monoxide levels in the fetal circulation include the formation of carboxyhemoglobin, which lessens oxygen delivery to the fetal tissues through a shift of the oxygen dissociation curve.[104,105]

These studies of the biologic effects of tobacco exposure on pregnancy outcomes have been complemented by a large body of epidemiologic research that has shown a myriad of adverse perinatal outcomes in women who use tobacco during pregnancy. Maternal smoking has been associated with infertility in case-control studies;[106-109] tubal dysfunction is strongly implicated as an causal factor in this setting.[107-110] Women who smoke during pregnancy appear to have an increased risk for ectopic pregnancy; the physiologic cause of this association may be related to impaired tubal transport of the ovum.[100,107,111] Preterm birth has been associated with maternal smoking during pregnancy.[112,113] Premature rupture of membranes, which accounts for approximately 30% of preterm births,[114] has been associated with maternal smoking. A reduction in the risk of preterm birth was noted in a study of women who quit smoking during their first trimester of pregnancy, compared with women who continued to smoke.[115]

Pregnant smokers are at increased risk for delivering low–birth weight infants. This association was recognized as early as 1957, when the incidence of low–birth weight infants less than 2500 g was reported to be twofold higher in women who smoked during pregnancy than in nonsmoking women.[116] Women who smoke during pregnancy deliver infants who are consistently 150 to 250 g lighter than those born to nonsmoking women.[117] As with preterm births, data support a beneficial effect of smoking cessation early in pregnancy on infant birth weight.[118] The biologic effects of smoking that underlie the association between tobacco exposure and birth weight are not fully known. Women who smoke are likely to gain less weight during pregnancy, which may have an adverse effect on fetal growth. The effect of chronic fetal hypoxia caused by nicotine may inhibit fetal growth. Changes in the structure of the placenta related to diminished uterine blood flow in the face of nicotine exposure, including placental infarcts, may influence fetal growth.[119]

Placental complications have been clearly associated with maternal smoking during pregnancy; these include placenta previa and abruptio placentae.[120-122] A relationship between the risk of abruptio placentae and the daily amount of cigarettes has been reported, with a risk of 23% noted in women smoking less than one pack of cigarettes a day during pregnancy, compared with a risk of 86% noted in those smoking more than one pack a day. A dose-response relationship between daily dose of cigarettes and risk of placenta previa has also been reported.[123] A study of the histology of the placentas showed decidual necrosis at the margin of the placenta more commonly in smoking than nonsmoking mothers;[121] this histologic lesion may be an initiation site for the separation of the placenta from the uterine wall that is the associated with abruption.

Sudden infant death syndrome (SIDS) is one of the leading causes of infant mortality. Although extensive research into etiologic factors has been undertaken, its cause is still not known. However, epidemiologic studies of both maternal smoking and ETS in the postnatal period have identified these as risk factors for SIDS;[124-126] other risk factors include sleeping in a prone position and not having been breast-fed.[127] The risk of SIDS was highest for infants whose mothers smoked both during and after pregnancy, with a threefold risk reported for those infants as compared with infants of nonsmoking mothers.[126] A dose-response relationship has been shown between the amount of cigarettes smoked during pregnancy and the risk for SIDS.[128] The relationship between maternal smoking and SIDS at the physiologic level may involve alterations of the central nervous system respiratory and hypoxic drives.[129]

Smoking Cessation During Pregnancy and After Birth

Many smoking cessation advocates have focused their efforts on reaching pregnant smokers—because of the major public health benefits of reducing smoking prevalence during pregnancy. Tobacco use is considered the most important potentially preventable cause of reproductive problems including preterm pregnancy, low birth weight, deaths from perinatal disorders, and SIDS. An added incentive to encouraging smoking cessation when women become pregnant is that they are more likely to quit during pregnancy than at any other time. The Surgeon General's Report on Women and Smoking estimates that eliminating maternal smoking during pregnancy could lead to a 10% reduction in all infant deaths and a 12% reduction in deaths from perinatal conditions.[14]

Smoking quit rates during pregnancy are relatively high. According to survey data from the mid-1980s, 39% of pregnant smokers quit either upon learning that they were pregnant or during the course of their pregnancy, with quitting more likely as education level increased.[130] Unfortunately, most mothers who quit return to smoking after birth; postnatal relapse rates range between 50% and 80% in the first year following delivery.[131] An extremely important risk factor for postpartum relapse appears to be socializing with or living with a smoking partner, which has a strong negative influence on maintenance of abstinence. Other factors include social support and the type of strategy used to resist smoking during pregnancy and in the postpartum period.[132,133] The continued development of strategies to decrease postpartum relapse will obviously have long-term health benefits to both mother and child.

TEENS—A SPECIAL PROBLEM
Why Teens Are a Particular Concern

Tobacco marketing and tobacco control efforts have typically targeted the young. Research has shown that adolescents are more susceptible to cigarette advertising and promotional activities than adults.[134-138] There is also evidence that adolescents are more susceptible than adults to nicotine addiction.[139,140] It is no surprise, therefore, that the majority (80% to 90%) of adult smokers began smoking during their teenage years[141,142] and that teenage smoking is frequently called "pediatric epidemic."[142]

The immediate health effects of smoking on teens include general decreased physical fitness, increased coughing and phlegm, greater susceptibility to and severity of respiratory illnesses, early development of artery disease, a slower rate of lung growth, and a reduced level of adult normal lung function.[98] The process of adolescent nicotine addiction and withdrawal is not fundamentally different from the process in adults.[139,142] However, adolescent smokers are more likely to develop severe levels of nicotine addiction than are individuals who start smoking at a later age, and therefore adolescents are more likely to develop the long-term health problems related to smoking.[143] This is particularly troublesome for adolescent girls because of the relationship between smoking and poor birth outcomes. Adolescents are not likely to be deterred by the prospect of the long-term health effects of smoking because they misunderstand the health risks related to smoking, they underestimate the power of nicotine addiction, and they believe they are invulnerable to these risks.[144-147]

Adolescent Smoking Incidence

In the 1940s, the incidence of cigarette smoking among 12- to 17-year-old boys was far higher than it was for girls. Female incidence rates started increasing in 1940, declined slightly during the early 1960s, and then sharply increased in the late 1960s when Philip Morris introduced Virginia Slims.[148] During that same period, male incidence declined.[149] Male and female incidence rates for teens have been similar since the mid-1970s.[150] Recent data show that 38.3% of middle school boys and 34.2% of middle school girls have tried smoking cigarettes. At the high school level, 65.3% of males and 62.5% of females have tried smoking.[141] It is estimated that every day, more than 6000 American teenagers younger than age 18 try smoking for the first time.[151]

Adolescent Smoking Prevalence

One of the standard measures of smoking prevalence is smoking in the past 30 days. Adolescent smoking prevalence is tracked at the state and national levels by the Monitoring the Future—the National Youth Tobacco Survey (MTF), which is sponsored by the National Institute on Drug Abuse (NIDA) and administered in schools throughout the country on an annual basis. Before 1975, female prevalence rates were lower than those of males. In 1975, females caught up to males and then surpassed them until the mid-1980s. Since the early 1990s, male rates have been slightly higher than female rates.[149] Figure 2-2 tracks the 30-day prevalence rate of cigarette smoking for twelfth-grade males and females since 1975.

Current adolescent smoking prevalence rates are also measured by the National Youth Tobacco Survey (NYTS), which was administered in 1999 and again in 2000. The NYTS is representative of all students in the 50 states and the District of Columbia. In addition, 13 states administered the survey in 2000. As in the MTF survey, tobacco use is defined as use

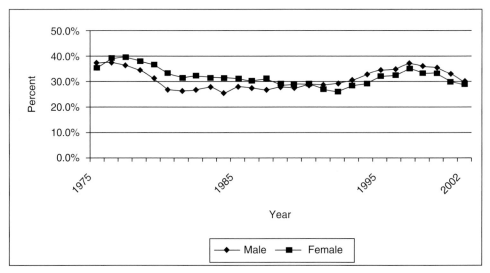

FIGURE 2-2
Thirty-day prevalence of cigarette smoking, by gender, 1975 to 2002. (From Johnston LD, O'Malley PM, Bachman JG: Teen smoking declines sharply in 2002, more than offsetting large increases in the early 1900s. Ann Arbor, Mich, *University of Michigan News and Information Services, 2002.*)

in the past 30 days. Figure 2-3 shows data from the national and state surveys in 2000. Smoking prevalence increases by age for both males and females. At the middle school level, the current smoking prevalence rate for boys was 11.7%; middle school girls' smoking prevalence was 10.2%. In high school, 28.8% of males smoked in the past 30 days, compared with 27.3% for females.[141]

Risk Factors for Adolescent Smoking

The Surgeon General describes adolescent tobacco use as part of a "syndrome of problem behaviors."[142] Smoking can be a means for teenagers to deal with the developmental tasks of adolescence,[152,153] such as establishing a self-image, developing feelings of maturity and autonomy, and identifying with a social group.[154] Risks for adolescent smoking can be attributed to the complex interaction of factors such as:

1. Personal attributes, including low educational aspirations, low self-esteem, anxiety, depression or other psychiatric diagnosis, low self-confidence, poor refusal skills, risk-taking and rebellious personality, use of alcohol and other illegal drugs, denial or minimization of the health consequences of smoking, and receptivity to advertising and the perception that tobacco serves a purpose [142,143,154-158]
2. Social influences, including perceived social norms and the attitudes and smoking behaviors of family and friends[143,147,154,156-159]
3. Environmental influences such as low socioeconomic status, low parental educational attainment, availability of tobacco products, and exposure to tobacco product advertising.[136,147,153-156,158,160]

Studies have found that girls who smoke are more self-confident, outgoing, rebellious, and socially skilled than are boys who smoke. Girls who are involved in organized social activities and who spend time with opposite-gender friends are more likely to smoke than are those who participate in sports or individual recreational activities.[154] Concerns about weight also put adolescent girls at high risk for smoking,[155,161-164] and industry advertising reinforces the association of smoking with thinness.[142]

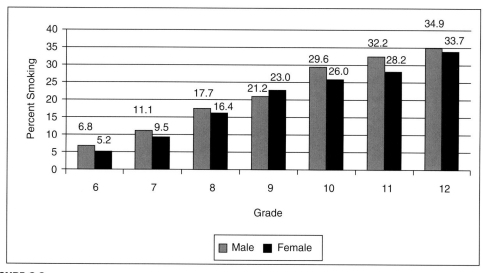

FIGURE 2-3
Thirty-day smoking prevalence by grade and gender, 2002. (From Farrelly MC, Vilsaint M, Lindsey DE, et al: Legacy first book report #7: cigarette smoking among youth: 2000 National Youth Tobacco Survey, Washington, DC, *American Legacy Foundation,* 2001.)

Prevention of Teen Smoking

Knowledge of the health risks related to tobacco use is not, in itself, a significant deterrent of adolescent smoking. Many studies have shown that providing information about smoking increases knowledge but does not prevent or delay cigarette smoking.[147]

Restricting legal access to tobacco is one way to discourage teens from smoking. Federal law prohibits selling tobacco to minors; many states and local jurisdictions have also enacted youth access laws. Sales clerks are required to request an identification card of a buyer, inspect the card, and calculate the age of the buyer. Enforcement of youth access laws is monitored by conducting compliance checks. This entails enlisting youth to attempt to buy tobacco and determining the proportion of successful buys. Clark and colleagues[165] analyzed a large sample of compliance check data and found that adolescent females are significantly more likely to be able to purchase tobacco illegally than are males.

The cost of smoking is another deterrent for teens, and tobacco taxes are one way to discourage their tobacco use.[97] Young people have been found to be particularly sensitive to tobacco price increases.[166] Increases in the price of tobacco have been found to decrease male smoking prevalence rates more than female rates.[167]

Because teenagers are vulnerable to advertising, one intervention approach is to restrict advertising. However, the evidence regarding the efficacy of advertising bans is mixed. Partial advertising bans appear to be less effective in reducing adolescent consumption of tobacco than are complete bans.[167] Mass media counteradvertising campaigns that target teens have shown more promise.[167,168]

School-based programs on tobacco have been implemented in many middle and high schools but have not, on their own, shown a long-term impact on youth tobacco use. Lantz and associates[167] reviewed these and found that the most promising programs are those based on developing skills to recognize and resist peer pressure to smoke. The best results are achieved when these types of programs are combined with other strategies that involve multiple community systems such as families, government, community organizations, churches, businesses, social service and health agencies, and law enforcement.[147,167,169] The Surgeon General estimates that educational strategies, combined with community and media-based activities, can postpone or prevent smoking onset in 20% to 40% of adolescents.[170]

Adolescent Smoking Cessation

National data show that more than half of adolescent smokers want to quit smoking, and there are no gender differences in the desire to quit. However, girls are more likely to have tried to quit than are boys.[141]

Research on youth cessation is scarce.[171] The few studies that exist show that 40% to 50% of adolescents who quit smoking did so with no outside intervention.[158] Teens with lower levels of use at baseline have been found to be more likely to quit than teens with higher use levels.[172,173] Therefore adolescents who smoke are more likely to quit if they do not become heavy smokers.

Studies of adolescent nicotine addiction report one to three out of five teen smokers are addicted to nicotine.[174] For adolescents who are addicted to nicotine, pharmacologic interventions such as bupropion, nicotine patches, nicotine inhalers, and nicotine nasal spray may be appropriate, but there have been few studies that have addressed the efficacy and safety of nicotine replacement for adolescents.[16]

The physician is in a unique role to reduce adolescent smoking prevalence. Clinical practice guidelines for treating tobacco use and dependence[60] recommend the following:

1. Clinicians should screen pediatric and adolescent patients and their parents for tobacco use and provide a strong message regarding the importance of totally abstaining from tobacco use.

2. Counseling and behavioral interventions shown to be effective with adults should be considered for use with children and adolescents. The content of these interventions should be modified to be developmentally appropriate.

3. When treating adolescents, clinicians may consider prescriptions for pharmacologic interventions such as bupropion or nicotine replacement when there is evidence of nicotine dependence and desire to quit tobacco use.

4. Clinicians in a pediatric setting should offer smoking cessation advice and interventions to parents to limit children's exposure to secondhand smoke.

CHEMOPREVENTION OF LUNG CANCER
Principles of Chemoprevention

Chemoprevention is the use of specific natural or synthetic agents to reverse, suppress, or prevent carcinogenic progression to invasive cancer.[175] Chemoprevention efforts in lung cancer have been based on two premises that are fundamental to chemoprevention in general: those of (1) field carcinogenesis, and (2) carcinogenesis as a multistep process. Field carcinogenesis in relation to lung cancer implies that the entire aerodigestive epithelium, which includes the respiratory epithelium, is a field that has been diffusely exposed to carcinogens, and that there were abnormalities of the epithelium from areas beyond the site of an original upper airway cancer, as well as the finding of multiple, distinct invasive cancers within cancer surgical specimens.[176] Epidemiologic support for the concepts of field carcinogenesis in the setting of lung cancer include studies that have shown increased risk of second primary aerodigestive cancers, including lung cancers, in persons with a prior diagnosis of lung cancer. Carcinogenesis as a multistep process involves an accumulation of changes at the molecular or genetic level that can lead to invasive cancer. The multistep nature of this process implies that premalignant phases offer opportunities to intervene with agents that can interrupt or reverse the carcinogenic process. In fact, it has been shown that histologically "normal" bronchoepithelium of smokers can harbor genetic alterations that have been related to lung carcinogenesis;[177] this implies an accumulation of genetic abnormalities in the bronchoepithelium in persons chronically exposed to tobacco that places them at risk for lung cancer.

There is a continued risk of lung cancer-related death in former smokers that decreases dramatically over the first decade after smoking cessation.[178] However, several large studies have shown that even 20 years after cessation, former smokers' risk of death from lung cancer may not reach that of never-smokers.[179-181] Of note, more than 50% of all new lung cancer cases are diagnosed today in *former smokers*.[182] Given that there are currently an estimated 40 to 50 million former smokers in the United States, strategies aimed at preventing the development of lung cancers have been actively pursued to decrease the extremely large public health burden of lung cancer–related morbidity and mortality. Several aspects of chemoprevention trial design are particularly relevant to lung cancer prevention. There are several clinical end points commonly used in lung cancer chemoprevention trials, including the development of a primary or a secondary lung cancer. However, because the development of invasive cancer such as lung cancer generally occurs years, if not decades, after exposure to lung carcinogens, other end points are needed for more rapid evaluation of promising chemoprevention agents. Thus the identification and development of intermediate or surrogate biomarkers of lung carcinogenesis have led to alternative end points in lung cancer chemoprevention trials. Intermediate biomarkers can be characterized as genotypic and phenotypic changes that occur during lung carcinogenesis that can be used as markers of risk for developing lung cancer as well as targets for modulation by chemopreventive agents. For lung carcinogenesis, there is an expanding list of potential biomarkers that are yet to be validated. These include histologic lesions such as bronchial metaplasia and dysplasia, genetic abnormalities such as loss of heterozygosity at chromosomes 3p (containing the locus for FHIT, a purported tumor suppressor gene) and 9p, mutations in p53 and Ras genes, epigenetic abnormalities such as hypermethylation of the promoter region of specific genes, and aberrant expression of growth receptor molecules such as epidermal growth factor receptor (EGFR) and the retinoid receptors RAR and RXR, and regulatory proteins such as cyclooxygenase-2 (COX-2).

An important concept in the use of intermediate biomarkers is that their natural history is not well understood in populations such as former smokers. Thus the potential for spontaneous regression over time must be controlled; this is accomplished by incorporating a placebo control arm in trials that use modulation of intermediate biomarkers as an end point.

The Retinoids

The investigations of several classes of agents for lung cancer chemoprevention have been based on epidemiologic studies that have shown increased rates of epithelial cancers in persons with low dietary and serum levels of certain vitamins and micronutrients. Both retinol (vitamin A) and its precursor, beta-carotene, have received epidemiologic support for their potential chemopreventive activity;[183-185] in addition, there has been in vitro and in vivo support for cancer inhibitory activity for retinol and synthetic retinoids.[186,187]

A single-arm (uncontrolled) study of etretinate in a cohort of heavy smokers showed a reduction in bronchial metaplasia index.[188] Unfortunately, regression of bronchial metaplasia was not reported in two randomized trials that used etretinate and isotretinoin.[189,190] However, smoking cessation was associated with regression of metaplasia. A study that showed encouraging results for retinoid supplementation was conducted with use of retinyl palmitate versus observation in patients after treatment for early stage (stage I) non–small-cell lung cancer. The end point was development of a second primary tumor (SPT). At a median follow-up of 46 months, there was a 39% incidence of versus 48% in the control arm.[191]

The Carotene and Retinol Efficacy Trial (CARET) evaluated beta-carotene and retinol in two populations at risk for lung cancer, including male asbestos workers and female and male cigarette smokers with a history of 20 or more pack-years (either current or former smoker within 6 years of cessation). This was a randomized trial that used a 2 by 2 factorial design. An increase in lung cancer in the cohort receiving study vitamins was noted, although it did not reach statistical significance. With further analysis, it appeared that the beta-carotene–supplemented cohort of current smokers had a 28% increase in rate of lung cancer.[192]

The surprising detrimental effect of beta-carotene in the CARET trial was in concert with findings of a large 2 by 2 factorial design study among Finnish male smokers who used beta-carotene and vitamin E in the Alpha Tocopherol Beta Carotene (ATBC) study. This study reported that the group taking beta-carotene supplements had an 18% increase in lung cancer as well as an 8% increase in total mortality.[193] There did not appear to be a benefit, in terms of lowering lung cancer risk, for a-tocopherol. It has been since hypothesized that oxidation products of beta-carotene formed in the presence of smoke may have procarcinogenic effects, with some in vitro and in vivo results supportive of this hypothesis.[194] These studies illustrate the importance of testing hypotheses derived from epidemiologic and laboratory data in the setting of large, randomized controlled trials, with careful consideration of potential and possibly unexpected interaction in the populations to be studied. Despite the less-than-encouraging results with retinoids in the earlier trials, there is continued interest in the development and testing of novel natural and synthetic retinoids as lung chemopreventive agents.

Micronutrients: Selenium

The trace element selenium is incorporated through dietary intake into a variety of body proteins. Geographic correlative data for the United States and worldwide have shown an inverse association between selenium levels in forage crops or diet and cancer mortality rates. For example, lower mortality for a number of cancers, including lung cancer, has been shown for people in the United States with moderate or high selenium in forage crops.[195] The potential for selenium supplementation to decrease the incidence of lung cancer was noted in a secondary end-point analysis in the Nutritional Prevention of Cancer Trial (NPCT), a large, randomized, placebo-controlled trial whose primary end point was incidence of secondary skin cancer.[196] This finding, in concert with epidemiologic data, has provided a rationale for the design of a large, randomized, placebo-controlled trial to evaluate the effect of selenium supplementation on the incidence of SPTs in early-stage lung cancer patients. A recent subset analysis of the NPCT has shown that the benefit of selenium in reducing lung cancer incidence is seen in persons with relatively low baseline plasma selenium levels.[197]

Novel, Targeted Agents in Lung Cancer Chemoprevention

With a greater understanding of the molecular pathogenesis of lung cancer as well as lung preneoplasia has come the development of many novel classes of agents that target specific cellular growth and regulatory pathways that may be differentially expressed on abnormal when compared with normal epithelium. Many of these agents are under development as therapeutics in the setting of established lung cancers. The following is a discussion of only several of a multitude of novel, highly targeted therapies that, because of improved side effect profiles and oral availability, make them extremely appealing to test in the lung chemoprevention arena.

Inhibitors of the Prostaglandin Pathway

One such class is the inhibitors of the prostaglandin pathway, which has been shown to be an important pathway in both lung cancer and in lung carcinogenesis. This class includes the cyclooxygenase inhibitors, of which nonsteroidal antiinflammatory drugs (NSAIDs) have nonselective effects in inhibiting cyclooxygenase enzymes and have shown in vitro and in vivo anticarcinogenic properties, inhibiting the development of multiple types of experimental epithelial cancers, including lung cancer.[198] The COX-2 isoform of the cyclooxygenase enzyme system has spurred interest as a target for lung carcinogenesis chemoprevention as well as treatment of established lung cancers in that it is an inducible enzyme that is not highly expressed in normal bronchial epithelium but is expressed in a significant percent of lung cancers, especially adenocarcinomas.[199] Selective COX-2 inhibitors such as Celecoxib are currently being studied in the context of lung cancer chemoprevention; relatively favorable side effect profiles make the cyclooxygenase inhibitors appealing for use in healthy, at-risk populations. Other agents that act to inhibit the prostaglandin pathway and that have shown antiproliferative activity in the in vitro models of lung carcinogenesis are the lipoxygenase inhibitors, which are being studied as chemopreventive agents in currently ongoing trials.

The Epidermal Growth Factor Receptor Inhibitors

The epidermal growth factor receptor (EGFR) is a cell membrane receptor that has an important role in cellular growth signal transduction pathways that lead to cell proliferation as well as programmed cell death (apoptosis). While present in normal epithelial cells including skin, corneal epithelium, and gastrointestinal tract epithelium, it is overexpressed in a number of cancers including non–small-cell lung cancer as well as lung premalignancy. In fact, overexpression of EGFR is noted in early preneoplastic lesions (basal cell hyperplasia) through squamous metaplasia and carcinoma in situ, in which EGFR is consistently heavily overexpressed.[200] The development of oral formulations of tyrosine kinase inhibitors of EGFR with favorable side effect profiles has afforded the opportunity to target this receptor and attempt to reduce the development of second primary aerodigestive tract tumors in persons who have had a primary lung cancer resected. The modulation of EGFR expression and the expression of other molecules in the cell growth and proliferative pathway can be used as intermediate biomarkers of effect to help evaluate the chemopreventive potential of EGFR inhibitors.

SCREENING AND EARLY DIAGNOSIS OF LUNG CANCER IN WOMEN

The highly lethal nature of lung cancer, which accounts for its ranking as the number one cause of cancer-related death for both women and men, can in large part be related to the difficulty in diagnosing lung cancer at an early stage. Lung cancer is often not symptomatic until it is in an advanced stage, at which point curability is rare. Some lung cancers are not curable even when diagnosed at an early stage, as a result of a biologic propensity for early micrometastases and inherent resistance to drug therapy. However, the improved survival of patients with early-stage lung cancers as a group, compared with patients with more advanced stage lung cancers, has been clearly shown; approximately 61% to 67% of persons with stage I lung cancers will be alive 5 years after diagnosis, compared with 1% to 13% for regionally advanced (stage III) and metastatic (stage IV) lung cancers.[201]

Although it is recognized that the ideal means for reducing lung cancer is through prevention efforts (i.e., eliminating smoking), there has thus been much effort in designing effective screening strategies that would allow for the detection of early-stage lung cancers. The importance of developing effective screening strategies for early-stage lung cancer is emphasized by studies that show that although the risk of lung cancer decreases once smoking cessation has been initiated, the risk unfortunately remains high during the first decade after smoking cessation. Additionally, several large studies have shown the risk of lung cancer in former smokers to approach—but never reach—that of never-smokers.[179-181] The earliest strategies implemented traditional chest radiography (CXR), with or without cytologic analysis of sampled sputum. More recent screening studies have used more sophisticated radiologic imaging techniques, such as helical low-dose computed tomographic (CT) scanning. The identification of molecular markers in sputum that are associated with the eventual development of lung cancer have contributed further to the development of screening strategies.

The measure of effectiveness of screening strategies has traditionally been the reduction of mortality because mortality is felt to represent the only outcome that is not subject to biases that include lead-time bias, length bias, and overdiagnosis.[202]

Standard Chest Radiography and Sputum Cytology in Screening for Lung Cancer

Despite these efforts, which began as early as 1951 and have included 10 prospective trials that used chest radiography, sputum cytology, or both, there are currently no well-accepted recommendations for screening for lung cancer. Nine of the 10 trials excluded women's participation. Focus has been placed on four of the ten trials because of their randomized controlled trial (RCT) design. The trials include three studies sponsored by the National Cancer Institute as well as a fourth study undertaken in Czechoslovakia[203-207] that used standard chest radiography, sputum cytology, or both to screen for persons with lung cancer. Both the Memorial Sloan Kettering Lung Project and the Johns Hopkins Lung Project evaluated the efficacy of screening for lung cancer in male smokers, comparing annual CXRs with sputum cytology in combination with CXRs; both studies showed no difference in patient outcome with the addition of sputum cytology to traditional imaging. These studies were not designed to address the value of CXRs for screening for lung cancer. The Mayo Lung Project compared a more intense, versus a less intense, program of chest radiography and sputum cytology in a randomized, prospective trial design in more than 9000 male smokers older than age 45. The screened group underwent CXRs and sputum cytology every 4 months. The control group was advised only to undergo yearly CXRs and sputum cytology. Although persons in the screened group showed improved survival, improved fatality, and improved staging and resectability of lung cancer, there was no difference between screened and control group in mortality from lung cancer. In fact, there was a small but not significant increase in lung cancer–related mortality (incidence multiplied by fatality) in the screened group. The fourth, the Czechoslovakian study, randomized more that 6000 male smokers to the study group, which underwent CXRs and sputum cytology every 6 months for 3 years, or the control group, which underwent CXRs and sputum cytology at 3 years. Both groups went on to CXRs at the end of the 4th, 5th, and 6th years. Although survival was greater in the study group, there was an insignificant increase in mortality in the study group.

The initial reports of these studies led to recommendations by organized medical bodies against screening for lung cancer. However, more recent reanalyses of these data have shed different light on these conclusions. Interpretations of the Mayo Lung Project and the Czechoslovakian trial have included analyses of other risk factors that may have imbalanced the study and control groups in the latter two trials. These include genetic predisposing factors and other environmental exposures such as asbestos and radon, and the influence of "overdiagnosis bias," where clinically nonrelevant lung cancers are found in a group of persons with competing morbid conditions, which may be an explanation for the trend toward increased mortality in the screened groups. Although reductions in mortality were not documented for the intensely screened experimental groups, there were meaningful improvements shown for the outcomes of lung cancer stage distribution, resectability, survival, and fatality, which may argue favorably for the use of screening CXRs for persons at high risk for lung cancer.[208]

Improvements in Screening Techniques
New Imaging Techniques

The use of more sensitive imaging techniques is being implemented in lung cancer screening studies. A recently reported trial used helical low-dose CT imaging of the chest in a non-randomized cohort of 1000 smokers older than 60 years of age and with a significant cigarette use history to detect small noncalcified lung nodules.[209] This trial, the Early Lung Cancer Action Project (ELCAP), was designed to define the curability rate based on the size of the nodules detected. All participants also underwent CXR imaging, thus allowing for the detection rate for lung nodules by spiral CT imaging to be compared with that for traditional CXR imaging. Women accounted for 46% of persons enrolled in the study. Although it used a noncomparative, single cohort rather than randomized control design, this study produced important results. It showed the superiority of helical low-dose CT scanning over CXR in the detection of noncalcified lung nodules (found in 233 persons by CT, compared with 68 persons by CXR). By an algorithm that included the use of an additional high-resolution CT scan to better assess the nodules and by assigning either a close follow-up program with reimaging of the nodules versus proceeding directly to biopsy, spiral CT imaging detected nearly six times more malignant nodules than did CXR (2.3% versus 0.4%). Of 28 nodules on which a biopsy was performed, 27 were malignant; thus only one biopsy was performed for a benign nodule. Resectability was shown for 26 of the 27 nodules detected by CT imaging. Importantly, the cost-effectiveness of this strategy thus far has been impressive—with the cost of less than $2000 per life-year saved.

Although these studies have shown promising results by using more sensitive techniques for detecting early-stage lung cancer, their implementation for routine screening for lung cancer awaits their validation in both larger and broader study populations. Other corollary issues that remain to be addressed include the optimal technique for biopsy of suspicious lesions and how to optimally manage patients with detected lung lesions.

Molecular Markers of Lung Cancer Risk

An extremely important issue is how to integrate molecular markers of lung cancer risk into developing strategies for the early detection of lung cancer. Although evaluating sputum by employing traditional cytology as previously described has not shown benefit for the early detection of lung cancer, specific genetic and epigenetic alterations in the bronchoepithelium have been shown to have predictive value in the diagnosis of lung cancer. Candidates for this type of molecular marker of risk include proteins that are differentially expressed in normal versus preneoplastic bronchoepithelium, the mutation of genes whose expression is involved in regulation of cellular proliferation and differentiation, and alterations of genetic and cellular elements that influence the transformation from normal to malignant tissue. A number of candidate biomarkers have been identified. As an example, the methylation status of the promoter region of genes affects their expression; aberrant methylation of the promoters of two genes, p16 and O6-methyl-guanine-DNA-methyl transferase, has been detected in DNA from archived sputum in 100% of patients with squamous cell lung cancer up to 3 years before diagnosis.[210] The protein hnRNP B1 is involved in mRNA processing; its expression has been reported through bronchial biopsy in 63.6% in bronchial dysplasia samples, compared with zero in normal bronchial epithelium.[211]

The incorporation of these and other potential biomarkers of lung carcinogenesis into more sensitive imaging protocols for lung cancer screening holds promise for improving our ability to detect lung cancer in its earliest stages, a strategy that may improve survival for those at risk for developing lung cancer.

REFERENCES

1. Greenlee RT, Hill-Harmon MB, Murray T, et al: Cancer statistics, 2001, *CA Cancer J Clin* 2001;51:15-36.

2. US Department of Health and Human Services: *The health consequences of smoking for women: A report of the surgeon general.* Washington, DC, US Department of Health and Human Services, Public Health Service, Office of the Assistant Secretary for Health, Office on Smoking and Health, 1980.

3. Wallace RA: "Lucky" or a sweet—or both! *Nation* 1929;123:305-307.

4. Fortune Magazine: The Fortune survey III: cigarettes. *Fortune Magazine* 1935;12:111-116.

5. Howe H: An historical review of women, smoking and advertising. *Health Education* 1984;15:3-9.

6. Burbank F: US lung cancer death rates begin to rise proportionally more rapidly for females than for males: a dose-response effect? *J Chronic Disease* 1972;25:473-479.

7. Gallup GH: *The Gallup Poll: public opinion 1935-1971. Volume one: 1935-1948.* New York, Random House, 1972.

8. Doll R, Hill AB: A study of the etiology of carcinoma of the lung. *BMJ* 1952;2:1271-1286.

9. Levin ML, Goldstein H, Gerhardt PR: Cancer and tobacco smoking: a preliminary report. *JAMA* 1950;143:336-338.

10. U.S. Department of Health, Education, and Welfare: *Smoking and health: report of the Advisory Committee to the Surgeon General of the Public Health Service.* U.S. Department of Health, Education, and Welfare, Public Health Service, Communicable Disease Center, 1964. DHEW Publication No. 1103.

11. Giovino GA, Schooley MW, Shu B-P, et al: Surveillance for selected tobacco-use behaviors: United States, 1900-1994. *MMWR* 1994;43:1-43.

12. Wingo, PA, Ries LAG, Giovino GA, et al: Annual report to the nation on the status of cancer, 1973-1996, with a special section on lung cancer and tobacco smoking. *J Natl Cancer Inst* 1999;91:675-690.

13. Parkin DM, Pisani P, Ferlay J: Global cancer statistics. *CA Cancer J Clin* 1999;49:33-64.

14. US Department of Health and Human Services: *Women and smoking: A report of the Surgeon General—2001.*

15. Mayne ST, Buenconsejo J, Janerich DT: Familial cancer history and lung cancer risk in United States nonsmoking men and women. *Cancer Epidemiol Biomarkers Prev* 1999;8:1065-1069.

16. Le Marchand L, Sivaraman L, Pierce L, Seifried A, et al: Associations of CYP1A1, GSTM1, and CYP2E1 polymorphisms with lung cancer suggest cell type specificities to tobacco carcinogens. *Cancer Res* 1998;58:4858-4863.

17. McWilliams J, Sanderson B, Harris E, et al: Glutathione S-transferase m1 (GSTM1) deficiency and lung cancer risk. *Cancer Epidemiol Biomarkers Prev* 1995;4:589-594.

18. Dressler CM, Fratelli C, Babb J, et al: Gender differences in genetic susceptibility for lung cancer. *Lung Cancer* 2000;30:153-60.

19. Seow A, Zhao B, Lee E, et al: Cytochrome P4501A2 (Cyp1A2) activity and lung cancer risk: a preliminary study among Chinese women in Singapore. *Carcinogenesis* 2001;22:673-677.

20. Corrigall WA, Franklin KBJ, Coen KM, et al: The mesolimbic dopaminergic system is implicated in the reinforcing effects of nicotine. *Psychopharmacology* 1992;107:285-289.

21. Crooks P, Dwoskin L: Contribution of CNS nicotine metabolites to the neuropharmacological effects of nicotine and tobacco smoking. *Biochem Pharmacol* 1997;54:743-753.

22. Izenwasser S, Cox BM: Inhibition of dopamine uptake by cocaine and nicotine: tolerance to chronic treatments. *Brain Res* 1992;573:119-125.

23. Spitz MR, Shi H, Yang F, et al: Case-control study of the D2 dopamine receptor gene and smoking status in lung cancer patients. *J Natl Cancer Inst* 1998;90:358-63.

24. Lerman C, Caporaso NE, Audrain J, et al: Evidence suggesting the role of specific genetic factors in cigarette smoking. *Health Psychology* 1999;18:14-20.

25. Staley JK, Krishnan-Sarin S, Zoghbi S, et al: Sex differences in [123I] beta-CIT SPECT measures of dopamine and serotonin transporter availability in healthy smokers and nonsmokers. *Synapse* 2001;41:275-284.

26. McQueen J, Wilson H, Dow R, et al: Oestradiol-17 increases serotonin transporter (SERT) binding sites and SERT mRNA expression in discrete regions of female rat brain. *J Physiol* 1996;495:114.

27. Morisette M, Paolo TD: Effect of chronic estradiol and progesterone treatments on ovariectomized rats on brain dopamine uptake sites. *J Neurochem* 1993;60:1876-1883.

28. US Department of Health and Human Services: *The health consequences of smoking: cancer, A report of the Surgeon General.* Rockville, MD, US Department of Health and Human Services, Public Health Service, Office on Smoking and Health, 1982. DHHS Publication No. (PHS) 82:50179.

29. Friedman GD, Tekawa I, Sadler M, et al: Smoking and mortality: the Kaiser Permanente experience. In Shopland DR, Burns DM, Garfinkel L, Samet JM, editors: *Changes in cigarette-related disease risks and their implication for prevention and control.* Smoking and tobacco control monograph 8. Rockville, MD: US Department of Health and Human Services, Public Health Service, National Institutes of Health, National Cancer Institute, 1997; 477-499. NIH Publication No. 97-4213.

30. Thun MJ, Day-Lally C, Myers DG, et al: Trends in tobacco smoking and mortality from cigarette use in cancer prevention I (1959 through 1965) and II (1982-1988). In Shopland DR, Burns DM, Garfinkel L, Samet JM, editors: *Changes in cigarette-related disease risks and their implication for prevention*

and control. Smoking and tobacco control monograph 8. Rockville, MD: US Department of Health and Human Services, Public Health Service, National Institutes of Health, National Cancer Institute, 1997; 305-382. NIH Publication No. 97-4213.

31. Schoenberg JB, Wilcox HB, Mason TJ, et al: Variation in smoking-related risk among New Jersey women. *Am J Epidemiol* 1989;130:688-95.

32. Osann KE, Anton-Culver H, Kurosaki T, et al: Sex differences in lung-cancer risk associated with cigarette smoking. *Int J Cancer* 1993;54:44-48.

33. Morabia A, Wynder EL: Cigarette smoking and lung cancer cell types. *Cancer* 1991;68:2074-2078.

34. Office of Health and Environmental Assessment, Environmental Protection Agency (EPA): *Respiratory health effects of passive smoking: lung cancer and other disorders*, Washington (DC), EPA, 1992.

35. Boffetta P, Agudo A, Ahrens W, et al: Multicenter case-control study of exposure to environmental tobacco smoke and lung cancer in Europe. *J Natl Cancer Inst* 1998;90:1440-1450.

36. Anderson KE, Carmella SG, Ye M, et al: Metabolites of a tobacco-specific lung carcinogen in nonsmoking women exposed to environmental tobacco smoke. *J Natl Cancer Inst* 2001;93:378-381.

37. Bennett WP, Alavanja MCR, Blomede B, et al: Environmental tobacco smoke, genetic susceptibility, and risk of lung cancer in never-smoking women. *J Natl Cancer Inst* 1999;91:2009-2014.

38. Wells AJ: Lung cancer from passive smoking at work. *Am J Public Health* 1998:88:1011-1012.

39. Doll R, Peto R: The causes of cancer: quantitative estimates of avoidable risks of cancer in the United States today. *J Natl Cancer Inst* 1981;66:1191-1308.

40. Samet JM, Lerchen ML: Proportion of lung cancer caused by occupation: a critical review. In Gee JBL, Morgan WKC, Brooks SM, editors: *Occupational lung disease*. New York, Raven Press, 1984.

41. Swanson GM, Burns PB: Cancer incidence among women in the workplace: a study of the association between occupation and industry and 11 cancer sites. *J Occup Environ Med* 1995:37:282-287.

42. Pohlabeln H, Boffetta P, Ahrens W, et al: Occupational risks for lung cancer among non-smokers. *Epidemiology* 2000;11:532-538.

43. Muscat JE, Stellman SD, Richie JP Jr., et al: Lung cancer risk and workplace exposures in black men and women. *Environ Res* 1998;76:78-84.

44. Jin F, Devesa SS, Zhang W, et al: Cancer incidence trends in urban Shanghai, 1972-1989. *Int J Cancer* 1993;53: 764-770.

45. He X, Chen W, Liu Z, et al: An epidemiologic study of lung cancer in Xian Wei Count, China: current progress, case-control study on lung cancer and cooking fuel. *Environ Health Perspect* 1991;94:9-13.

46. Metayer C, Wang Z, Kleinerman RA, et al: Cooking oil fumes and risk of lung cancer in women in rural Gansu, China. *Lung Cancer* 2002;35:111-117.

47. Gao YT, Blot WJ, Zheng W, et al: Lung cancer among Chinese women. *Int J Cancer* 1987;40:604-609.

48. Zhu B, Giovino GA, Mowery PD, et al: The relationship between cigarette smoking and education revisited: implications for categorizing persons' educational status. *Am J Pub Health* 1996;86:1582-1589.

49. National Center for Health Statistics: *Fertility, family planning, and women's health: New data from the 1995 National Survey of Family Growth*. Vital Health Statistics. Series 23, No. 19. Hyattsville, MD, US Department of Health and Human Services, Public Health Service, Centers for Disease Control and Prevention, National Center for Health Statistics, 1997.

50. Breslau N, Kilbey M, Andreski P: Nicotine dependence, major depression and anxiety in young adults. *Arch Gen Psychiatry* 1991;48:1069-1074.

51. Covey LS, Hughes DC, Glassman AH, et al: Ever-smoking, quitting, and psychiatric disorders: evidence from the Durham, North Carolina, Epidemiologic Catchment Area. *Tob Control* 1994;3:222-227.

52. Hofer TP, Katz SJ: Healthy behaviors among women in the United States and Ontario: the effect on use of preventive care. *Am J Pub Health* 1996;86:1755-1759.

53. Istvan J, Matarazzo JD: Tobacco, alcohol and caffeine use: a review of their interrelationships. *Psychol Bull* 1984;95:301-326.

54. Lyons RA, Lo SV, Littlepage BN: Perception of health amongst ever-smokers and never-smokers: a comparison using the SF-36 Health Survey Questionnaire. *Tob Control* 1994;3:213-215.

55. Hughes JR, Hatsukami DK, Mitchell JE, et al: Prevalence of smoking among psychiatric outpatients. *Am J Psychiatry* 1986;143:993-997.

56. Carney RM, Rich MW, te Velde A, et al: The relationship between heart rate, heart rate variability, and depression in patients with coronary artery disease. *J Psychosom Res* 1988;32:159-165.

57. Kendler KS, Neale MC, MacLean CJ, et al: Smoking and major depression: a causal analysis. *Arch Gen Psychiatry* 1993;50:36-43.

58. Pomerleau CS, Pomerleau OF: The effects of a psychological stressor on cigarette smoking and subsequent behavioral and physiological responses. *Psychophysiology* 1987;24:278-285.

59. Masterson E, O'Shea B: Smoking and malignancy in schizophrenia. *Br J Psychiatry* 1992;145:429-432.

60. Fiore MC, Bailey WC, Cohen SJ, et al: *Treating tobacco use and dependence*: clinical practice guideline. Rockville, MD, US Department of Health and Human Services, Public Health Service, June 2000.

61. McBride CM, Lozano P, Curry SJ, et al: Use of health services by children of smokers and non-smokers in a health maintenance organization. *Am J Pub Health* 1998;88:897-902.

62. Ettner SL: The timing of preventive services for women and children: the effect of having a usual source of care. *Am J Pub Health* 1996;86:1748-1754.

63. Shiffman S: Tobacco "chippers": individual differences in tobacco dependence. *Psychopharmacology* 1989;97:539-547.

64. Benowitz NL, Jacob P III, Jones RT, et al: Interindividual variability in the metabolism and cardiovascular effects of nicotine in man. *J Pharmacol Exp Ther* 1982;221:368-372.

65. Wesnes K, Warburton DM: Smoking, nicotine and human performance. *Pharmacol Ther* 1983;21:189-208.

66. Alexander BK, Hadaway PF: Opiate addiction: the case for an adaptive orientation. *Psychol Bull* 1982;92:367-381.

67. Hajek P, West R, Wilson J: Regular smokers, lifetime very light smokers, and reduced smokers: comparison of psychosocial and smoking characteristics in women. *Health Psychol* 1995;14:195-201.

68. Kawachi I, Troisi RJ, Rotnitzky AG, et al: Can physical activity minimize weight gain in women after smoking cessation? *Am J Pub Health* 1996;86:999-1004.

69. Hennrikus DJ, Jeffery RW, Lando HA: Occasional smoking in a Minnesota working population. *Am J Pub Health* 1996;86:1260-1266.

70. Cigarette smoking—attributable mortality and years of potential life lost: United States, 1990. *MMWR* 1993;42:645-649.

71. Emery S, Gilpin EA, Ake C, et al: Characterizing and identifying "hard-core" smokers: implications for further reducing smoking prevalence. *Am J Pub Health* 2000;90:387-394.

72. Pierce JP, Farkas AJ, Gilpin EA: Beyond stages of change: the quitting continuum measures progress towards successful smoking cessation. *Addiction* 1998;93(2):277-286.

73. American Psychiatric Association: *Diagnostic and statistical manual of mental disorders,* 4th ed. Washington, DC: American Psychiatric Association, 1994.

74. Breslau N, Kilbey M, Andreski P: Nicotine withdrawal symptoms and psychiatric disorders: findings from an epidemiologic study of young adults. *Am J Psychiatry* 1992;149:464-469.

75. Cohen S, Lichtenstein E, Prochaska JO, et al: Debunking myths about self-quitting: evidence from 10 prospective studies of persons who attempt to quit smoking by themselves. *Am Psychol* 1989;44:1355-1365.

76. Gilpin E, Pierce JP, Goodman J, et al: Reasons smokers give for stopping smoking: do they relate to success in stopping? *Tob Control* 1992;1:256-263.

77. Curry S, Wagner EH, Grothaus LC: Intrinsic and extrinsic motivation for smoking cessation. *J Consult Clin Psychol* 1990;58:310-316.

78. Lando HA, Pirie PL, Hellerstedt WL, et al: Survey of smoking patterns, attitudes, and interest in quitting. *Am J Prev Med* 1991;7:18-23.

79. Cummings KM, Sciandra R, Davis S, et al: Response to anti-smoking campaign aimed at mothers with young children. *Health Education Res* 1989;4:429-437.

80. Orleans CT, Rimer BK, Crisinziio S, et al: *Smoking patterns and quitting motives, barriers and strategies among older smokers aged 50-74: a report for the American Association of Retired Persons.* Philadelphia, Fox Chase Cancer Center, 1990.

81. Fiore MC, Novotny TE, Pierce JP, et al: Methods used to quit smoking in the United States: do cessation programs help? *JAMA* 1990;263:2760-2765.

82. Fiore MC, Bailey WC, Cohen SJ, et al: *Smoking cessation:* clinical practice guideline no. 18. AHCPR Publication No 96-0692. Rockville, MD, US Dept of Health and Human Services, Public Health Service, Agency for Health Care Policy and Research, 1996.

83. Hollis JF, Lichtenstein E, Vogt T, et al: Nurse-assisted counseling for smokers in primary care. *Ann Intern Med* 1993;118:521-525.

84. Zhu S-H, Melcer T, Sun J, et al: Smoking cessation with and without assistance: a population-based analysis. *Am J Prev Med* 2000;18:3005-3011.

85. Prochaska JO, DiClementa CC: Stages and processes of self-change of smoking: toward an integrative model of change. *J Consult Clin Psychol* 1983;51:390-395.

86. Hymowitz N, Cummings KM, Hyland A, et al: Predictors of smoking cessation in a cohort of adult smokers followed for five years. *Tob Control* 1997;6:S57-S62.

87. Office on Smoking and Health, National Center for Chronic Disease Prevention and Health Promotion, Centers for Disease Control and Prevention: *Dispelling the myths about tobacco: a community toolkit for reducing tobacco use among women.* Atlanta, CDC, 2001.

88. Jeffery RW, French SA: Socioeconomic status and weight control practices among 2- to 45-year-old women. *Am J Pub Health* 1996;86:1005-1010.

89. Seidman DF, Covey LS, editors: *Helping the hard-core smoker: a clinician's guide.* Mahwah, NJ, Lawrence Erlbaum Associates, 1999.

90. Bernstein M, Morabia A, Heritier S, Katchatrian N: Passive smoking, active smoking, and education: their relationship to weight history in women in Geneva. *Am J Pub Health* 1996;86:1267-1272.

91. National Center for Health Statistics. *Fertility, family planning, and women's health: new data from the 1995 National Survey of Family Growth.* Vital Health Statistics. Series 23, No. 19. Hyattsville, MD: U.S. Department of Health and Human Services, Public Health Service, Centers for Disease Control and Prevention, National Center for Health Statistics, 1997.

92. Windsor RA, Lowe JB, Perkins LL, et al: Health education for pregnant smokers: its behavioral impact and cost benefit. *Am J Public Health* 1993; 83:201-206.

93. Kendrick JS, Zahniser SC, Miller N, et al: Integrating smoking cessation into routine public prenatal care: the Smoking Cessation in Pregnancy Project. *Am J Public Health* 1995;85:217-222.

94. Sugarman JR, Brenneman G, LaRoque W, et al: The urban American Indian oversample in the 1988 National Maternal and Infant Health Survey. *Public Health Rep* 1994;109:243-250.

95. Floyd RL, Rimer BK, Giovino GA, et al: A review of smoking in pregnancy: effects on pregnancy outcomes and cessation efforts. *Annu Rev Public Health* 1993;14:379-411.

96. Ventura SJ, Martin JA, Taffel SM, et al: Advance report of final natality statistics, 1993. *Mon Vital Stat Rep* 1995;44:1-83.

97. USDHHS: *Preventing tobacco use among young people: A report of the Surgeon General.* Atlanta, US Department of Health and Human Services, Public Health Service, Centers for Disease Control and Prevention, National Center for Chronic Disease Prevention and Health Promotion, Office on Smoking and Health, 1994.

98. Luck W, Nau H, Hanesen R, et al: Extent of nicotine and cotinine transfer to the human fetus, placenta and amniotic fluid of smoking mothers. *Dev Pharmacol Ther* 1985;8:384-395.

99. Gindoff PR, Tidey GF: Effects of smoking on female fecundity and early pregnancy outcome. *Semin Reprod Endocrinol* 1989;7:305-313.

100. Mattison DR, Singh H, Takizawa K, et al: Ovarian toxicity of benzo(a) pyrene and metabolites in mice. *Reprod Toxicol* 1989;3:115-125.

101. Blackburn CW, Peterson CA, Hales HA, et al: Nicotine, but not cotinine, has a direct toxic effect of ovarian function in the immature gonadotropin-stimulated rat. *Reprod Toxicol* 1994;8:325-331.

102. Lambers D, Clark K: The maternal and fetal physiologic effects of nicotine. *Semin Perinatol* 1996;20:115-126.

103. Barnwell SL, Sastry BVR: Depression of amino acid uptake in human placental villus by cocaine, morphine, and nicotine. *Trophoblast Res* 1983;1:101-120.

104. Hill EP, Hill JR, Power GG, et al: Carbon monoxide exchanges between the human fetus and mother: a mathematical model. *Am J Physiol* 1977;232:H311-323.

105. Benowitz NL: Nicotine replacement therapy during pregnancy. *JAMA* 1991;266:3174-3177.

106. Cramer DW, Scheff I, Schoenbaum SC, et al: Tubal infertility and the intrauterine device. *N Engl J Med* 1985;312:941-947.

107. Phipps WR, Cramer DW, Schiff I, et al: The association between smoking and female infertility as influenced by cause of the infertility. *Fertil Steril* 1987;48:377-382.

108. Joesoef MR, Beral V, Aral SO, et al: Fertility and use of cigarettes, alcohol, marijuana, and cocaine. *Ann Epidemiol* 1993;3:592-594.

109. Tzonou A, Hsieh CC, Tichopoulos D, et al: Induced abortions, miscarriages, and tobacco smoking as risk factors for secondary infertility. *J Epidemiol Community Health* 1993;47:36-39.

110. Beral V, Rolfs R, Joesoef MR, et al: Primary infertility: characteristics of women in North America according to pathological findings. *J Epidemiol Community Health* 1994;48:576-579.

111. Stergachis A, Scholes D, Daling JR, et al: Maternal cigarette smoking and the risk of tubal pregnancy. *Am J Epidemiol* 1991;133:332-337.

112. Kyrklund-Blomberg NB, Cnattingius S: Preterm birth and maternal smoking: risks related to gestational age and onset of delivery. *Am J Obstet Gynecol* 1998;179:1051-1055.

113. Meis PJ, Michielutte R, Peters TJ, et al: Obstetrics: factors associated with preterm birth in Cardiff, Wales: I. univariable and mutivariable analysis. *Am J Obstet Gynecol* 1995;173:590-596.

114. Hadley C, Main D, Gabbe S: Risk factors for preterm premature rupture of the fetal membranes. *Am J Perinatol* 1990;7:374-379.

115. Mainous AG, Hueston WJ: The effect of smoking cessation during pregnancy on preterm delivery and low birthweight. *J Fam Pract* 1994;38:262-266.

116. Simpson W: A preliminary report of cigarette smoking and the incidence of prematurity. *Am J Obstet Gynecol* 1957;73:808-815.

117. US Department of Health and Human Services: *The health benefits of smoking cessation: a report of the surgeon general,* 1990.

118. MacArthur C, Knox E: Smoking in pregnancy: effects of stopping at different stages. *Br J Obstet Gynaecol* 1988;95:551-555.

119. Naeye R: Effects of maternal cigarette smoking on the fetus and placenta. *Br J Obstet Gynaecol* 1978;85:732-737.

120. Meyer M, Tonascia J: Perinatal events associated with maternal smoking during pregnancy. *Am J Epidemiol* 1976;1103:464-476.

121. Naeye R: Abruptio placentae and placenta previa: frequency, perinatal mortality and cigarette smoking. *Obstet Gynecol* 1980;55:701-794.

122. Chelmow D, Andrew DE, Baker ER: Maternal cigarette smoking and placenta previa. *Obstet Gynecol* 1996;87:703-706.

123. Monica D, Lilja C: Placenta previa, maternal smoking and recurrence risk. *Acta Obstet Gynecol Scand* 1995;74:341-345.

124. Schoendorf KC, Kiely JL: Relationship of sudden infant death syndrome to maternal smoking during and after pregnancy. *Pediatrics* 1992;90:905-908.

125. Mitchell EA, Ford RP, Stewart BJ, et al: Smoking and the sudden infant death syndrome. *Pediatrics* 1993;91:893-896.

126. Klonoff-Cohen HS, Edelstein SL, Lefkowitz ES, et al: The effect of passive smoking and tobacco exposure through breast milk on sudden infant death syndrome. *JAMA* 1995;273:795-798.

127. Willinger M, Hoffman HJ, Hartford RB: Infant sleep position and the risk for sudden infant death syndrome: report of a meeting held January 13 and 14, 1994, National Institutes of Health, Bethesda, MD. *Pediatrics* 1994;93:814-819.

128. Malloy MH, Hoffman HJ, Peterson DR: Sudden infant death syndrome and maternal smoking. *Am J Public Health* 1992;82:1380-1382.

129. Hasan S, Simakajornboon N, MacKinnon Y, et al: Prenatal cigarette smoke exposure alters protein kinase C and nitric oxide synthetase expression within the neonatal rat brainstem. *Neurosci Lett* 2001;301:135-138.

130. Fingerhut L, Kleinman J, Hendrick J: Smoking before, during, and after pregnancy. *Am J Pub Health* 1990;80:541-545.

131. Ockene J: Smoking among women across the life span: prevalence, interventions, and implications for cessation research. *Ann Behav Med* 1993;15:135-48.

132. McBride CM, Pirie PL: Postpartum smoking relapse. *Addict Behav* 1990;15:165-168.

133. McBride CM, Pirie PL, Curry SJ: Postpartum relapse to smoking: a prospective study. *Health Educ Res* 1992;3:381-390.

134. Evans N, Farkas A, Gilpin E, et al: Influence of tobacco marketing and exposure to smokers on adolescent susceptibility to smoking. *J Natl Cancer Instit* 1995;18:1538-1545.

135. Sargent JD, Dalton M, Beach M: Exposure to cigarette promotions and smoking uptake in adolescents: evidence of a dose-response relation. *Tob Control* 2000;9:163-168.

136. Sargent JD, Dalton M, Beach M, et al: Effect of cigarette promotions on smoking uptake among adolescents. *Prev Med* 2000;30:514-515.

137. Pierce JP, Choi WS, Gilpin EA, et al: Tobacco industry promotion of cigarettes and adolescent smoking. *JAMA* 1998;279: 511-515.

138. Pierce JP, Gilpin EA: A historical analysis of tobacco marketing and the uptake of smoking by youth in the United States: 1890-1977. *Journal of Health Psychology* 1995;14:500-508.

139. DiFranza JR, Rigotti NA, McNeill AD, et al: Initial symptoms of nicotine dependence in adolescents. *Tob Control* 2000;9:313-319.

140. Zickler P. Adolescents, women, and whites more vulnerable than others to becoming nicotine dependent. *NIDA Notes* 2001;16:2.

141. Office on Smoking and Health, National Center for Chronic Disease Prevention and Health Promotion, American Legacy Foundation, CDC Foundation, Macro International, State Youth Tobacco Survey Coordinators: Youth Tobacco Surveillance—United States, 2000. In CDC Surveillance Summaries, November 2, 2001. *MMWR* 2001;50(No SS-4):1-84.

142. Elders MJ, Perry CL, Ericksen MP, et al: The report of the surgeon general: preventing tobacco use among young people. *Am J Pub Health* 1994;84:543-547.

143. SAMHSA: *Reducing tobacco use among youth: community-based approaches, a guideline for prevention practitioners.* Center for Substance Abuse Prevention, USDHHS Publication No. (SMA)97-3146, 1997.

144. Romer D, Jamieson P: Do adolescents appreciate the risks of smoking?: evidence from a national survey. *J Adolesc Health* 2001;29:12-21.

145. Arnett JJ: Optimistic bias in adolescent and adult smokers and nonsmokers. *Addict Behav* 2000;25:625-632.

146. Milam JE, Sussman S, Ritt-Olson A, et al: Perceived invulnerability and cigarette smoking among adolescents. *Addict Behav* 2000;25:71-80.

147. Botvin GH, Epstein JA, Botvin EM: Adolescent cigarette smoking: prevalence, causes, and intervention approaches. *Adolesc Med* 1998;9:299-313.

148. Pierce JP, Lee L, Gilpin EA: Smoking initiation by adolescent girls, 1944 through 1988, an association with targeted advertising. *JAMA* 1994;271: 629-630.

149. Burns DM, Johnston LD: Overview of recent changes in adolescent smoking behavior. In National Cancer Institute: *Changing adolescent smoking prevalence.* Smoking and Tobacco Control Monograph No. 14. Bethesda, MD, US Department of Health and Human Services, National Institutes of Health, National Cancer Institute, NIH Pub. No. 02-5086, 2001.

150. Anderson CM, Burns DM: Pattern of adolescent initiation rates over time: national and California data. In National Cancer Institute: *Changing adolescent smoking prevalence.* Smoking and Tobacco Control Monograph No. 14. Bethesda, MD, US Department of Health and Human Services, National Institutes of Health, National Cancer Institute, NIH Pub. No. 02-5086, 2001.

151. Giovino GA: Epidemiology of tobacco use among US adolescents. *Nicotine Tob Res* 1999;1:S31-S40.

152. Peltcher JR, Schwarz DF: Current concepts in adolescent smoking. *Curr Opin Pediatr* 2000;12:444-449.

153. Moolchan RT, Ernst M, Henningfield JE: A review of tobacco smoking in adolescents: treatment implications. *J Am Acad Child Adolesc Psychiatry* 2000;39:682-693.

154. French SA, Perry CL: Smoking among adolescent girls: prevalence and etiology. *J Am Med Womens Assoc* 1996;51:25-28.

155. Voorhees CC, Schreiber GB, Schumann BC, et al: Early predictors of daily smoking in young women: the National Heart, Lung and Blood Institute Growth and Health Study. *Prev Med* 2002;34:616-624.

156. Kaufman NJ, Brian MS Castrucci C, et al: Predictors of change on the smoking uptake continuum among adolescents. *Arch Pediatr Adolesc Med* 2002;156:581-587.

157. Flay BR, Petraitis J, Hu FB: Psychosocial risk and protective factors for adolescent tobacco use. *Nicotine Tob Res* 1999;1:S59-65.

158. Fritz DJ: Adolescent smoking cessation: how effective have we been? *J Pediatr Nurs* 2000;15:299-306.

159. Bauer UE, Johnson TM: Predictors of tobacco use among adolescents in Florida, 1998-1999. In National Cancer Institute: *Changing Adolescent Smoking Prevalence.* Smoking and Tobacco Control Monograph No 14. Bethesda, MD, US Department of Health and Human Services, National Institutes of Health, National Cancer Institute, NIH Pub. No. 02-5086, 2001.

160. Altman DG, Levine DW, Coeytaux R, et al: Tobacco promotion and susceptibility to tobacco use among adolescents aged 12 through 17 years in a nationally representative sample. *Am J Public Health* 1996;86:1590-1593.

161. Boles SM, Johnson PB: Gender, weight concerns, and adolescent smoking. *J Addict Dis* 2001;20:5-14.

162. Tomeo CA, Field EA, Berkey CS: Weight concerns, weight control behaviors, and smoking initiation. *Pediatrics* 1999;104:918-924.

163. French SA, Perry CL, Leon GR, Fulkerson JA: Weight concerns, dieting behavior, and smoking initiation among adolescents: a prospective study. *Am J Public Health* 1994;84:1818-1820.

164. Clark PI, Natanblut SL, Schmitt CL, et al: Factors associated with tobacco sales to minors, lessons learned from the FDA compliance checks. *JAMA* 2000;284:729-734.

165. Chaloupka FJ, Grossman M: *Price, tobacco control policies and youth smoking.* National Bureau of Economic Research working paper 5740. NBER, 1996.

166. Chaloupka FJ, Pacula RL: Sex and race differences in young people's responsiveness to price and tobacco control policies. *Tob Control* 1999;8:373-377.

167. Lantz PM, Jacobson PD, Warner KE, et al: Investing in youth tobacco control: a review of smoking prevention and control strategies. *Tob Control* 2000;9:47-63.

168. Sly DF, Hopkins RS, Trapido E, Ray S: Influence of a counteradvertising media campaign on initiation of smoking: the Florida "truth" campaign. *Am J Public Health* 2001;91:233-238.

169. Wakefield M, Chaloupka F. Effectiveness of comprehensive tobacco control programmes in reducing teenage smoking in the USA. *Tob Control* 2000;9:177-186.

170. USDHHA. *Reducing tobacco use: a report of the Surgeon General.* Atlanta, US Department of Health and Human Services, Centers for Disease Control and Prevention, National Center for Chronic Disease Prevention and Health Promotion, Office on Smoking and Health, 2000.

171. Sussman S, Lichtman K, Ritt A, et al: Effects of thirty-four adolescent tobacco use cessation and prevention trials on regular users of tobacco products. *Subst Use Misuse* 1999;34:1469-1503.

172. Sargent JD, Mott LA, Stevens M: Predictors of smoking cessation in adolescents. *Arch Pediatr Adolesc Med* 1998;152:388-393.

173. Ershler J, Leventhal H, Fleming R, et al: The quitting experience for smokers in sixth through twelfth grades. *Addict Behav* 1989;14:365-378.

174. Colby SM, Tiffany ST, Shiffman S, et al: Are adolescent smokers dependent on nicotine? a review of the evidence. *Drug Alcohol Depend* 2000;59 (Suppl 1): S83-S95.

175. Sporn MB, Dunlop NM, Newton DL, et al: Prevention of chemical carcinogenesis by vitamin A and its synthetic analogues (retinoids). *Fed Proc* 1976;35:1332-1338.

176. Slaughter DP, Soutwick HW, Smejkal W: Field cancerization in oral stratified squamous epithelium. *Cancer* 1953;6:963-968.

177. Mao L, Lee JS, Kurie JM, et al: Clonal genetic alterations in the lungs of current and former smokers. *J Natl Cancer Inst* 1997;89:857-862.

178. Halpern MT, Gillespie BW, Warner KE: Patterns of absolute risk of lung cancer mortality in former smokers. *J Natl Cancer Inst* 1993;85:457-464.

179. Hammond EC: Smoking in relation to the death rates of one million men and women. *Natl Cancer Inst Monogr* 1966;19:127-204.

180. Doll R, Peto R: Mortality in relation to smoking: 20 years' observations on male British doctors. *Br Med J* 1976;2:1525-1536.

181. Rogot E, Murray J: Cancer mortality among nonsmokers in an insured group of US veterans. *J Natl Cancer Inst* 1980;65:1163-1168.

182. Tong L, Spitz MR, Fueger JJ, et al: Lung carcinoma in former smokers. *Cancer* 1996;78:1004-1010.

183. Kark JD, Smith AH, Switzer BR, et al: Serum vitamin A (retinol) and cancer incidence in Evans County, Georgia. *J Natl Cancer Inst* 1981;66:7-16.

184. Nomura AM, Stemmermann GN, Heilburn LK, et al: Serum vitamin levels and risk of cancer of specific sites of men of Japanese ancestry in Hawaii. *Cancer Res* 1985;45:2369-2372.

185. Gerster H: Anticarcinogenic effect of common carotenoids. *Int J Vitam Nutr Res* 1993;63:93-121.

186. Lotan R: Effects of vitamin A and its analogs (retinoids) on normal and neoplastic cells. *Biochem Biophys Acta* 1980;605:33-91.

187. Lippman S, Kessler J, Meyskens FL: Retinoids as preventive and therapeutic anticancer agents. *Cancer Treat Rep* 1987;71:391-405, 493-515.

188. Misset JL, Mathe G, Santelli G, et al: Regression of bronchial epidermoid metaplasia in heavy smokers with etretinate treatment. *Cancer Detect Rev* 1986;9:167-170.

189. Arnold AM, Browman GP, Levine MN, et al: The effect of the synthetic retinoid etretinate on sputum cytology: results form a randomized trial. *Br J Cancer* 1992;65:737-743.

190. Lee JS, Lippman SM, Benner DE, et al: Randomized placebo-controlled trial of isotretinoin in chemoprevention of bronchial squamous metaplasia. *J Clin Oncol* 1994;12:937-945.

191. Pastorino U, Infante M, Maioli M, et al: Adjuvant treatment of stage I lung cancer with high-dose vitamin A. *J Clin Oncol* 1993;11:1216-1222.

192. Omenn GS, Goodman GE, Thornquist M, et al: Effects of combination of beta-carotene and vitamin A on lung cancer and cardiovascular disease. *N Engl J Med* 1996;334:1150-1155.

193. The α-Tocopherol, Beta-Carotene Prevention Study Group: The effect of vitamin E and ß-carotene on the incidence of lung cancer and other cancers in male smokers. *N Engl J Med* 1994;330:1029-1035.

194. Wang X, Liu C, Bronson RT, et al: Retinoid signaling and activator protein-1 expression in ferrets given ß-carotene supplements and exposed to tobacco smoke. *J Natl Cancer Inst* 1999;91:60-66.

195. Shamberger RJ, Willis C: Selenium distribution and human cancer mortality. *CRC Crit Rev Clin Lab Sci* 1971;2:211-221.

196. Clark LC, Combs GF Jr, Turnbull BW, et al: Effects of selenium supplementation for cancer prevention in patients with carcinoma of the skin: a randomized controlled trial. *JAMA* 1996;276;1957-1963.

197. Reid ME, Duffield-Lillico AJ, Garland L, et al: Selenium supplementation and lung cancer incidence: an update of the nutritional prevention of cancer trial. *Cancer Epidemiol Biomarkers Prev* 2002;11:1285-1291.

198. Duperron C, Castonguay A: Chemopreventive efficacies of aspirin and sulindac against lung tumorigenesis in A/J mice. *Carcinogenesis* 1997;18:1001-1006.

199. Hasturk S, Kemp B, Kalapurakal SK, et al: Expression of cyclooxygenase-1 and cyclooxygenase-2 in bronchial epithelium and nonsmall cell lung carcinoma. *Cancer* 2002;94:1023-1031.

200. Franklin WA, Veve R, Hirsch FR, et al: Epidermal growth factor receptor family in lung cancer malignancy. *Semin Oncology* 2002;29:3-14.

201. Mountain CF: The international system for lung cancer staging. *Semin Surg Oncol* 2000;18:106-115.

202. Hulka BS: Cancer screening: degrees of proof and practical application. *Cancer* 1988;62:1776-1780.

203. Fontana RS, Sanderson DR, Taylor WF, et al: Early lung cancer detection: results of the initial (prevalence) radiologic and cytologic screening in the Mayo Clinic study. *Am Rev Respir Dis* 1984;130:561-565.

204. Melamed MR, Flehinger BJ, Zaman MB, et al: Screening for early lung cancer: results of the Memorial Sloan-Kettering study in New York. *Chest* 1984;86:44-53.

205. Tockman M: Survival and mortality from lung cancer in a screened population: the Johns Hopkins study. *Chest* 1986;89:325S-326S.

206. Kubrik A, Polak J: Lung cancer detection: results of a randomized prospective study in Czechoslovakia. *Cancer* 1986;57:2428-2437.

207. Kubrik A, Parkin DM, Khlat M, et al: Lack of benefit from semi-annual screening for cancer of the lung: follow-up report of a randomized controlled trial on population of high-risk males in Czechoslovakia. *Int J Cancer* 1990;45:26-33.

208. Strauss GM, Gleason RE, Sugarbaker DJ: Screening for lung cancer: another look; a different view. *Chest* 1997;111:754-768.

209. Henschke CI, McCauley DI, Yankelevitz DF, et al: Early Lung Cancer Action Project: overall design and findings from baseline screening. *Lancet* 1999;354:99-105.

210. Palmisano WA, Divine KK, Saccomanno G, et al: Predicting lung cancer by detecting aberrant promoter methylation in sputum. *Cancer Res* 2000;60:5954-5958.

211. Sueoka E, Sueoka N, Goto Y, et al: Heterogeneous nuclear ribonucleoprotein B1 as early cancer biomarker for occult cancer of human lungs and bronchial dysplasia. *Cancer Res* 2001;61:1896-1902.

CHAPTER 3

Breast Cancer Risk Factors and Prevention

Karen Todd Lane
Helena R. Chang

Breast cancer is the most common cancer among American women. It is estimated that more than 175,000 new invasive cases are being diagnosed each year. In women, breast cancer is the second major cause of cancer death, with an estimated 44,000 deaths per year. At time of diagnosis, 85% to 90% of women will have disease that is clinically limited to the breast or regional nodes with an overall 5-year survival of 79%.[1] Although early diagnosis is critical to maximize the likelihood of long-term survival, breast cancer prevention is the ultimate goal.

INCIDENCE AND MORTALITY

The average lifetime risk of a woman developing breast cancer in the United States is 12% (1 in 8 women). A woman has a 3.5% lifetime risk of dying from breast cancer (1 in 29).[2] The incidence and mortality of breast cancer increases with age. Table 3-1 shows the risk of developing breast cancer by age. Seventy-seven percent of women with newly diagnosed breast cancer are older than 50 years of age. Breast cancer is less common in younger women, with an incidence of one case per 100,000 for women ages 20 to 24. Women younger than 30 years of age make up 0.3% of the total of new breast cancer cases per year. Women between the ages of 30 and 39 account for 4.8% of new cases of breast cancer per year. Women between 40 and 49 and between 50 and 59 have a drastically increased rate of developing breast cancer. Each group accounts for 18% of all cancer cases. This percentage further rises to 20.3% for women in the age range of 60 to 69. The highest number of new breast cancer cases occurs in women ages 70 to 79 (24.2%). Women over the age of 80 account for 14% of newly diagnosed breast cancers per year[3] (see Table 3-1).

As a result of the prevalence of breast cancer increasing in different age groups, breast cancer mortality rates in the population increase with increasing age. The mortality rate for women younger than 40 years of age is 25 per 100,000. This is in contrast to women older than 70 years of age, who have a mortality rate of at least 125 per 100,000.[3] Although mortality rates have been shown to increase for women as they age, breast cancer survival rates appear to be worse in younger women. Women who develop breast cancer younger than age 45 have a 5-year survival rate of 79% (all stages combined). The five-year survival rate increases to 84% for women ages 45 to 64 and to 87% for women ages 65 and over. It is believed that younger women have more aggressive tumors and are less responsive to hormonal therapy, which may contribute to their lower survival rates in this age group.[3]

Table 3-1
Risk of Developing Breast Cancer by Age[5]

Age (years)	Incidence per Year
<30	0.3%
30-39	4.8%
40-49	18%
50-59	18%
60-69	20.3%
70-79	24.2%
>80	14%

Incidence in Different Ethnic Groups

Breast cancer is the most commonly occurring cancer in all groups of US women except for Vietnamese-American women, who have a higher rate of cervical cancer. Between 1988 and 1992, the highest annual age-adjusted incidence of invasive breast cancer was in non-Hispanic White women (115.7/100,000), followed by Native American women (105.6/100,000) and African-American women (95.4/100,000). The lowest incidence rates were seen in Korean-American, American Indian of New Mexico, Vietnamese-American, and Chinese-American women. Japanese-American, Alaskan Native, Filipino-American, and Hispanic women had intermediate incidence rates.[4]

Although most women present with early operable breast cancer, African-American women have been shown to have a higher rate of stage II to IV breast cancer when compared with White women (Table 3-2).[5]

This corresponds to higher mortality rates in African-American women when compared with White women, despite a lower incidence of breast cancer in this group.[1] The 5-year survival for African-American women with breast cancer is 71%, compared with a 5-year survival of 86% for White women.[4] The reason for African-American women presenting at a later stage than White women is unclear, although access to health care and to mammography is thought to play a role. It has been proposed that African-American women may be more likely to have estrogen receptor–negative tumors or that these tumors may be more aggressive and difficult to treat.

Table 3-2
Rate of Breast Cancer by Stage—White Women vs. Black Women[3]

Stage	White Women	Black Women
II	27.2%	31.4%
III	5.3%	7.3%
IV	3.6%	6.5%

RISK FACTORS
Reproductive Factors
Menarche and Menstrual Cycles

Women with an earlier age of menarche have been shown to have an increased risk of breast cancer (Box 3-1). It is estimated that breast cancer risk is decreased by about 10% per 2-year delay of menarche.[6] Butler assessed the associations of early menarche, rapid initiation of regular ovulatory cycles, short cycle length, and more days of flow with the risk of developing breast cancer in 1505 controls and 1647 cases. Younger age at menarche (age 12) and regular cycles within 2 years of menarche increased breast cancer risk (odds ratio [OR] = 1.5 and 1.7, respectively). These associations were stronger in thinner women (body mass index < 22 kg/m^2) than heavier women (body mass index > 28.8 kg/m^2).[6] These data are difficult to interpret because they relied on the patients' recollections of period regularity and initiation of ovulation. There may be a difference in the way women recently diagnosed with breast cancer remember their menstrual histories, when compared with controls.

The characteristics of a woman's menstrual cycle have also been studied in association with breast cancer risk. In one prospective study, menstrual cycles less than 26 days or greater than 31 days during the ages of 18 to 22 were predictive of reduced breast cancer risk. Another study showed that shorter cycle length at age 30 was associated with a reduced breast cancer risk.[1] The importance of these results is unclear.

Age at First Birth

The risk of breast cancer has been shown to increase with an increase in a woman's age at her first full-term pregnancy. This is thought to be due to the pregnancy-induced maturation of mammary cells, which makes them less susceptible to carcinogenic transformation or a long-lasting hormonal change. In a study by Chie and associates, two case-control studies were analyzed to determine any association between age at any full-term pregnancy and breast cancer

---

BOX 3-1 Breast Cancer Risk Factors

Reproductive Factors
Early menarche
Late maternal age at first pregnancy
Decreased parity
Lack of breast-feeding
Endocrine
Oral contraceptives
Hormone replacement
Older than 45 with 75% dense breast tissue in mammogram
Atypical hyperplasia of the breast
Dietary
Alcohol consumption
Obesity
Genetic/Familial
Family member with breast cancer (Table 3-3)
Breast cancer familial syndrome (Table 3-4)
Family history of ovarian cancer

risk. Between 1988 and 1996, information was available on 9891 cases and 12,271 controls. The age of first pregnancy had a greater effect on the risk of developing breast cancer than did subsequent births. The OR for women with first full-term pregnancy at age 30 was 1.36, compared with women under 30, whose OR was 1.18.[7] In the Cancer and Steroid Hormone (CASH) study, a twofold increase in breast cancer risk was found when comparing first full-term pregnancy at age 30 years or older with first birth before age 20 (OR = 1.8).[8]

Although full-term pregnancy at an early age has been associated with a reduced risk of breast cancer, the role of pregnancy termination in relation to the risk of breast cancer is unclear. A case-control study by Newcomb and associates evaluated 6888 women with breast cancer, compared with 9529 controls, to determine breast cancer risk in relation to spontaneous or induced abortions. There was a weak association between breast cancer and pregnancy termination (relative risk [RR] = 1.12).[9] This may be due to a different hormonal milieu in women with pregnancy termination, compared with women who have a full-term pregnancy. However, the data for this study were collected from telephone interviews, and underreporting of induced abortions is possible.

Parity

The CASH study showed that there was a decrease in breast cancer risk with increasing parity.[8] The high levels of circulating hormones during pregnancy result in differentiation of the terminal duct–lobular unit (TDLU), which is the major site of malignant transformation in the breast. This process of differentiation of the TDLU is protective against breast cancer development, and its effect is permanent.[8]

Breast-feeding

Breast-feeding is considered important for infant growth and development. The effect of breast-feeding on maternal health has not been proven. Byers and associates reported a protective effect of breast-feeding against breast cancer.[10] This is most consistent for premenopausal breast cancer.[11] In a study by Minami and colleagues, various maternal factors played a role in determining which infant feeding method was used. Women with late age of menarche and high body mass index were more likely to breast-feed, compared with women with late age of first child, higher educational level, and maternal history of breast cancer. The authors conclude that these factors need to be considered when attempting to evaluate the relationship between breast-feeding and breast cancer.[12]

Lipworth and associates performed a review of the literature from 1966 to 1998 to ascertain the relationship between breast-feeding and the risk of breast cancer. Almost all studies were found to be of the case-control type and varied according to classification of breast-feeding history. The overall results showed a weak protective effect of breast-feeding against breast cancer. Some studies showed that long-term breast-feeding had a stronger effect in reducing breast cancer risk.[13] The cause of the protective effect of breast-feeding has been postulated to be due to reduced estrogen levels, removal of estrogens through the breast fluid, excretion of carcinogens from the breast during breast-feeding, changes in the mammary epithelial cells that reflect maximum differentiation, and delay of reestablishment of ovulation. Overall, breast-feeding appears to be of minimal importance in reducing the risk of developing breast cancer.

Endocrine

Endogenous

It has been recognized that one of the most important risk factors for developing breast cancer is a woman's lifelong exposure to her endogenous hormones. Andrieu and associates looked at various reproductive factors and the risk of developing breast cancer in 2948 cases and 4170 controls. A significant decreased risk for development of breast cancer was seen in women who had menarche at the age of 15 or older, compared with women who had menarche at age 12 or younger ($p < .001$). Menopause before the age of 50 was shown to decrease the risk of breast cancer (OR = 0.60).[14] Factors such as early menstruation (before age 12) and late menopause (after age 55) are being considered as risk factors contributing to breast cancer development.

Ovarian ablation has been considered as adjuvant therapy for the treatment of breast cancer; however, its role in prevention is less clear. Women who have bilateral oophorectomy at ages 50 to 54 years had a relative risk of developing breast cancer of 1.34, compared with women undergoing bilateral oophorectomy at ages 45 to 49 years. Women with artificial menopause induced before age 45 had a relative risk of developing breast cancer of 0.77.[15] No randomized trial has assessed the role of oophorectomy in decreasing the risk of developing breast cancer. Further, oophorectomy may result in coronary artery disease or osteoporosis, especially in young women. The risks and benefits must be weighed before recommending this approach to any individual.

Exogenous
Oral contraceptives
There is still controversy regarding the role of oral contraceptives in the development of breast cancer. Despite contradictory studies, the overall data suggest that oral contraceptive use results in an increased risk of breast cancer in premenopausal but not postmenopausal women.[8]

A case-control study of injectable and oral contraceptive use and breast cancer by Shapiro and associates examined 419 patients with breast cancer and 1625 controls. Between 1994 and 1997, the overall relative risk for oral contraceptive use was 1.2. Among women younger than 35, the relative risk was 1.7 and was unrelated to the duration or recency of use. The use of injectable progesterone did not increase the risk of developing breast cancer. Because of the low likelihood of a woman younger than 25 years of age developing breast cancer, the expected number of cases of breast cancer in young women who use oral contraceptives will be very small.[16]

Grabrick and associates studied a cohort of 426 breast cancer families to evaluate the risk of oral contraceptive use in women with a family history of breast cancer. The use of oral contraceptives was associated with a significantly increased risk of breast cancer among sisters and daughters of women with breast cancer (RR = 3.3). This increased risk was most evident for oral contraceptive use before 1975, when higher doses of estrogen and progesterone were used. Therefore further study with newer lower-dosage formulations of oral contraceptives is necessary before drawing any conclusions regarding increased risk.[17]

Hormone replacement therapy
Hormone replacement therapy does increase the risk of breast cancer, but some studies have shown that these tumors have a more favorable prognosis.[1] Several metaanalyses of the existing studies have been performed that show a relation between the duration of hormone replacement therapy use and breast carcinoma risk. Recent metaanalyses showed an increase in breast cancer risk of 2.3% for each year that a woman used a postmenopausal hormone.[8] The Nurses' Health Study followed postmenopausal women for 725,550 woman-years and found a total of 1935 invasive cancers. An increased risk was found in users of estrogen

replacement or combined estrogen-progesterone replacement (RR = 1.32 and 1.41, respectively). For hormone users of 5 years or more, the RR was 1.46.[8]

Chiechi and associates looked at risk factors for the development of breast cancer that would influence a woman's use of postmenopausal hormone replacement therapy. Obesity is associated with an increased risk of postmenopausal breast cancer, and the risk is linked to elevated endogenous hormonal levels of obese women. Obesity is associated with an increased aromatization of androgens and higher levels of circulating sex steroids. Upper body (android) obesity but not lower body (gynoid) obesity is associated with higher levels of estradiol and testosterone and an increased risk of breast cancer. Therefore hormone replacement therapy may be contraindicated in women with android obesity.[18]

Women age 45 or older whose mammograms show at least 75% dense breast tissue have a fivefold increased risk of developing breast cancer. These women may not be candidates for hormone replacement therapy. High endogenous estrogen levels may also increase the risk of breast cancer. One study found that doubling estradiol levels resulted in a threefold increase in breast cancer risk. The authors recommend measuring endogenous estrogen levels before starting a postmenopausal woman on hormone replacement therapy.[18]

Alcohol consumption increases breast cancer risk with a dose-related effect. Several studies show that drinking 5 g of alcohol per day increased the risk of developing breast cancer. Alcohol increased the blood concentration of estradiol in women taking exogenous hormones. Hormone replacement therapy may further increase the risk of developing breast cancer in women with significant alcohol intake.[18]

Benign breast disease such as proliferative lesions or atypical hyperplasia increases the risk of breast cancer. As hormone replacement therapy stimulates the occurrence of benign breast disease, it may in turn increase the risk of breast cancer. Exogenous estrogen may therefore add further risk in these patients. Lastly, family history of breast cancer should be considered when counseling a woman about the use of hormone replacement.[18]

Ross and associates looked at the effect of hormone replacement therapy on breast cancer risk. In a case-control study, 1897 women with breast cancer and 1637 controls ages 55 to 72 were evaluated over a 4½-year period. Hormone replacement therapy was associated with a 10% higher breast cancer risk for each 5 years of use (OR = 1.10). Risk was substantially higher for combined estrogen-progesterone replacement than for estrogen alone (OR = 1.24 vs. 1.06). The authors concluded that the addition of progestin to hormone replacement therapy markedly increases the risk of breast cancer relative to estrogen use alone.[19]

In summary, postmenopausal hormone replacement therapy halves the risk of coronary heart disease and osteoporosis but increases the risk of breast cancer by 30% to 40%.[2] Although the benefits of hormone replacement therapy appear to outweigh the risks in the majority of women, this is not the case in women who are at increased risk for the development of breast cancer. Every woman should receive individual counseling about the use of hormone replacement therapy.

Fertility drugs

Infertility is one of the factors that are felt to increase the risk of breast cancer. Several studies have attempted to determine whether there is a link between fertility drugs and the development of breast cancer. These studies can be difficult to evaluate because of the small number of cancer cases reported in women receiving infertility treatment and the confounding factors such as nulliparity, age at first birth, and family history. Potashnik and associates performed a historic-prospective cohort study of 1197 women who underwent treatment at an infertility clinic between 1960 and 1984. Of 20 breast cancers diagnosed, 16 cases were detected among the 780 women who had been exposed to follicle-stimulating medications. The increased incidence was not statistically significant when compared with the general population (standardized incidence ratio = 1.65, 95% confidence interval [CI], 0.94-2.68).[20] The authors concluded that women exposed to fertility drugs did not have an increased risk for developing breast cancer when compared with unexposed infertile women or the general population. However, the mean age at the end of the study was 44 years. The true effects of fertility drugs may not be seen until these women are in their sixties. There were no data on patient's family history or use of oral contraceptives, which are risk factors for the development of breast cancer.

Ricci and associates performed a case-control study of 3415 women with breast cancer and 2916 controls. Fifty (1.5%) cases and 53 (1.8%) controls reported a history of infertility (OR = 0.8). Sixteen (0.5%) cases and 11 (0.4%) controls reported using fertility drugs (OR = 1.2). The authors concluded that the use of fertility drugs did not increase the risk of developing breast cancer.[21] It is important to note that the data for this study were obtained by questionnaire, and perhaps there was a difference in how infertility was defined by the women participating in the study or the duration of time that fertility drugs were taken. Also, because the number of patients in this study was very small, it is difficult to draw any conclusions.

Finally, Venn and associates looked at a cohort of 29,700 women—20,656 were exposed to fertility drugs, and 9044 were not—who underwent in vitro fertilization (IVF). There were a total of 143 cases of breast cancer, but this overall incidence was no greater than expected in both the exposed and unexposed groups (standardized incidence ratios = 0.91 and 0.95 respectively). However, the incidence of breast cancer was significantly higher within the first 12 months of exposure to fertility drugs with IVF than expected (standardized incidence ratio = 1.96). The authors hypothesize that the reason for this may be due to the patient's receiving intensive medical care during the infertility treatment that identifies the tumor or that the fertility drugs may promote the development of preexisting tumors.[22] Inasmuch as the numbers are small, the reason for this early increase in the incidence of breast cancer in women receiving fertility drugs and IVF is unclear.

Dietary
Alcohol Intake
Previous studies have shown that an increased breast cancer risk is associated with chronic alcohol intake.[23] It has been postulated that this increased risk is due to alcohol-related changes in estrogen activity. Other theories maintain that alcohol activates carcinogens or that the metabolism of carcinogens contained in alcohol is impaired by alcohol-related liver dysfunction.

The association between increased breast cancer risk and alcohol intake is stronger for postmenopausal women. Various studies have shown an increase in estrogen concentrations in the blood or urine after moderate alcohol intake.[23] Alcohol increases the aromatization of androgen to estrogen in fat and skin. This may counteract some of the effects of menopausal symptoms in women.

Alcohol also causes hyperinsulinemia, which can stimulate expression of insulin-like growth factor receptor in mammary tissue. This would result in estrogen-independent growth in precancerous lesions in the years leading up to menopause when estrogen levels are falling. It has been postulated that many of the precancerous lesions undergo spontaneous involution at menopause as estrogen levels fall. These lesions then enter a dormant state from which they can be reactivated by promoting factors such as alcohol. The alcohol-related hyperinsulinemia might counteract the spontaneous regression of these precancerous lesions that occurs at menopause. The growth of these lesions may be changed from estrogen-dependent to autonomous growth.

Garland and associates evaluated alcohol consumption prospectively in relation to breast cancer risk in 116,671 women enrolled in 1989. During a follow-up period of 6 years, 445 cases of invasive breast cancer developed. Only drinking more than 6 drinks per week at ages 23 to 30 was associated with an increased risk (RR = 1.72; p = .05).[24] However, most women enrolled in this study were light to moderate drinkers; thus these numbers are too low to draw any significant conclusions about heavy alcohol use and the risk of breast cancer in premenopausal women.

Dietary Fat

The role of dietary fat in the etiology of breast cancer in unclear. Fat may increase endogenous hormone levels of estrogen and progesterone. A randomized trial of dietary intervention to reduce fat intake did show a reduction in mammographic density.[1] Holmes and associates looked at 88,795 women free of cancer in 1980 and followed up for 14 years in the Nurses' Health Study. The relative risk of breast cancer for an incremental increase in fat intake was measured by a food frequency questionnaire. There was no significant difference in the relative risk of breast cancer in women who consumed 20% or less fat, compared with women consuming 30% to 35% fat (RR = 1.15).[25] This question remains to be answered.

Obesity

Obesity has been evaluated as a risk factor for the development of breast cancer. Obesity is associated with decreased risk of premenopausal breast cancer and increased risk of post-menopausal breast cancer.[1] Mezzetti and associates conducted a case-control study on 2569 breast cancer patients and 2588 controls in attempts to determine potentially modifiable risk factors for breast cancer. Obesity as measured by a body mass index greater than 26.6 kg/m^2 was associated with an increased incidence of breast cancer (OR = 1.22) in post-menopausal women.[26] Trentham-Dietz and associates looked at 5031 women aged 50 to 79 years who were newly diagnosed with invasive breast cancer and compared them with 5255 similarly aged controls. Women in the top quintile groups for height at age 20, recent weight, and recent body mass index had significantly increased risks of breast cancer (p < .001). It appears that weight gain in postmenopausal women increases the risk of development of breast cancer.[27]

Physical Activity

It is known that physical activity can interrupt the menstrual cycle and perhaps lower a woman's cumulative exposure to estrogen. A study by Thune and associates looked at 25,624 women between the ages of 20 and 54 who answered a questionnaire about physical activity to determine the role of exercise in the development of breast cancer. Physical activity was graded from 1 to 4, which ranged from sedentary activities to vigorous exercise. The risk of developing breast cancer was reduced in women who exercised vigorously, compared with sedentary women (RR = 0.63).[28] This effect was more pronounced for premenopausal then postmenopausal women. Mezzetti and associates also found that low levels of physical activity were associated with increased risk of breast cancer in both premenopausal and postmenopausal women (OR = 1.5).[26] Physical activity may result in decreased body mass index, which reduces fat stores and the aromatization of androgens to estrogens. Therefore these factors may not be independent.

In contrast, Rockhill and associates studied 116,671 nurses aged 25 to 42 in the Nurses' Health Study II to determine whether physical activity played a role in the development of breast cancer. Questionnaires were mailed every 2 years from 1989 to 1995. There was no difference in the development of breast cancer in women who engaged in strenuous activity, compared with women who did not engage in such activity (RR = 1.1).[29] A later study by Rockhill, which looked at 121,701 women aged 30 to 55, concluded that women who engaged in 7 or more hours of vigorous physical activity per week had a slightly reduced risk of breast cancer, when compared with women who engaged in less than 1 hour of exercise weekly (RR = 0.82).[30]

It is difficult to determine the accuracy of self-reporting associated with accumulating data from a questionnaire. Women may have overestimated their level of physical activity. Therefore it is difficult to draw any significant conclusions from these studies.

Genetic Familial
Affected Relative
Studies have shown that a woman with a first-degree relative with breast cancer has a risk of developing breast cancer that is 1.7 to 4.0 times that of the general population.[31] Familial breast cancer can be defined as two or more cases of breast cancer within a family (Table 3-3). Family members with early onset of tumors and bilateral cancers increase a woman's risk of developing breast cancer. The genetic factors in these cases are probably multifactorial. These cases may arise from environmental and genetic interaction.[32]

Breast and Ovarian Familial Syndromes
Breast and ovarian cancer may occur as part of several familial cancer syndromes. Li-Fraumeni syndrome, which results from a p53 mutation, is a rare condition associated with brain tumors, soft tissue sarcomas, and breast cancer in families. Hereditary nonpolyposis colon cancer (Lynch syndrome) results in colon cancer in family members and endometrial cancer in females. Breast and ovarian carcinoma are both higher in families with Lynch syndrome than in the general population. Cowden's syndrome, associated with a PTEN gene

Table 3-3
Affected Relatives and the Risk of Breast Cancer[51,52]

Family Member	Relative Risk
Mother before age 60	2.0
Mother after age 60	1.4
First-degree relative	1.2-3.0
Premenopausal	3.1
Premenopausal (bilateral)	8.5-9.0
Postmenopausal	1.5
Postmenopausal (bilateral)	4.0-5.4
Two first-degree relatives	4.6

Table 3-4
Breast Cancer Familial Syndromes[33]

Syndrome	Gene Mutation	Manifestations	Risk
Li-Fraumeni	P53	Brain tumors, sarcomas Breast cancer, leukemia	50%-89%
Cowden	CD1	Bilateral breast cancer Thyroid cancer, hamartomas	30%-40%
Lynch	hMLH1	Hereditary nonpolyposis colorectal cancer, endometrial cancer	Not available
	hMSH2	Breast cancer, ovarian cancer	
BRCA1	185de1AG	Breast cancer, ovarian cancer	60%-85%
BRCA2	6174de1T	Breast cancer, ovarian cancer	60%-85%

mutation, results in distinctive skin manifestations and increased incidence of breast and thyroid cancer (Table 3-4).

In contrast to these rare syndromes, BRCA1 and BRCA2 account for 50% or more of all breast and ovarian cancer families.[33]

Ovarian Cancer As a Risk for Breast Cancer

Sutcliffe and associates performed a prospective cohort analysis of 2304 women with a strong family history of ovarian cancer (two or more first-degree relatives with ovarian cancer), comparing the number of incident breast cancers with the expected based on population incidence rates. The RR for developing breast cancer for women younger than 50 years of age was 3.74 and 1.79 for women 50 years of age or older. These trends were both statistically significant when compared with expected population incidence ($p = .02$ and $p = .034$).[34] Thus it seems that a family history of ovarian cancer does increase a patient's risk of developing breast cancer. However, it is unclear from this study whether the cases of ovarian cancer had similar risk factors for the development of breast cancer when compared with the general population (i.e., age at menarche, parity, age of first pregnancy, family history).

Table 3-5
Molecular Aspects of BRCA Genes[53]

Aspect	BRCA1	BRCA2
Year of discovery	1994	1995
MRNA size	7-8 kb	10-12 kb
Chromosomal location	17q21	13q12-13

BRCA 1 and BRCA 2

All the breast cancer susceptibility genes are autosomal dominant. Two breast cancer susceptibility genes have been identified: BRCA1 and BRCA2. BRCA1 maps to chromosome 17q21, and ovarian cancer is also linked to the same gene in these breast, cancer families. BRCA2 maps to chromosome 13q12-13, and ovarian cancer is also a prominent finding in BRCA2-linked families (Table 3-5).[33]

Women with mutations in either of these genes have a lifetime risk of breast cancer of 60% to 85% and a lifetime risk of ovarian cancer of 15% to 40%. Characteristics associated with increased likelihood of carrying the BRCA1 or BRCA2 gene, or both, are early-onset breast cancer, breast and ovarian cancer, and Ashkenazi Jewish ancestry.

In families with known mutations in BRCA1 and BRCA2, genetic testing can separate women who carry the familial mutation from those who do not. The patient first should receive genetic counseling before testing to give her information about the probability that she carries a mutation in BRCA1 or BRCA2 and the risks and benefits of testing. BRCA mutations are rare in non–Ashkenazi Jewish populations and account for fewer than 5% of the diagnosed breast cancers.[2]

The number of breast cancer cases in a family correlates with the discovery of a mutation in affected members of the family. The more breast cancer cases occurring on one side of the family, the more likely a mutation will be found. However, for families with only breast cancer, more than half may be due to factors other than BRCA1 or BRCA2 mutations. Therefore before genetic testing is performed, women must be told that the absence of these genes does not rule out another genetic or environmental risk factor for breast or ovarian carcinoma.[33] Approximately 8% to 10% of all breast cancers are inherited, and approximately 50% of all inheritable breast cancers are associated with the BRCA1 gene. Thirty-two percent of all inheritable breast cancers are associated with the BRCA2 gene.

The majority of breast cancers associated with BRCA1 are invasive ductal carcinomas; however, there is an excess number of medullary carcinomas. BRCA1-associated cancers usually have a poor histologic grade associated with a significantly high mitotic index. Most of these tumors are hormone receptor negative. For BRCA2-associated tumors, there is not the same increased incidence of medullary type tumors, but the histologic grade is also poor. Several studies have looked at prognosis in women with BRCA-associated breast cancer. The results are conflicting, and more studies are needed to determine whether survival is different in women with familial breast cancer.[31]

Table 3-6
BRCA1 and BRCA2 Mutations in Various Ethnicities[54]

Population	BRCA1 Mutations	BRCA2 Mutations
Ashkenazi Jews	185de1AG; 5382insC	6174de1T
Icelanders		999de15
Dutch	2804de1AA, del510; de13835	5573insA
Norwegians	1136insA	
Swedes	Q563X; 3166ins5; 1201del1; 2594delC	4486delG
African-Americans	M1775R; 1832del5; 5296del4	

Individuals at risk

In the United States, the Ashkenazi Jewish population has three mutations that are present at higher frequencies than in other populations (2% of the Ashkenazi Jewish population carries these mutations). Two mutations are in the BRCA1 gene and one in the BRCA2 gene. For BRCA1, the founder mutation, 185delAG, is responsible for 21% of breast cancers in this population. The 6174delT founder mutation is responsible for 8% of breast cancers associated with BRCA2. The penetrance of these mutations is about 50% for breast cancer and 20% for ovarian cancer.[33] Different mutations occur in various ethnic groups (Table 3-6).

The markers for the presence of a breast cancer predisposition gene in a cluster of cancers in multiple family members are: young age of onset relative to general population, occurrence of same type of cancer more than once in one individual, and multiple cases of cancer in addition to the breast and ovarian cancers in several individuals.[35] It is important that all women undergo pretest genetic counseling. Only women with at least a 20% probability of being a BRCA carrier should be tested.[31] Factors influencing the probability that a woman with breast cancer carries a BRCA mutation include any blood relative younger than 50 years of age with breast cancer, any blood relative with ovarian cancer, a woman with bilateral breast cancer or ovarian and breast cancer, or breast cancer diagnosed younger than age 40.[31]

When to test

Affected women in families with a strong family history of breast or ovarian cancer, or both, should be tested first. It is informative if the person with a specific cancer is tested for the presence of a genetic mutation. The other family members can then be tested for the particular mutation. When unaffected relatives are known to have a negative result on the specific mutation, they can be ensured that they are not carriers.[33] Without a known genetic mutation, a negative test in unaffected individuals does not rule out the possibility that they may have an as yet undiscovered gene.[33] Further, if there is a mutation but the proband does not yet have a diagnosis of breast cancer, it is difficult to interpret the results with full confidence.

Malone and associates looked at BRCA2 mutations in young women with a personal breast-cancer history before age 35 (n = 203) versus women diagnosed before age 45 *and* with a first-degree relative with breast cancer (n = 225). In women with a first-degree relative with breast cancer, 4.9% had BRCA2 mutations. Within this group, women diagnosed before the age of 30 had a BRCA2 mutation frequency of 15.4%. For women diagnosed before the age of 35, the BRCA2 frequency was greatest for women diagnosed with breast cancer before the age of 30 (4.4%).[36] When both groups of patients were combined, BRCA2 occurred most frequently in women with four or more relatives with breast cancer (10%). The frequency of BRCA2 mutations was lower than that for BRCA1 mutations in both the women diagnosed before age 35 (3.4% vs. 5.9%) and women diagnosed before age 45 *and* with first-degree relatives (4.9% vs. 7.1%). The overall frequency of mutation of either gene was 9.8%.[36] The authors' conclusion is that BRCA1 and BRCA2 screening will have its greatest impact when targeted to specific at-risk populations.

Jernstrom and associates looked at various reproductive factors in women who carry the BRCA1 or BRCA2 mutation. Age at menarche, menstrual cycle length, age at first full-term pregnancy and nulliparity did not significantly differ between BRCA1 mutation carriers and noncarriers. Women from non-BRCA1/BRCA2 hereditary breast cancer families were older at menarche, but this was not found to be significant.[37]

The histologic characteristics of breast cancers caused by BRCA1 and BRCA2 mutations differ from sporadic breast cancers. High-grade tumors tend to occur more often among BRCA1 mutation carriers than among controls. The biology of BRCA1-induced tumors also differs from sporadic tumors. They are more frequently steroid receptor negative and DNA-aneuploid, and they have a higher S-phase fraction than controls.[32] BRCA1 tumors are more likely to be atypical medullary or medullary type with features of lymphocytic infiltrate. These tumors also demonstrate a higher frequency of p53 mutations but a decreased incidence of c-erbB-2 overexpression.[38]

Implications of testing

Benefits of genetic testing for cancer include reduced anxiety of facing unknown cancer risk, increased information about cancer in a family, possible positive influence on family interactions, motivation for screening and prevention, identifying at-risk family members, avoiding unnecessary testing or surgery, and providing informed children and possibly family planning. The test is not without risks, which include employment discrimination, insurance discrimination, negative family interactions, cost of testing, anxiety associated with mutation status, possible false-positive or false-negative results, and confusion from uninformative results.[32]

Genetic testing has implications for the entire family. It is not a diagnostic test. It can identify individuals at risk for hereditary breast and ovarian cancer and identify noncarriers in a family with a known mutation, but it does not predict when the cancer will be found clinically. Further, the effectiveness of preventive interventions in women with a positive test varies widely.[32] A positive test may push for a decision about preventative measures that are imperfect at the present time. A positive test can therefore result in increased anxiety for the individual tested and her family. A positive test may have some social implications. A negative test does not change the risk of the development of sporadic cancer. Genetic testing does not detect all mutations.

Ethical and legal issues

Genetic testing for breast cancer predisposition has shown that there is an increased interest in testing by women of higher social class, and interest is proportionate to the level of anxiety.[35] There is a question of at what age this testing should be offered. Testing of children is only done for those conditions in which medical management would be altered. This is an area of controversy because many of the cancer syndromes are late-onset disorders for which there may be a cure by the time the cancer may be diagnosed.

There are no clear guidelines for insurance companies to use genetic information. Many argue that, like all other medical tests, genetic testing will have to be declared when one seeks insurance.[35] This could create a group of people that is uninsurable. This question will have to be answered in the coming decades as the human genome project continues. Refer to Chapter 11 for further discussion of legal issues.

Management of patients with a gene mutation

Current recommendations for women with excessive risk of developing breast cancer are early surveillance, chemoprevention, prophylactic mastectomy, and modified lifestyle. Monthly breast self-examination should begin early in adult life, with annual or semiannual breast examination by a health professional beginning between age 25 and 30. Annual mammogram should be started between age 25 and 35, depending on the particular family history of each individual. Another option is to start mammographic screening 5 to 10 years before the age of disease in the youngest relative with breast cancer and annually after age 35 for all carriers.

Chemoprevention is currently being investigated for women with BRCA1 and BRCA2 mutations. There has not been a clearly approved chemopreventive regimen in this group of patients. Current therapies under investigation include tamoxifen, raloxifene, and soy protein.

Prophylactic mastectomy in this group of patients is also under investigation. Observational data from the Mayo Clinic found a 90% reduction in breast cancer cases in women who underwent prophylactic mastectomy, compared with the expected number of cancers predicted.[33] Schrag and associates compared prophylactic mastectomy with no prophylactic surgery among women who carry mutations in the BRCA1 or BRCA2 gene. The average 30-year-old woman, carrying BRCA1 or BRCA2 mutations, gained from 2.9 to 5.3 years of life expectancy from prophylactic mastectomy.[39] This gain declined with age until women at age 60 had minimal benefit. Each woman must weigh the risks and benefits of prophylactic mastectomy. Negative factors include psychological distress; altered quality of life; continued, although significantly reduced risk of breast cancer; and morbidity of surgery. The positive effects include reduced risk of morbidity and mortality associated with breast cancer, decreased anxiety for developing breast cancer, and reduced morbidity from surveillance and possible adjuvant therapy for treating breast cancer.[31]

Jernstrom and associates performed a case-control study of 189 BRCA1 case-control pairs and 47 BRCA2 case-control pairs to assess the effect of pregnancy on the development of breast cancer in BRCA1 and BRCA2 carriers. Carriers of the BRCA1 and BRCA2 mutations who had children were significantly more likely to develop breast cancer by age 40 than carriers who were nulliparous (OR = 1.61 and 2.13). Early pregnancy did not protect the carriers from the development of breast cancer. This could have important implications in counseling women who carry BRCA1 and BRCA2 mutations.[37]

Environmental
Ionizing Radiation

Radiation is found in the environment from natural sources and includes cosmic rays as well as terrestrial radiations influenced by the distribution of radioactive elements in the soil and by internally deposited radionucleotides such as radon. The effects of low exposure are difficult to assess. Single large-dose exposures such as from the atomic bomb blasts or from repeated radiation therapy (such as mantle radiation therapy for Hodgkin's disease) are established causes of breast cancer. A linear dose response is observed. The age at exposure also appears to influence the relative risk with decreasing risk with increasing age of exposure. The highest risk is observed for women exposed between ages 10 and 20. There is little risk for women exposed at age greater than 40.[40]

Several studies have looked at occupational exposure to radiation and the risk of breast cancer. Airline attendants, radium dial workers, and radiologic technologists have not been shown to have an increased breast cancer risk. Even in areas of industrial accidents, exposure to low-dose radiation has not been shown to increase breast cancer risk.[40]

There have been data to suggest that there is an association between the treatment of Hodgkin's lymphoma with mantle radiation and the development of breast cancer.[41]

Other External Factors

Environmental exposure to chemicals, specifically organochlorines, has been studied with respect to the risk of breast cancer. This class of compounds includes pesticides and industrial chemicals. Some of these compounds are weakly estrogenic and are excreted in the breast milk, which means that the ductal cells are directly exposed to these chemicals. The population is exposed to the organochlorines through ingestion of fish, meat, and dairy products.[40] Ecological, occupational, and population-based case-control studies have all failed to show a significant increase in breast cancer risk in women exposed to these chemicals.[40]

PREVENTION
Primary Prevention
Prophylactic Mastectomy

Specific considerations for prophylactic mastectomy may include personal history of unilateral breast cancer, one first-degree relative with bilateral premenopausal breast cancer, two first-degree relatives with premenopausal breast cancer, and lobular carcinoma in situ (LCIS). Hartmann and associates performed a retrospective cohort analysis of 639 women who underwent bilateral prophylactic mastectomy at the Mayo Clinic between 1960 and 1993. A reduction of 90% in the risk of breast cancer was seen in women with a moderate to high-risk family history.[42]

Prophylactic mastectomy is an option for reducing the risk of breast cancer. Despite prophylactic mastectomy, breast cancer can develop in the residual breast glandular tissue. Breast tissue is widely distributed over the anterolateral chest wall and axilla, and residual nonvisible breast tissue may remain after mastectomy.

Subcutaneous versus simple mastectomy

Both a subcutaneous and a simple mastectomy have been used to reduce an individual's risk of breast cancer. The subcutaneous mastectomy preserves the nipple-areolar complex and a small amount of retroareolar breast tissue for vascular supply. Because of the residual breast tissue, there could be a greater risk of developing breast cancer than after a simple (or total) mastectomy. The latter one is the preferred type of mastectomy for patients who seek surgical prophylaxis.

Chemoprevention

Chemoprevention of cancer has recently been shown to be possible and has opened a new area of therapy for women at high risk for breast cancer. It is important to minimize the adverse side effects in the development of new protocols that are used on healthy individuals. Several compounds are being actively studied for use as chemopreventative agents.

Tamoxifen

The use of tamoxifen in the prevention of breast cancer stems from review of trials and meta-analyses which noted that tamoxifen reduced the incidence of contralateral breast cancer in women being treated for breast cancer by 50%. Other incidental findings demonstrated that tamoxifen reduced osteoporosis, did not increase coronary artery disease, but did increase endometrial cancer rates. These studies led to several randomized clinical trials to determine whether tamoxifen could be used to prevent breast cancer in women at increased risk (history of LCIS, atypical hyperplasia, family history).[43]

The Breast Cancer Prevention Trial (BCPT) randomized 13,000 women with a 5-year risk of breast cancer of 1.7% or more to tamoxifen (20 mg per day) or placebo. After a mean follow-up of 4 years, tamoxifen reduced the incidence of breast cancer by 49%, compared to the incidence with placebo.[2] Tamoxifen also reduced the risk of noninvasive breast cancer by 50%. The effect on osteoporosis was shown by a 19% reduction in hip, radius, and spine fractures in women taking tamoxifen. There was no difference in the rate of ischemic heart disease in women given placebo versus tamoxifen.[43] Tamoxifen has considerable risks, such as endometrial cancer (relative risk = 2.5), thromboembolic events such as deep venous thrombosis (relative risk = 1.6) and pulmonary embolism (relative risk = 3), cataracts, and hot flashes. Therefore the risks and benefits must be weighed for each individual patient. Further, there is some controversy regarding tumors that develop in women given tamoxifen as chemoprevention. Perhaps these tumors are more aggressive and not suitable for tamoxifen as adjuvant therapy.[43] Because of this and other adverse effects of tamoxifen, women at less than a 5-year breast cancer risk of 1.7 percent are not candidates for tamoxifen in preventing breast cancer.

Raloxifene (Evista), a selective estrogen receptor modulator, is currently used for preventing osteoporosis in women. A recent European study of 7705 women showed that raloxifene reduced the risk of developing breast cancer fourfold.[43] A National Surgical Adjuvant Breast and Bowel Project (NSABP) randomized study that compares tamoxifen and raloxifene (STAR) in 22,000 postmenopausal women at high risk for breast cancer is under way.[1,43]

Retinoids

Natural retinoids play a role in cellular proliferation and differentiation but are not tolerated well in clinical situations. A less toxic vitamin A analog, fenretinide (4-HPR), is being studied for use as chemoprevention in women at high risk for breast cancer. Although its mechanism of action remains unclear, fenretinide appears to inhibit the insulin-like growth factor (IGF) system in breast cancer, thus resulting in inhibition of tumor growth. It also appears to work by inducing apoptosis. A phase III trial aimed at reducing contralateral breast cancer randomized 2972 women with stage I breast cancer or ductal carcinoma in situ (DCIS) to receive fenretinide or placebo for 5 years. Overall, there was no difference between the two groups at a median follow-up of 5 years. However, premenopausal women had a 35% reduction in the rate of local recurrence with no reduction in postmenopausal women. Plasma IGF levels were lower in premenopausal women only.[44] Recently, a pilot study combining tamoxifen and fenretinide in at-risk women showed this combination to be well-tolerated. Further studies are under way in premenopausal women.

Secondary Prevention
Screening the General Population

Screening for breast cancer is aimed at detecting the disease before it is clinically apparent. Diseases for which screening is worthwhile must be serious, prevalent, and treatable, and the screening tool must be safe, sensitive, cost-effective, and practical. There also must be a preclinical phase during which the disease is detectable and the treatment results are better than waiting for symptoms to appear. Breast cancer screening meets all of these criteria. Screening tests include mammography, clinical breast examination, and breast self-examination, which are all widely available, noninvasive, and affordable.[45]

Mammography

Evidence of mortality reduction from breast cancer screening in women ages 50 to 69 has led to agreement on screening in these women. The results of a randomized controlled trial in the late 1970s revealed a 35% reduction in mortality in women ages 50 to 64. When to stop screening is controversial. The incidence of breast cancer rises considerably with each decade of life so that the incidence for a 70-year-old woman is four times that for a 40-year-old woman. Mammography for women older than 65 shows a higher positive predictive value for abnormal findings, higher yield on breast biopsy, and higher cancer detection rates than for younger women. One randomized control study has shown a reduction in relative risk of breast cancer death in women aged 65 to 74 who participated in screening (RR = 0.68).[45] As women older than 70 vary more greatly in their overall health status, most clinicians recommend routine screening for women up to the age of 70 and screening based on clinical judgment thereafter. We believe all women older than 70 years of age in good overall health should continue to receive yearly screening mammograms. The steep rise in cancer incidence with age despite the modest relative risk reduction means an overall benefit from continuing the screening process.[45]

At the other end of the spectrum is the debate over when to start breast cancer screening. In this group of women under the age of 50, the benefits of screening must be weighed against the risks. Based on randomized controlled trials, there appears to be a delay in reduction in breast cancer mortality 10 years after the initiation of screening. The data from eight randomized controlled trials at 10 to 18 years of follow-up in women ages 40 to 49 at entry showed an 18% reduction in women who were screened. The National Institutes of Health (NIH) consensus meeting in 1996 suggested that the data were insufficient to warrant yearly mammography for women in their forties. Despite this controversy, the American Cancer Society has published its guidelines and currently recommends annual mammograms for women ages 40 to 49.[46]

In women younger than 50, the breast density is much higher, and some argue that mammography is less likely to detect early breast cancer at a curable stage. The incidence of breast cancer is low in women younger than 50; therefore it has been argued that fewer women in this group will benefit from screening.[2] However, 18% of breast cancers are detected in women in their forties, and the same percent is detected in women in their fifties. At present, the benefit of screening mammography in women ages 40 to 49 is thought to outweigh the risks.

It is important for the patient to understand that mammography is not without false results. False-positive examinations are a potential risk that lead to unnecessary anxiety and the risks of invasive procedure. Approximately 10% of all mammograms in the United States are read as abnormal. The cumulative risk of a false-positive result of breast cancer was evaluated in a retrospective study of 2400 women aged 40 to 69 years. There was a false-positive mammogram rate of 23.8%, and the rate was found to be higher in women aged 40 to 49, compared with women aged 50 or older.[46]

False-negative examinations are associated with false reassurance and a subsequent delay in evaluation. Up to 25% of all invasive breast cancers are not detected by mammography in women ages 40 to 49 years. This is compared with 10% not detected by mammography in women ages 50 to 69 years. The risks of false-positives and false-negatives are higher in younger women as a result of the lower sensitivity and specificity in this age group.[46]

Clinical breast examination

Clinical breast examination and breast self-examination are also part of the screening for breast cancer. Between 41% and 67% of women report performing breast self-examinations monthly. There is no strong evidence of a survival benefit from breast self-examination. There is no strong recommendation for or against inclusion of breast self-examination in the screening program. Sirovich and associates state that adolescent and young women should not be encouraged to perform breast self-examinations because the incidence of breast cancer is so low in these groups. If a woman is performing breast self-examinations, it is important that she be taught the correct way to examine the breast for a benefit to be seen.[45]

Recent randomized control studies have shown that 3% to 24% of breast cancers are missed by mammography but are detected by clinical breast examination. The proportion of these tumors is higher in women under the age of 50. However, no study has shown an additional survival benefit from including the clinical breast examination in a mammographic screening program.[45]

Screening Populations at High Risk

Mammography

Intensive screening for women at high risk for breast cancer works by detecting breast cancer at an earlier, more treatable stage. There are no data available with respect to the effectiveness of screening in women who are carriers for the BRCA1 or BRCA2 mutations. Screening is effective for women older than 50 because of the significant incidence of breast cancer in this patient population. The threshold size for detecting breast tumors by mammography is 1 to 2 mm (20 doublings), whereas a tumor of 1 cm or larger is likely to be detected by palpation. The time from tumor inception to mammographic detection has been calculated to be approximately 6.8 years. The time from mammographic detection to palpation adds another 3.4 years. Therefore there is a greater than 3-year window for mammography to detect a breast cancer before it will be found on physical examination.[47]

Breast cancer will develop in 19.1% of carriers of the BRCA1 or BRCA2 gene before the age of 40 and in 50% of these women before the age of 50. The rate of growth of breast cancer is faster in younger women and the breast parenchyma is denser, which makes mammographic detection more difficult. The time from tumor inception to mammographic detection in younger women is 2.7 years. The time from mammographic detection to palpation in this group of women is an additional 1.35 years. This is a substantially shorter time period than is seen in older women. There is also the additional problem that as many as 33% of tumors in women younger than 40 years of age may not be detected on mammography as a result of the density of the breast tissue.[47]

It is likely that breast cancers in women who are carriers for the BRCA1 mutation will grow quickly because of the individual's young age and the genetic mutation. In summary, young women with BRCA1 or BRCA2 mutations may have faster growing tumors that are more difficult to identify by mammography as a result of the density of the breast. A proportion of these women will be diagnosed at a later stage with larger tumors and possible metastatic lesions. These women should be aggressively screened in attempts to detect these tumors at an early stage.[47] Currently, screening for women who carry a genetic mutation involves yearly clinical breast examinations between the ages of 25 and 30 and yearly mammograms, starting no later than age 35.[35]

Other modalities for high-risk women

The sensitivity of magnetic resonance imaging (MRI) is 91% to 98% in detecting breast cancer and is being evaluated in high-risk women. It is an attractive modality because of the excellent soft tissue resolution and lack of ionizing radiation. Furthermore, the tomographic imaging prevents tissue overlap. The tumor enhancement seen with gadolinium injection is due to the increased vascularity seen with malignancy. MRI may be helpful in identifying the extent of the tumor, especially the involvement of the chest wall and nipple, which may be useful in the surgical planning. It has also been suggested that MRI may be useful to assess residual disease after primary excision.[48]

Tilanus-Linthorst and associates looked at 109 women with more than a 25% risk of breast cancer and no evidence of tumor on previous mammography. She found that MRI detected breast cancer in three patients (2.8%) that were occult at mammography. Although this may advance the detection of early breast cancers, the cost was found to be considerable.[49]

Olson and associates looked at 40 women with biopsy-proven adenocarcinoma metastatic to the axillary lymph nodes with no evidence of primary cancer. MRI of the breast identified a primary breast lesion in 28 of 40 women (70%). Forty-seven percent of patients had breast conservation therapy. The authors concluded that MRI might identify occult tumors and facilitate breast conservation.[50]

It is important to note that MRI cannot identify microcalcifications, which are important in the identification of DCIS. Another limitation is that there are changes in the T1 value during the menstrual cycle; therefore patients should be scanned between the sixth and sixteenth day of the cycle to reduce false-positives.[49] Finally, although MRI is a sensitive method, it is very expensive and impractical for routine screening.

When and how often

Little information is available to determine the effectiveness of close monitoring of high-risk women. In the NSABP-P1 study that compared tamoxifen and placebo in reducing breast cancer risk in high-risk women, clinical breast examination was performed women every 6 months in high-risk in addition to their yearly mammograms. In the 6599 women who received a placebo, 175 invasive breast cancers developed, and 27% of these patients were found to have positive lymph nodes. Despite screening with breast examination every 6 months and mammography every year, cancer was not detected in these high-risk women until they had regional disease.[42] It is difficult to determine what the best screening program for these women should be. It is important to remember that intensive screening does not work by preventing breast carcinoma but by detecting breast carcinoma at an earlier, more treatable stage.

SUMMARY

Breast cancer prevention is the ultimate goal in the treatment of this disease, which affects a significant number of women in the United States each year. Clearly recognized risk factors include early menarche, age 30 or older at first birth, nulliparity, prolonged hormone replacement therapy, proliferative breast disease or atypical hyperplasia, and prolonged exposure to radiation therapy. Genetic factors include affected first-degree relative or multiple relatives, familial cancer syndromes, family history of ovarian cancer, and BRCA1 and BRCA2 mutations. Less clear associations have been made between breast cancer and breast-feeding, oral contraceptive use, fertility drugs, alcohol intake, obesity, and exposure to organochlorines.

Primary prevention currently includes tamoxifen for many women at high risk for breast cancer although each woman is assessed individually before starting treatment with this medication. Prophylactic mastectomy may be the treatment of choice for some high-risk women, especially those with a personal history of breast cancer or multiple relatives with the disease. It is important that women understand that this does not completely eliminate their risk of developing breast cancer. Newer chemopreventive agents such as raloxifen, retinoids, and soy protein are currently under investigation to determine their effectiveness in preventing breast cancer, particularly in high-risk patients.

Breast cancer screening in the general population should involve yearly mammograms and clinical breast examinations starting at age 40. For those women at higher risk, the screening recommendations are less clear, but close surveillance is necessary. Women who carry the BRCA1 or BRCA2 mutations should begin clinical breast examinations between the ages of 25 and 30. Annual mammography should begin no later than age 35. Other modalities of screening such as MRI are currently under investigation.

REFERENCES

1. Alberg AJ, Lam AP, Helzlsouer KJ: Epidemiology, prevention, and early detection of breast cancer. *Curr Opin Oncol* 1999;11:435-441.

2. Armstrong K, Eisen A, Weber B: Assessing the risk of breast cancer. *N Engl J Med* 2000;342:564-570.

3. Ries LAG, Kosary CL, Hankey BF, et al, editors: *SEER cancer statistics review 1973-1996: tables and graphs.* Bethesda, MD, NCI 1999, 1-14.

4. Hunter CP: Epidemiology, stage at diagnosis, and tumor biology of breast carcinoma in multiracial and multiethnic populations. *Cancer* 2000;88:1193-1202.

5. Wolff AC, Davidson NE: Early operable breast cancer. *Curr Treat Options Oncol* 2000;1:210-220.

6. Butler LM, Potischman NA, Newman B, et al: Menstrual risk factors and early-onset breast cancer. *Cancer Causes Control* 2000;11:451-458.

7. Chie WC, Hsieh CC, Newcomb PA, et al: Age at any full-term pregnancy and breast cancer risk. *Am J Epidemiol* 2000;151:715-722.

8. Pathak DR, Osuch JR, He J: Breast carcinoma etiology: current knowledge and new insights into the effects of reproductive and hormonal risk factors in black and white populations. *Cancer* 2000;88:1230-1238.

9. Newcomb PA, Storer BE, Longnecker MP, et al: Pregnancy termination in relation to risk of breast cancer. *JAMA* 1996;275:283-287.

10. Byers T, Graham S, Rzepka T, et al: Lactation and breast cancer: evidence for a negative association in premenopausal women. *Am J Epidemiol* 1985;121:664-674.

11. Mettlin C: Breast cancer risk factors: contributions to planning breast cancer control. *Cancer* 1992;69:1904-1909.

12. Minami Y, Ohuchi N, Fukao A, et al: Determinants of infant-feeding method in relation to risk factors for breast cancer. *Prev Med* 2000;30:363-370.

13. Lipworth L, Bailey LR, Trichopoulos D: History of breast-feeding in relation to breast cancer risk: a review of the epidemiologic literature. *J Natl Cancer Inst* 2000;92:302-312.

14. Andrieu N, Prevost T, Rohan TE, et al: Variation in the interaction between familial and reproductive factors on the risk of breast cancer according to age, menopausal status, and degree of familiality. *Int J Epidemiol* 2000;29:214-223.

15. Henderson IC: Risk factors for breast cancer development. *Cancer* 1993;71:2127-2140.

16. Shapiro S, Rosenberg L, Hoffman M, et al: Risk of breast cancer in relation to the use of injectable progestogen contraceptives and combined estrogen/progestogen contraceptives. *Am J Epidemiol* 2000;151:396-403.

17. Grabrick DM, Hartmann LC, Cerhan JR, et al: Risk of breast cancer with oral contraceptive use in women with a family history of breast cancer. *JAMA* 2000;284:1791-1798.

18. Cheichi LM, Secreto G: Factors of risk for breast cancer influencing post-menopausal long-term hormone replacement therapy. *Tumori* 2000;86:12-16.

19. Ross RK, Paganini-Hill A, Wan PC, et al: Effect of hormone replacement therapy on breast cancer risk: estrogen versus estrogen plus progestin. *J Natl Cancer Inst* 2000;92:328-332.

20. Potashnik G, Lerner-Geva L, Genkin L, et al: Fertility drugs and the risk of breast and ovarian cancers: results of a long-term follow-up study. *Fertil Steril* 1999;71:853-859.

21. Ricci E, Parazzini F, Negri E, et al: Fertility drugs and the risk of breast cancer. *Human Reprod* 1999;14:1653-1655.

22. Venn A, Watson L, Bruinsma F, et al: Risk of cancer after use of fertility drugs with in-vitro fertilization. *Lancet* 1999;354:1586-1590.

23. Stoll BA: Alcohol intake and late-stage promotion of breast cancer. *Eur J Cancer* 1999;35:1653-1658.

24. Garland M, Hunter DJ, Colditz GA, et al: Alcohol consumption in relation to breast cancer risk in a cohort of United States women 25-42 years of age. *Cancer Epidemiol Biomarkers Prev* 1999;8:1017-1021.

25. Holmes MD, Hunter DJ, Colditz GA, et al: Association of dietary intake of fat and fatty acids with risk of breast cancer. *JAMA* 1999;281:914-820.

26. Mezzetti M, LaVecchia C, Decarli A, et al: Population attributable risk for breast cancer: diet, nutrition, and physical exercise. *J Natl Cancer Inst* 1998;90:389-394.

27. Trentham-Dietz A, Newcomb PA, Egan KM, et al: Weight change and risk of postmenopausal breast cancer (United States). *Cancer Causes Control* 2000;11:533-542.

28. Thune I, Brenn T, Lund E, et al: Physical activity and the risk of breast cancer. *N Engl J Med* 1997;336:1269-1275.

29. Rockhill B, Willett WC, Hunter DJ, et al: Physical activity and breast cancer risk in a cohort of young women. *J Natl Cancer Inst* 1998;90:1155-1160.

30. Rockhill B, Willett WC, Hunter DJ, et al: A prospective study of recreational physical activity and breast cancer risk. *Arch Intern Med* 1999;159:2290-2296.

31. Gauthier-Villars M, Gad S, Caux V, et al: Genetic testing for breast cancer predisposition. *Surg Clin North Am* 1999;79:1171-1185.

32. Holli K: Hereditary breast cancer. *Acta Oncologica Suppl* 1999;13:29-32.

33. Clark S, Iglehart JD: Genetic counseling for breast cancer. *Adv Surg* 1999;33:199-214.

34. Sutcliffe S, Pharoah PDP, Easton DF, Ponder BAJ: Ovarian and breast cancer risks to women in families with two or more cases of ovarian cancer. *Int J Cancer* 2000;87:110-117.

35. Eeles RA: Screening for hereditary cancer and genetic testing, epitomized by breast cancer. *Eur J Cancer* 1999;35:1954-1962.

36. Malone KE, Daling JR, Neal C, et al: Frequency of BRCA1/BRCA2 mutations in a population-based sample of young breast carcinoma cases. *Cancer* 2000;88:1393-1402.

37. Jernstrom HCB, Johannsson OT, Loman N, et al: Reproductive factors in hereditary breast cancer. *Breast Cancer Res Treat* 1999;58:295-301.

38. Phillips KA: Immunophenotypic and pathologic differences between BRCA1 and BRCA2 hereditary breast cancers. *J Clin Oncol* 2000;18:107-112.

39. Schrag D, Kuntz KM, Garber JE, et al: Decision analysis-effects of prophylactic mastectomy and oophorectomy on life expectancy among women with BRCA1 or BRCA2 mutations. *N Engl J Med* 1997;336:1465-1471.

40. Laden F, Hunter DJ: Environmental risk factors and female breast cancer. *Annu Rev Public Health* 1998;19:101-123.

41. Clemons M, Loijens L, Goss P: Breast cancer risk following irradiation for Hodgkin's disease. *Cancer Treat Rev* 2000;26:291-302.

42. Hartmann LC, Sellers TA, Schaid DJ, et al: Clinical options for women at high risk for breast cancer. *Surg Clin North Am* 1999;79:1189-1203.

43. Osborne MP: Chemoprevention of breast cancer. *Surg Clin North Am* 1999;79:1207-1219.

44. Decensi A, Costa A: Chemoprevention strategies for specific cancers. *Eur J Cancer* 2000;36:694-709.

45. Sirovich BE, Sox HC: Breast cancer screening. *Surg Clin North Am* 1999;79:961-987.

46. Primic-Zakelj M: Screening mammography for early detection of breast cancer. *Ann Oncol* 1999;10:S121-S127.

47. Hughes KS, Papa MZ, Whitney T, et al: Prophylactic mastectomy and inherited predisposition to breast carcinoma. *Cancer* 1999;86:2502-2516.

48. Rankin SC: MRI of the breast. *Br J Radiol* 2000;73:806-818.

49. Tilanus-Linthorst MMA, Obdeijn IMM, Bartels KCM, et al: First experiences in screening women at high risk for breast cancer with MR imaging. *Breast Cancer Res Treat* 2000;63:53-60.

50. Olson JA, Morris EA, Van Zee KJ, et al: Magnetic resonance imaging facilitates breast conservation for occult breast cancer. *Ann Surg Oncol* 2000;7:411-415.

51. Winchester DP: Putting prophylactic mastectomy in proper perspective. *CA Cancer J Clin* 1995;45:261-304.

52. Harris JR, Lippman ME, Veronesi U, et al: Breast cancer. *N Engl J Med* 1992;327:319-328.

53. Kamb A, Skolnick MH: Identification of the BRCA1 breast cancer gene and its clinical implications. In DeVita VT, Hellman S, Rosenberg SA, editors: *Important advances in oncology.* Philadelphia, Lippincott-Raven, 1996, 23-35.

54. Neuhasen SL: Ethnic differences in cancer risk resulting from genetic variation. *Cancer* 1999;86:2575-2582.

CHAPTER 4

Colorectal Cancer

Charles P. Theuer

INTRODUCTION

Colorectal cancer (CRC) is highly curable in its early stages, before it spreads to regional lymph nodes or distant sites. Furthermore, the detection and removal of colonic polyps, the precursor of invasive cancer, is easily accomplished and can nearly eliminate the risk of CRC. Unfortunately, although one in 20 Americans develop CRC, most Americans do not engage in the practice of colorectal screening. As a result, the majority of patients present with metastatic disease to regional lymph nodes or distant sites, resulting in an overall survival rate of less than 50%.

This chapter discusses colorectal carcinogenesis, current screening guidelines, and the various factors—both environmental and genetic—that increase the risk of developing CRC, Secondary prevention—detecting colorectal neoplasia at a subclinical stage—is one focus. Methods of reducing the incidence of colorectal neoplasia—primary prevention—are also emphasized.

General Anatomy

The human colon and rectum are storage and absorptive organs. The colon is approximately 4 feet in length and is subdivided into the cecum, ascending colon, hepatic flexure, transverse colon, splenic flexure, descending colon, and sigmoid colon, which is continuous with the rectum (Figure 4-1). The cecum, ascending colon, and hepatic flexures are considered the right colon. Branches of the superior mesenteric artery supply these and the transverse colon. The splenic flexure, descending colon, and sigmoid colon are considered the left colon. These and the rectum are supplied by branches of the inferior mesenteric artery. Hemorrhoidal branches from the iliac arteries also supply the rectum. The cecum is 7 to 8 cm in diameter and is the widest portion of the colon. The colon progressively diminishes in size and is narrowest at the sigmoid colon, which is 2 to 3 cm in diameter. This size discrepancy accounts for the fact that neoplasia of the right colon may grow to a large size without causing symptoms of obstruction. These lesions frequently result in anemia from chronic bleeding and pain from invasion of pericolonic structures. In contrast, sigmoid lesions lead to obstructive symptoms at far smaller tumor sizes.

Histology

The colonic wall consists of four layers: mucosa, submucosa, muscularis propria, and serosa (Figure 4-2). The colon and rectum contain flat mucosa punctuated by numerous straight, normally unbranched, symmetric tubular crypts that form the glands of Lieberkuhn and extend into the underlying lamina propria. Mainly goblet mucous cells line the crypts. The mucosal surface is covered with absorptive cells that contain microvilli. Surface cells and those in the upper half of epithelial crypts are relatively mature and

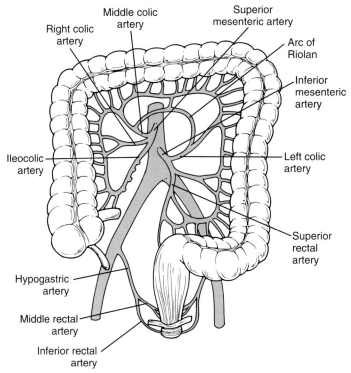

FIGURE 4-1
Arterial blood supply of colon and rectum. (From Schwartz S, et al: *Principles of Surgery, ed 6,* New York, McGraw-Hill, 1994.)

well-differentiated; those in the lower half are proliferating and less well-differentiated. Once formed, cells migrate upward from the crypt to the surface in 4 to 6 days. Abnormalities in crypt cell division are the earliest detectable signs of colonic neoplasia.

The simple columnar epithelium is anchored by a fine basement membrane and supported by the connective tissue of the lamina propria. The lamina propria is normally infiltrated by a variety of leukocytes. The mucosa is separated from the submucosa by the thin muscularis mucosae, which is arrayed in indistinct circular and longitudinal layers. The colon is encircled by lymphatic channels located in the submucosa and the muscularis mucosae. The mucosa has a rich vascular supply but no lymphatics. As a result, superficial cancers that do not penetrate the muscularis mucosae cannot metastasize via the lymphatic route. The submucosa is surrounded by the inner circular and outer longitudinal muscles. The entire colon is surrounded by the visceral peritoneal membrane (serosa) except for a portion of the cecum, ascending, and sigmoid colon. The majority of the rectum also lacks a serosa, the glistening outer surface of the colon.

Treatment of Colorectal Cancer

Surgical resection remains the primary curative modality for the treatment of CRC. Cure rates of 90% are expected in localized disease (node-negative). Cure rates of 60% (using surgery and adjuvant chemotherapy) are expected for regional (node-positive disease). Surgery also plays a role as a palliative modality in patients with obstruction or bleeding who have distant metastases. Infrequently, surgery to resect favorable hepatic metastases in patients without other evidence of metastases is employed, with a 30% 5-year rate. Chemotherapy

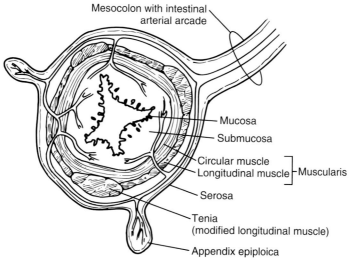

FIGURE 4-2
Anatomy of the colonic wall. (From Kodner IJ: Colostomy and ileostomy. *Ciba Clinical Symposia* 1978;30:5.)

(5-fluorouracil and leucovorin) has proved to be beneficial as an adjuvant therapy for node-positive patients who undergo curative resection. Palliative chemotherapy is frequently employed for unresectable metastatic disease and occasionally produces dramatic results. Radiation therapy is used for local control either preoperatively or postoperatively in cases of advanced rectal cancer. Radiation also can be used palliatively for localized bone metastases. Despite advances in colorectal treatment, the real victory lies in the prevention and early detection of colorectal neoplasia. The phrase "an ounce of prevention is worth a pound of cure" is particularly applicable to colorectal carcinogenesis.

PROGNOSTIC FACTORS

Stage of disease at presentation is the most significant prognostic factor in CRC. Dukes proposed an initial staging system that grouped cancers into those that penetrated the mucosa and submucosa but not the muscularis propria (Dukes' A), those that penetrated the muscularis propria (Dukes' B), and those associated with lymphatic spread (Dukes' C). SEER (Surveillance, Epidemiology, and End Results, a program of the National Cancer Institute) groups patients according to localized, regional, and distant disease. Patients with localized disease (node-negative) have a 90% 5-year survival and are generally treated with surgery alone. Patients with regional disease (node-positive disease or direct extension of the cancer into another organ) have a 5-year survival of 60% and are generally treated with surgery and adjuvant chemotherapy. Patients with distant metastases have a 5-year survival of less than 10% despite treatment with conventional therapies. Currently, staging using the TNM system allows for very precise staging of CRC (Table 4-1).

Histologic grade has been shown repeatedly to be an independent prognostic factor by multivariate analyses. Specifically, these studies have demonstrated that "high tumor grade" is an adverse prognostic factor, compared with "low grade."[1-13] Tumor invasion into submucosal vessels, either lymphatic or venous, has been shown to be associated with a significantly increased risk of regional lymph node and liver metastases, respectively.[14-19] In light of the clinical and biologic importance of this feature, the American

Table 4-1
TNM Classification of Colorectal Carcinoma

pT	Microscopic description of depth of primary tumor on pathologic examination
PTx	Minimum requirements to assess the primary tumor cannot be met
PT_0	No evidence of primary tumor
pT_{is}	In situ carcinoma (intraepithelial or invasive into muscularis mucosae and/or lamina propria only)
pT_1	Tumor invades through muscularis mucosae into submucosa
pT_2	Tumor invades into but not through muscularis propria
pT_3	Tumor invades through muscularis propria subserosa or into nonperitonealized pericolonic or perirectal tissue
pT_4	Tumor invades directly into other organs or structures and/or perforates the visceral peritoneum of the specimen
PN	Regional lymph node status on pathologic examination
pN_x	Minimum requirements to assess the regional lymph nodes cannot be met
PN_0	No regional lymph node metastasis found
pN_1	Metastasis in 1-3 pericolonic or perirectal lymph nodes
pN_2	Metastasis in 4 or more pericolonic or perirectal lymph nodes
pN_3	Metastasis in lymph node along the course of a major named vascular trunk (iliocolic; right, middle, or left colic; inferior mesenteric; superior rectal {hemorrhoidal}; and/or internal iliac arteries but not sigmoid arteries) and/or metastasis in apical lymph node(s) when marked by the surgeon
PM	Distant metastasis after definitive regional therapy
pM_x	Minimum requirements to assess distant metastasis cannot be met
PM_0	No distant metastasis found
pM_1	Distant metastasis documented by pathologic examination (including external or common iliac lymph nodes)

Stage Groupings	T	N	M
Stage 0	T_{is}	0	0
Stage I	1 or 2	0	0
Stage II	3 or 4	0	0
Stage III	Any	1, 2 or 3	0
Stage IV	Any	Any	1

From Hamilton SR: Pathology and biology of colorectal neoplasia. In Young GP, Rozen P, Levin B, editors: *Prevention and early detection of colorectal cancer.* Philadelphia, WB Saunders, 1996, 3-21.

Joint Committee on Cancer Prognostic Factors Consensus Conference has recommended that the T1 category be modified to include T1a (no evidence of lymphatic or venous invasion) and T1b (lymphatic or venous invasion is present).[20] Elevated carcinoembryonic antigen (CEA) levels (>5.0 ng/ml) have been shown to have an adverse impact on prognosis that is independent of tumor stage.[21-26] Several studies have shown by multivariate analysis that perineural invasion is an independent indicator of poor prognosis.[1,8,27-30] Other markers that have been associated with prognosis include host lymphoid response to the tumor,[31-33] allelic loss of the long arm of chromosome 18,[34] and K-*ras* mutation.[35] Further study of these markers is needed before they will be accepted for routine clinical staging.

EPIDEMIOLOGY

Data indicate that 51,200 women develop colon cancer and 24,600 develop rectal cancer annually in the United States; 15,800 women die of colon cancer, and 4,000 women die of rectal cancer each year.[36] Colorectal cancer represents the third most common cancer in women and the third most common cause of cancer death among women (following lung and breast cancer). Among U.S. women, age-adjusted annual incidence rates vary by ethnicity/race: Blacks (46/100,000) > Whites (38/100,000) > Asians (21-34/100,000) > Latinos (25/100,000) > American Indians (15/100,000).[37] Alaskan Natives have the highest reported rates (67/100,000). The overall age-adjusted annual death rate is 11/100,000. Ethnic/racial death rates parallel incidence rates: Blacks (20/100,000) > Whites (15/100,000) > Asians (6-12/100,000) > Latinos (8/100,000). Alaskan Natives also have the highest death rates (24/100,000) from colon cancer.

The prevalence of CRC in women varies with age. The prevalence in patients younger than 39 years of age is 1 in 2000, between the ages of 40 and 59 is 1 in 147, and between the ages of 60 and 79 is 1 in 31. During their lifetime, 1 in 17 women will develop CRC; the prevalence is slightly less than that for men at all age intervals. However, the lifetime risk is nearly identical because women outlive men.

The overall 5-year survival rate from CRC is higher in Whites (62%) than Blacks (52%)[37] because White women are more likely to have cancers detected at favorable stages (localized stage: 38% versus 32%; regional stage: 37% versus 35%; distant stage: 19% versus 25%). Stage-stratified survival, however, is also higher among White women than Black women (localized stage: 92% versus 86%; regional stage: 64% versus 60%; distant stage: 8% versus 5%). The explanation for superior stage-stratified survival among White women is not understood and persists even after careful histologic comparisons of tumors from Whites and Blacks.[38] Population-based survival data among Latinos and Asians are currently unavailable but are being actively acquired by the National Cancer Institute. In recent years the survival rate among women with CRC has increased.[39] From 1986 to 1993 the overall 5-year survival in Whites and Blacks (63% and 53%, respectively) was superior to the overall survival in these groups from 1974 to1976 (50% and 46%, respectively). Survival is proportional to stage, and increased survival statistics may reflect an increase in the detection of early stage cancers through screening. Screening allows the detection of cancers before the spread to regional lymph nodes or distant sites, when cure is the rule rather than the exception.

ETIOLOGY

The genetically defined hereditary CRC syndromes, familial adenomatous polyposis coli (FAP) and hereditary nonpolyposis CRC (HNPCC), account for only 2% to 3% of all cases of CRC (Figure 4-3). Family kindred studies indicate that many families meet criteria for familial CRC but do not have known germline mutations. The contributions of recessive traits (susceptibility genes) and combinations of genes (gene-gene interactions) are difficult to assess through family linkage studies. Individuals in these families likely harbor combinations of prevalent but low-penetrance susceptibility genes that have not been identified at this time. These cases as well as the majority of CRCs (which are termed "sporadic") are the result of gene-environment interactions that currently are incompletely understood.

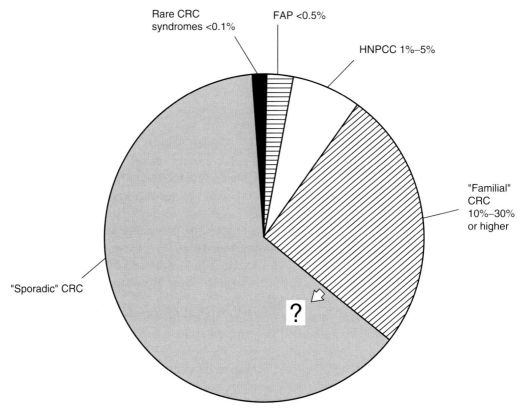

FIGURE 4-3

Familial causes of colorectal cancer. The rare colorectal cancer (CRC) syndromes include the hamartomatous polyposis conditions and other extremely rare diseases. Familial adenomatous polyposis coli (FAP) accounts for approximately 0.5% of cases, and hereditary nonpolyposis colorectal cancer (HNPCC) for 1% to 5%. Epidemiologic studies suggest that familial CRC outside the well-defined syndromes involved 10% to 30% of cases. Pedigree studies that include adenomatous polyps suggest that this proportion is much higher and that familial factors, probably inherited, may be present in the majority of colonic neoplasms. (From Burt RW, Petersen GM: Familial colorectal cancer: diagnosis and management. In Young GP, Rozen P, Levin B, editors: *Prevention and early detection of colorectal cancer.* Philadelphia, WB Saunders, 1996.)

Nature Versus Nurture

Colon cancer is the result of a complex series of events that represents the end result of the effects of environmental factors upon an individual's inherited susceptibility.[40] This interaction produces somatic mutations that accumulate over time and cause neoplastic transformation of normal colonic epithelium into premalignant adenomatous polyps and ultimately into invasive disease (Figure 4-4). The relative influences of genetic constitution and environmental exposure in the causation of cancer have been debated for decades.

A prominent epidemiologic characteristic of CRC is the great variation in incidence among countries throughout the world, encompassing sixfold to sevenfold differences in risk.[41] Geographic differences, time trend analyses, and migrant population studies indicate that environmental influences play an overwhelming role in cancer causation. For example, studies of Japanese migrating to Hawaii reveal excessive CRC risk for first-generation (Issei) and second-generation (Nisei) who were among groups that regularly consumed only Western-style meals.[42] Among Australian immigrants and their descendants,

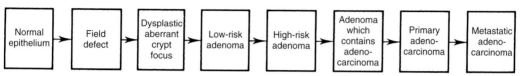

FIGURE 4-4

Model for the morphogenesis of colorectal adenocarcinoma. (From Hamilton SR: Pathology and biology of colorectal neoplasia. In Young GP, Rozen P, Levin B, editors: *Prevention and early detection of colorectal cancer.* Philadelphia, WB Saunders,1996.)

incidence rates rapidly reach those of the host country, sometimes within the migrating generation.[43] Data on large-bowel cancer among the Polish-born in Australia, most of whom migrated shortly after World War II, reveal a shift in CRC mortality rates toward the higher Australian mortality rates.[44] These studies suggest that events in adult life associated with migration can visibly alter bowel cancer risk in approximately 20 years.

The relative contributions of environmental and heritable factors were assessed in an analysis of cohorts of twins from Sweden, Denmark, and Finland.[45] This study indicates a strong influence of heritable factors in the development of CRC. Female monozygotic twins of affected women with CRC had a 16% probability of also having CRC. This represented a fourteenfold elevated risk, compared with a monozygotic twin of a woman without CRC. Heritable factors were estimated to account for 35% of all cases of CRC in the cohort. The majority of CRCs, however, were predicted to result from environmental exposures. Although the data indicated that environmental exposures are responsible for the development of the majority of CRCs, the high proportion of cancers related to hereditary factors indicate that further research to understand gene-environment interactions and susceptibility gene polymorphisms is necessary. These susceptibility genes are relatively common genes that carry only a moderate risk—so-called high-prevalence, low-penetrance genes. Many of these susceptibility genes appear to be involved in the metabolism or activation of carcinogens.[46]

Diet

Although diet plays a significant role in colon carcinogenesis, it has been difficult to quantify and isolate those individual macronutrients and micronutrients that contribute to carcinogenesis. This difficulty is partly related to differences in the design and methodology of studies performed to evaluate this subject, including the type of dietary questionnaire administered, differences in demographics of study cohorts, confounding effects of other dietary components, selection and recall bias, sample size, and duration of follow-up.

Both case-control and cohort studies indicate that fat and red meat intake are associated with CRC incidence.[47-52] The Nurses' Health Study prospectively studied a cohort of 88,751 female United States nurses aged 30 to 55 years by questionnaire every 2 years for 12 years.[48] This study found a twofold increase in colon cancer among women in the highest quintile, compared with women in the lowest quintile of animal fat intake. Multivariate analyses indicated that risk was associated with red meat intake rather than fat. Red meat intake has also been implicated in colon cancer causation by large prospective studies in Iowa and the Netherlands.[49,50] Findings from the largest American cohort of more than 700,000 men, however, indicate that neither fat nor red meat are associated with colon cancer risk.[51] This study, like many negative studies, has been criticized on the basis of questionnaire design and the nature of end points used. These findings highlight the inconsistencies found in many studies that assess risk from questionnaires and are unable to corroborate intake using alternative measures.

Research to determine what component of red meat contributes to colon carcinogenesis implicates heterocyclic amines produced by cooking meats at high temperatures (frying, broiling, barbecuing).[52,53] Heterocylic amine production can be minimized by cooking at lower temperatures: baking, stewing, poaching, microwaving, and oven roasting.

Dietary fiber intake is felt to be inversely associated with CRC risk. Burkitt observed very low rates of CRC among Africans and proposed that a high-fiber diet protects against CRC.[54] Insoluble fibers, such as wheat-bran fiber, are thought to protect against CRC by binding carcinogens in the gut, diluting concentrations of bile acids, and binding to bile acids to promote their fecal excretion.[55] A metaanalysis of 13 case-control studies, representing 9 countries, reported an inverse relationship between high-fiber foods and CRC, after considering the effects of gender and age.[56] Observational studies suggest that the ingestion of red meat and dietary fat increases the risk of CRC, whereas the ingestion of vegetables, dietary fiber, and certain micronutrients lowers the risk.[47,57-59] These results are not seen in all studies, however. Both the Nurses' Health Study and the Health Professionals' Follow-up Study failed to find that cereal fiber prevented colon cancer.[60,61]

Large prospective randomized trials have assessed the impact of a low-fat, high-fiber diet. The Toronto Polyp Prevention Trial reported no significant difference in recurrence after 2 years between subjects in the intervention group and those in the control group who reported ingesting 25% and 33% of calories from fat and 35 to 16 g of fiber per day, respectively.[62] In the Australian Polyp Prevention Project, none of the interventions (a reduction in dietary fat, use of a wheat-bran fiber supplement, and supplementation with beta carotene) resulted in a statistically significant reduction in the risk of recurrence of polyps after 4 years.[63] The American Polyp Prevention Trial found that adopting a diet that is low in fat and high in fiber, fruits, and vegetables does not influence the risk or recurrence of colorectal adenomas.[64] The Phoenix Colon Cancer Prevention Physicians' Network found that a high wheat-bran diet (13.5 g per day) did not protect against recurrent colorectal adenoma.[55] These studies have been criticized because patients in the intervention group maintained a diet very similar to that of the control group.[65,66] In addition, CS, although the most sensitive test for the detection of colonic polyps, is imperfect and misses approximately 20% of polyps, especially those that are less than 5 mm in diameter and are located in the right colon. Both the intervention and control groups of these randomized trials used CS to verify the absence of polyps at study entry; these groups may have been contaminated by a sizable proportion of polyps present at entry but not detected until the follow-up examination, when they may have increased in size. This contamination will bias toward the null hypothesis, namely that the intervention did not reduce the incidence of new polyps. In summary, there is no evidence in randomized trials that fiber prevents CRC. It is likely, however, that the effects of dietary fiber can only be appreciated with longer follow-up than that reported in current randomized trials.

Tobacco has been associated with adenoma formation in prospective studies. These studies estimate that 20% of adenomas are attributable to smoking.[67] Physical inactivity and high body mass index are also associated with increased CRC risk in both men and women.[68,69] The incidence of both adenomas and invasive cancers is higher in groups with physical inactivity and high body mass indices. Increasing physical activity and maintaining lean body weight have not been proven to modify one's risk of colonic neoplasia but seem worthwhile goals.

CARCINOGENESIS, ONCOGENES, AND TUMOR-SUPPRESSOR GENES

Colorectal cancer represents the end result of the accumulation of a series of genetic changes to DNA that can best be described as the process of carcinogenesis. Factors responsible for carcinogenesis have been classified in very general terms as those responsible for the initiation and those responsible for promotion.

Initiation is the process by which the DNA of the colonocyte is damaged. In general terms, DNA damage may result from viruses, irradiation, or chemical mutagens. A cell containing a mutated gene will not necessarily clonally expand into a cancer. Other factors are necessary to allow the mutated cell to multiply. These "promoters" do not damage DNA but rather allow the expansion of mutated cells. In addition, by increasing proliferation, promoters sensitize mutated cells to further initiating events, thus perpetuating clonal expansion of mutated cells with multiple DNA mutations. Initiation and promotion are linked processes. Mechanisms of DNA repair exist to correct mutated DNA, and mechanisms of programmed cell death (or apoptosis) eliminate mutated cells. Initiating events that inactivate genes that regulate cell cycle checkpoints (such as the p53 gene), however, favor cellular proliferation of cells containing mutated DNA that might normally be channeled for apoptosis.

Molecular Genetics

The transition of normal colonocyte to invasive cancer is incompletely understood. Recent discoveries have allowed an understanding of many of the genetic changes involved. Identification of the germline mutations responsible for the familial predisposition to CRC in hereditary CRC syndromes has illuminated the process of carcinogenesis. Moreover, the genes responsible for these familial syndromes are also frequently mutated in sporadic CRC.

Carcinogenesis is the result of many genetic changes that represent "gain-of-function" mutations in proto-oncogenes and "loss-of-function" mutations in tumor suppressor genes.[70-73] Proto-oncogenes represent normal cellular genes. The majority of proto-oncogenes encode proteins that regulate cell growth and differentiation. They encode proteins that function within the cell nucleus, cell membrane, or extracellular matrix. Oncogenes are mutated counterparts of normal proto-oncogenes. Oncogenes act in a dominant manner to promote malignancy and, in a genetic sense, are gain-of-function mutations. Because of their dominant nature, oncogene mutations are always acquired mutations. They are not perpetuated in the germline.

Proto-oncogenes may be activated by three general mechanisms. First, point mutations may alter the function of the protein product. The *ras* family of proto-oncogenes (H-*ras*, K-*ras* and N-*ras*) each encode a guanosine triphosphatase. Activation of *ras* proto-oncogenes by point mutation is seen in 50% of CRC cases. Mutated *ras* proteins are less able to interact with other cellular proteins that regulate *ras* activity. Hence, mutant ras proteins remain turned "on" and unable to regulate cellular pathways involved in proliferation and differentiation, releasing other proteins from regulatory control and thereby altering signaling pathways and gene regulation. Second, chromosomal translocations may alter the flanking sequences around a proto-oncogene that allow unregulated transcription and increase expression of the protein product. This mechanism is responsible for activation of the *myc* gene in Burkitt's lymphoma by juxtaposition with immunoglobulin gene sequences following chromosomal translocation. Proto-onocgene activation by gene amplification, as is seen frequently in the case of the HER-2-*neu* gene in cases of breast and gastrointestinal cancer, is a final mechanism by which overexpression of a gene product may occur.

Tumor Suppressor Genes

The existence of familial cancer syndromes indicates that the ability of cells to form a tumor is a recessive trait. The malignant phenotype of a human cancer cell line can be suppressed by fusion to normal diploid human cells.[74,75] Hybrids that retain both sets of parental chromosomes are suppressed; tumorigenic clones arise only after loss of specific normal diploid chromosomes containing specific tumor suppressor genes that maintain cell differentiation.[76] Knudson's observations of the age-specific incidence of retinoblastoma led him to propose a "two-hit theory of mutagenesis."[77-79] He proposed that familial retinoblastoma resulted from mutation in a retinoblastoma susceptibility locus that contains a tumor suppressor gene. Knudson proposed that an individual with the inherited form of the disease inherited a germline mutation in a retinobalstoma susceptibility locus from one parent. This mutation was insufficient for tumorigenesis. A second acquired, or somatic, mutation was necessary for tumor formation. Given the likelihood of a somatic mutation occurring in at least one retinal cell during development, this hypothesis explained that the autosomal dominant inheritance pattern of the disease was a result of recessive genetic determinants.

Molecular genetics have demonstrated that the concept of loss of heterozygosity (LOH) is consistent with Knudson's hypothesis (Figure 4-5). The allelic loss of heterozygosity seen in human cancer is characterized by the loss of chromosomal segments. Genes (one from each parent) in human cells have distinct sequences or polymorphisms. These genes may be amplified using polymerase chain reaction and cut into fragments with restriction endonucleases. The fragmented DNA can be detected using a radiolabeled DNA probe. Normal diploid cells contain two unique DNA fragments: two restriction fragment length polymorphisms (RFLPs), representing genes from each parent. Tumors frequently contain chromosomal deletions. RFLPs from tumor will contain only a single band and thus manifest loss of heterozygosity. Knudson's hypothesis predicts that the retained copy should be inactivated by a more localized or subtle mutation. Tumor suppressor genes are frequent victims of LOH. The resultant cell has only one copy of a regulatory gene, which may then be mutated and inactivated, thereby allowing cellular proliferation. Several tumor suppressor genes inactivated in human CRC are mutated by a combination of allelic loss and more subtle mutation of the retained allele.

Colon Carcinogenesis

A discussion of the prevention of colon cancer requires an understanding of the process of colorectal carcinogenesis. Colorectal carcinogenesis (see Figure. 4-6) involves the change of normal colonic mucosa into an invasive lesion through a set of successive incremental steps.[40] Rarely, cancer may develop de novo or involve the development of cancer from dysplastic epithelium, as in chronic ulcerative colitis. The majority of colon cancers, however, are sporadic and develop from preexisting benign polyps (adenomas), which in turn are thought to arise from dysplastic epithelium or aberrant crypt foci, or from both.

Sporadic CRC develops as the result of a series of morphologic alterations to the colonic mucosa.

The colonic epithelium renews itself every 4 to 6 days. Colonocytes are constantly shed from the tip of the villi. The colonocytes of the crypts actively divide to replace the colonocytes that are shed at the surface. New cells constantly arise in the lower half of the crypt through mitosis of undifferentiated cells. A circadian rhythm of proliferation has been observed under normal physiologic conditions. Rate of renewal can be quantified by several techniques: by counting mitotic figures; by determining the fraction of cells in *S* phase of

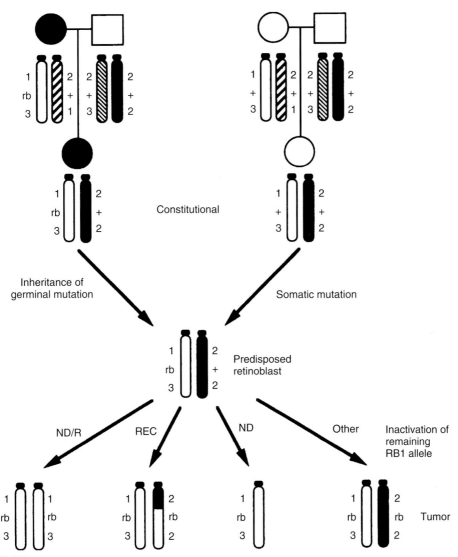

FIGURE 4-5

Chromosomal mechanisms that result in loss of heterozygosity for alleles at the retinoblastoma locus at chromosome band 13q14. In the inherited form of the disease, the child inherits a copy of chromosome 13 from her affected mother. This copy of chromosome 13 carries a recessive mutation at the RB1 locus (this allele is designated *rb*). The other copy of chromosome 13 from her father has no mutation at the RB1 locus (designated +). Thus each of the girl's cells contains one mutated and one wild-type RB1 allele (the genotype of the cells is rb/+). A retinoblastoma can arise after the loss or inactivation of the remaining wild-type retinoblastoma allele by one of the mechanisms shown. In the noninherited (sporadic) form of the disease, a recessive mutation arises somatically at one retinoblastoma allele in a developing retinal cell. Subsequently, a retinoblastoma will develop if the remaining RB1 allele in this predisposed cell is inactivated by one of the mechanisms shown: ND/R—mitotic recombination; ND—nondisjunction; and other (e.g., localized mutation). The two parental copies of chromosome 13 present in each cell of an individual can be distinguished by study of restriction fragment length polymorphisms (RFLPs) at loci flanking the RB1 locus chromosome 13q (the polymorphic alleles are designated "1" and "2"). (Modified with permission of Elsevier Press from Cavenee WK, Koufos A, Hansen MF: Recessive mutant genes predisposing to human cancer. *Mutat Res* 1986;168:3-14.)

the cell cycle; or by quantification of immunohistochemical staining for cell cycle–associated proteins, especially proliferating cell nuclear antigen or those proteins expressed during apoptosis.[80-84]

Initial carcinogenic changes represent disregulation of growth. The zone of proliferation expands from the basal portion of the colorectal crypt into the upper portions (Figure 4-6). These changes are not detectable on histopathologic examination but are characterized by changes in markers of proliferation, differentiation, and apoptosis. These cell cycle alterations are first manifest histologically as a dysplastic aberrant crypt focus. Human aberrant crypt foci (ACF) demonstrate two patterns, one more reminiscent of hyperplastic crypts (and polyps) and those that are dysplastic and therefore premalignant. ACF do not appear to represent precursors to carcinoma except in a minority of cases in which dysplasia is evident.[85-88] The frequency of ACF in normal-appearing mucosa appears to increase with cancer risk. The mucosa of patients harboring CRC shows increased numbers of ACF, compared with mucosa of unaffected individuals, and patients with FAP harbor hundreds of ACF within a few centimeters of colon.[88,89] ACF are larger in diameter than surrounding crypts and have thicker epithelium and increased cellularity (Figures 4-7 and 4-8). Unregulated growth results in the expansion of cells of the dysplastic aberrant crypt into adenomatous polyps (Figure 4-9). These polyps are small but macroscopic, consisting of tubular architecture and low-grade dysplasia. Adenomas are considered the most certain precursor lesion for invasive colon cancer.[90-92] A minority of these small polyps progress, with the development of higher grades of dysplasia and villous architecture, along with further increases in size.

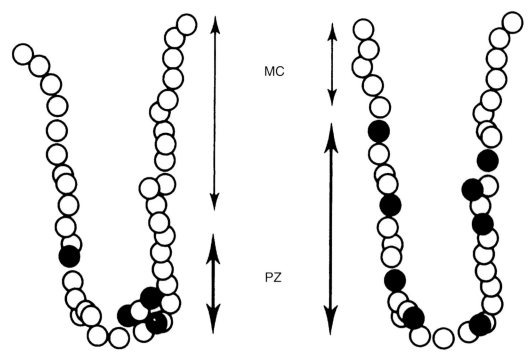

FIGURE 4-6
Schematic representation of hyperproliferation in mucosa at increased risk for cancer. *MC,* mature cell compartment; *PZ,* proliferative cell zone. Filled circles indicate nuclei in *S* phase, normally only in the crypt base *(left);* in the hyperproliferative crypt *(right),* the dividing nuclei are also found in the MC. (From Margovich MJ: Precancer markers and prediction of tumorigenesis. In Young GP, Rozen P, Levin B, editors: *Prevention and early detection of colorectal cancer.* Philadelphia, WB Saunders, 1996.)

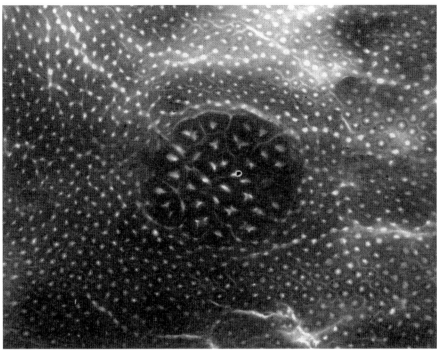

FIGURE 4-7
Aberrant crypt focus in *en face* macroscopic view of colonic mucosal sheet stained with methylene blue. The aberrant crypts in the focus are larger in diameter than the surrounding crypts and have thicker epithelium with increased cellularity. (From Hamilton SR: Pathology and biology of colorectal neoplasia. In Young GP, Rozen P, Levin B, editors: *Prevention and early detection of colorectal cancer.* Philadelphia, WB Saunders, 1996.)

Several lines of evidence converge to support the proposal that the majority of CRC develops from adenomatous polyps. First, histologic analyses of many CRCs reveal residual adenomas in many cases (Figure 4-10). Second, foci of invasive cancer are found in nearly 3% of adenomas, thus suggesting that the larger adenoma is the precursor lesion in these cases. Third, studies assessing the relationship between patient age and histologic grade of mucosal polyps indicate that advancing atypia correlates to increased patient age. Patients with adenomas are 8 to 11 years younger than those with CRC,[93] and patients with FAP will inevitably develop CRC. The most compelling evidence substantiating the adenoma-carcinoma sequence comes from the National Polyp Study. The cohort of more than 1000 patients who had therapeutic CS (with polypectomy) experienced a 76% to 90% lower incidence of CRC than unscreened groups.[94]

Autopsy studies indicate that one third to one half of Americans develop tubular adenomas in their lifetimes.[95-97] Most of these are less than 1 cm in diameter.[93,94] Only approximately 1 in 10 becomes malignant.[95] Adenomas occur more commonly in men than in women.[98] By their mid-fifties, 22% of women have one or more adenomas, compared with 41% of men.[95] Polyp incidence is directly proportional to age, and by age 80 nearly half of each sex has polyps.[96]

Adenomas are distributed throughout the colon and rectum. The majority of adenomatous polyps (two thirds) are found proximal to the splenic flexure.[95] Neoplastic polyps account for 73% of all polyps in the right colon. This is reversed in the distal colon, where

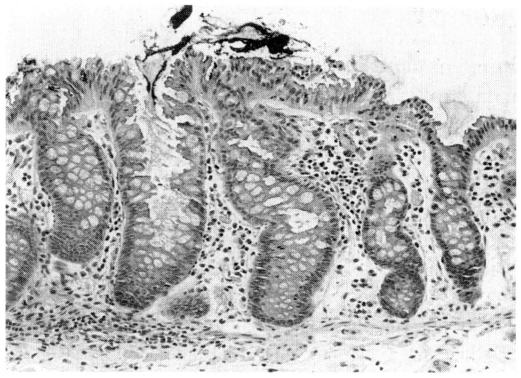

FIGURE 4-8
Longitudinal histologic section of a five-gland ACF from a patient with resectable colonic cancer. India ink dots mark ACF in the gross specimen and help to track them through the histologic processing (hematoxylin and eosin staining, original magnification × 100). (From Margovich MJ: Precancer markers and prediction of tumorigenesis. In Young GP, Rozen P, Levin B, editors: *Prevention and early detection of colorectal cancer.* Philadelphia, WB Saunders, 1996.)

nonneoplastic polyps (hyperplastic polyps and polypoid mucosa) represent 65% of all polyps in the rectum. Older women have a higher frequency of proximal polyps than do younger women. Larger polyps, which are at higher risk of malignant degeneration, are also seen more frequently proximal to the splenic flexure of older women.[99-101] In a study of 3371 adenomas in 1867 patients, high-grade dysplasia was found in only 2% of adenomas that were 0.1 to 0.5 cm and in 24% of those that were 2.1 to 2.5 cm.[102] Even small polyps may harbor malignancy; carcinoma occurred in 1.2% of 2229 neoplastic colorectal polyps smaller than 5 mm excised endoscopically.[100] This point emphasizes the importance of endoscopic removal of all adenomatous polyps regardless of size.[103]

The majority of polyps smaller than 5 mm do not progress to invasive cancer.[104] In fact, most adenomas smaller than 5 mm remain unchanged in size and morphology over the long term.[105] The precise time course of the adenoma to carcinoma pathway is unclear and certainly depends on adenoma size. With increasing size, a polyp has greater chance of developing villous architecture and greater atypia. Data from both the National Polyp Study and the St. Mark's Hospital study,[92,106,107] which described the long-term observation of unresected colorectal adenomas, support an average time course of approximately 10 years for the progression from a small adenoma to a cancer in average-risk individuals. In the case of polyps found in patients with HNPCC, the time course appears to be significantly shortened.

Most cases of advanced invasive adenocarcinoma are unaccompanied by evidence of a precursor polyp; the invasive component of the neoplastic growth obliterates the precursor polyp (Figures 4-11 and 4-12). Just as the chances of malignancy within a polyp are related

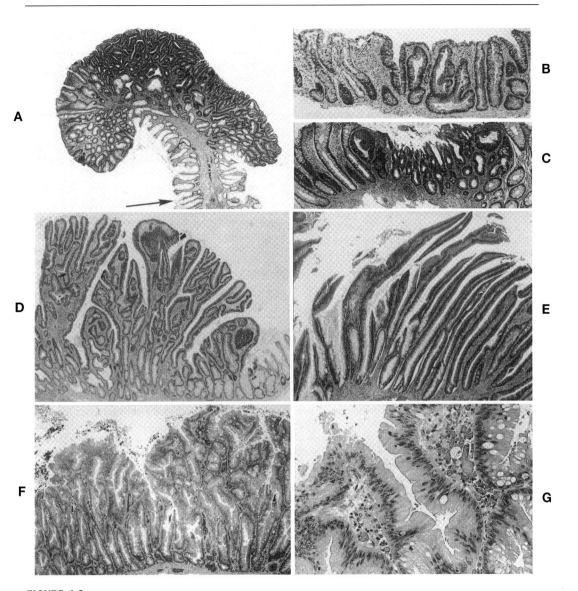

FIGURE 4-9

Examples of configurations and types of colorectal adenomas. **A,** Small polypoid tubular adenoma on a stalk. The head of the adenoma is characterized by irregular glands lined by adenomatous epithelium. The stalk *(arrow)* is composed of submucosa containing large blood vessels and nonneoplastic mucosa with crypt distortion and hypermucinous epithelium, representing so-called transitional mucosa. **B,** Flat tubular adenoma. Abrupt transition from nonneoplastic epithelium to adenomatous epithelium is evident. The adenomatous glands on the right side of the photomicrograph are distorted and have enlarged caliber. There is no protrusion of the dysplastic glands above the surrounding mucosal surface. The adenomatous epithelium has scattered residual goblet cells. **C,** Depressed adenoma. The luminal surface of the small adenoma is lower than the luminal surface of the surrounding mucosa. **D,** Tubulovillous adenoma. The adenoma protrudes above the surrounding mucosal surface. The luminal surface has finger-like protrusions but also glandular structures. **E,** Villous adenoma. The luminal surface is characterized by finger-like extensions of lamina propria that support the adenomatous epithelium. **F** and **G,** Serrated adenoma. **F,** The serrated mucosal architecture with stellate glandular structures is evident and resembles a hyperplastic polyp. **G,** The adenomatous nature of the epithelium is evident. (From Hamilton SR: Pathology and biology of colorectal neoplasia. In Young GP, Rozen P, Levin B, editors: *Prevention and early detection of colorectal cancer.* Philadelphia, WB Saunders, 1996.)

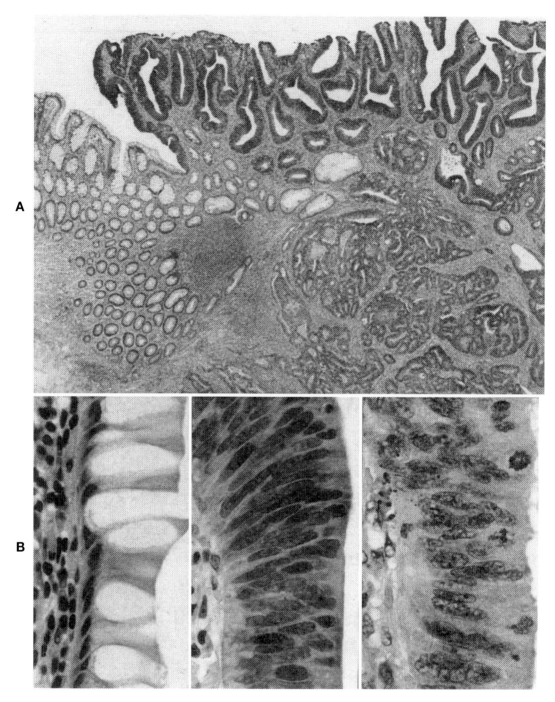

FIGURE 4-10

Adenocarcinoma arising in an adenoma. **A,** Architectural features. The mucosa has ovoid crypts of relatively uniform size in this tangential area. By contrast, the adenoma (A) has irregular glands that vary in size, whereas the glands of the adenocarcinoma (Ca) invade the submucosa and are strikingly complex. **B,** Epithelial morphology and cytologic features. *Left:* The epithelium of the colorectal mucosa has small regular nuclei located basally in the cells. Abundant mucus is present in the cytoplasm of goblet cells. *Middle:* The epithelium of the adenoma is markedly hypercellular with enlarged, stratified, hyperchromatic nuclei, representing high-grade dysplasia. Cytoplasmic mucin is scant. *Right:* The malignant epithelium of the carcinoma has enlarged ovoid nuclei with a strikingly irregular chromatin pattern, including areas of clearing and condensation along the nuclear membrane. Nucleoli are evident. Only scattered cytoplasmic mucin vacuoles are present. (From Hamilton SR: Pathology and biology of colorectal neoplasia. In Young GP, Rozen P, Levin B, editors: *Prevention and early detection of colorectal cancer.* Philadelphia, WB Saunders, 1996.)

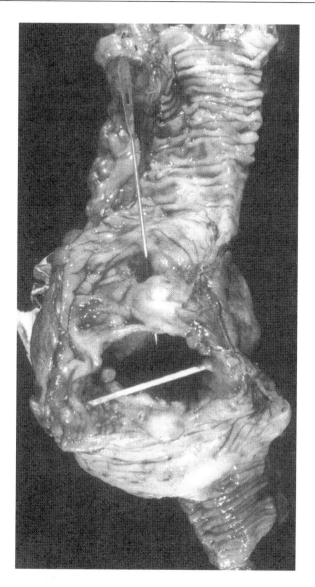

FIGURE 4-11
Endophytic excavated mucinous adenocarcinoma of the proximal ascending colon. The carcinoma (held open by stick) has a hollowed-out appearance as a result of extrusion of the mucinous material into the lumen. A fistula (metal probe) extends into the mucosa of the ascending colon. (From Hamilton SR: Pathology and biology of colorectal neoplasia. In Young GP, Rozen P, Levin B, editors: *Prevention and early detection of colorectal cancer.* Philadelphia, WB Saunders, 1996.)

to polyp size, the potential for metastatic spread is related to the size of the primary cancer. As the primary malignancy grows, individual cells that have greater access to the microcirculation and enhanced ability to proliferate at a distant site (Figure 4-13) develop. This fact emphasizes that CRC screening has dual roles: to detect adenomatous polyps that can be removed before the development of malignancy and to detect cancers when they are small and curable by surgical extirpation.

Hyperplastic Polyps

The adenomatous polyp can be a precursor of invasive cancer,[107] and it is therefore important to resect and retrieve any polyp found during endoscopy.[108] In contrast, hyperplastic

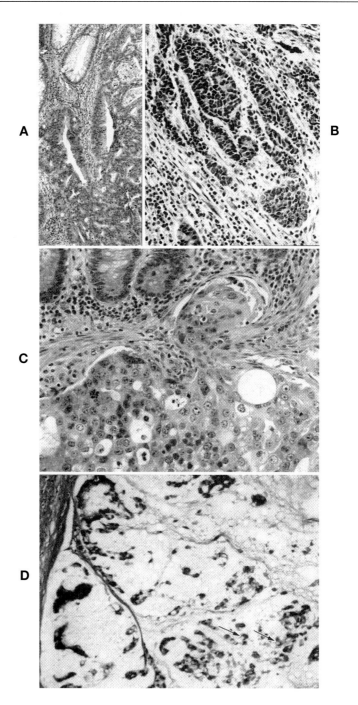

FIGURE 4-12
Spectrum of histopathology of colorectal carcinomas. **A**, Typical moderately differentiated, gland-forming adenocarcinoma. **B**, Poorly differentiated carcinoma of small cell type. **C**, Poorly differentiated carcinoma of large cell type. **D**, Mucinous or colloid adenocarcinoma with abundant extracellular mucin forming pools that contain malignant epithelium. A few signet ring cells *(arrows)*, which are characterized by a cytoplasmic mucin vacuole that displaces the nucleus, are evident. (From Hamilton SR: Pathology and biology of colorectal neoplasia. In Young GP, Rozen P, Levin B, editors: *Prevention and early detection of colorectal cancer.* Philadelphia, WB Saunders, 1996.)

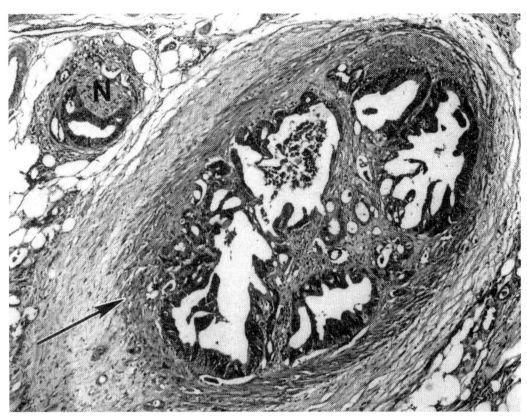

FIGURE 4-13
Vascular and perineural involvement by rectal adenocarcinoma. The muscular wall *(arrow)* of a small vein occluded by adenocarcinoma is evident. Adenocarcinoma infiltrates the perineural space of a nearby small nerve (N). (From Hamilton SR: Pathology and biology of colorectal neoplasia. In Young GP, Rozen P, Levin B, editors: *Prevention and early detection of colorectal cancer.* Philadelphia, WB Saunders, 1996.)

polyps (HPs) are regarded as nonneoplastic lesions without malignant potential.[109] The epithelial cells of HPs are morphologically well-differentiated, and cell replication is confined, as in normal mucosa, to a proliferative zone in the lower epithelial crypt.[110,111] Adenomatous polyps tended to have a red surface color, whereas HPs are more likely to be associated with a white surface color. Their presence does not alter CRC screening guidelines. It is not completely clear, however, that HPs are entirely benign.[112] HPs share common lifestyle risk factors with colorectal adenomas and carcinomas.[113] Further, the coexistence of hyperplastic, adenomatous, and carcinomatous tissue within single polyps has been reported,[114-116] and one study found adenomatous tissue within 13% of HPs.[117] Several studies also indicate that HPs may be a marker of additional neoplasia in other regions of the colon. A study of 129 patients who underwent flexible sigmoidoscopy and subsequent full CS indicated that HPs predicted proximal neoplasia to a degree comparable to adenomatous polyps. Of patients without polyps in the distal colon, 15% had proximal neoplasia, whereas 32% and 37% of patients with HPs and adenomatous polyps, respectively, had proximal colonic neoplasia.[118] Imperiale found that patients with distal HPs had a 2.6 times greater chance of proximal colonic neoplasia, compared with patients without HPs. Other prospective data of patients found to have HPs on initial endoscopy, however, indicated that these patients had a high risk of developing further HPs but did not have an increased risk of developing adenomatous polyps.[119] Adenomatous and HPs did not predict each other's occurrence. This suggests that hyperplastic and adenomatous polyps reflect different biologic processes.[119] In summary, HPs are not considered neoplastic or markers of neoplasia at the current time. Further study will address whether the presence of HPs should warrant more frequent CRC screening.

Molecular Genetics of Colorectal Carcinogenesis

Progressive molecular events occur during the progressive disregulation of growth known as colorectal carcinogenesis. Hypomethylation of DNA, which activates gene expression, precedes the allelic loss of tumor suppressor genes in most cases.[120] Loss of heterozygosity in CRC is seen frequently on chromosomes 1, 5, 8, 17, 18, and 22. These losses imply the inactivation of tumor suppressor genes. Included among these are the APC (adenomatous polyposis coli), MCC (mutated in colorectal cancer), DCC (deleted in colorectal cancer), and p53 genes. Somatic mutation of APC loci is noted in most cases of sporadic CRC. APC mutations appear to be early events in the adenoma-carcinoma sequence, inasmuch as mutations have been found in adenomas as small as 0.5 cm in diameter.[121] Vogelstien proposes that APC mutation is an early initiating event in colorectal carcinogenesis.[69] The MCC gene is a candidate tumor suppressor gene that was identified on chromosome 5 during the search for the APC gene. Somatic mutations in the MCC gene are found in only approximately 10% of colorectal carcinomas.[122,123] Mutation of the DCC gene, found on chromosome 18q, is noted frequently in CRC. Affected individuals frequently demonstrate loss of heterozygosity at the DCC locus and abnormal expression of the preserved allele.[124-127] The p53 gene is the gene most commonly mutated in human cancer overall. In the case of CRC, loss of heterozygosity of the 17p chromosome, containing p53, has been demonstrated in 75% of cancers, although it is rarely seen in adenomatous polyps.[128,129] The allelic loss is confined to the invasive portion of neoplastic growth.[130] Analyses of the remaining allele in cases of 17p loss of heterozygosity indicated missense mutations in many cases.[131] Colorectal cancers without loss of heterozygosity of chromosome 17 demonstrate missense mutations in the majority of both copies of p53 genes.[132] P53 events appear to occur predominantly beyond the adenoma stage in the carcinogenesis pathway.[69] Mutations in the K-*ras* oncogene are found in half of all CRCs and in a similar proportion of larger polyps. They are rarely noted in smaller polyps, indicating that this mutation is associated with the transition to invasive disease.[69,133] Figure 4-14 indicates the current understanding of the progression of genetic changes in sporadic CRC.

Hereditary Colorectal Cancer

CRC has a large familial component, compared with most human cancer. As much as 35% of the disease may arise is individuals with an inherited genetic predisposition (see Fig. 4-3). Only approximately 2% to 3% of CRCs, however, can be attributed to particular familial syndromes at this time. The two known syndromes are considered "polyposis" and "nonpolyposis" types although each still involves the development of CRC from precursor polyps. These familial CRC syndromes have important distinctive clinical features, and study of these syndromes has led to the identification of their genetic determinants.

Familial Adenomatous Polyposis Coli

FAP, an autosomal, dominant inherited disease that affects approximately 1 in 7000 individuals, is defined by the presence of 100 or more polyps within the colon and rectum. FAP is rare and accounts for less than 1% of all CRC cases. Patients with FAP develop colorectal

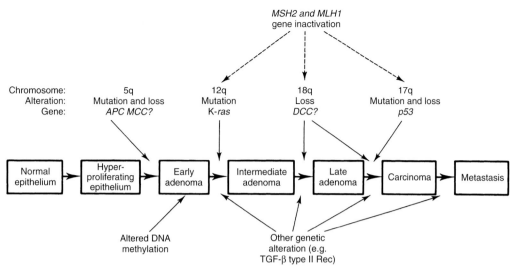

FIGURE 4-14

A genetic model of colorectal cancer. Evidence from clinical and histopathologic studies supports the notion that the majority of colorectal cancers arise from adenomatous polyps over a period of years or even decades. The inherited and somatic genetic alterations found at various stages of colorectal tumorigenesis are indicated, with a specific gene affected, its chromosomal location, and the nature of the alteration in the gene noted. Many of the genetic alterations are discussed in more detail in the text. However, it should be noted that although most cancers display several of the alterations indicated in the figure, only a subset display all of the indicated defects. Inactivation of DNA damage repair genes (e.g., MSH2 and MLH1) in those with HNPCC may lead to more rapid acquisition of mutations in oncogenes such as K-*ras* and in tumor suppressor genes such as p53, TGF-β type II receptor (TGF-β type II rec) and DDC. Although 15% to 20% of sporadic colorectal cancers demonstrate evidence of mismatch repair defects, the specific gene defects underlying this phenotype are not yet known. (Figure modified from Fearon, ER, Vogelstein B: A genetic model for colorectal tumorigenesis. *Cell* 1990;61:759.)

adenomas at puberty and typically develop a "carpet of polyps" throughout the colon and rectum (Figure 4-15). Although the adenomas are not individually life-threatening, their large numbers virtually guarantee that some will progress to cancer. Hence, individuals with FAP all will develop CRC, at a mean age of 42 years.

FAP patients may develop extracolonic manifestations: periampullary adenoma and carcinoma, congenital hypertrophy of the retinal pigment epithelium (CHRPE), fundic gland polyps, adenoma and carcinoma of the stomach, papillary thyroid cancer, hepatoblastoma, osteoma of the skull and mandible, epidermal cysts, desmoid tumor, and medulloblastoma. Osteomas, epidermal cysts, and desmoid tumors form the basis for the designation of Gardner's syndrome, and the combination of hereditary colon cancer and medulloblastoma is referred to as *Turcot's syndrome*.[134,135]

The identification of the gene responsible for FAP was the result of efforts of geneticists and epidemiologists. Genetic linkage analyses demonstrated tight linkage of the disease to markers on the long arm of chromosome 5.[136-139] Subsequent molecular studies of FAP led to the identification of the responsible gene, adenomatous polyposis coli gene (APC), in 1991.[140-144] FAP patients inherit a germline mutation in one copy of the APC gene. Studies in humans and mice with analogous mutations of the murine homologue of APC suggest that the rate-limiting step in tumor initiation is a somatic mutation of the wild-type APC allele from the unaffected parent.

The majority of APC mutations result in truncated proteins that lack varying portions of the C-terminus. Certain truncations are associated with unique clinical features. For

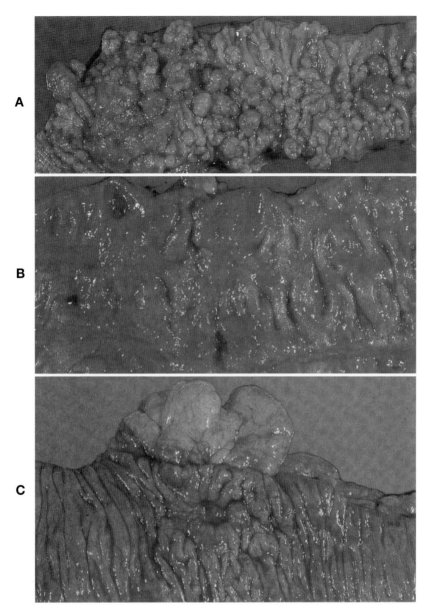

FIGURE 4-15
Gross specimens of colorectal carcinoma in patient with, **A**, familial adenomatous polyposis, **B**, ulcerative colitis, and, **C**, sporadic neoplasia. (From Hamilton SR: Pathology and biology of colorectal neoplasia. In Young GP, Rozen P, Levin B, editors: *Prevention and early detection of colorectal cancer.* Philadelphia, WB Saunders, 1996.)

example, truncation mutations between codons 463 and 1387 are associated with congenital hypertrophy of the retinal pigment epithelium (CHRPE; Figure 4-16).[144] Likewise, colonic manifestations have been shown to vary with the position of the mutation.[145] Phenotype is also modulated by environmental influences and gene-gene interactions. Individuals with identical truncation lesions (identical genotypes) may develop dissimilar clinical features (phenotypes).

Truncating mutations upstream of codon 157 are associated with an attenuated form of FAP in which patients develop a relatively small number of polyps.[146] This syndrome had

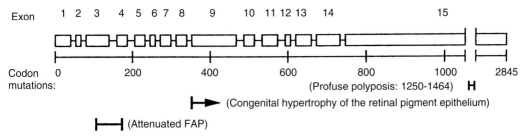

FIGURE 4-16
Diagram of the adenomatous polyposis coli (APC) gene. As reviewed in the text, a correlation between the clinical phenotype and the location of APC mutations has been noted in profuse-type familial adenomatous polyposis, congenital hypertrophy of the retinal pigment epithelium (CHRPE), and attenuated familial adenomatous polyposis. (Reprinted with permission from Reale MA, Fearon ER: Molecular genetics of hereditary colorectal cancer. *Hem/Onc Annals* 1994;2:129.)

previously been designated the hereditary flat adenoma syndrome.[147] Patients with attenuated APC usually have fewer than 100 colonic adenomas, and the development of CRC is delayed until a mean age in the fifth decade. Nevertheless, APC mutation (with severely truncated gene products) is responsible for the syndrome of attenuated FAP.

Gene testing for FAP is a clinically useful tool in the approach to families with this syndrome. Genetic testing became feasible with the development of the in vitro synthesized-protein assay,[148] which was introduced commercially in 1994 (Figure 4-17). This test can identify an APC gene mutation in 80% of affected family members with FAP.[148] When the mutation in a kindred is known, direct gene testing can differentiate, with nearly 100% accuracy, affected family members from those who are unaffected by FAP. Interestingly, 25% of FAP cases occur in families without a family history of CRC. These patients presumably develop a germline APC mutation in utero.

When used appropriately, APC gene testing can confirm the diagnosis of FAP at the molecular level, justify surveillance with CS of those at risk, and aid in surgical management and family planning.[149-152] A study of APC gene testing, however, found that the physicians' interpretation of the test was incorrect in nearly one third of cases (32%) and would have led to misinforming patients. Physicians did not realize that a test in which no mutation was detected could represent a false-negative result in a pedigree in which the APC gene mutation had not been previously identified in an affected family member. Ordering genetic counseling before the test and obtaining informed consent for testing are considered essential,[153,154] but neither was done in more than 80% of the cases. Twenty percent of clinically unaffected patients considered at risk underwent presymptomatic testing before the APC mutation was identified in an affected family member, which would have established the usefulness of testing. The authors concluded that the use of genetic counseling before testing would eliminate many of these procedural errors.[155]

Screening in individuals at risk for FAP is critical. Routine colon screening for adenomatous polyps by annual flexible sigmoidoscopy should begin in puberty and may be decreased in frequency to every 3 years after age 40. Patients with demonstrated gene mutation or those who develop clinical FAP should be referred for proctocolectomy. Chemoprevention is not an acceptable preventative strategy for FAP at this time. Surveillance for gastric, duodenal and periampullary adenomas should begin at the time of diagnosis of colonic polyposis and continue every 1 to 3 years afterward.[156]

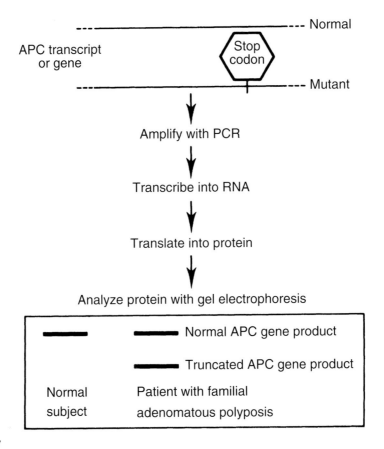

FIGURE 4-17

Schematic representation of APC mutation detected by the in vitro synthesized protein assay (also known as the protein truncation test). The APC gene is divided into overlapping segments encompassing the entire coding region of the gene. These regions are amplified with specifically designed PCR primers that place the necessary transcriptional and translational regulatory sequences at the 5′ end of the PCR product. Radiolabeled APC protein is synthesized in vitro from these surrogate genes in a simple one-step coupled transcription-translation reaction (illustrated as two steps). Truncating mutations can be then identified when smaller protein products are visualized after gel electrophoresis and autoradiography. The stop codon represents a typical APC mutation resulting in premature truncation of the protein product (e.g., a small insertion or deletion resulting in a frameshift in protein translation). (Reprinted with permission from Powell SM, Petersen GM, Krush AJ, et al: Molecular diagnosis of familial adenomatous polyposis. *N Engl J Med* 1993;329:1982.)

Hamartomatous Polyposis Syndromes

Peutz-Jeghers syndrome is an autosomal-dominant inherited disorder characterized by multiple gastrointestinal hamartomas and mucocutaneous melanin pigmentation.[157] The gene responsible for Peutz-Jeghers syndrome is located on chromosome 19.[158-160] Although the polyps in Peutz-Jeghers syndrome are not adenomatous, patients with this syndrome have a significantly elevated risk of developing CRC.[161,162] Screening in at-risk individuals should begin in the second decade of life. Once the diagnosis is made, both upper and lower endoscopy is indicated every 3 to 5 years to detect and remove large, abnormal, or bleeding polyps. Small bowel radiographs should be performed at similar intervals.[156]

Familial juvenile polyposis syndrome is another autosomal dominant polyposis syndrome that is characterized by multiple gastrointestinal polyps.[162-164] Although the polyps are typically benign, affected patients have an increased risk of developing CRC at an early age (mean age of 40 years). Unaffected family members also appear to be at an increased risk of congenital hypertrophy of the retinal pigment epithelium.[165-166] Screening in at-risk individuals should begin in the second decade of life. Once the diagnosis is made, both upper and lower endoscopy is indicated every 3 to 5 years to detect and remove large, abnormal, or bleeding polyps. Small bowel radiographs should be performed at similar intervals.[156]

Hereditary Nonpolyposis Colorectal Cancer

Henry Lynch observed a high rate of CRC in families in the Midwest in the 1950s.[167] These families were remarkable for a high prevalence of right-sided colon cancers that occurred at a relatively early age (younger than 50) and occurred in multiple generations. These components of the Lynch syndromes have been incorporated in the Amsterdam criteria: the presence of histologically verified CRC in at least three relatives (one of whom is a first-degree relative of the other two), the presence of the disease in at least two successive generations, and an age at onset of CRC of younger than 50 years in one of the relatives. In addition, the various polyposis syndromes must be excluded.[168]

HNPCC is characterized by early-onset cancers occurring in the mid-forties as opposed to the seventies, as is seen with sporadic CRC. Many studies indicate a predominance of proximal disease, and 70% of cancers occur proximal to the splenic flexure.[169-170] The proximal location of tumors in the syndrome, however, may be specific to the family kindred under study; population-based studies have identified families with primarily left-sided cancers.[171] Patients are at increased risk for synchronous and metachronous CRC. Approximately 30% of patients develop a metachronous carcinoma within 10 years of their initial cancer if treated with less than subtotal colectomy. The histology of CRC in patients with HMPCC is characterized by an excess of mucoid, signet ring cell, poorly differentiated medullary features, and lymphocytic infiltration. Interestingly, HNPCC patients with CRC have superior stage-stratified survival compared with patients with sporadic CRC.[172,173] HNPCC kindreds are at increased risk of gastric, ovarian, pancreatic, hepatobiliary, ureteral, renal pelvis, endometrial, and breast cancer. Patients with extracolonic cancers are considered to have the Lynch II syndrome.[167]

Cancers of patients with HNPCC demonstrate errors in replication of DNA. Affected individuals inherit a mutated copy of a gene involved in DNA repair. DNA repair is not impaired in normal cells of HNPCC patients because cells retain an unaffected copy of the involved gene from an unaffected parent. However, during tumorigenesis, the remaining wild-type allele is inactivated by somatic mutation in colonocytes, and affected cells acquire a "mutator" phenotype and accumulate mutations in a rapid fashion. These errors lead to genetic mutations and also to the introduction or deletion of additional single or dinucleotides at areas of the genome (called microsatellites) that contain mononucleotide or dinucleotide repeats. These new alleles are evident at multiple microsatellite foci, suggesting a genomic defect of the replication or repair of these simple repeated sequences. The microsatellite instability (MSI), or replication error (RER) phenotype, is seen in 10% to 20% of sporadic CRC cases but is present in nearly every case of HNPCC.

Genetic linkage analyses of individual families in Europe, North America, and New Zealand allowed the identification of the genetic determinants of HNPCC. The recognition that microsatellite instability in tumors from these families was similar to that observed in yeast harboring mutations in mismatch repair genes prompted the search for mutated human mismatch repair genes. Thus far five human mismatch repair genes have been identified: MSH2, MLH1, PMS1, PMS2, and GTBP (also called MSH6).[174-182] Germline mutations occurring in MSH2 and MLH1 account for the majority (greater than 90%) of HNPCC kindreds.

Individuals with HNPCC, unlike FAP, have a similar number of polyps as patients at average risk for CRC. However, adenomas in cases of HNPCC acquire mutations at a rate of two or three orders of magnitude higher than in normal cells. The resultant accumulation of mutations in oncogenes and tumor suppressor genes results in a rapid progression to invasive disease. HNPCC patients thus appear to have an accelerated rate of development of invasive cancer from adenomatous polyps. This contrasts with FAP patients who appear to develop invasive cancer from adenomatous polyps at a rate similar to that seen in sporadic CRC.

Germline HNPCC mutations are found in approximately 1% to 2% of population-based studies of CRC patients. A much larger proportion of CRC patients (12%) demonstrate microsatellite instability.[169,181-183] Algorithms that predict that chance of harboring a germline mismatch repair gene mutation have been developed. These algorithms focus on the identification of individuals likely to be RER-positive and can then be studied further for specific germline mismatch repair gene mutations. Aaltonen and associates evaluated the frequency of HNPCC in Finland by screening 509 CRC patients for the RER phenotype.[184] Tumors from 63 (12%) patients were RER-positive, and 10 of these patients harbored germline MSH2 or MLH1 mutations. The authors recommended RER testing for all CRC patients who meet one or more of the following criteria: a family history of colorectal or endometrial cancer, an age at diagnosis of younger than 50 years, and a history of multiple colorectal or endometrial cancers. Another study calculated the probability of finding a germline mutation by using a model that incorporated age at diagnosis, fulfillment of Amsterdam criteria, and incidence of one family member having both colorectal and endometrial cancer. Those with a high probability of mutation can forgo RER determination and proceed directly to MSH2 and MLH1 mutation analysis with denaturing gradient gel electrophoresis of amplified genomic DNA. Those with a lower probability were recommended to undergo RER testing and then specific mismatch repair gene mutation testing if they were RER-positive.[185]

Patients with the HNPCC syndrome should begin colonoscopic screening at a far younger age than patients at average risk for CRC. Lynch and associates recommend full CS every 2 years starting at age 25 for patients and first-degree relatives of patients with HNPCC.[183] They further advocate annual CS once a specific germline mutation is identified because of the problem of accelerated carcinogenesis.[172,186] Subtotal colectomy is recommended for the management of CRC without distant metastases. Yearly screening of the rectum remains essential in these patients. Prophylactic subtotal colectomy should be considered for patients who will not be compliant with annual CS, have confirmed germline mutation in a mismatch repair gene, or have adenomas and the HNPCC syndrome.[187-189]

Inflammatory Bowel Disease

Ulcerative colitis (UC) is a disease characterized by colorectal mucosal inflammation whose cause is unclear. Patients with UC are at increased risk for developing colorectal carcinoma.[190] The pathophysiology of CRC in patients with UC differs from that of "sporadic" CRC. CRC developing in the setting of chronic UC does not manifest as the adenomatous polyp-to-invasive cancer pathway. Rather, dysplasia develops in the setting of chronic inflammation (Figure 4-18). The early molecular changes in the development of UC associated with CRC include the development of genomic instability as manifested by DNA aneuploidy and microsatellite instability. APC gene mutation, seen in most cases of sporadic CRC, is rarely identified in UC-associated cancers. Mutations in p53 are typically thought to occur later in the pathway of sporadic CRC. In contrast, in patients with UC, this mutation appears to occur earlier in the pathway toward dysplasia and cancer.

The risk of developing CRC in patients with UC is related to three factors: duration of disease, anatomic extent of disease, and age at onset.[190-194] Increasing duration of disease is generally accepted to be a risk factor for the development of CRC in UC patients. The increased risk begins 10 years after the initial attack. Estimates of cumulative risk vary dramatically, depending on the source population under study, from 1.8% at 20 years to 43% after 35 years.[191-194] Earlier reports exaggerated the danger of malignant changes because they were based upon retrospective studies of patients who had been referred to tertiary centers.[195,196] The cumulative risk of developing CRC in patients with UC has been stated to increase 5% to 10% for every decade of duration of disease after 10 years.[190-196] Patients with total colitis (generally defined as disease proximal to the hepatic flexure) have higher cumulative risk estimates than patients with limited disease. Ekbom reported population-based data that indicate standardized incidence ratios of 1.7 (95%, confidence interval [CI] 0.8-3.2), 2.8 (95%, CI 1.6-4.4), and 14.8 (95%, CI 11.4-18.9) for patients with disease limited to the rectum, extending beyond the rectum but no further than the hepatic flexure, and extending proximal to the hepatic flexure, respectively.[197] Thus patients with left-sided colitis have CRC risk only slightly higher than the overall population. Age at diagnosis has been associated with an increased risk of CRC. Younger patients (<15 years) appear to be at highest cumulative risk.[197,198] Studies have not clearly identified whether the presence of primary sclerosing cholangitis, disease activity, or pharmacologic therapy alters the risk of CRC in UC patients.

Total proctocolectomy eliminates the risk of CRC in patients with UC. Patients may elect to have a permanent ileostomy or may have an ileoanal anastomosis following proctocolectomy. Proctocolectomy with ileoanal anastomosis removes the entire colon and rectum and creates a neorectum from the small bowel. This pouch is anastomosed to the rectum following removal of the rectal mucosa. Sphincter function is preserved but patients have frequent bowel movements, occasional sexual dysfunction (males), and nighttime soiling, and are at risk for pouchitis. The end ileostomy is generally chosen in older patients or those with poor sphincter function to minimize problems associated with frequent bowel movements and potential fecal incontinence. Patients who undergo ileoanal pouch anastomosis may develop CRC if the rectal mucosa is incompletely removed at surgery. This mucosa remains at risk for the development of CRC, and surveillance following proctocolectomy is advocated by many. Some physicians recommend total proctocolectomy for patients with greater than 8 to 10 years of extensive disease. Total proctocolectomy greatly affects patient lifestyle. In cases where the UC is severe, total proctocolectomy with either ileoanal anastomosis or permanent ileostomy may be a welcome improvement in lifestyle. However, many patients without severe UC are reluctant to accept the lifestyle changes associated with total proctocolectomy.

Screening for CRC in UC patients has become part of routine clinical care to determine which patients should consider proctocolectomy to prevent the development of CRC. Colonoscopy is done to detect frank cancer but mainly is done to detect premalignant dysplasia. The presence of high-grade dysplasia, whether or not associated with a macroscopic lesion, appears to be highly predictive of the presence of concurrent cancer or the

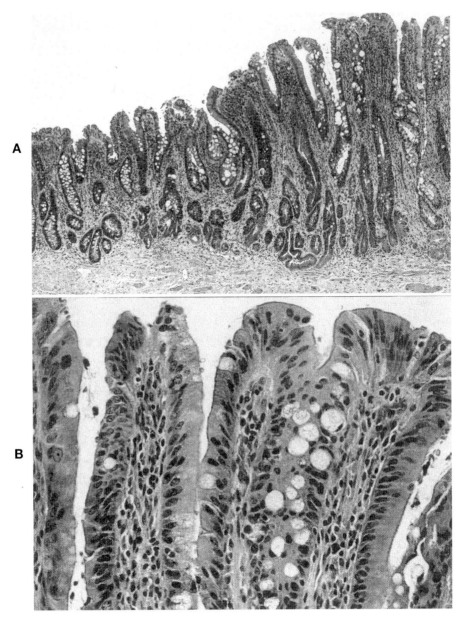

FIGURE 4-18
Histopathology of epithelial dysplasia is a patient with ulcerative colitis. **A,** The area of dysplasia is thicker than the surrounding mucosa, which shows evidence of inactive ulcerative colitis as manifested by crypt distortion, chronic inflammation of the lamina propria, and reactive epithelial changes. **B,** The dysplastic epithelium includes scattered goblet cells. (From Hamilton SR: Pathology and biology of colorectal neoplasia. In Young GP, Rozen P, Levin B, editors: *Prevention and early detection of colorectal cancer.* Philadelphia, WB Saunders, 1996.)

development of CRC[199,200] and mandates colectomy. Patients with low-grade dysplasia are at relatively high risk for developing high-grade dysplasia or cancer, and some may have concurrent cancer. It will eventually affect 80% of subjects and waxes and wanes in the colitic population.[201,202]

Unfortunately, a negative CS does not reliably exclude CRC in the setting of UC. The development of CRC in the setting of chronic inflammation in UC is insidious. Lesions are flat and difficult to distinguish from chronic inflammation. It is also clear that the repeated colonoscopic surveillance may overlook invasive cancer until is has become advanced and incurable. Patients may develop CRC soon after a negative surveillance CS.[203]

Dysplasia is used as a marker for CRC in these patients but is an imperfect surrogate. Colorectal cancer in UC can arise de novo without associated dysplastic lesions.[204] Ransohoff and associates noted that only 50% of colectomy specimens harbored dysplasia distant from the cancerous lesion.[205] Cancers in these patients will be missed by a screening test that uses high-grade dysplasia as a surrogate for invasive cancer (unless the biopsy specimen happens to be taken at the actual site of the cancer). Dysplasia, even when present, may be undetected. Dysplastic lesions in UC occur in a patchy distribution and may be missed even with multiple random biopsies. A prospective study form London found that carcinoma developed in 13 of the 186 patients with extensive colitis with a history of disease for 10 years or more, despite regular surveillance. Of the total 16 carcinomas in these 13 patients, 11 were Dukes' stage A, 3 Dukes' stage B, 1 Dukes' stage C, and 1 was inoperable.[206] Colonoscopy has not been proven to lower the mortality from CRC in patients with UC.[207] Aggregate studies of surveillance programs indicate that 41% of CRCs detected were node-positive.[208] It appears that the screening procedure did in fact diagnose the cancers present but that the diagnosis was frequently at a late stage at which survival was not optimal. The overall yield was also poor; only one cancer per 476 examinations was detected. This yield is lower than the yield of routine screening (every 5 years) in the United States.

Recommendations for screening include annual CS with biopsies every 10 cm for patients with disease extending beyond the sigmoid for greater than 8 years. For patients with left-sided colitis, CS may start after 12 to 15 years of symptoms. Surveillance should be repeated every 1 or 2 years. Colectomy is recommended for patients with repeated evidence of low-grade dysplasia in the absence of acute inflammation, high-grade dysplasia, or cancer. Colectomy should also be considered in patients with colitis that is refractory to medical management and in those patients who will not comply with surveillance. Based on the results of previous studies, at least 56 biopsies should be performed to have greater than 95% chance of detecting dysplasia if it is present.[209-211] It is important that patients understand that colectomy is an alternative to CS. Many UC patients are lost to follow-up, and the poorly compliant patient may be best served by proctocolectomy. Those patients who undergo ileoanal pouch should consider surveillance of the pouch anastomosis.

The risk of CRC is also increased in long-standing Crohn's colitis.[212] The increased risk of cancer is similar to that of UC of equivalent duration and anatomic extent. A similar protocol for surveillance for UC should be implemented in these patients. Segmental colectomy/proctectomy should be employed when disease is limited to regions of the colon or rectum.[213-215]

Screening Tests for Colorectal Neoplasia

The majority of cases of CRC do not occur in patients at increased risk for the disease. Most CRCs (70%-80%) develop in patients without a family or personal history of colorectal neoplasia or a history of inflammatory bowel disease. Screening tests and guidelines have been developed to detect colonic neoplasia in patients at "average risk" for the disease. Each of these screening tests has advantages and disadvantages that require examination before recommending them to patients. Each test is considered individually because each is frequently employed individually in clinical practice for the screening of colorectal neoplasia.

Fecal Occult Blood Testing

In 1993, a randomized controlled trial in Minnesota indicated that annual fecal occult blood testing (FOBT) was effective in reducing CRC mortality by 33%.[216] Population-based trials in England and Denmark subsequently showed 15% and 18% mortality reductions with biennial screening, respectively.[217,218] A follow-up report from the Minnesota Colon Cancer Control Study indicated a 33% and 18% reduction in CRC mortality with annual and biennial screening, respectively,[219] and indicated that FOBT also reduced the incidence of CRC.[220] Control patients in these studies were not screened at all. A portion of the reduction in mortality from FOBT screening has been attributed to chance detection resulting from CS following a positive fecal occult blood test.[221-223] Indeed the logical control group to isolate the effect of FOBT would have been a group of patients randomly selected to receive CS in equal number to those prompted by a positive fecal occult blood test. It is also important to note that FOBT was performed in patients following dietary restrictions (no red meat, fresh fruit, iron preparations, vitamin C, aspirin, or other nonsteroidal anti-inflammatory agents [NSAIDs] during the 3 days when the samples were taken) using six guaiac-impregnated Hemoccult slides from three consecutive fecal samples. Slides were rehydrated before testing. This protocol is far different than the typical FOBT done following the annual rectal examination in a doctor's office. Even in study settings, the positive predictive value of FOBT for CRC is as low as 2%. Clearly FOBT alone is an inadequate screening test for the detection of colonic neoplasia. In fact, patients with a positive FOBT in whom iron deficiency anemia and active bleeding have been excluded have been shown to be more likely to harbor upper gastrointestinal lesions than colonic lesions.[224] Compared with other screening modalities, the cases of colorectal neoplasia that FOBT does identify are likely to be cancers and not premalignant polyps.

Flexible Sigmoidoscopy

The development of fiberoptic endoscopy revolutionized CRC screening. Flexible sigmoidoscopy was the first endoscopic procedure found to clearly reduce colorectal mortality. In 1992, Selby and associates reported a case-control study from Northern California Kaiser Permanente Hospitals, where they analyzed the performance of sigmoidoscopy during the 10-year period before the diagnosis of CRC.[225] They found that only 8.8% of CRC patients had a screening sigmoidoscopy, as compared with 24.2% of patients without CRC; flexible sigmoidoscopy provided a 60% reduction in CRC mortality. The negative association of cancer with sigmoidoscopy remained strong with screening intervals from prior sigmoidoscopy to cancer diagnosis of as long as 10 years.

Flexible sigmoidoscopy combined with FOBT is an approved method of colorectal screening (Table 4-2).[226] Flexible sigmoidoscopy is an excellent test for the detection of neoplasia distal to the splenic flexure. It does not, however, survey the majority of the colon. Patients in whom adenomas are identified on sigmoidoscopy are recommended to have a total colonic evaluation to assess the right side of the colon. Advocates of total colonic evaluation, however, point out that most patients with right-sided cancers do not have left-sided polyps.[227-233] Imperiale and associates found that 62% of more than 2000 patients with advanced proximal neoplasms had either no distal lesion or only HPs, which would not have warranted CS according to current guidelines.[232] Lieberman in a similar study found that 52% of veterans with proximal neoplasia had no lesions in the distal colon that would have warranted CS according to current guidelines.[233] Relying upon flexible sigmoidoscopy to detect CRC has been compared to performing unilateral mammography for the detection of breast cancer.[234] These patients must rely on FOBT, which has limited sensitivity for detecting neoplasia,[234] to serve as an indicator of proximal polyps or curable cancers.

Table 4-2
American Cancer Society Guidelines for Screening and Surveillance for Early Detection of Colorectal Polyps and Cancer*

Risk Category	Recommendation[+]	Age to Begin	Interval
Average Risk			
All people 50 years or older who are not in the categories below	One of the following: FOBT plus flexible sigmoidoscopy[±] or TCE[§]	Age 50 Age 50	FOBT every year and flexible sigmoidoscopy every 5 years Colonoscopy every 10 years or DCBE every 5-10 years
Moderate Risk			
People with single, small (< 1 cm) adenomatous polyps	Colonoscopy	At time of initial polyp diagnosis	TCE within 3 years after initial polyp removal; if normal, as per average risk recommendations (above)
People with large (> 1 cm) or multiple adenomatous polyps of any size	Colonoscopy	At time of initial polyp diagnosis	TCE within 3 years after initial polyp removal; if normal, TCE every 5 years
Personal history of curative-intent resection of colorectal cancer	TCE[¶]	Within 1 year after resection	If normal, TCE in 3 years; If still normal, TCE every 5 years
Colorectal cancer of adenomatous polyps in first-degree relative younger than 60 years or in two or more first-degree relatives of any ages	TCE	Age 40 or 10 years before the youngest case in the family, whichever is earlier	Every 5 years
High Risk			
Family history of familial adenomatous polyposis	Early surveillance with endoscopy, counseling to consider genetic testing, and referral to a specialty center	Puberty	If genetic test positive or polyposis confirmed, consider colectomy; otherwise; endoscopy every 1-2 years
Family history of hereditary nonpolyposis colon cancer	Colonoscopy and counseling to consider genetic testing	Age 21 years	If genetic test positive or if patient has not had genetic testing, colonoscopy every 2 years until age 40 years, then every year
Inflammatory bowel disease	Colonoscopies with biopsies for dysplasia	8 years after the start of pancolitis; 12-15 years after the start of left-sided colitis	Every 1-2 years

*Approximately 70%-80% of cases are from average-risk individuals, approximately 15%-20% are from moderate-risk individuals, and 5%-10% are from high-risk individuals.
+Digital rectal examination should be done at the time of each sigmoidoscopy, colonoscopy, or DCBE.
±Annual FOBT has been shown to reduce mortality from colorectal cancer, so it is preferable to no screening; however, the ACS recommends that annual FOBT be accompanied by flexible sigmoidoscopy to further reduce the risk of colorectal cancer mortality.
§TCE includes either colonoscopy or DCBE. The choice of procedure should depend on the medical status of the patient and the relative quality of the medical examinations available in a specific community. Flexible sigmoidoscopy should be performed in those instances in which the rectosigmoid colon is not well-visualized by DCBE. DCBE would be performed when the entire colon has not been adequately evaluated by colonoscopy.
¶This assumes that a perioperative TCE was done.
DCBE = double-contrast barium enema; FOBT = fecal occult blood testing; TCE = total colon examination.

Advocates of sigmoidoscopy point out its lower incidence of complications; improved cost-effectiveness, assuming a short polyp dwell time; widespread availablity because it can be performed without sedation in the primary care setting or by paramedical personnel in the community setting; and lack of need for oral bowel preparation. It is clear the ability of a flexible sigmoidoscopic-based screening program to detect colonic neoplasia is inferior to that of one employing CS.

Barium Enema

Barium enema (BE) is a recommended CRC screening test. Patients at average risk for CRC are recommended to undergo total colonic evaluation using either air-contrast barium enema (ACBE) every 5 to 10 years or CS every 10 years (without annual fecal occult blood test). Barium enema can be done as a single-contrast study using barium alone or as an ACBE, where the barium is evacuated and air is instilled into the colon to allow the delineation of mucosal abnormalities. Single-contrast barium enema is not recommended for polyp detection because large mucosal abnormalities are difficult to detect. ACBE is a recommended screening test, although single-contrast enemas are sometimes substituted by radiologists in cases involving elderly or debilitated patients who may be less able to tolerate the discomfort associated with instillation of air into the colon and rectum.

Patients require cleansing of the colon before a barium enema. Patients usually are instructed to take clear liquid and are given oral cathartics (polyethylene glycol or oral phosphosoda) on the day before the study. They may be given enemas. Patients are not sedated for the procedure. The patient lies prone, and a soft 2-cm balloon tip catheter is inserted into the rectum. Liquid barium is instilled, and the table is rolled to the left and right and then tilted upright to allow the barium to move by gravity to the proximal colon. In the case of the ACBE, air is then instilled to assist the progress of the barium and to provide a double-contrast examination. Radiographs are then taken with the patient rolled so as to allow different portions of the colon to be dependent, thus making all mucosal surfaces visible. Patients are discharged following the examination, which takes 30 to 40 minutes. They pass barium for 1 to 2 days and are given laxatives to facilitate evacuation and prevent fecal impaction. Barium enema images the entire colon in most complete examinations. The laxative preparation is critical to avoid the classic "retained fecal matter, cannot rule out polyps" report.

The proportion of polyps detectable by barium enema is related to the size of the adenomas. Winawer and associates studied patients with a history of colonic polyps with paired CS and ACBE examinations.[235] Findings on ACBE were positive in only 39% of the colonoscopic examinations in which one or more adenomas were detected. The effectiveness of ACBE was related to polyp size. ACBE detected 32% of polyps from CS examinations in which the largest adenomas detected were 0.5 cm or less, 53% for those in which the largest adenomas detected were 0.6 to 1.0 cm, and 48% for those in which the largest adenomas detected exceeded 1.0 cm. Of the 139 paired examinations with positive results on barium enema and negative results on CS, less than 10% had adenomas on CS reexamination. The rate of false-positives on barium enema (14%) was higher than the rate of true-positives (13%). Some have argued that the polyps missed by barium enema are small and unlikely to harbor malignancy. Although the presence of dysplasia is clearly related to polyp size,[236] the ability of ACBE to detect even larger polyps is concerning.

Barium enema appeared particular futile in the Winawer study assessing polyp detection.[235] However, its ability to detect cancer is also imperfect. The overall sensitivity for CRC is approximately 80% to 85%. The ACBE appeared to be as sensitive as CS for the diagnosis of advanced cancer. Unfortunately, the detection of advanced cancer is much less important because of poor cure rates. The main difference between barium enema and CS was the failure of barium enema to detect Dukes' A lesions. In a study comparing the two modalities, the ability of CS to detect Dukes' A lesions was three times higher in the CS group.[237] The detection of these lesions is critical because treatment is associated with cure (and a 5-year survival of more than 90%).

Barium enema has the advantage of identifying the exact location of the lesion. Colon length is affected by insufflation used during endoscopy; as well, looping of the endoscope may cause an endoscopist to consider a lesion to be much further into the colon than it really is. These errors can be avoided to some degree by correlating colonic landmarks (e.g., the liver and splenic shadows) rather than by relying entirely on the depth of the colonoscope at the time of lesion identification. Barium enema has the advantage that it does not require conscious sedation and is far less expensive. A comparison of costs in Pennsylvania[238] indicated that barium enema was one third the cost of CS in the office ($121 vs. $502) and in the hospital setting ($211 vs. $767). Barium enema has also been found to be very cost effective when measured as years of life gained from screening intervention divided by screening costs. Wagner consistently found BE alone or BE combined with FOBT to be the most cost-effective measures. It is important to note that ACBE alone did not result in the greatest gain of years of life per 100,000 screened. However, its lower costs resulted in a lower ratio of years of life gained for lifetime costs of screening.[239]

Colonoscopy

Colonoscopy (CS) is the most effective means of detecting and treating colonic neoplasia. The removal of adenomas detected at CS substantially decreases the incidence of CRC.[94] In the absence of any obstructing lesion, an expert can perform complete CS in 98% of examinations and in 95% of all patients who present for CS. Studies from community hospitals indicate that full CS can be accomplished 90% of the time.[240] Total CS may be more difficult in women than men, but a previous hysterectomy does not seem to adversely affect the ability to perform CS.[241] Age has been assumed to be an independent risk factor for complications from CS. Patients older than 65 years have been shown to have a slightly increased incidence of bleeding following polypectomy in comparison with younger patients. The presence of cardiac, pulmonary, liver, or kidney disease or prior abdominal or pelvic surgery has not been associated with an increased risk of complications.[242] Overall, the risk of perforation and of problems associated with the use of conscious sedation is less than 0.2%.[243]

Although CS is the "gold standard" in the evaluation of colorectal neoplasia, it too is an imperfect test. The sensitivity for CRC is estimated to be 95%, not 100%.[244] The sensitivity for small polyps is lower. Adenomas smaller than 1 cm in diameter escape detection 10% to 20% of the time.[245,246] Rex and associates studied back-to-back colonoscopies in 183 patients and found that the overall miss rate for polyps was 24%. Right-sided polyps smaller than 5 mm were most likely to be missed. Importantly, however, miss rates for adenomas larger than 1 cm (which are more likely to harbor invasive disease) were low.[244]

Colonoscopy is also the only screening modality able to detect flat lesions. Flat adenomas[247] predominate in what seems to be a variant of FAP[248] and may be an uncommon precursor to sporadic cancers. Adenomas recognizable only by erythema or irregular mucosal folds accounted for 36% of adenomas detected among 1000 Britons who underwent CS.[249]

Virtual Colonoscopy

Advances in three-dimensional (3-D) computer graphics, coupled with technical improvements in high-resolution computed tomographic (CT) imaging, have aided the development of interactive 3-D visualization of the colon and rectum. Spiral CT colonography (or virtual CS) refers to the acquisition of transaxial spiral CT images, with interactive display of a variety of 2-D and 3-D imaging tools to evaluate the colonic mucosa for neoplasia. One such 3-D tool, perspective volume rendering, gives rise to virtual CS (VCS), the computer-simulated, 3-D endoscopic visualization of the colonic mucosa.

VCS requires meticulous bowel preparation on the day before the CT scan. On the day of examination a small rubber catheter is placed into the rectum, and room air or carbon dioxide is pumped into the rectum to distend the colon to the maximal level tolerated by the patient. Patients are not sedated. Manual insufflation of room air is simple to administer and generally results in prolonged distension. This is valuable for extended spiral CT scanning but may be moderately uncomfortable for the patient. In contrast, carbon dioxide is rapidly absorbed by the colon, which improves patient comfort but might result in less prolonged distension. In either case, glucagon is usually given to combat colonic spasm in response to distension.

Patients are scanned in a workstation equipped with software for three-dimensional rendering. Using this software, a single radiologist generates both antegrade and retrograde endoluminal virtual endoscopic navigations of the colon. On average, the time required for virtual CS is 20 minutes for CT scanning, 30 minutes for image manipulation, and 10 minutes for interpretation.[250,251]

False-positive reading may result from solid stool simulating a neoplastic lesion. Residual stool may also obscure polyps. Residual fluid cannot be aspirated and solid stool cannot be lavaged as is the case with CS. Hence thorough bowel cleansing is essential for virtual CS. Novel approaches to bowel preparation for virtual CS use cathartics followed by an oral iodonated contrast agent before the CT examination. The goal of these combined agents is to first liquefy the stool and then opacify the residual fluid to permit visualization of submerged polyps as low-attenuation structures in a pool of high-attenuation fluid. Published reports should be forthcoming.

VCS has a number of advantages over CS. With VCS, the examination is performed without sedation in less time than conventional CS and involves little risk of complications. The radiologist, using a number of static and dynamic display options, can examine and reexamine segments of the colon after the procedure has been performed. The localization of lesion is precise, and both sides of the bowel folds can be scrutinized. The disadvantages of VCS include the need for bowel cleansing and infusion of gas to distend the colon. Scanning hardware is expensive, and the interpretation of the images is relatively difficult and time-consuming. Retained stool or fluid or contracted segments of colon interfere with the detection of neoplasia. Suctioning retained fluid or lavaging adherent solid stool, options that are available in conventional CS, cannot be done in VCS.

Several institutions are investigating virtual CS for the detection of colorectal neoplasia. The earliest study by Hara and associates described 70 patients with a prior or current history of colonic polyps.[252] In this study, a total of 115 polyps were evaluated independently by two radiologists. The study-reported sensitivities were 67% and 73%, respectively, for adenomas ≥ 10 mm in diameter, 56% and 69% for adenomas 5 to 10 mm in diameter, and 25% and 27% for adenomas ≤ 5 mm. More recently, Fenlon and associates reported results of 100 patients at high risk for colorectal neoplasia in whom 115 polyps were found with CS.[253] All patients were studied with CT colonography immediately before the conventional CS. The entire colon was visualized in 87% and 89% of patients evaluated with VCS and CS, respectively. VCS demonstrated a sensitivity of 91% for the detection of polyps ≤ 10 mm, 82% for polyps 6 to 9 mm, and 55% of polyps 1 to 5 mm.

An important question is whether the low rate of sensitivity for the detection of polyps between 1 and 5 mm in diameter is acceptable. There is controversy about what constitutes a clinically significant polyp with regard to size.[254-256] Although many would argue for the removal of all adenomatous polyps, whatever their size, the prevalence of polyps less than 10 mm in diameter in people older than 50 years of age is high (30% to 50%). Removal of all such polyps for the prevention of CRC would be a formidable challenge. Moreover, in the subgroup of patients with adenomatous polyps that are 10 mm or smaller, the probability of cancer is low, and the likelihood of any single lesion progressing to cancer is also small. Some have thus argued that a policy of identifying and removing only polyps above a specific threshold for size, as opposed to a policy of universal polypectomy, could result in a similar reduction in mortality but at lower risk and cost.[257]

The sensitivity of VCS for the detection of CRC is, as expected, much higher. Virtual CS (VCS) appears to be a preferred study for obstructing cancers that prevent full CS. In a series of 29 patients suspected of having CRC, VCS helped to identify all 29 occlusive carcinomas and demonstrated 2 cancers and 24 polyps in the colon proximal to the cancer.[258] Even though a distal occlusive carcinoma prevented complete evaluation of the proximal colon with either CS or barium enema in all patients, a complete colonic evaluation was possible in 90% of patients examined with VCS.

For VCS to be substituted for an established method of CRC screening, it first must be shown to be as safe, acceptable, available, and cost-effective as the method it is replacing. VCS is more painful than CS and still requires a bowel preparation, which many patients consider as the most troublesome part of CRC screening. Those patients with lesions (which may be 30% to 50% of all patients) will need a repeat bowel cleansing to undergo conventional CS to evaluate and remove lesions identified on VCS. In summary, the prohibitive cost and questionable sensitivity for polyps make VCS an impractical screening test at the present time.

Screening Recommendations

The American Cancer Society (ACS) has recommended screening for CRC since 1980.[259] The 1997 recommendation calls for everyone older than age 50 who is at "average risk" to be screened with annual FOBT and sigmoidoscopy every 5 years or total colon examination, either by CS (every 10 years) or by double-contrast barium enema (every 5 to 10 years).[226] "Average risk" is defined by exclusion as individuals without a personal or family history of CRC, adenomatous polyps, or inflammatory bowel disease.[226] Between 70% and 80% of all CRCs occur among patients at "average risk."

Many patients elect flexible sigmoidoscopy and FOBT. Those who have a left-sided adenomatous polyp or a positive FOBT should receive full CS. Those who have a normal flexible sigmoidoscopy and FOBT need to understand that they have a 2% to 3% chance of harboring undetected advanced proximal neoplasia, including cancer. Colonoscopy provides the best opportunity for identifying and removing neoplastic lesions. This study should be repeated every 10 years if normal initially. ACBE is an alternative means of total colonic examination to CS with markedly lower sensitivity for colonic neoplasia (especially small and flat lesions). Both require full bowel preparation, but double-contrast barium enema (DCBE) does not allow for the sampling or removal of abnormalities. DCBE is done without sedation and is much less comfortable than CS. Retained stool may be misinterpreted as neoplasia and prompt CS, including a repeat full bowel preparation. Because the balloon used for barium enema limits evaluation of the distal rectum, some advocate flexible sigmoidoscopy in addition to DCBE to avoid missing distal lesions. DCBE advantages include lower cost and smaller risk of complications. It is best reserved for cases where CS is unavailable or contraindicated. FOBT is unnecessary for patient screening using a method of total colonic evaluation.

Colonoscopy should be used in any patient with inflammatory bowel disease or a personal or family history of colonic neoplasia. Patients should repeat screening in 3 years following an initial examination to clear the colon and rectum of benign neoplasia. A shorter interval may be necessary in cases of multiple adenomas, excision of an adenoma with invasive cancer, incomplete removal of a sessile adenoma, or a suboptimal examination secondary to a poor bowel preparation.[156] If the 3-year survey is normal, many clinicians revert to an every-5-year screening program. Patients who have endoscopic removal of malignant polyps should have repeat endoscopy at 3 to 6 months and again 1 year later before reverting to 3-year screening intervals.

Patients with one or two first-degree relatives with colonic neoplasia are at increased risk for CRC, even if they do not harbor germline mutations characteristic of FAP or HNPCC. These patients should begin screening at age 40, or 10 years younger than the age of the family member with the earliest diagnosed familial CRC, whichever is earlier.[156] These patients require colonoscopic surveillance.

Use of Screening Tests for CRC

Colorectal cancer screening is severely underused in the United States. In 1997, the Behavioral Risk Factor Surveillance System reported the percentage of respondents aged 50 or greater who reported having had CRC screening tests within recommended intervals.[260] Whereas 20.9% of women had FOBT during the preceding year (as opposed to 18.3% of men), only 26.7% had sigmoidoscopy or proctoscopy within the preceding 5 years (as opposed to 35.1% of men). The proportion of respondents who reported having had either test increased with each age group until age 70 to 79, then decreased among persons aged 80 or more years of age. In general, elderly patients were more likely to use screening: 31.6%, 37.0%, and 33.2% of patients 80 and older, 70 to 79, and 60 to 69 years of age, respectively, used sigmoidoscopy or proctoscopy within the preceding 5 years, compared with 23.6% of those aged 50 to 59.

Those with higher levels of education were more likely to use CRC screening, with 22.8% and 35.9% of college graduates using FOBT and sigmoidoscopy or proctoscopy, respectively, compared to 16.2% and 27.5% of those who did not finish high school. Screening use was also related to income. Those earning more than $75,000 were more likely to use FOBT (23.0%) and sigmoidoscopy or proctoscopy (36.8%) than those earning less than $10,000 per year (16.1% and 23.0%, respectively). Both Whites and Blacks reported the highest use of CRC screening. Twenty percent of both Whites and Blacks used FOBT, and approximately 30% used some form of endoscopy. Asians were much less likely to participate, with only 11.5% reporting FOBT and 25.9% reporting endoscopy. Native Americans also infrequently used CRC screening: 12.1% used FOBT within the prior year, and 24.4% used some form of endoscopy. Respondents identifying themselves as of Hispanic origin were less likely to report having had either test than were respondents who identified themselves as non-Hispanic. By state, the proportion of respondents who reported having had FOBT during the preceding year ranged from 9.2% (Mississippi) to 28.4% (Maine). The proportion of respondents who reported having had sigmoidoscopy or proctoscopy during the preceding 5 years ranged from 15.5% (Oklahoma) to 41.5% (District of Columbia). The single most important factor identified was whether subjects had health care coverage: 20.6% and 31.4% of respondents, respectively, with health insurance had FOBT or endoscopy within the appropriate interval. However, only 8.2% and 16.3% of uninsured individuals, respectively, had appropriate screening.

The telephone survey overestimated screening test use because it did not differentiate between screening and diagnostic testing. In other words, patients who underwent endoscopy to evaluate rectal bleeding were not excluded. Severe underuse reflects patient and provider barriers. Patient barriers include lack of knowledge of screening recommendations, access to health care, anticipated discomfort, and embarrassment. Provider barriers include lack of knowledge of screening recommendations, ability to perform the procedure, and time to counsel patients. Activities to increase awareness of CRC screening include the ACS and Centers for Disease Control and Prevention (CDC) establishment of the National Colorectal Cancer Roundtable, a collaboration of state health departments, professional and medical societies, private industry, consumers, and cancer survivors to promote CRC screening and awareness. In 1998, the Health Care Financing Administration expanded Medicare coverage to include CRC screening. For average-risk people 50 years of age or older, coverage is provided for annual FOBT and sigmoidoscopy or CS every 4 years; for high-risk persons, coverage will be provided for CS every 2 years. ACBE may be substituted for either sigmoidoscopy or CS if requested in writing by the provider. Many commercial plans also cover CRC screening.

Asians and Latinos have a much higher proportion of left-sided cancers than do Whites or Blacks.[261] Latinos and Asians are also much less likely to use colorectal screening than Whites or Blacks.[260] The use of sigmoidoscopy, which can be performed by paramedical personnel outside of medical facilities, should be strongly advocated in these groups. Recommendations to screen with flexible sigmoidoscopy before age 65 and CS after age 65 should be studied in these groups.[262]

Cost-effectiveness

Colorectal cancer treatment costs more than $6.5 billion per year; the cost of treatment is second only to breast cancer ($6.6 billion per year).[263,264] The primary goal of cost-effectiveness analysis is to guide decisions about whether the cost of an intervention is justified compared with the alternative use of available resources. Cost-effectiveness ratios are frequently expressed in dollars spent per year of life saved. The lower the expenditure spent to save a year of life, the better the cost-effectiveness of a particular program. In the United States, well-accepted interventions, including mammography, hypertension control, and hemodialysis, have cost-effectiveness ratios under $40,000 to $60,000 per year of life saved. Therefore $40,000 to $60,000 per year of life saved is generally the American benchmark for cost-effectiveness, and interventions with ratios less than this are considered cost-effective.[265-267]

Mathematical models of colorectal screening consistently indicate that screening using any of the recommended programs is cost effective starting at age 50 and continuing to age 85.[268-274] Colorectal cost-effectiveness is inversely related to CRC incidence rates; groups with high rates have lower cost-effectiveness ratios. In the United States, CRC incidence varies dramatically among ethnic and racial groups.[275] However, screening of each of the four major racial or ethnic groups in America (Blacks, Whites, Asians, and Latinos) is cost effective starting at age 50.

PRIMARY PREVENTION OF CRC
Chemoprevention

Chemoprevention is a form of primary prevention. It involves the use of specific chemical agents to prevent, inhibit, or reverse carcinogenesis. Chemoprevention can occur at any point in the carcinogenesis pathway, either early—during the formation of an adenoma—or late—during the progression of a villous adenoma to invasive cancer. Chemopreventive agents are given to prevent cancer, not to treat invasive disease. This review focuses on compounds, rather than dietary manipulations, administered to prevent colorectal carcinogenesis.

Chemoprevention agents must share certain properties to be useful. They are designed for chronic consumption by healthy patients and therefore must have few if any side effects at an efficacious dose. They should be inexpensive. They should require convenient dosages (one-a-day oral doses) to encourage patient compliance.

Colorectal chemoprevention clinical trials are complicated by the impracticality of the logical end point—the development of cancer. The duration of studies required, sample sizes necessary, cost, and ethical considerations make the use of CRC development as an end point untenable. Instead, surrogate end points are used to establish effectiveness. Acceptable criteria for surrogate end-point biomarkers include fitting the expected biologic mechanisms, reliable and quantitative assessment, easy measurement, and correlation with decreased cancer incidence. To be valid, however, surrogate end point biomarkers need to accurately represent events involved in the process of carcinogenesis. When an intervention such as a chemopreventive agent is used, there should be a clear relationship between the agent, modulation of the biomarker, and the development of cancer. Surrogate end points for cancer should ideally be validated in the context of clinical studies that use cancer as the ultimate end point. The surrogate end point biomarker must also occur at sufficient incidence to allow statistically significant differences between control and test subjects to be determined. Colorectal carcinogenesis trials frequently assess adenoma incidence in groups at increased risk for CRC as the primary end point. The use of adenoma as an end point allows for shorter, smaller, and less expensive trials.

Investigators have searched for alternative end points with shorter latency than the development of adenomas. The potential utility of proliferation indices is suggested by the association of CRC with hyperproliferation in colonic epithelial mucosa. This association has led to the investigation of proliferation biomarkers such as DNA labeling, proliferation cell nuclear antigen (PCNA), and Ki-67 as intermediate biomarkers by correlating their levels with increasing severity of dysplasia in adenomas.

Markers of proliferation, however, may not correlate with actual neoplasia. Sandler and associates obtained rectal mucosal biopsy specimens from 333 participants in a randomized controlled chemoprevention trial of calcium supplementation to determine whether labeling index was correlated with concurrent or future colorectal neoplasia.[276] They found that a labeling index assayed using PCNA immunohistochemistry did not predict future neoplasia, although it was weakly associated with the presence of current adenomas. They concluded that although it may be attractive to include measurement of intermediate markers in large controlled trials, better-proven and more reliable intermediates, such as adenomas, should be relied upon until it is possible to be more confident about the performance of intermediate markers.

The list of potential chemopreventive agents will grow dramatically in the upcoming years. In vitro assays that assess the ability of compounds to prevent mutagenesis of CRC cell lines have been developed. Promising agents undergo preclinical studies in rodents. Agents are given to rodents who develop colorectal neoplasia as a result of either a germline knockout mutation (e.g., mice who lack the murine APC gene) or the administration of a carcinogen (e.g., intraperitoneal dimethylhydrazine). In the later case, the appropriate carcinogen dose and treatment schedule are selected to ensure that the effectiveness of the chemopreventive agent can be evaluated accurately and not masked by carcinogen toxicity. Animals are typically given between 40% and 80% of the maximum tolerated dose of a potential chemopreventive agent and then sacrificed, and the prevalence of colorectal neoplasia is assessed. Frequently, aberrant crypt foci are chosen as a surrogate end-point biomarker to optimize the power of statistical analyses. Promising agents are considered for clinical trials.

Chemopreventive Agents

Aspirin and nonsteroidal antiinflammatory agents

Aspirin (ASA) and NSAIDs are the most widely studied agents for the chemoprevention of CRC. These agents inhibit cyclooxygenase-1 (COX-1) and cyclooxygenase-2 (COX-2), enzymes involved in prostaglandin synthesis. COX-1 is constitutively expressed by mucosal cells. In contrast, COX-2 is undetectable in normal tissues but is induced by cytokines, growth factors, and mitogens and therefore contributes to the synthesis of prostaglandins in inflamed and neoplastic tissues.[277,278] COX-2 is elevated in up to 90% of sporadic CRCs and 40% of colonic adenomas but is not elevated in normal colonic epithelium. Increased levels of COX-2 are found in patients with FAP and in experimentally induced colon tumors in rodents.

The NSAIDs indomethacin and piroxicam consistently prevent carcinogen-induced intestinal cancer in animals. The anticancer effect is reversible; the incidence of tumors increases shortly after the agent is discontinued.[279] Furthermore, knocking out the COX-2 gene or administering pharmacologic inhibitors of COX-2 in murine models of FAP significantly reduces the number of intestinal polyps.[280]

A series of case-control studies demonstrated a 40% to 50% reduction in the risk of colonic neoplasia among patients who took aspirin.[281] Prospective cohort studies indicated that long-term NSAID nearly halved the risk of CRC.[282-285] A population-based retrospective study indicated that NSAID use was associated with a 39% reduction in CRC. The duration of use but not daily dose of NSAIDs appears to be an important factor for chemoprevention. The protective effect is shared by most NSAIDs and is not confined to a small number of these drugs.[286]

Randomized trials of NSAIDs used to prevent colorectal neoplasia have involved patients with FAP and also patients at average risk for CRC. In patients with FAP, 6 months of twice-daily treatment with celecoxib, a COX-2 inhibitor, reduced the number of polyps by 28% and reduced the polyp burden (sum of polyp diameters) by 31% without increased adverse events.[287] Similar results were seen in trials using sulindac in FAP patients.[288,289] No patient had complete resolution of polyps. The benefit of NSAIDs was transient; an increase in the number and size of polyps has been noted in patients 3 months after NSAIDs were discontinued.[287,289] The agents neither eliminate the polyp predisposition nor prevent the development of CRC in FAP patients.[290] The current standard of care of FAP patients remains surgical removal of the colon and rectum.

The use of NSAIDs in patients at average or moderate increased risk of CRC is tenable and has been prospectively studied. Low-dose aspirin, however, was not found to be associated with a substantial reduction in the incidence of CRC during 5 years of randomized treatment and 12 years of follow-up.[291,292] It is possible that the negative findings of this study may be the result of the short treatment period (5 years) and short duration of follow-up (12 years). Prospective studies indicate that little or no risk reduction is evident until 10 or more years of aspirin use.[293] Selective COX-2 inhibitors have been shown in an endoscopically controlled study to cause less injury to the mucosa of the upper gastrointestinal tract than nonselective NSAIDs.[283] These agents are currently being studied in nonpolyposis patients.

Calcium

Dietary patterns have repeatedly been associated with the risk of CRC neoplasia. Diets high in fruits and vegetables are associated with lower risk, whereas diets high in animal fat and red meat are associated with higher risk.[294] The potential chemopreventive activity of calcium was originally suggested by epidemiologic studies that reported an inverse relationship between intake of vitamin D and calcium and CRC.[295,296] Animal and in vitro data indicated that excess amounts of free bile acids and unabsorbed fatty acids promote carcinogenesis by irritating and damaging the colonic mucosa, which induces compensatory proliferation. Indeed, the concentration of serum deoxycholic acid correlates with the presence of colorectal adenomas.[297] Newmark and associates proposed that calcium binds to bile acids in the gut, inhibiting their proliferative and carcinogenic effects.[298] Animal studies indicate that calcium inhibits dietary fat–promoted colon carcinogenesis.[299,300]

Calcium is also involved in cellular differentiation, proliferation, apoptosis, and intracellular and intercellular signaling. Before the development of human colonic neoplasms, colonic epithelial cells showed altered growth and differentiation. Colonic crypt proliferation is inhibited by increased extracellular calcium in vitro. The growth inhibition induced by high levels of extracellular calcium is lost at a stage in tumor development before cells become malignant.[301] The suggested protective role of calcium in vitro is corroborated by its ability to reduce the proliferative activity of the colonic mucosa in animal models[300-302] and in high-risk groups with hereditary colon cancer.[303] Some, but not all, studies in humans who consumed high-calcium diets or receiving calcium supplements have shown a decreased proliferation of colorectal epithelial cells and favorable changes in bile acid composition. In some studies, calcium supplementation normalized the distribution of proliferating cells in the colonic crypt without affecting the rate of proliferating cells in the colorectal mucosa.[304] The potential beneficial effects of calcium have not been uniformly observed, however, [296] and studies of the effects of calcium on the rectal mucosa have not always demonstrated a reduction in the rate of proliferation.[305]

Randomized trials have yielded encouraging data. Patients supplemented with 1200 mg of nonfat dairy products demonstrated decreased numbers of proliferating cells throughout the crypts in comparison with controls.[306] These changes were small but statistically significant. In addition, biopsy specimens from the supplemented group showed significantly reduced expression of the dedifferentiation marker cytokeratin AE1.

A randomized double-blind trial of 930 patients supplemented with either 1200 mg of calcium carbonate or placebo found a moderate but significant reduction (relative risk of .85) in the development of colorectal polyps over a 4-year period.[307] The protective effect of calcium was observed as early as 1 year after supplementation began, thus suggesting that calcium acts very early in the pathway of colorectal carcinogenesis.

Difluoromethylornithine

The majority of chemopreventive agents studied at this time represent agents used in routine clinical practice. Rapid progress in the field of chemoprevention makes it likely that unfamiliar agents will soon enter clinical trials. At this time, difluoromethylornithine (DFMO), a polyamine synthesis inhibitor, represents one such agent with significant promise for CRC chemoprevention.[308]

The strong association between high levels of polyamines and rapid proliferation in eukaryotes was recognized 30 years ago.[309,310] Polyamine contents are often elevated in rodent and human neoplastic cells or tissues. This is particularly true in the case of colorectal neoplasia in comparison with normal adjacent mucosa.[311-313] DFMO inhibits ornithine decarboxylase (ODC), the first enzyme in mammalian polyamine synthesis. Ornithine decarboxylase is one target gene for the transcriptional transactivation by the *c-myc* oncogene,[314,315] and it was predicted that inhibition of polyamine synthesis would be a successful strategy for cancer treatment.[316] DFMO is a cytostatic drug, thus causing a reduction in the rate of cell proliferation in the absence of cell death. The mechanism of cancer prevention by DFMO probably involves more than simple inhibition of cell proliferation. Studies in animals suggest that DFMO acts late in models of chemical carcinogenesis and affects the transition of noninvasive tumors to invasive cancers.[317] DFMO suppresses both the increased polyamine content and tumorigenesis in a murine model of FAP.[318]

Side effects from DFMO include gastrointestinal upset and reversible hearing changes. These have not been observed, however, at the doses proposed for long-term chemoprevention.[308] Treatment of humans with DFMO causes suppression of the polyamines putrescine and spermidine content in colonocytes because the intracellular pools of these compounds depend on ODC activity.[319] DFMO lowers polyamines in rectal mucosa and does so in a dose-dependent manner without a rebound increase in polyamine levels after discontinuation of the drug.[320,321] The end points of this study were polyamine levels, not colonic neoplasia. However, a recent case-control study of patients with colon cancer indicates that increases in mucosal polyamine levels are significantly associated with risk (odds ratio, 4.8).[322] This study provides compelling evidence for validating polyamines as biomarkers for identifying high-risk individuals and as intermediate end points in colon cancer prevention trials.

Although DFMO is a potent inhibitor of epithelial carcinogenesis, it does not completely suppress tumorigenesis in animal models. Consequently, combination therapy of DFMO with other agents is being undertaken. A clinical trial that combines DFMO with the NSAIA sulindac is under way at this time.

Folate

Folate is a micronutrient that is essential for regenerating the amino acid methionine, the methyl donor for DNA methylation, and for producing the purines and pyrimidines necessary for DNA synthesis.[323] Folate-deficient rats demonstrate heightened sensitivity to carcinogens.[324] Low dietary folate intake has emerged as a possible risk factor for colorectal neoplasia in case-control studies.[325-330] Prospective studies, two in men and one in women, suggest that inadequate intake of folate increases colon cancer risk.[331-334] The Nurses' Health Study found that folate from dietary sources alone was related to a modest reduction in risk for colon cancer.[332] The benefit of long-term multivitamins containing folate was present across all levels of dietary intakes and pronounced after 15 years of use. The long time needed for a clinical benefit to become evident suggests that folate acts early in the pathway of colorectal carcinogenesis. The Health Professionals' Study cohort also suggested that folate supplementation was inversely related to colon cancer risk, whereas dietary folate was not.[333] Neither dietary nor supplemental folate protected against the development of colorectal adenomas during short-term study (less than 4 years).[334,335]

Epidemiologic studies have consistently indicated an inverse relationship between intake of fruits and vegetables or their antioxidant nutrients (vitamins C and E and carotenoids) and cancers at various sites.[336] Multivitamin components other than folate have been evaluated in several case-control and cohort studies. These studies have failed to discover any protective effect of beta-carotene or vitamins A, C, D, or E against colorectal neoplasia.[332,337,338] There are several reasons why studies that focus on a specific micronutrient may provide conflicting results. Dissimilar populations may be studied; the diet of one population may be frankly deficient in a certain micronutrient. Alternatively, a certain population may have a higher susceptibility to the carcinogenic effects of micronutrient deficiency. In the case of folate metabolism, for example, a functional polymorphism in the folate-metabolizing enzyme methylene tetrahydrofolate reductase has been associated with a 50% reduction in colon cancer risk.[339] Another population may be more likely to engage in behavior (e.g., smoking) that interacts with micronutrient intake. Most important, the period of follow-up may be insufficient to assess the effectiveness of an intervention over several decades.[340]

Hormone Replacement Therapy

Case-control studies indicate an inverse relationship between hormone replacement therapy (HRT) and colonic neoplasia.[341-343] Two recent metaanalyses found an aggregate reduction in the risk of CRC of 15% to 20% with HRT.[344,345] The suggested protective effect was greatest in more recently published studies and greatest among current or recent users and among users of more than 5 years, compared with short-term users.[344] The mechanism by which HRT may reduce colorectal risk remains unclear. HRT use may alter bile acid composition to decrease the proportion of secondary bile acids that may promote carcinogenesis[346] and modulate cancer risk through upregulation of estrogen receptor gene expression.[347] Definitive evidence that HRT reduces CRC risk awaits the report of data from randomized clinical trials.

Other Agents

New chemopreventive agents are being actively sought. Urosidal (a modulator of bile acid composition)[348] and oltipraz (an inducer of the mutagen-detoxification enzyme glutathione S-transferase)[349] are being evaluated in animals and humans. Additional agents are being sought that have the ability to prevent mutagenesis of cultured cells. Those agents effective at preventing mutagenesis at low doses proceed through animal and then clinical evaluations.

In summary, prospective trials indicate that aspirin and other NSAIDs, supplemental calcium and folate, and postmenopausal HRT each have a protective effect on the development of CRC. The value of these chemopreventive agents, however, has not been confirmed in double-blind, placebo-controlled randomized studies. These trials are essential to prove effectiveness and also to determine the potential side effects of long-term ingestion of any chemopreventive agents. This consideration applies to both drug therapies (aspirin, NSAIDs, HRT) and micronutrient supplementation (calcium). Until these studies are completed, colorectal chemoprevention cannot be accepted as a standard medical practice. Patients who elect to use a chemopreventative agent must understand that such use does not in any way alter the need for secondary prevention according to published guidelines depending on risk stratification.

REFERENCES

1. Chapuis PH, Dent OF, Fisher R, et al: A multivariate analysis of clinical and pathological variables in prognosis after resection of large bowel cancer. *Br J Surg* 1985;72:698-702.

2. Newland RC, Dent OF, Lyttle MN, et al: Pathologic determinants of survival associated with colorectal cancer with lymph node metastases: a multivariate analysis of 579 patients. *Cancer* 1994;73:2076-2082.

3. Scott NA, Wieand HS, Moertel CG, et al: Colorectal cancer, Dukes' stage, tumor site, preoperative plasma CEA level, and patient prognosis related to tumor DNA ploidy pattern. *Arch Surg* 1987;122:1375-1379.

4. Wiggers T, Arends J, Volovics A: Regression analysis of prognostic factors in colorectal cancer after curative resections. *Dis Colon Rectum* 1988;31:33-41.

5. Freedman L, Macaskill P, Smith A: Multivariate analysis of prognostic factors for operable rectal cancer. *Lancet* 1984;11:733-736.

6. Griffin MR, Bergstralh EJ, Coffey RJ, et al: Predictors of survival after curative resection of carcinoma of the colon and rectum. *Cancer* 1987;60:2318-2324.

7. Fisher ER, Sass R, Palekar A, et al: Dukes' classification revisited: findings from the national surgical adjuvant breast and bowel projects (Protocol R-01). *Cancer* 1989;64:2354-2360.

8. Hermanek P, Guggenmoos-Holzmann I, Gall FP: Prognostic factors in rectal carcinoma, a contribution to the further development of tumor classification. *Dis Colon Rectum* 1989;32:593-599.

9. Ruschoff J, Bittinger A, Neumann K, et al: Prognostic significance of nucleolar organizing regions (NORs) in carcinomas of the signoid colon and rectum. *Pathol Res Pract* 1990;186:85-91.

10. Robey-Cafferty SS, el-Naggar AK, Grignon DJ, et al: Histologic parameters and DNA ploidy as predictors of survival in stage B adenocarcinoma of colon and rectum. *Mod Pathol* 1990;3:261-266.

11. Bottger TC, Potratz D, Stockle M, et al: Prognostic value of DNA analysis in colorectal carcinoma. *Cancer* 1993;72:3579-3587.

12. Deans GT, Patterson CC, Parks GT, et al: Colorectal carcinoma: importance of clinical and pathological factors in survival. *Ann R Coll Surg Engl* 1994;76:59-64.

13. D'Eredita G, Seerio G, Neri V, et al: A survival refression analysis of prognostic factors in colorectal cancer. *Aust N Z J Surg* 1996;66:445-451.

14. Cooper HS: Surgical pathology of endoscopically removed malignant polyps of the colon and rectum. *Am J Surg Pathol* 1983;7:613-623.

15. Cranley JP, Petras RE, Carey WD, et al: When is endoscopic polypectomy adequate therapy for colonis polyps containing invasive cancer? *Gastroenterology* 1988;91:419-427.

16. Richards WO, Webb WA, Morris SJ, et al: Patient management after endoscopic removal of the cancerous colon adenoma. *Ann Surg* 1987;207:665-670.

17. Coverlizza S, Risio M, Ferrari A, et al: Colorectal adenomas containing invasive carcinoma: pathologic assessment of lymph node metastatic potential. *Cancer* 1989;64:1937-1947.

18. Muller S, Chesner IM, Egan MJ, et al: Significance of venous and lymphatic invasion in malignant polyps of the colon and rectum. *Gut* 1989;30:1385-1391.

19. Cooper HS, Deppisch LM, Gourly WK, et al: Endoscopically removed malignant colorectal polyps: clinicopathologic correlations. *Gastroenterology* 1995;108:1657-1665.

20. Compton C, Fenoglio-Preiser CM, Pettigrew N, et al: American Joint Committee on Cancer Prognostic Factors Consensus Conference: Colorectal working group. *Cancer* 2000;88:1739-1757.

21. Wanebo HJ, Rao B, Pinsky CM, et al: Preoperative carcinoembryonic antigen level as a prognostic indicator in colorectal cancer. *N Engl J Med* 1978;299:448-451.

22. Wolmark N, Fisher B, Wieand HS, et al: The significance of preoperative carcinoembryonic antigen levels in colorectal cancer. *Ann Surg* 1984;199:375-382.

23. Onetto M, Paganuzzi M, Secco GB, et al: Preoperative carcinoembryonic antigen and prognosis in patients with colorectal cancer. *Biomed Pharmacother* 1985;39:392-395.

24. Scott NA, Wieand HS, Moertel CG, et al: Colorectal cancer, Dukes' stage, tumor site, preopeative plasma CEA level, and patient prognosis related to tumor DNA ploidy pattern. *Arch Surg* 1987;122:1375-1379.

25. Wiggers T, Arends J, Volovics A: Regression analysis of prognostic factors in colorectal cancer after curative resections. *Dis Colon Rectum* 1988;31:33-41.

26. Harrison LE, Guillem JG, Paty P, et al: Preoperative carcinoembryonic antigen predicts outcomes in node-negative colon cancer patients: a multivariate analysis of 572 patients. *J Am Coll Surg* 1997;185:55-59.

27. Mulcahy HE, Skelly MM, Husain A, et al: Long-term outcome following curative surgery for malignant large bowel obstruction. *Br J Surg* 1996;83:46-50.

28. Knusen JB, Nilsson T, Sprechler M, et al: Venous and nerve invasion as prognostic factors in postoperative survival of patients with resectable cancer of the rectum. *Dis Colon Rectum* 1983;26:613-617.

29. Michelassi F, Block GE, Vannussi L, et al: A 5- to 21-year follow-up and analysis of 250 patients with rectal adenocarcinoma. *Ann Surg* 1988; 208:379-389.

30. Shirouzu K, Isomoto H, Kakegawa T: Prognostic evaluation of perineural invasion in rectal cancer. *Am J Surg* 1993;165:233-237.

31. Jass JR: Lymphocytic infiltration and survival in rectal cancer. *J Clin Pathol* 1986;39:585-589.

32. Halvorsen TB, Seim E: Association between invasiveness, inflammatory reaction, desmoplasia and survival in colorectal cancer. *J Clin Pathol* 1989;42:162-166.

33. Nori D, Merimsky O, Saw D, et al: Tumor ploidy as a risk factor for disease recurrence and short survival in surgically treated Dukes' b2 colon cancer patients. *Tumour Biol* 1996;17:75-80.

34. Jen J, Kim H, Piantadosi S, et al: Allelic loss of chromosome 18q and prognosis in colorectal cancer. *N Engl J Med* 1994;331:213-221.

35. Kato M, Ito Y, Kobayashi S, et al: Detection of DCC and Ki-ras gene alterations in colorectal carcinoma tissue as prognostic markers for liver metastatic recurrence. *Cancer* 1996;77:1729-1735.

36. Landis SH, Murray T, Bolden S, et al: Cancer statistics, 1998. *CA Cancer J Clin* 1998;48:6-30.

37. Parker SL, Davis KJ, Wingo PA: Cancer statistics by race and ethnicity. *CA Cancer J Clin* 1998;48:31-48.

38. Chen VW, Fenoglio-Preiser CM, Wu XC, et al: Aggressiveness of colon carcinoma in Blacks and Whites. *Cancer Epidemiol Biomarkers Prev* 1997;6:1087-1093.

39. Ries LAG, Kosary CL, Hankey BF, editors: *SEER Cancer Statistics Review, 1973-1994.* NIH Publication No. 97-2789. Bethesda, MD, National Cancer Institute, NIH, 1997.

40. Fearon ER, Vogelstein B: A genetic model for colorectal tumorigenesis. *Cell* 1990;61:759-767.

41. Muir C, Waterhouse J, Mack T, editors: *Cancer in the Five Continents,* vol 5. Lyon, France, International Agency for Research on Cancer, scientific publication number 88, 1992.

42. Haenszel W, Berg JW, Segi M, et al: Large-bowel cancer in Hawaiian Japanese. *J Natl Cancer Inst* 1973;6:1765-1779.

43. McMichael AJ, Giles G: Cancer in migrants to Australia: extending the descriptive epidemiological data. *Can Res* 1988;48:751-756.

44. Staszewski J, McCall MG, Stenhouse NS: Cancer mortality in 1962-66 among Polish migrants to Australia. *Br J Cancer* 1971;25:599-610.

45. Lichtenstein P, Holm NV, Verkasalo PK, et al: Environmental and heritable factors in the casusation of cancer. *N Engl J Med* 2000;343:78-85.

46. Keefe K, Meyskens FL Jr: Cancer prevention. In Abeloff MD et al, editors: *Clinical Oncology.* New York, Churchill Livingstone, 2000.

47. Giovanucci E, Rimm EB, Stampfer MJ, et al: Intake of fat, meat, and fiber in relation to risk of colon cancer in men. *Cancer Res* 1994;54:2390-2397.

48. Willett WC, Stampfer MJ, Colditz GA, et al: Relation of meat, fat, and fiber intake to the risk of colon cancer in a prospective study among women. *N Engl J Med* 1990;264:2648-2653.

49. Goldbohm RA, van den Brandt PA, van't Veer P, et al: A prospective cohort study on the relation between meat consumption and the risk of colon cancer. *Cancer Res* 1994;54:718-723.

50. Bostick RM, Potter JD, Kushi LH, et al: Sugar, meat, and fat intake, and non-dietary risk factors for colon cancer incidence in Iowa women (United States). *Cancer Causes Control* 1994;5:38-52.

51. Thun MJ, Calle EE, Namboodiri MM, et al: Risk factors for fatal colon cancer in a large prospective study [see comments]. *J Natl Cancer Inst* 1992;84:1491-1500.

52. Voskuil DW, Kmpman E, Grubben MJ, et al: Meat consumption and preparation and genetic susceptibility in relation for colorectal adenomas. *Cancer Lett* 1997;114:309-311.

53. Sugimura T: Carcinogenicity of mutagenic heterocylic amines formed during the cooking process. *Mutat Res* 1985;150:33-41.

54. Burkitt DP: Some neglected leads to cancer causation. *J Natl Cancer Inst* 1971;47:913-919.

55. Alberts DS, Martinez ME, Roe DJ, et al: Lack of effect of a high-fiber cereal supplement on the recurrence of colorectal adenomas. *N Engl J Med* 2000;342:1156-1162.

56. Howe GR, Benito E, Castelleto R, et al: Dietary intake of fiber and decreased risk of cancers of the colon and rectum: evidence from the combined analysis of 13 case-control studies [see comments]. *J Natl Cancer Inst* 1992;84:1887-1896.

57. Potter JD: Colorectal cancer: molecules and populations. *J Natl Cancer Inst* 1999;91:916-932.

58. Giovannucci E, Stampfer MJ, Colditz GA, et al: Multivitamin use, folate, and colon cancer in women in the Nurses' Health Study. *Ann Intern Med* 1998;129:517-524.

59. Martinez ME, Willett WC: Calcium, vitamin D, and colorectal cancer: a review of the epidemiologic evidence. *Cancer Epidemiol Biomarkers Prev* 1998;7:163-168.

60. Fuchs CS, Giovannucci EL, Colditz GA, et al: Dietary fiber and the risk of colorectal cancer and adenoma in women. *N Engl J Med* 1999;340:169-176.

61. Platz EA, Giovannucci E, Rimm EB, et al: Dietary fiber and distal colorectal adenomas in men. *Cancer Epidemiol Biomarkers Prev* 1997;6:661-670.

62. McKeown-Eyssen GE, Bright-See E, Bruce WR, et al: A randomized trial of a low fat high fibre diet in the recurrence of colorectal polyps. *J Clin Epidemiol* 1994;47:525-536.

63. MacLennan R, Macrae F, Bain C, et al: Randomized trial of intake of fat, fiber, and beta carotene to prevent colorectal adenomas: the Australian Polyp Prevention Project. *J Natl Cancer Inst* 1995;87:1760-1766.

64. Schatzkin A, Lanza E, Corle D, et al: Lack of effect of a low-fat high-fiber diet on the recurrence of colorectal adenomas. *N Engl J Med* 2000;342:1149-1155.

65. Ornish D: High-fiber diet and colorectal adenomas. *N Engl J Med* 2000;343:736.

66. Davis BM: High-fiber diet and colorectal adenomas. *N Engl J Med* 2000;343:736.

67. Giovanucci E, Martinez ME: Tobacco, colorectal cancer, and adenomas: a review of the evidence. *J Natl Cancer Inst* 1996;88:1717-1730.

68. Martinez ME, Giovanucci E, Spiegelman D, et al: Leisure-time physical activity, body size, and colon cancer in women: Nurses' Health Study Research Group. *J Natl Cancer Inst* 1997;89:948-955.

69. Giovanucci E, Ascherio A, Rimm EB, et al: Physical activity, obesity, and risk for colon cancer and adenoma in men. *Ann Intern Med* 1995;122:327-334.

70. Cunningham C, Dunlop MG: Genetics of colorectal cancer. *Br Med Bull* 1994;50:640-655.

71. Weinberg RA: Oncogenes, antioncogenes, and the molecular bases of multistep carcinogenesis. *Cancer Res* 1989;49:3713-3721.

72. Vogelstein B, Fearon ER, Hamilton SR, et al: Genetic alterations during colorectal tumor development. *N Engl J Med* 1988;319:525-532.

73. Weinberg RA: Oncogenes and tumor suppressor genes. *Cancer J Clin* 1994;44:160-170.

74. Ephrussi B, Davidson RL, Weiss MC, et al: Malignancy of somatic cell hybrids. *Nature* 1969;224:1314-1316.

75. Harris H: The analysis of malignancy by cell fusion: the position in 1988. *Cancer Res* 1988;48:3302-3306.

76. Stanbridge EJ, Der CJ, Doerson CJ, et al: Human cell hybrids: analysis of transformation and tumorigenicity. *Science* 1982;215:252-259.

77. Knudson AG Jr: Antioncogenes and human cancer. *Proc Natl Acad Sci USA* 1993;90:10914-10921.

78. Knudson AG Jr: Hereditary cancer, oncogenes, and anti-oncogenes. *Cancer Res* 1985;45:1437-1443.

79. Knudson AG Jr: Mutation and cancer: statistical study of retinoblastoma. *Proc Natl Acad Sci USA* 1971;68:820-823.

80. Goodllad RA, Levi S, Lee CY, et al: Morphometry and cell proliferation in endoscopic biopsies: evaluation of a technique. *Gastroenterology* 1991;101:1235-1241.

81. Maskens AP, Deschner EE: Tritiated thymidine incorporation into epithelial cells of normal-appearing colorectal mucosa of cancer patients. *J Natl Cancer Inst* 1977;58:1221-1224.

82. Welberg JWM, De Vries EGE, Hardonk MJ, et al: Proliferation rate of colonic mucosa in normal subjects and patients with colonic neoplasms: a refined immunohistochemical method *J Clin Pathol* 1990;43:453-456.

83. Kubben FJGM, Peeters-Haesevoets A, Engels LGJB, et al: Proleferating cell nuclear antigen (PCNA): a new marker to study human colonic cell proliferation. *Gut* 1994;35:530-535.

84. Korsmeyer SJ: Bcl-2 initiates a new category of oncogenes: regulators of cell death. *Blood* 1992;80:879-886.

85. Jen J, Powell SM, Papadopoulos N, et al: Molecular determinants of dysplasia in colorectal lesions. *Cancer Res* 1994;54:5523.

86. Fearon ER: K-ras gene mutation as a pathogenetic and diagnostic marker in human cancer. *J Natl Cancer Inst* 1993;85:1978.

87. Smith AJ, Stern HS, Penner M, et al: Somatic APC and K-ras mutations in aberrant crypt foci from human colons. *Cancer Res* 1994;54:5527-5530.

88. Pretlow TP, Barrow BJ, Ashton WS, et al: Aberrant crypts: putative neoplastic foci in colonic mucosa. *Cancer Res* 1991;51:1564-1567.

89. Roncucci L, Medline A, Bruce WR: Classification of aberrant crypt foci and microadenomas in human colon. *Cancer Epidemiol Biomarkers Prev* 1991;1:57-60.

90. Risio M, Coverlizza S, Ferrari A, et al: Immunohistochemical study of epithelial cell proliferation in hyperplastic polyps, adenomas, and adenocarcinomas of the large bowel. *Gastroenterology* 1988;94:899-906.

91. Enblad P, Busch C, Carlsson U, et al: The adenoma-carcinoma sequence in rectal adenomas: support by the expression of blood group substances and carcinoma antigens. *Am J Clin Pathol* 1988;90:121-130.

92. Nitta Y, Suzuki K, Kohli Y, et al: Early progression stage of malignancy of human colon border-line adenoma as revealed by immunohistochemical demonstration of increased DNA-instability. *Eur J Histochem* 1993;37:207-218.

93. Kozuka S, Nogaki M, Ozeki T, et al: Premalignancy of the mucosal polyp in the large intestine: estimation of the periods required for malignant transformation of mucosal polyps. *Dis Colon Rectum* 1975;18:494-500.

94. Winawer SJ, Zauber AG, Ho MN, et al: Prevention of colorectal cancer by colonoscopic polypectomy. *N Engl J Med* 1993;329:1977-1981.

95. Rickert RR, Auerbach O, Garfinkel MA, et al: Adenomatous lesions of the large bowel: an autopsy survey. *Cancer* 1979;43:1847-1857.

96. Arminski TC, McLean DW: Incidence and distribution of adenomatous polyps of the colon and rectum based on 1000 autopsy examinations. *Dis Colon Rectum* 1964;7:249-261.

97. Blatt LJ: Polyps of the colon and rectum: incidence and distribution. *Dis Colon Rectum* 1961;4:277-282.

98. Rex DK, Lehman GA, Ulbright TM, et al: Colonic neoplasia in asymptomatic persons with negative fecal occult blood tests: influence of age, gender, and family history. *Am J Gastroenterol* 1993;88:825-831.

99. Bernstein MA, Feczko PJ, Halpert RD, et al: Distribution of colonic polyps: increased incidence of proximal lesions in older patients. *Radiology* 1985;155:35-38.

100. Eide TJ, Stalsberg H: Polyps of the large intestine in northern Norway. *Cancer* 1978;42:2839-2848.

101. Eide TJ: Risk of colorectal cancer in adenoma-bearing individuals within a defined population. *Int J Cancer* 1986;38:173-176.

102. O'Brien MJ, Winawer SJ, Zauber AG, et al: The National Polyp Study: patient and polyp characteristics associated with high-grade dysplasia in colorectal adenomas. *Gastroenterology* 1990;98:371-379.

103. Waye JD, Lewis BS, Frankel A, et al: Small colon polyps. *Am J Gastroenterol* 1988;83:120-122.

104. Hoff G, Foerster A, Vatn MH, et al: Epidemiology of polyps in the rectum and colon: recovery and evaluation of unresected polyps 2 years after detection. *Scand J Gastroenterol* 1986;21:853-862.

105. Ueyama T, Kawamoto K, Iwashita I, et al: Natural history of minute sessile colonic adenomas based on radiographic findings: is endoscopic removal of every colonic adenoma necessary? *Dis Colon Rectum* 1995;38:268-272.

106. Muto T, Bussey HJR, Morson BC: The evolution of cancer of the colon and rectum. *Cancer* 1975;36:2251-2270.

107. Morson BC: Evolution of cancer of the colon and rectum. *Cancer* 1974;34:845-849.

108. Atkin WS, Morson BC, Kuzick J: Long-term risk of colorectal cancer after excision of rectosigmoid adenomas. *N Engl J Med* 1992;326:658-662.

109. Fenoglio CM, Lane N: The anatomic precursor of colorectal carcinoma. *Cancer* 1974;34:819-823.

110. Troncale F, Hertz R, Lipkin M: Nucleic acid metabolism in proliferating and differentiating colon cells of man and in neoplastic lesions of the colon. *Cancer Res* 1971;31:463-467.

111. Hayashi T, Yatani R, Apostol J: The pathogenesis of hyperplastic polyps of the colon: a hypothesis based on ultrastructural and in vitro cell kinetics. *Gastroenterology* 1974;66:347-356.

112. Fraser GM, Niv Y: Editorial: hyperplastic polyp and colonic neoplasia: is there an association? *J Clin Gastroenterol* 1993;16:278-280.

113. Martinez ME, McPherson RS, Levin B, et al: A case-control study of dietary intake and other lifestyle risk factors for hyperplastic polyps. *Gastroenterology* 1997; 113:423-429.

114. Bengoecha O, Martinez-Penuela JM, Larrinaga B, et al: Hyperplastic polyposis of the colorectum and adenocarcinoma in a 24-year old man. *Am J Surg Pathol* 1987;11:323-327.

115. Urbanski SJ, Kossakowska AE, Marcon N, et al: Mixed hyperplastic adenomatous polyps: an underdiagnosed entity. *Am J Surg Pathol* 1984;8: 551-556.

116. Cooper HS, Patchefsky AS, Marks G: Adenomatous changes within hyperplastic colonic epithelium. *Dis Colon Rectum* 1979;22:152-156.

117. Estrada RE, Spujt HJ: Hyperplastic polyps of the large bowel. *Am J Surg Pathol* 1980;4:127-133.

118. Foutch PG, DiSario JA, Pardy K, et al: The sentinel hyperplastic polyp: a marker for synchronous neoplasia in the proximal colon. *Am J Gastroenterol* 1989;84:1482-1485.

119. Bensen SP, Cole BF, Mott LA, et al: Colorectal hyperplastic polyps and risk of recurrence of adenomas and hyperplastic polyps. *Lancet* 1999; 354:1873-1874.

120. Goelz SE, Vogelstein B, Hamilton SR, et al: Hypomethylation of DNA from benign and malignant human colon neoplasms. *Science* 1985;228:187-190.

121. Powell SM, Zilz N, Beazer-Barclay Y, et al: APC mutations occur early during colorectal tumorigenesis. *Nature* 1992;359:235-237.

122. Nishisho I, Nakamura Y, Miyoshi Y, et al: Mutations of chromosome 5q21 genes in FAP and colorectal cancer patients. *Science* 1991;253: 665-669.

123. Kinzler KW, Nilbert MC, Vogelstein B, et al: Identification of a gene located at chromosome 5q21 that is mutated in colorectal cancers. *Science* 1991;251:1366-1370.

124. Fearon ER, Cho KR, Nigro JM, et al: Identification of a chromosome 18q gene that is altered in colorectal cancers. *Science* 1990;247:49-56.

125. Hedrick L, Cho KR, Fearon ER, et al: The DCC gene product in cellular differentiation and colorectal tumorigenesis. *Genes Dev* 1994;8:1174-1183.

126. Cho KR, Oliner JD, Simons JW, et al: The DCC gene: structural analysis and mutations in colorectal carcinomas. *Genomics* 1994;19:525-531.

127. Itoh F, Hinoda Y, Ohe M, et al: Decreased expression of DCC mRNA in human colorectal cancers. *Int J Cancer* 1993;53:260-263.

128. Delattre P, Olschwang S, Law DJ, et al: Multiple genetic alterations distinguish distal from proximal colorectal cancer. *Lancet* 1989;2:353-356.

129. Kikuchi-Yanoshita R, Konishi M, Ito S, et al: Genetic changes of both p53 alleles associated with the conversion from colorectal adenoma to early carcinoma in familial adenomatous polyposis and non-familial adenomatous polyposis patients. *Cancer Res* 1992;52:3965-3971.

130. Fearon ER, Hamilton SR, Vogelstein B: Clonal analysis of human colorectal tumors. *Science* 1987;238:193-197.

131. Baker SJ, Fearon ER, Nigro JM, et al: Chromosome 17 deletions and p53 gene mutations in colorectal carcinomas. *Science* 1989;244:217-221.

132. Ohue M, Tomita N, Monden T, et al: A frequent alteration of p53 gene in carcinoma in adenoma of colon. *Cancer Res* 1994;54:4798-4804.

133. Miyaki M, Seki M, Okamoto M, et al: Genetic changes and histopathological types in colorectal tumors from patients with adenomatous polyposis. *Cancer Res* 1990;50:7166-7173.

134. Lynch HT, Smyrk T: Hereditary non-polyposis colorectal cancer (Lynch syndrome). *Cancer* 1996;78:1149-1167.

135. Hamilton SR, Liu B, Parsons RE, et al: The molecular basis of Turcot's syndrome. *N Engl J Med* 1995;332:839-847.

136. Bodmer WC, Bailey J, Bodner H, et al: Localization of the gene for familial adenomatous polyposis on chromosome 5. *Nature* 1987; 328:614.

137. Leppert M, Dobbs M, Scambler P, et al: The gene for familial polyposis coli maps to the long arm of chromosome 5. *Science* 1987;238:1411.

138. Nakamura Y, Lathrop M, Leppert M, et al: Localization of the genetic defect in familial adenomatous polyposis within a small region of chromosome 5. *Am J Hum Genet* 1988;43:638.

139. Khan MP, Tops CM, Brock M, et al: Close linklage of a highly polymorphic marker (D5S37) to familial adenomatous polyposis (FAP) and confirmation of FAP location on 5q21–q22. *Hum Genet* 1989;79:183-188.

140. Groden J, Thliveris A, Somowitz W, et al: Identification and characterization of the familial adenomatous coli gene. *Cell* 1991;66:589.

141. Kinzler KW, Nilbert MC, Su L, et al: Identification of FAP locus genes from chromosome 5q21. *Science* 1991;253:661.

142. Nishisho I, Nakamura Y, Miyoshi Y, et al: Mutations of chromosome 5q21 genes in FAP and colorectal cancer patients. *Science* 1991;253:665.

143. Smith KJ, Johnson KA, Bryan RM, et al: The APC gene product in normal and tumor cells. *Proc Natl Acad Sci USA* 1993;90:2846.

144. Olschwang S, Tiret A, Laurent-Puig P, et al: Restriction of ocular fundus lesions to a specific subgroup of APC mutations in adenomatous polyposis coli patients. *Cell* 1993;75:959.

145. Leppert M, Burt R, Hughes JP, et al: Genetic analysis of an inherited predisposition to colon cancer in a family with a variable number of adenomatous polyps. *N Engl J Med* 1990;322:904.

146. Spirio L, Olschwang S, Groden J, et al: Alleles of the APC gene: an attenuated form of familial polyposis. *Cell* 1993;75:951.

147. Burt RW, Samowitz WS: The adenomatous polyp and the hereditary polyposis syndromes. *Gastroenterol Clin North Am* 1988;17:657.

148. Powell SM, Petersen GM, Krush AJ, et al: Molecular diagnosis of familial adenomatous polyposis. *N Engl J Med* 1993;329:1982-1987.

149. Petersen GM, Slack J, Nakamura Y: Screening guidelines and premorbid diagnosis of FAP using linkage. *Gastroenterology* 1991;100:1658-1664.

150. Petersen GM, Brensinger JD: Genetic testing and counseling in FAP. *Oncology* 1996;10:89-94.

151. Petersen GM: Genetic counseling and predictive genetic testing in FAP. *Semin Colon Rectal Surg* 1995;6:55-60.

152. Petersen GM, Botd PA: Gene tests and counseling for colorectal cancer risk: lessons from familial polyposis. In *Hereditary breast, ovarian, and colon cancer*. Journal of the National Cancer Institute monograph No.17. Washington, DC, Government Printing Office, 1995, 67-71. (NIH publication 94-03837.)

153. Wertz DC, Fanos JH, Reilly PR. Genetic testing for children and adolescents: who decides? *JAMA* 1994;272:875-881.

154. Statement of the American Society of Clinical Oncology: genetic testing for cancer susceptibility, adopted on February 20, 1996. *J Clin Oncol* 1996;14:1730-1736.

155. Giardiello FM, Brensinger JD, Petersen GM, et al: The use and interpretation of commercial APC gene testing for familial adenomatous polyposis. *N Engl J Med* 1997;336:823-827.

156. Markowitz AJ, Winawer SJ: Screening and surveillance for colorectal cancer. *Semin Oncol* 1999;26:485-498.

157. Jeghers H, McKusick VA, Kats KH: Generalized intestinal polyposis and melanin spots of the oral mucosa, lips and digits: a syndrome of diagnostic significance. *N Engl J Med* 1949;241:993-1005.

158. Jenne DE, Reimann H, Nezu J, et al: Peutz-Jeghers syndrome is caused by mutation in a novel serine threonine kinase. *Nat Genet* 1998;18:38-43.

159. Hemminki A, Markie D, Tomlinson I, et al: A serine/threonine kinase gene defective in Peutz-Jeghers syndrome. *Nature* 1998;391:184-187.

160. Giardiello FM, Welsh SB, Hamilton SR, et al: Increased risk of cancer in the Peutz-Jeghers syndrome. *N Engl J Med* 1987;316:1511-1514.

161. Spigelman AD, Murday V, Phillips RKS: Cancer and the Peutz-Jeghers syndrome. *Gut* 1989; 30:1588-1590.

162. Watanabe A, Nagashima H, Motoi M, et al: Familial juvenile polyposis of the stomach. *Gatroenterology* 1979;77:148-151.

163. Grotsky HW, Rickert RR, Smith WD, et al: Familial juvenile polyposis coli: a clinical and pathologic study of a large kindred. *Gastroenterology* 1982;82:494-501.

164. Sachatello CR, Pickren JW, Grace JT Jr: Generalized juvenile gastrointestinal polyposis: a hereditary syndrome. *Gastroenterology* 1970;58:699-708.

165. Haggitt RC, Reid BJ: Hereditary gastrointestinal polyposis syndromes. *Am J Surg Pathol* 1986;10: 871-887.

166. Jarvinen H, Franssila KO: Familial juvenile polyposis coli: increased risk of colorectal cancer. *Gut* 1984;25:792-800.

167. Lynch HR, Smyrk RC, Watson P, et al: Genetics, natural history, tumor spectrum, and pathology of hereditary nonpolyposis colorectal cancer. *Gastroenterology* 1993;104:1535.

168. Vasern HFA, Mecklin J-P, Khan PM, et al: The International Collaborative Group on Hereditary Non-Polyposis Colorctal Cancer (ICG-HNPCC). *Dis Colon Rectum* 1991;34:424-425.

169. Aarnio M, Mecklin JP, Aaltonen LA, et al: Lifetime risk of different cancers in hereditary nonpolyposis colorectal cancer (HNPCC) syndrome. *Int J Cancer* 1995;64:430-433.

170. Dunlop MG, Farrington SM, Carothers AD, et al: Cancer risk associated with germline DNA mismatch repair gene mutations. *Hum Mol Genet* 6:105-110, 1997.

171. Peel DJ, Ziogas A, Fox EA, et al: Characterization of Hereditary Nonpolyposis Colorectal Cancer families from a population-based series of cases. *J Natl Cancer Inst* 2000;92:1517-1522.

172. Lynch HT, Smyrk T, Lynch J. An update of HNPCC (Lynch syndrome) *Cancer Genet Cytogenet* 1997;93:84-99.

173. Watson P, Lin K, Rodriguez-Bigas MA, et al: Colorctal cancer survival among hereditary nonpolyposis colorectal cancer family members. *Cancer* 1998;83:259-266.

174. Fishel R, Lescoe MK, Rao MRS, et al: The human mutator gene homolog MSH2 and its association with hereditary nonpolyposis colon cancer. *Cell* 1993;75:1027.

175. Leach FS, Nicolaides NC, Papadopoulos N, et al: Mutations of a mutS homolog in hereditary nonpolyposis colorectal cancer. *Cell* 1993;75:1215.

176. Bronner CE, Baker SM, Morrison PT, et al: Mutation in the DNA mismatch repair gene homolog hMLH1 is associated with hereditary nonpolyposis colon cancer. *Nature* 1994;368:258.

177. Kolodner RD, Hall NR, Lipford J, et al: Structure of the human MLH1 locus and analysis of a large hereditary nonpolyposis colorectal carcinoma kindred for MLH1 mutations. *Cancer Res* 1995;55:242.

178. Papadopoulos N, Nicolaides NC, Wei Y-F, et al: Mutation of a mutL homolog in hereditary colon cancer. *Science* 1994;263:1625.

179. Nicolaides NC, Papadopoulos N, Lui B, et al: Mutations of two PMS homologues in hereditary nonpolyposis colorectal cancer. *Nature* 1994; 371:75.

180. Drummond JT, Li GM, Longley MJ, et al: Isolation of an hMSH2-p160 heterodimer that restores DNA mismatch repair to tumor cells. *Science* 1995;268:1909.

181. Palombo R, Gallinari P, Iaccarino I, et al: GTBP, a 160-kilodalton protein essential for mismatch-binding activity in human cells. *Science* 1995;268:1912.

182. Papadopoulos N, Nicolaides NC, Liu B, et al: Mutations of GTBP in genetically unstable cells. *Science* 1995;268:1915.

183. Lynch HT, Smyrk TC: Hereditary colon cancer. *Semin Oncol* 1999;26:478-484.

184. Aaltonen LA, Salovaara R, Kristo P, et al: Incidence of hereditary nonpolyposis colorectal cancer and the feasibility of molecular screening for the disease. *N Engl J Med* 1998;338:1481-1487.

185. Wijnen JT, Vasen HFA, Khan M, et al: Clinical findings withimpications for genetic testing in families with clustering of colorectal cancer. *N Engl J Med* 1998;339:511-518.

186. Jass JR: Colorectal adenoma progression and genetic change: is there a link? *Ann Med* 1995;27:301-306.

187. Lynch HT: Is there any role for prophylactic subtotal colectomy among hereditary nonpolyposis colorectal cancer germline mutation carriers? *Dis Colon Rectum* 1996;39:109-110.

188. Church JM: Prophylactic colectomy in patients with hereditary nonpolyposis colorectal cancer. *Ann Med* 1996;28:479-482.

189. Kristo P, et al: Incidence of hereditary nonpolyposis colorectal cancer and the feasibility of molecular screening for the disease. *N Engl J Med* 1998;338:1481-1487.

190. Lewis JD, Deren JJ, Lichtenstein GR: Cancer risk in patients with inflammatory bowel disease. *Gastroenterol Clin North Am* 1999;28:459-477.

191. Gyde SN, Prior P, Allan RN, et al: Colorectal cancer in ulcerative colitis: a cohort study of primary referrals from three centers. *Gut* 1988;29: 206-217.

192. Henricksen C, Kreiner S, Binder V: Longterm prognosis in ulcerative colitis—based on results from a regional patient group from the county of Copenhagen. *Gut* 1985;26:158-156.

193. Katzka I, Brody RS, Morris E, et al: Assessment of colorectal cancer risk in patients with ulcerative colitis: experience from a private practice. *Gastroenterology* 1983;85:22-29.

194. Axon ATR: Cancer surveillance in ulcerative colitis—a time for reappraisal. *Gut* 1994;35:587-589.

195. Langholz E, Munkholm P, Davidsen M, et al: Colorectal cancer risk and mortality in patients with ulcerative colitis. *Gastroenterology* 1992;103: 1444-1451.

196. Kewenter J, Ahlman H, Hulten L: Cancer risk in ulcerative colitis. *Ann Surg* 1978;15: 824-828.

197. Ekbom A, Helmick C, Zack M, et al: Ulcerative colitis and colorectal cancer: a population-based study. *N Engl J Med* 1990;323:1228-1233.

198. Devroede GJ, Taylor WF, Sauer WG, et al: Cancer risk and life expectancy of children with ulcerative colitis. *N Engl J Med* 1971;285: 17-21.

199. Blackstone MO, Riddell RH, Rogers BHG, et al: Dysplasia-associated lesion or mass (DALM) detected by colonoscopy in longstanding ulcerative colitis: an indication for colectomy. *Gastroenterology* 1990;99:1021-1031.

200. Bernstein CN, Shanahan F, Weinstein WM: Are we telling the patients the truth about surveillance colonoscopy in ulcerative colitis. *Lancet* 1994;343:71-74.

201. Lynch DAF, Lobo AJ, Sobala GM, et al: Failure of colonoscopic surveillance in ulcerative colitis. *Gut* 1983;34:1075-1080.

202. Lashner BA, Silverstein MD, Hanaver SB: Hazard rates for dysplasia and cancer in ulcerative colitis. *Dig Dis Sci* 1989;34:1536-1541.

203. Wollrich AJ, DaSilva MD, Korelitz BI: Surveillance in the routine mangement of ulcerative colitis: the predictive value of low-grade dysplasia. *Gastroenterology* 1992;103:431-483.

204. Gyde S: Screening for colorectal cancer in ulcerative colitis: dubious benefits and high costs. *Gut* 1990;31:1089-1092.

205. Ransohoff DF, Riddell RH, Levin B: Ulcerative colitis and colonic cancer. Problems in assessing the diagnostic usefulness of mucosal dysplasia. *Dis Colon Rectum* 1985;28:383-388.

206. Lennard-Jones JE, Melville DM, Morson BC, et al: Precancer and cancer in extensive ulcerative colitis: findings among 401 patients over 22 years. *Gut* 1990;31:800-806.

207. Provenzale D, Kowdley KV, Arora S, et al: Prophylactic colectomy or surveillance for chronic ulcerative colitis?: a decision analysis. *Gastroenterology* 1995;109:1188-1196.

208. Nugent FW, Haggitt RC, Gilpin PA: Cancer surveillance in ulcerative colitis. *Gastroenterology* 1991;100:1241-1248.

209. Manning AP, Bulgim OR, Dixon MF, et al: Screening by colonoscopy for colonic epithelial dysplasia in inflammatory bowel disease. *Gut* 1987;28:1489-1494.

210. Rubin CE, Haggitt RC, Burmer GC, et al: DNA aneuploidy in colonic biopsies predicts future development of dysplasia in ulcerative colitis. *Gastroenterology* 1992;103:1611-1620.

211. Jonsson B, Ahsgren L, Andersson LO, et al: Colorectal cancer surveillance in patients with ulcerative colitis. *Br J Surg* 1994;81:689-691.

212. Gillen CD, Walmsley RS, Prior P, et al: Ulcerative colitis and Crohn's disease: a comparison of the colorectal cancer risk in extensive colitis. *Gut* 1994;35:1590-1592.

213. Greenstein AJ, Sachar DB, Smith H, et al: A comparison of cancer risk in Crohn's disease and ulcerative colitis. *Cancer* 1981;48:2742-2745.

214. Ekbom A, Helmick C, Zack M, et al: Increased risk of large bowel cancer in Crohn's disease with colonic involvement. *Lancet* 1990;336:357-359.

215. Sachar DB: Cancer in Crohn's disease: Dispelling the myths. *Gut* 1994;35:1507-1508.

216. Mandel JS, Bond JH, Church TR, et al: Reducing mortality from colorectal cancer by screening for fecal occult blood: Minnesota Colon Cancer Control Study. *N Engl J Med* 1993;328:1365-1371.

217. Hardcastle JD, Chamberlain JO, Robinson MH, et al: Randomised controlled trial of faecal-occult-blood screening for colorectal cancer. *Lancet* 1996;348:1472-1477.

218. Kronborg O, Fenger C, Olsen J, et al: Randomised study of screening for colorectal cancer with faecal-occult-blood test. *Lancet* 1996;348:1467-1471.

219. Mandel JS, Church TR, Ederer F, et al: Colorectal cancer mortality: effectiveness of biennial screening for fecal occult blood. *J Natl Cancer Inst* 1999;91:434-437.

220. Mandel JS, Church TR, Bond JH, et al: The effect of fecal occult-blood screening on the incidence of colorectal cancer. *N Engl J Med* 2000;343:1603-1607.

221. Ederer F, Church TR, Mandel JS: Fecal occult blood screening in the Minnesota study: role of chance detection of lesions. *J Natl Cancer Inst* 1997;89:1423-1428.

222. Ahlquist DA, Moertel CG, McGill DB: Screening for colorectal cancer [letter]. *N Engl J Med* 1993;329:1351.

223. Lang CA, Ransohoff DF: Fecal occult blood screening for colorectal cancer: is mortality reduced by chance selection for screening colonoscopy? *JAMA* 1994;271:1011-1013.

224. Rockey DC, Koch J, Cello JP: Relative frequency of upper gastrointestinal and colonic lesions in patients with positive fecal occult-blood tests. *N Engl J Med* 1998;339:153-159.

225. Selby JV, Friedman GD, Quesenberry CP Jr, et al: A case-control study of screening sigmoidoscopy and mortality from colorectal cancer. *N Engl J Med* 1992;326:653-657.

226. Byers T, Levin B, Rothenberger D, et al: American Cancer Society Guidelines for screening and surveillance for early detection of colorectal polyps and cancer: update 1997. *CA Cancer J Clin* 1997;47:154-160.

227. Atkin WS, Cuzick J, Northover JM, et al: Prevention of colorectal cancer by once-only sigmoidoscopy. *Lancet* 1993;341:736-740.

228. Foutch PG, Mai HD, Pardy K, et al: Flexible sigmoidoscopy may be ineffective for secondary prevention of colorectal cancer in asymptomatic, average-risk men. *Dig Dis Sci* 1991;36:924-928.

229. Rex DK, Lehman GA, Ulbright TM, et al: Colonic neoplasia in asymptomatic persons with negative fecal occult blood tests: influence of age, gender, and family history. *Am J Gastroenterol* 1993;88:825-831.

230. Read TE, Read JO, Butterly LF: Importance of adenomas 5 mm or less in diameter that are detected by sigmoidoscopy. *N Engl J Med* 1997;336:8-12.

231. Dinning JP, Hixson LJ, Clark LC: Prevalence of distal colonic neoplasia associated with proximal colon cancers. *Arch Intern Med* 1994; 154:853-856.

232. Imperiale TF, Wagner DR, Lin CY, et al: Risk of advanced proximal neoplasms in asymptomatic adults according to the distal colorectal findings. *N Engl J Med* 2000;343:169-174.

233. Lieberman DA, Weiss DG, Bond JH, et al: Use of colonoscopy to screen asymptomatic adults for colorectal cancer. *N Engl J Med* 2000;343: 162-168.

234. Bhattacharya I, Sack EM: Screening colonoscopy: the cost of common sense. *Lancet* 1996;347: 1744-1745.

235. Winawer SJ, Stewart ET, Zauber AG, et al: A comparison of colonoscopy and double-contrast barium enema for surveillance after polypectomy. *N Engl J Med* 2000;342:1766-1772.

236. O'Brien MJ, Winawer SJ, Zauber AG, et al: The National Polyp Study: patient and polyp characteristics associated with high-grade dysplasia in colorectal adenomas. *Gastroenterology* 1990;98: 371-379.

237. Rex DK, Rahmani EY, Haseman JH, et al: Relative sensitivity of colonoscopy and barium enema for detection of colorectal cancer in clinical practice. *Gastroenterology* 1997;112:17-23.

238. Karasick S, Ehrlich SM, Levin DC, et al: Trends in use of barium enema examination, colonoscopy, and sigmoidoscopy: is use commensurate with risk of disease? *Radiology* 1995;195:777-784.

239. Wagner JL, Tunis S, Brown M, et al: Cost-effectiveness of colorectal cancer screening in average-risk adults. In Young GP, Rozen P, Levin B, editors: *Prevention and early detection of colorectal cancer*. Philadelphia, WB Saunders, 1996, 21-56.

240. Freeman B, Engel JJ, Fine MS, et al: Colonoscopy to the cecum: how often do we get there? experience in a community hospital. *Am J Gastroenterol* 1993;88:789.

241. Waye JD, Bashkoff E: Total colonoscopy: is it always possible? *Gastrointest Endosc* 1991;37: 152-154.

242. DiPrima RE, Barkin JS, Blinder M, et al: Age as a risk factor in colonoscopy: fact versus fiction. *Am J Gastroenterol* 1988;83:123-125.

243. Rankin GB: Indications, containdications and complications of colonoscopy. In Sivak MV, editor: *Gastrointestinal endoscopy*. Philadelphia, WB Saunders, 1987, 873-878.

244. Rex DK, Cutler CS, Lemmel GT, et al: Colonoscopic miss rates of adenomas determined by back-to-back colonoscopies. *Gastroenterology* 1997;112:24-28.

245. Hixson LJ, Fennerty MB, Sampliner RE, et al: Prospective blinded trial of the colonoscopic miss-rate of large colorectal polyps. *Gastrointest Endosc* 1991;37:125-127.

246. Neugut AI, Jacobson JS, Ahsan H, et al: Incidence and recurrence rates of colorectal adenomas: a prospective study. *Gastroenterology* 1995;108:402-408.

247. Adachi M, Muto T, Morioka Y, et al: Flat adenoma and flat mucosal carcinoma (IIIb type)—a new precursor of colorectal carcinoma? *Dis Colon Rectum* 1988;31:236-243.

248. Lynch HT, Smyrk TC, Watson P, et al: Hereditary flat adenoma syndrome: a variant of familial adenomatous polyposis? *Dis Colon Rectum* 1992;35:411-421.

249. Rembacken BJ, Fujii T, Cairns A, et al: Flat and depressed colonic neoplasms: a prospective study of 1000 colonoscopies in the UK. *Lancet* 2000;355:1211-1214.

250. Fenlon HM, Nunes DP, Schroy PC, et al: A comparison of virtual and conventional colonoscopy for the detection of colorectal polyps. *N Engl J Med* 1999;341:1496-1503.

251. Bronk JA, McFarland EG, Satava R: Virtual colonoscopy. *Contemporary Surgery* 2000;56:310-321.

252. Hara AK, Johnson CD, Reed JE: Detection of colorectal polyps with CT colography: initial assessment of sensitivity and specificity. *Radiology* 1997;205:59-65.

253. Rex DK, Vining D, Kopecky KK: An initial experience with screening for colon polyps using spiral CT with and without CT colography (virtual colonoscopy). *Gastrointest Endosc* 1999;50:309-313.

254. Stryker SJ, Wolff BG, Culp CE, et al: Natural history of untreated colonic polyps. *Gastroenterology* 1987;93:1009-1011.

255. Waye JD, Lewis BS, Frankel A, et al: Small colon polyps. *Am J Gastroenterol* 1988;83:120-122.

256. Nusko G, Mansmann U, Partzsch U, et al: Invasive carcinoma in colorectal adenomas: multivariate analysis of patient and adenoma characteristics. *Endoscopy* 1997;29:626-631.

257. Glick S, Wagner JL, Johnson CD: Cost-effectiveness of double-contrast barium enema in screening for colorectal cancer. *AJR Am J Roentgenol* 1998;170:629-636.

258. Fenlon HM, McAneny DB, Nunes DP, et al: Occlusive colon carcinoma: virtual colonoscopy in the preoperative evaluation of the proximal colon. *Radiology* 1999;210:423-428.

259. Eddy D: Guidelines for the cancer-related checkup: recommendations and rationale. *CA Cancer J Clin* 1980;30:3-50

260. Screening for colorectal cancer: United States, 1997. *MMWR* 1999;48:116-121.

261. Theuer CP, Taylor TH, Anton-Culver H: Screening for colorectal cancer. *N Engl J Med* 2000;343:1652-1261.

262. Levin TR, Palitz A, Grossman S, et al: Predicting advanced proximal colonic neoplasia with screening sigmoidoscopy. *JAMA* 1999;281:1611-1617.

263. Smith TJ, Hillner BE, Desch CE: Efficacy and cost-effectiveness of cancer treatment: rational allocation of resources based on decision analysis. *J Natl Cancer Inst* 1993;85:1460-1474.

264. Schuette HL, Tucker TC, Brown ML, et al: The costs of cancer care in the United States: implications for action. *Oncology (Huntingt)* 1995;9:19-22.

265. Garber AM, Phelps CE: *Economic foundations of cost-effectiveness analysis working paper no. 4164.* Palo Alto, CA, National Bureau of Economic Research, 1992.

266. Garber AM, Phelps CE: Economic foundations of cost-effectiveness analysis. *J Health Econ* 1997;16:1-31.

267. Russell LB: Some of the tough decisions required by a national health plan. *Science* 1989;246:892-896.

268. Eddy DM: Screening for colorectal cancer. *Ann Intern Med* 1990;113:373-384.

269. Lieberman DA: Cost-effectiveness model for colon cancer screening. *Gastroenterology* 1995;109:1781-1790.

270. United States Office of Technology Assessment: *Cost and effectiveness of colorectal cancer screening in the elderly: background.* Publication BP-H-74. Washington, DC, United States Government Printing Office, 1990.

271. United States Office of Technology Assessment: *Cost and effectiveness of colorectal cancer screening average-risk adults.* Washington, DC, United States Government Printing Office, 1995.

272. Wagner JL, Herdman RC, Wadhwa S: Cost effectiveness of colorectal cancer screening in the elderly. *Ann Intern Med* 1991;115:807-817.

273. Wagner JL, Tunis S, Brown M, et al: Cost-effectiveness of colorectal cancer screening in average-risk adults. In Young GP, Rozen P, Levin B, editors: *Prevention and early detection of colorectal cancer.* Philadelphia, WB Saunders, 1996, 21-56.

274. Glick S, Wagner JL, Johnson CD: Cost-effectiveness of double-contrast barium enema in screening for colorectal cancer. *AJR Am J Roentgenol* 1998;170:629-636.

275. Theuer CP, Wagner JL, Taylor TH, et al: Racial and ethnic colorectal cancer patterns affect the cost-effectiveness of colorectal screening in the United States. *Gastroenterology* 2001;120(4):848-856.

276. Sandler RA, Baron JA, Tosteson TA, et al: Rectal mucosal proliferation and risk of colorectal adenomas: results from a randomized controlled trial. *Cancer Epidemiol Biomarkers Prev* 2000;9:653-656.

277. Subbaramaiah K, Telang N, Ramonetti JT, et al: Transcription of cyclooxygenase-2 is enhanced in transformed mammary epithelial cells. *Cancer Res* 1996;56:4424-4429.

278. Herschman HR: Prostaglandin synthase 2. *Biochem Biophys Acta* 1996;1299:125-140.

279. Reddy BS, Maruyama H, Kelloff G: Dose-related inhibition of colon carcinogenesis by dietary

piroxicam, a nonsteroidal antiinflammatory drug, during different stages of rat colon tumor development. *Cancer Res* 1987;47:5340-5346.

280. Oshima M, Dinchuk JE, Kargman SL, et al: Suppression of intestinal polyposis in APCd716 knockout mice by inhibition of cyclooxygenase-2 (Cox-2). *Cell* 1996;87:803-809.

281. DuBois RN, Giardello FM, Smalley WE: Nonsteroidal anti-inflammatory drugs, eicosanoids, and colorectal cancer prevention. *Gastroenterol Clin North Am* 1996;25:773-791.

282. Thun MJ, Namboodiri MM, Clark WH Jr: Aspirin use and reduced risk of fatal colon cancer. *N Engl J Med* 1991;325:1593-1596.

283. Bjarnason I, Macpherson A, Rotman H, et al: A randomized, double-blind, crossover comparative endoscopy study on the gastroduodenal tolerability of a highly specific cyclooxygenase-2 inhibitor, flosulide, and naproxen. *Scand J Gastroenterol* 1997;32:126-130.

284. Giovannucci E, Rimm EB, Stampfer MJ, et al: Aspirin use and the risk for colorectal cancer and adenoma in male health professionals. *Ann Intern Med* 1994;121:241-246.

285. Giovannucci E, Egan KM, Hunter DJ, et al: Aspirin use and reduced risk of fatal colon cancer in women. *N Engl J Med* 1995;333:609-614.

286. Smalley W, Ray WA, Daugherty J, et al: Use of nonsteroidal anti-inflammatory drugs and incidence of colorectal cancer: a population-based study. *Arch Intern Med* 1999;159:161-166.

287. Steinbach G, Lynch PM, Phillips RKS, et al: The effect of celecoxib, a cyclooxygenase-2 inhibitor, in familial adenomatous polyposis. *N Engl J Med* 2000;342:1946-1952.

288. Giardello FM, Hamilton SR, Krush AJ, et al: Treatment of colonic and rectal adenomas with sulindac in familial adenomatous polyposis. *N Engl J Med* 1993;328:1313-1316.

289. Labayle D, Fischer D, Vielh P, et al: Sulindac causes regression of rectal polyps in familial adenomatous polyposis. *Gastroenterology* 1991;101:635-639.

290. Keller JJ, Offerhaus GJ, Polak M, et al: Rectal epithelial apoptosis in familial adenomatous polyposis patients treated wiith sulindac. *Gut* 1999;45:822-828.

291. Gann PH, Manson JE, Glynn RJ, et al: Low-dose aspirin and incidence of colorectal tumors in a randomized trial. *J Natl Cancer Inst* 1993;85:1220-1224.

292. Sturmer T, Glynn RJ, Lee I-M, et al: Aspirin use and colorectal cancer: post-trial follow-up data from the Physicians' Health Study. *Ann Intern Med* 1998;128:713-720.

293. Giovanucci E, Egan KM, Hunter DJ, et al: Aspirin and the risk of colorectal cancer in women. *N Engl J Med* 1995;333:609-614.

294. 294. Sandler RS: Epidemiology and risk factors for colorectal cancer. *Gastroenterol Clin North Am* 1996;25:717-735.

295. Garland L, Shekelle RB, Barrett-Conner E, et al: Dietary vitamin D and calcium and risk of col-

orectal cancer: a 19-year prospective study in men. *Lancet* 1985;1:307-309.

296. Bostick RM, Potter JD, Sellers TA, et al: Relationship of calcium, vitamin D, and dairy food intake to incidence of colon cancer among older women: the Iowa Women's Health Study. *Am J Epidemiol* 1993;137:1302-1307.

297. Bayerdorffer E, Mannes GA, Richter WO, et al: Increased serum deoxycholic acids levels in men with colorectal adenomas. *Gastroenterology* 1993;104:145-151.

298. Newmark HL, Wargovich MJ, Bruce WR: Colon cancer and dietary fat, phosphate, and calcium: a hypothesis. *J Natl Cancer Inst* 1984;72:1323-1325.

299. Pence BC: Role of calcium in colon cancer prevention: experimental and clinical studies. *Mutat Res* 1993;290:87-95.

300. Pence BC, Buddingh F: Inhibition of dietary fat-promoted colon carcinogenesis in rats by supplemental calcium or vitamin D3. *Carcinogenesis* 1988;9:187-190.

301. Buset M, Lipkin M, Winawer S, et al: Inhibition of human epithelial cell proliferation in vivo and in vitro by calcium. *Cancer Res* 1986;46:5426-5430.

302. Wargovich MJ, Eng VWS, Newmark HL, et al: Calcium ameliorates the toxic effects of deoxycholic acid on colonic epithelium. *Carcinogenesis* 1983;4:1205-1207.

303. Lipkin M, Newmark H: Effect of added dietary calcium on colonic epithelial-cell proliferation in subjects at high risk for familial colonic cancer. *N Engl J Med* 1985;313:1381-1384.

304. Bostick RM, Fosdick L, Wood JR, et al: Calcium and colorectal epithelial cell proliferation in sporadic adenoma patients: a randomized, double-blinded placebo-controlled clinical trial *J Natl Cancer Inst* 1995;87:1307-1315.

305. Baron JA, Tosteson TD, Wargovich MJ, et al: Calcium supplementation and rectal mucosal proliferation: a randomized controlled trial. *J Natl Cancer Inst* 1995;87:1303-1307.

306. Holt PR, Atillasoy EO, Gilman J et al: Modulation of abnormal colonic epithelial cell proliferation and differentiation by low-fat dairy food: a randomized controlled trial. *JAMA* 1998;28:1074-1079.

307. Baron JA, Beach M, Mandel JS, et al: Calcium supplements for the prevention of colorectal adenomas. *N Engl J Med* 1999;34:101-107.

308. Meyskens FL, Gerner EW: Development of difluoromethylornithine (DFMO) as a chemopreventive agent. *Clin Cancer Res* 1999;5:945-951.

309. Pohjanpelto P, Raina A: Identification of a growth factor produced by human fibroblasts in vitro as putrescine. *Nat New Biol* 1972;235:247-249.

310. Russell DH: The roles of the polyamines, putrescine, spermidine and spermine in normal and malignant tissues. *Life Sci* 1973;13:1635-1647.

311. Hixson LJ, Garewell HS, McGee D, et al: Ornithine decarboxylase and polyamines in colorectal neoplasia and adjacent mucosa. *Cancer Epidemiol Biomarkers Prev* 1993;2:369-374.

312. Rozhin J, Wilson PS, Bull AW, et al: Ornithine decarboxylase activity in the rat and human colon. *Cancer Res* 1984;44:3226-3230.

313. Tempero M: Bile acids, ornithine decarboxylase, and cell proliferation in colon cancer: a review. *Dig Dis* 1986;4:49-56.

314. Bello-Fernandez C, Packham G, Cleveland JL: The ornithine decarboxylase gene is a transscriptional target of c-Myc. *Proc Natl Acad Sci USA* 1993;90:7804-7808.

315. Pena A, Reddy CD, Wu S, et al: Regulation of human ornithine decarboxase expression by the c-Myc.Max protein complex. *J Biol Chem* 1993;268:27277-27285.

316. McCann PP, Pegg AE, Sjoerdsma A, editors: Inhibition of polyamine metabolism: biological significance and basis for new therapies. New York, Academic Press, 1987.

317. Slaga TJ: Multiskin carcinogenesis: a useful model for the study of the chemoprevention of cancer. *Acta Pharmacol Toxicol* 1984;55(Suppl 2):107-124.

318. Su LK, Kinzler KW, Vogelstein B, et al: Multiple intestinal neoplasia caused by a mutation in the murine homolog of the *APC* gene. *Science* 1992;256:668-670.

319. Meyskens FL, Gerner E, Emerson S, et al: A randomized double-blind placebo controlled Phase IIb trial of difluoromethylornithine for colon cancer prevention. *J Natl Cancer Inst* 1986;77: 1309-1313.

320. Meyskens FL, Boyle JO, Meyskens FL, et al: Polyamine contents in rectal and buccal mucosae in humans treated with oral difluoromethylornithine. *Cancer Epidemiol Biomarkers Prev* 1992;1:131-135.

321. Meyskens FL Jr, Emerson SS, Pelot D, et al: Dose de-escalation chemoprevention trial of alpha-difluoromethyl ornithine in patients with colon polyps. *J Natl Cancer Inst* 1994;86:1122-1130.

322. Wang W, Liu LQ, Higuchi CM: Mucosal polyamine measurements and colorectal cancer risk. *J Cell Biochem* 1996;63:252-257.

323. Giovannucci E, Stampfer MJ, Colditz GA, et al: Multivitamin use, folate, and colon cancer in women in the Nurses' Health Study. *Ann Intern Med* 1998;129:517-524.

324. Cravo ML, Mason JB, Dayal Y, et al: Folate deficiency enhances the development of colonic neoplasia in dimethylhydrazine-treated rats. *Cancer Res* 1992;52:2002-2006.

325. Benito E, Stiggelbout A, Bosch FX, et al: Nutritional factors in colorectal cancer risk: a case-control study in Majorca. *Int J Cancer* 1991;49:161-167.

326. Benito E, Cabeza E, Morena V, et al: Diet and colorectal adenomas: a case-control study in Majorca. *Int J Cancer* 1993;55:213-219.

327. Freudenheim JL, Graham S, Marshall JR, et al: Folate intake and carcinogenesis of the colon and rectum. *Int J Epidemiol* 1991;20:368-374.

328. Ferraroni M, La Vecchia C, D'Avanzo B, et al: Selected micronutrient intake and the risk of colorectal cancer. *Br J Cancer* 1994;70:1150-1155.

329. Giovannucci E, Stampfer MJ, Colditz GA, et al: Folate, methionine, and alcohol intake and risk of colorectal adenoma. *J Natl Cancer Inst* 1993;85:875-884.

330. Meyer F, White E: Alcohol and nutrients in relation to colon cancer in middle-aged adults. *Am J Epidemiol* 1993;138:225-236.

331. Giovannucci E, Stampfer MJ, Colditz GA, et al: Folate, methionine, and alcohol intake and risk of colorectal adenoma. *J Natl Cancer Inst* 1993;85:875-884.

332. Giovannucci E, Stampfer MJ, Colditz GA, et al: Multivitamin use, folate, and colon cancer in women in the Nurses' Health Study. *Ann Intern Med* 1998;129:517-524.

333. Giovannucci E, Rimm EB, Ascherio A, et al: Alcohol, low-methionine–low-folate diets and risk of colon cancer in men. *J Natl Cancer Inst* 1995;87:265-273.

334. Glynn SA, Albanes D, Pietinen P, et al: Colorectal cancer and folate status: a nested case-control study among male smokers. *Cancer Epidemiol Biomarkers Prev* 1996;5:487-494.

335. Baron JA, Sandler RS, Haile RW, et al: Folate intake, alcohol consumption, cigarette smoking, and risk of colorectal adenomas. *J Natl Cancer Inst* 1998;90:57-62.

336. Block G, Patterson B, Subar A: Fruit, vegetables and cancer prevention: a review of the epidemiologic evidence. *Nutr Cancer* 1992;18:1-29.

337. Giovanucci E, Stampfer MJ, Colditz GA et al: Multivitamin use, folate, and colon cancer in women in the Nurses' Health Study. *Ann Intern Med* 1998;129:517-24.

338. Malila N, Virtanmo J, Viranen M, et al: The effect of alpha-tocopherol and beta-carotene supplementation on colorectal adenomas in middle-aged male smokers. *Cancer Epidemiol Biomarkers Prev* 1999;8:489-493.

339. Hennekens CH, Buring JE, Manson JE, et al: Lack of effect of long-term supplementation with beta carotene on the incidence of malignant neoplasms and cardiovascular diasease. *N Engl J Med* 1996;334:1145-1149.

340. Ma J, Stampfer NJ, Giovanucci E, et al: Methylenetetrahydrofolate reductase polymorphism, dietary interactions, and risk of colorectal cancer. *Cancer Res* 1997;57:1098-1102.

341. Potter JD, Bostick RM, Grandits GA, et al: Hormone replacement therapy is associated with lower risk of adenomatous polyps of the large bowel: the Minnesota Cancer Prevention Research Unit case-control study. *Cancer Epidemiol Biomarkers Prev* 1996;5:779-784.

342. Fernandez E, La Vecchia C, Braga C, et al: Hormone replacement therapy and risk of colon and rectal cancer. *Cancer Epidemiol Biomarkers Prev* 1998;7:329-333.

343. Kampman E, Potter JD, Slattery ML, et al: Hormone replacement therapy, reproductive history, and colon cancer: a multicenter, case-control study in the United States. *Cancer Causes Control* 1997;8:146-158.

344. Hebert-Croteau N: A meta-analysis of hormone replacement therapy and colon cancer in women. *Cancer Epidemiol Biomarkers Prev* 1998;7:653-659.

345. Grodstein F, Newcombe PA, Stampfer MJ: Postmenopausal hormone therapy and the risk of colorectal cancer: a review and meta-analysis. *Am J Med* 1999;106:574-582.

346. McMichael AJ, Potter JD: Reproduction, endogenous and exogenous sex hormones, and colon cancer: a review and hypothesis. *J Natl Cancer Inst* 1980;65:1201-1207.

347. Issa JPJ, Ottaviano YL, Celano P, et al: Methylation of the oestrogen receptor CpG island links ageing and neoplasia in human colon. *Nat Genet* 1994;7:536-540.

348. Earnest DL, Holubec H, Wali RK, et al: Chemoprevention of azoxymethane-induced colonic carcinogenesis by supplemental dietary ursodeoxycholic acid. *Cancer Res* 1994;54:5071-5074.

349. Rao CV, Rivenson A, Latiwalla M, et al: Chemopreventive effect of oltipraz during different stages of experimental colon carciogenesis induced by azoxymethane in male F344 rats. *Cancer Res* 1993;53:2502-2506.

Skin Cancer

Part I: Nonmelanoma Skin Cancer
Vandana S. Nanda

Part II: Cancer of the Skin
James Jakowatz

PART I: NONMELANOMA SKIN CANCER
INCIDENCE, MORTALITY, AND MORBIDITY

Cancer of the skin (including melanoma and nonmelanoma skin cancer) accounts for more than 40% of all cancers and is the most common skin cancer. The incidence of non-melanoma skin cancer (NMSC) is increasing rapidly; basal cell carcinoma (BCC) and squamous cell carcinoma (SCC) of the skin are the most common malignant neoplasms in the Caucasian population. In the United States, the incidence of these cancers is estimated to be increasing by 2% to 3% yearly.[1]

In the United States, approximately 480,000 persons were diagnosed with NMSC in 1983, and approximately 200,000 SCCs and 800,000 BCCs were diagnosed in 1999. Currently, 1.3 million cases of NMSCs are diagnosed annually in the United States. Because doctors are not required to report NMSCs to the Cancer Registry, the number is not as accurate as it is for other types of cancers. BCCs account for more than 95% of all NMSCs and are associated with significant morbidity (loss of function and disfigurement). Fortunately, mortality from these cancers is low.[2,3] Deaths do occur because of particularly aggressive or multiple tumors or the absence of early treatment. The American Cancer Society predicted that there would be approximately 2200 deaths from NMSC in 2002[4] (Table 5-1 lists approximated statistics for 2001). Death rates for NMSCs are associated with sex, race, and geographic location in a similar but weaker manner than melanomas are.

The annual NMSC incidence rate increased from 233 per 100,000 among Caucasians in 1983 to an estimated 726 to 933 per 100,000 in 1994. In Australia, the reported annual incidence is even higher, at 1000 to 2000 per 100,000[5,6] with an increase of 11% in BCC and 51% in SCC between 1985 and 1990.[7] The ratio of BCC to SCC among Caucasians in the United States, Australia, and the United Kingdom is approximately 4:1.[1,8] A recent U.S. study suggests that the current annual incidence of BCC is 350 per 100,000 population for females and 480 per 100,000 for males. A study confined to Hawaii resulted in slightly higher annual figures of 293 per 100,000 for females and 576 per 100,000 for males.[2]

Basal cell carcinomas occur almost exclusively on hair-bearing skin. The majority of patients are elderly; have fair skin (tan poorly and burn easily); are of Celtic ancestry; and have red or blond hair, blue eyes, and a significant amount of cumulative sun exposure.[9-11] Half of all BCCs are found on the face and not always on areas of maximum solar exposure. Lesions are commonly seen near the inner canthus and in the nasolabial fold. In addition to effects of ultraviolet light (UV) exposure, a relationship to embryologic closure lines may exist.

Table 5-1
Approximated Skin Cancer Statistics (US 2001)

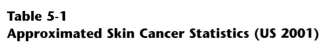

	Basal Cell Carcinoma and Squamous Cell Carcinoma	Malignant Melanoma
Annual incidence	1.3 million	47,000
Annual mortality	9000	7700

Source: American Cancer Society (URL: http://www3.cancer.org/cancerinfo/load)

BCCs are initially seen as slow-growing, shiny or translucent raised papules or nodules. Small dilated blood vessels can be seen on the surface. The center may ulcerate as the lesion accelerates its growth. A typical rolled pearly border is appreciated (Figure 5-1). A number of nodular BCCs may contain pigment (Figure 5-2) and therefore be confused with malignant melanoma. An easily missed variant is the morpheaform BCC, which presents as a firm, scarlike area, usually in nasolabial folds (Figure 5-3). The pearly raised edge and central ulceration are usually absent. This lesion tends to be more extensive on palpation. Morpheaform BCC has a higher incidence of local and regional spread than other types. BCCs in the central face recur more frequently than do those on other sites, and a higher proportion of these lesions are the morpheaform variant.

A recent critical review and metaanalysis of the evidence-based literature assessing risk of developing a subsequent NMSC with a prior history of NMSC showed that the risk of developing a BCC after a previous BCC is 44% at 3 years. The same report demonstrated that the risk of a recurrent SCC is a much lower 18% at three years. The mean three year cumulative risk of developing a BCC with a prior history of SCC is 43%. Because BCCs

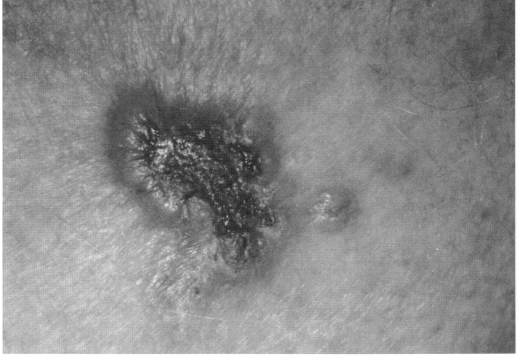

FIGURE 5-1
A typical basal cell carcinoma with a pearly rolled border.

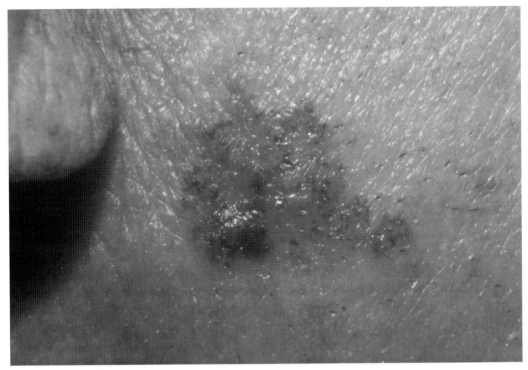

FIGURE 5-2
A pigmented basal cell carcinoma easily confused with malignant melanoma.

represent 85% of all NMSCs, this is not surprising. The 3-year cumulative risk doubles in patients with two or more NMSCs.[1]

SCC is a malignant neoplasm that originates from epidermal keratinocytes with a capacity for metastatic spread. SCC is mostly seen in the Caucasian population with increased cumulative lifetime sunlight exposure. Chung and associates reported a forty-fivefold increase in NMSC in the Japanese population in Kauai, Hawaii, compared with the Japanese population in Japan.[12] The incidence of SCC but not BCC correlated directly with the amount of sun exposure in a study done on Maryland watermen (Caucasians who make a living fishing in the Chesapeake Bay).[13] The close correlation between chronic cumulative sun exposure and SCC is also demonstrated in a 12,000-patient population-based study.[14] Geographically, the incidence of skin cancer in Caucasians increases the closer they live to the equator, thus supporting the role of sunlight in carcinogenesis. The true incidence of basal and squamous cell tumors is difficult to determine accurately because many cancer registries combine both tumors in one category. A majority of these NMSCs are treated in private offices, with consequent underreporting. A recent U.S. study by Weinstock and associates calculated the current incidence of SCC to be 59 per 100,000 in males.[2] A European study demonstrated a that the incidence of SCC in females in Switzerland tripled between 1976 and 1992.[15] Mortality from NMSC is low, compared with melanoma, and most deaths are attributed to SCC rather than BCC. In the United States, the 1991 age-adjusted mortality rate for NMSC was 0.44 per 100,000 population.[16]

SCC arises on sun-damaged skin. The typical patient is an elderly male, and the most usual sites are dorsum of hand, arm, face, and neck. The lesion presents as a firm, indurate, often crusty, scaly nodule (Figure 5-4). SCC may develop in scars and adjacent to chronic ulcerations. Carcinoma of the lip almost always involves the lower lip (Figure 5-5). SCC of the oral mucosa occurs in parts of the world where chewing tobacco or betel nuts is com-

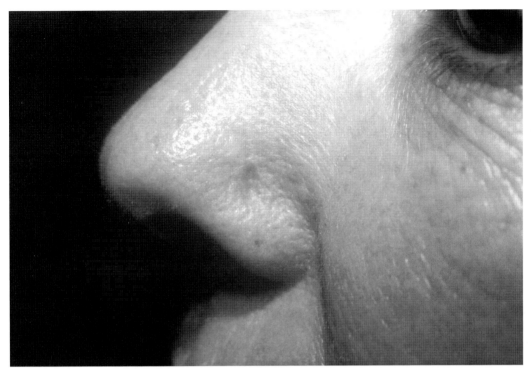

FIGURE 5-3
A morpheaform basal cell, a firm scarred-like plaque.

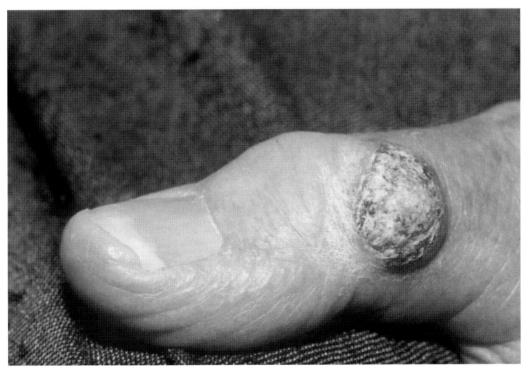

FIGURE 5-4
Squamous cell carcinoma, a crusty scaly nodule.

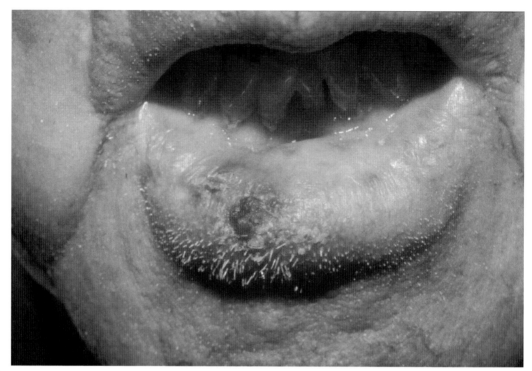

FIGURE 5-5
Squamous cell of the lower lip.

mon. Alcohol may also have a synergistic effect. Verrucous carcinoma of the oral mucosa is seen in smokers who also are heavy users of alcohol.

The risk of metastatic spread varies according to the type of damage associated with the SCC. Moller and associates have reported very different rates of metastases from different types of SCC. From lip lesions the rate is 11%, from lesions adjacent to chronic scars and ulcerations 10% to 30%, and from actinic lesions 3%.[17] The 3-year cumulative risk of developing SCC after an SCC is 18%, and 6% after a prior BCC.[1] SCC has the ability to metastasize and cause death. All patients who have had a pathologically proven SCC should be observed closely and educated about sun exposure and the use of sunscreens.

RISK FACTORS

Animal models used in studying cutaneous carcinogenesis previously relied heavily on chemical carcinogens. In the past few decades the role of natural sunlight as a cutaneous carcinogen in humans has become important, and laboratory workers' attention has turned to ultraviolet radiation (UVR) studies. In addition, the role of papillomaviruses, oncogenes, immunodeficiency status, and depletion of the ozone layer as carcinogens or co-carcinogens is also currently being studied (Table 5-2).

Ultraviolet Radiation

Fear of increased UVB radiation from ozone depletion in the stratosphere has caused research on the relationship between the sun and skin cancer to escalate. The principal action spectrum in sunlight is UVB (280-320 nm). There is general consensus that the most important factor involved in NMSC pathogenesis is ultraviolet radiation[16,18] (the closer one

Table 5-2
Agents Capable of Inducing Skin Cancer

Initiators	Promoters
Polycyclic aromatic hydrocarbons (tar)	Phenol
Quinolones	Phorbol esters
Nitrogen mustard	Anthralin
Psoralens	Benzoyl peroxide
Ultraviolet radiation (mainly UVB)	Ultraviolet radiation (mainly UVB)

lives to the equator, the greater the risk of developing skin cancer)[19] and clear evidence that a quantitative relationship exists between cumulative lifetime sun exposure and the risk of developing NMSC.[14,20] BCCs are generally associated with intermittent low-level exposure, whereas SCC is generally thought to be associated with continual exposure to high levels of UVR.[21] The dramatic increase of NMSC in several inherited diseases characterized by increased sensitivity to UVR damage, including xeroderma pigmentosum and albinism, supports the significance of UVR in the development of NMSC.

Exposure to UVR has been estimated to account for approximately 90% of NMSC.[21] UVB radiation (290-320 nm) induces both photochemical damage and systemic immunosuppression. In the laboratory, Ziegler and associates[22] and Nomura and associates[21] demonstrated the role of UVB in the induction of mutations in the p53 gene and in the development of actinic keratosis and SCC of human skin. Originally it was thought that UVB induces cutaneous neoplasms solely by its direct transforming effect on the DNA of the host cell. However, it was later recognized that UVB induces a state of immunodeficiency that is best shown by the inability of the UVB-irradiated mice to mount a protective immune response against highly immunogenic tumors that are UVB-induced.[23] There exists a link between UVB-induced immune dysfunction and cutaneous carcinogenesis.

Both in mice and in humans there is evidence that Langerhans cells are the main targets in the UVB-induced immunosuppression. The number, function, and phenotype of Langerhans cells is altered. Several cytokines are produced by UVB-triggered keratinocytes. IL-10 plays a role in UVB-induced immunsuppression of Langerhans cells. More recently, erythematogenic doses or chronic low doses of UVA have been shown to induce a state of immunosuppression similar to that seen with UVB. Cell DNA has been clearly identified as the prime target of UVB and pyrimidine dimers as the primary event in photocarcinogenesis. A tumor suppressor gene (p53) mutation consisting of C-to-T and C-to-A single-based pair changes at dipyrimidine sequences and tandem double CC-to-TT mutations is known to be associated with UVR exposure.[21] Both UVR (200-400 nm) and UVA (320-400 nm) induced pyrimidine dimers in epidermal DNA. Forty percent to 56% of NMSCs contain p53 mutations. The p53 mutations characteristic of sun exposure have also been described in histologically normal sun-exposed skin, and so the significance of these mutations is unclear.[24]

Ozone Layer

Ozone is formed by the reaction of a single oxygen atom with a doublet oxygen molecule. The oxygen atom is created when the oxygen molecule absorbs high-energy solar UVR and splits into two oxygen atoms. These unstable single atoms react with oxygen molecules to form ozone. Ozone is found mostly in the stratosphere, the part of the atmosphere from 10 to 30 miles above the surface of the earth.[25] The ozone level in the stratosphere varies directly with UVR output. Sunspot activity causes the sun's UVR output to change every 11 years.[19]

UVR represents 5% of the total solar energy that reaches the Earth and comprises UVC (200-280 nm), UVB (280-320 nm), and UVA (320-400 nm). UVB is 10% of UVR. The oxygen and ozone molecules in the stratosphere absorb 100% of UVC and 90% of UVB. UVA is not significantly affected by the ozone layer. In recent years there has been considerable concern about the depletion of the ozone layer by environmental chemicals, mainly chlorofluorocarbons (CFCs). CFCs are being released from modern-day products, such as aerosol sprays, air conditioners, refrigerants, and cleaning agents. These chemicals or their derivatives catalyze the conversion of ozone back to the oxygen molecule, thereby decreasing the ozone level. The most severe depletion of ozone over the southern hemisphere occurred in winter of 1993.[26,27] Moan and Dahlbeck have calculated that a 10% ozone depletion will translate in a 16% to 18% increase in the incidence of SCC in both sexes in Norway, and a 19% rise in melanoma in males and 32% increase in melanoma in females.[28] Current mathematical models suggest that it will take more than 50 years to appreciate the full effect of the depletion of the ozone layer in increasing all forms of skin cancer.[20]

Type of Skin

Fair-skinned individuals who burn easily and tan poorly are at greatest risk for developing cancerous and precancerous lesions of the skin. Darkly pigmented persons and those who tan well are significantly less likely to develop lesions.[29] The protective role of skin pigmentation is well-demonstrated in the dark skin of individuals of Afro-Caribbean ethnic descent, in which cutaneous malignancy is relatively rare. Studies of albinos demonstrate the efficacy of melanin as a photoprotective agent. In the African countries, albinos have a very high incidence of cutaneous malignancy (i.e., actinic keratoses and SCC, which occur almost exclusively on sun-exposed sites).[30]

Tanning History

Tanned skin is cherished in the Western world as a sign of luxury and good health. After World War II, dress codes changed, allowing women to obtain more sun exposure, and increased outdoor leisure and professional activities became more popular. In the last 20 to 30 years, the use of artificial sources of light to induce a tan has greatly increased. Home-tanning lamps, which emitted a larger proportion of UVB radiation (280-320 nm), were available in the 1950s. Commercial sunbeds, which emit an even larger proportion of UVA radiation (320-400 nm), have been available since the 1970s. Because both intermittent low exposure to UVB radiation and chronic exposure to UVB and UVA radiation affect the development of BCC and SCC, respectively, it is important to obtain the tanning history of an individual when assessing risk of NMSC. An individual who tans poorly and burns easily is especially at risk for sun-induced skin problems, both photoaging and cancer. These processes may be heightened by the use of tanning beds or suntan lamps.

Occupational Exposure

One of the earliest examples of occupational SCC is scrotal malignancy in chimney sweeps secondary to contact with carcinogens in soot. Petroleum, shale oils, and creosote oils are also recognized as causes of skin cancer and an occupational hazard in cotton spinners.[20] BCCs can arise in burns caused by a hot metal chip or a welding spark.[31] Excessive exposure to UV light, however, is the main etiologic factor in the development of NMSC. Ramani and associates demonstrated an increased incidence of skin cancer in World War II veterans stationed in the Pacific, compared with those who served in Europe.[32] Occupations that increase chronic cumulative lifetime sun exposure, as shown in a study of Maryland watermen, also demonstrate UVR as a significant risk factor for development of skin cancer.[13] Outdoor sports and increasing recreational sun exposure are likely to increase the incidence of NMSC in women.

Ionizing Radiation

X-irradiation may give rise to BCCs and SCCs. As with most carcinogens, the latency for development of the carcinomas is usually long,[11] and the minimum amount of exposure necessary for carcinoma formation has not been determined.[31] DNA damage probably plays a critical role, similar to in UVR-induced carcinoma. X-irradiation radiation was used for benign conditions, including tinea capitis, hirsutism, and acne. Grenz-ray therapy also was a popular treatment for many benign inflammatory conditions of the skin. In a Swedish study, no increase in NMSC or melanoma was reported even in individuals who received a high cumulative does of Grenz rays.

Other Exposures

Arsenic

Exposure arsenic has been thought to play a role in cutaneous and visceral carcinogenesis; inorganic arsenic appears to be more carcinogenic than organic arsenic. Sources of arsenic have included well water, medicines, cough remedies, insecticides, mining, and smelting. In the presteroid era, arsenic was used as therapy, making a high proportion of arsenic-induced malignancy iatrogenic.[20] Arsenic exposure usually causes multiple lesions of Bowen's disease or SCC in situ. Clinically, these lesions appear to be irregular red-pink scaly plaques, mostly found on the trunk. Keratoses of the palms and soles and basal and SCCs have also been reported.[31]

Tar

Tar has been used in topical treatments in psoriasis and other inflammatory skin diseases. It is recognized as a carcinogen and is used in experimental systems to induce skin cancer in animals. A recent report found no increased skin cancer in patients who had used tar for psoriasis over a long period of time.[20]

Phototherapy with Psoralens and Ultraviolet A

The use of oral psoralen with UVA (PUVA) for psoriasis and other dermatologic disorders was popularized in the mid-1970s. From the beginning it was recognized as a potential carcinogen. U.S. studies by Stern and associates have demonstrated a 13 times higher risk of SCC in patients receiving high doses of UVA versus lower doses.[33] Also very disturbing is a U.S. report that recorded metastatic spread of PUVA-induced SCC in 7 of 1389 patients during long-term follow-up.[34] Initial studies in Europe produced less worrisome results, but more recent studies have recorded an 18% incidence of SCC in patients receiving high-dose PUVA. PUVA lentigos are large, stellate freckles and are seen commonly on light-exposed skin. Some degree of atypia is noted histopathologically.[20]

Therapeutic Ultraviolet B Radiation and Skin Cancer

Ultraviolet B radiation is recognized as a significant carcinogen. Therapeutic artificial UVB is frequently used routinely in psoriasis and other dermatoses, but there are insufficient reports of skin cancer in patients treated with UVB to evaluate the risk of therapeutic UVB in the development of skin cancer. Further study on use of this treatment is needed.

Smoking

Cigarette smoking is the single greatest preventable cause of morbidity in the United States. The external manifestations and consequences of smoking are not well-studied. Karagas and associates performed a multicenter prospective study on the risk of a second NMSC.[35] These studies showed the risk of a second SCC to be higher in current smokers and to a lesser extent in former smokers than in nonsmokers. Risk increased with the number of cigarettes smoked and the duration of smoking. No clear evidence between smoking and BCC was noticed. A study of 107,900 nurses found that current smokers had a 50% increase in the risk of SCC of the skin, compared with those who had never smoked.[36] Smoking coupled with UVR is also a major risk factor for lip cancer. Other adverse effects of smoking include poor wound healing, increased wrinkling, sallow complexion, and some association with other inflammatory skin disorders.

Association with Human Papilloma Virus

Human papilloma virus (HPV) infection has been implicated in some SCCs, notably cervical and anal. The role of HPV in the pathogenesis of NMSC is relatively well-established for development of NMSC in immunosuppressed individuals but is less so for skin cancers in the immunocompetent host. HPV DNA has been associated with some cutaneous SCCs, especially in immunocompromised transplant recipients, patients on chronic immunosuppressives, and epidermodysplasia verruciformis (EV),[37-39] an inherited disorder of cell-mediated immunity known for failure to control infection with certain cutaneous HPVs. Patients with EV develop numerous flat, atypical warts; 40% to 60% of these lesions may undergo malignant transformation after patients reach age 30.[40] EV HPV types 5 and 8 carry a high risk for development of SCCs, but the available data consist only of small- to medium-sized case reports. Detection of HPV in cutaneous samples technically is difficult because of numerous HPV types and limited number of primer sets.

Renal transplant recipients who are iatrogenically immunosuppressed develop numerous warts and are at high risk for NMSC cancers, especially in sun-exposed areas.[40] Systemic corticosteroids alone do not appear to predispose to an increased incidence of cutaneous neoplasia.[31] De Villiers and associates detected HPV in 90% of in situ and invasive SCCs and in 35% of histologically normal tissues in skin samples from benign and malignant lesions from 25 renal transplant recipients.[41]

Human immunodeficiency virus (HIV)-infected individuals are known to have difficulty in controlling HPV infection. They are also reported to have NMSC, but whether they are at higher risk than the general population is not clear. NMSC lesions in this setting have not been extensively analyzed for HPV DNA.[40]

The prevalence of HPV in NMSC or histologically normal tissue from immunocompetent hosts is not known. Case reports document the presence of HPV[40] in neoplastic lesions of fingers, nail beds,[42] and palmar plantar regions in immunocompetent individuals. The etiologic role of HPV in the development of cutaneous neoplasia in the immunosuppressed and immunocompetent individuals is unclear, but it appears that viral infection may play a role in oncogenesis.

Genetic and Familial

Mutations in oncogenes or tumor suppressor genes lead to many types of cancers by activation of oncogenes or inactivation of tumor suppressor genes. Several genes involved in skin cancer development have been identified in a few rare hereditary diseases of the skin. For example, xeroderma pigmentosum, an autosomal recessive disease, is caused by a mutation of genes involved in DNA repair. A high incidence of both nonmelanoma and melanoma skin cancers is reported in these patients, beginning in early childhood. The lack of DNA repair capacity makes these patients susceptible to skin cancer.

Basal cell nevus syndrome, also known as Gorlin's syndrome, is a rare autosomal dominant disorder that results in early development of BCCs, other tumors, and developmental abnormalities. Mutations of a gene on chromosome 9q22.3 have recently been identified. This gene is thought to be a tumor suppressor gene that is inactivated in 33% to 68% of sporadic BCCs.[40] The role of chromosome 9q22 mutations in the pathogenesis of BCC is not clear.

The *ras* family of oncogenes involved in signal transduction is also mutated in 10% to 40% of skin cancers.[23] Glutathione S-transferase 1 (GSTM1) is another gene implicated in increased susceptibility to skin cancer. Alleles of this gene code for isoenzymes that are responsible for detoxifying reactive oxygen species that could result from UVR or chemical damage.[23]

There are a number of different genetic pathways involved in the development of NMSC. Further studies are necessary to clarify the biology underlying the pathogenesis of these tumors.

PREVENTION

Primary Prevention

Primary prevention involves blocking the development of the malignancy itself. The challenge for primary care practitioners is to effectively apply the available information and technologies to alter high-risk behaviors and to ensure early detection. Because skin cancer affects more Americans than any other type of cancer and skin cancer (nonmelanoma and melanoma) accounts for 40% of all cancer cases and 2% of all cancer deaths, primary prevention efforts are aimed at educating the masses and detecting premalignant lesions early.

A sun-sensible approach to skin cancer prevention should be communicated not only to adults but also to children starting with elementary age groups. Children are prime targets for prevention education because sun overexposure in early childhood may affect the development of skin cancer later in life.[43,44] Preventive habits acquired during a child's formative years are less resistant to change than those acquired as an adult.[43] In evaluating two age-appropriate curricula developed at the University of Arizona, a positive effect on preschoolers' knowledge and comprehension of sun safety was found.[43] Studies of adolescents' use of sunscreen indicate that 29% to 70% have never used it or do not regularly use sunscreen, even though they may understand the rationale for its use.[45] Plomer and associates have shown that a simple intervention directed at the staffs of child care centers can have an impact on knowledge and attitudes of directors and on the use of sunscreens.[46]

Recommendations for primary prevention of skin cancers include the following: (1) avoid outdoor activities in the middle of the day (11:00 AM to 3:00 PM) when 75% of the sun's daily ultraviolet rays are transmitted; (2) use hats and clothing to block sun exposure; and (3) use sunscreens with a sun protection factor of 15 or greater on exposed skin. Because lesions of NMSC primarily occur on parts of the body with direct chronic UV exposure, eliminating or decreasing solar exposure should help prevent skin cancer. Educating both the physicians and patients about the early signs and symptoms of photodamage will enhance prevention efforts. Alert physicians are more likely to counsel on safe sun habits.[47]

Precancerous actinic keratoses (AKs) are rough, scaly, pink to red or skin-colored lesions on sun-exposed skin (Figure 5-6). They are slow-growing and usually do not have symptoms or signs other than patches or blemishes on the skin. They often regress and recur. The presence of AKs indicates overexposure to ultraviolet light. AKs are much more

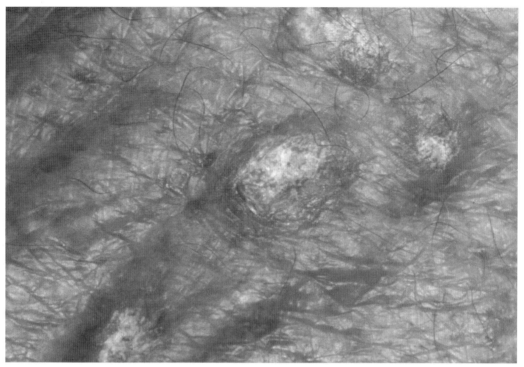

FIGURE 5-6
Actinic keratoses are premalignant papules that are often tender, red, and scaly.

prevalent and rapid in their onset following UV exposure than are skin cancers. Women develop fewer AKs than men do because they are less likely to be exposed to the sun.[48] Clinically actinic or solar keratoses are seen predominantly on the face, hands, and forearms of white-skinned individuals. The lower lip is also a common site. To the patient, AKs may appear as nonhealing wounds. In Australia 40% of people over age 40 will have one or more AKs, and 2% to 3% will have an NMSC.[49] AKs may infrequently develop into SCC. The risk is estimated to be approximately 6% to 15%. Naylor and associates have demonstrated that the regular use of a high–sun protection factor (SPF) sunscreen over a 2-year period can significantly reduce cutaneous neoplasia, as indicated by its suppression of precancerous lesions.[48]

Identification of Premalignant Lesions

Three of four Americans visit a physician's office or clinic an average of three times every year and so have the opportunity to receive preventive services. The primary care doctor, who is more likely than the dermatologist to have regular contact with patients, is often responsible for a patient's first skin screening. However, increasing demands, shorter office visits, and lack of reimbursement for preventive care often lead to infrequent counseling about skin cancer and lack of routine skin examinations by primary care doctors. In addition, many of these physicians find themselves inadequately trained to counsel on skin cancer and perform skin examinations. Dolan and associates showed that a brief skin cancer education intervention aimed at primary care physicians did not significantly affect cancer control attitudes, knowledge, beliefs, or behaviors.[47] The authors concluded that a more intensive intervention may be necessary to show a stronger impact on attitudes and knowledge about skin cancer among primary care physicians.

Skin cancer screening

Skin damage and photoaging is observed most frequently in the Caucasian population. In individuals who burn easily and tan poorly (skin types I-III; Table 5-3), the extent of sun damage depends on the degree of sun exposure. The Celtic populations that have settled in the United States or Australia tend to show photoaging in their early twenties.[47] Screening for premalignant lesions depends on the extent of damage to each individual. Annual screening should begin for people in the early twenties if sun damage is extensive. More frequent follow-up may be required.

Sunscreens

The damaging effects of solar radiation result from absorption of UVR by DNA, RNA, proteins, and cell organelles present in cells in the epidermis, dermis, and the cutaneous vasculature. These effects depend on duration, frequency, and intensity of exposure. Photoprotection and prevention of skin damage can be achieved by reducing the impact of UV light on the skin surface. There are four basic principles governing attenuation of UVR: (1) absorption and filtration of UVR at the stratum corneum level to prevent penetration further into the epidermis and dermis; (2) scattering radiation; (3) reflection of radiation using barrier agents such as titanium dioxide (TiO_2) or zinc oxide (ZnO); and (4) inactivation or destruction of free radicals that are produced in the skin when exposed to UVR.[50] There are many methods of photoprotection of the skin. Chemical sunscreens in the form of creams, lotions, or gels contain a known quantity of a UV-absorbing chemical that absorbs, scatters, or reflects the radiation and prevents penetration into the skin. These sunscreen chemicals can absorb both UVA and UVB radiation. Because no one chemical has excellent broad-spectrum absorption in both the UVA and the UVB range, sunscreens are formulated with several chemicals to provide broad-spectrum UVA and UVB coverage (Table 5-4).[51] Examples of physical but chemical sunscreens that scatter and reflect light in the UVA and UVB region are the TiO_2 and ZnO compounds. Other photoprotective methods involve use of special synthetic fabrics. Artificial tanning of the skin appears to have photoprotective effects as well.

The SPF value of a sunscreen formulation depends on the total amount and uniformity of application to the skin per unit area. The SPF value is based on uniform application of 100 mg or 100 mL per 50 cm^2 of skin. This provides 2 mg/cm^2 or 2 mL/cm^2 for basic photoprotection. The SPF is defined as the ratio of the dose of UVR required to

Table 5-3
Sun Reactive Skin Phototypes

Skin Phototype	Unexposed Skin Color (Buttock)	Sun Sensitivity	Suntan Ability
I	Pale white	Very sensitive Burns easily	None Never tan
II	White	Very sensitive Burns easily	Tan minimally with difficulty
III	White	Quite reactive Burns moderately	Tans moderately
IV	Beige	Moderately reactive Burns minimally	Tans easily
V	Brown or tanned	Minimal Rarely burns	Tans profusely
VI	Dark brown or black	Never burns	Tans profusely

Table 5-4
Chemical Components of UVB- and UVA-Absorbing Sunscreens

UV-Absorbing Chemical	Absorption Range UVB/UVA
Paraaminobenzoic acid (PABA)-related chemical	UVB
Salicylates	UVB
Cinnamates	UVB
Benzophenones	UVB and UVA
Avobenzone, PARSOL 1789	UVA
Anthranilates	UVA
ZnO, TiO$_2$	UVB and UVA

produce one minimal erythema dose (MED) on protected skin after application of 2 mg/cm^2 of product to the dose of UVR to produce one MED on unprotected skin.

$$SPF = UVR \text{ dose on protected skin}/UVR \text{ dose on unprotected skin}$$

The SPF number value is a factor that can be used to calculate the amount of time to get a sunburn. For example, if an individual usually gets a sunburn in 10 minutes at noon, an adequate application of enough quantity uniformly applied of SPF value of 15 would allow 150 minutes of sun exposure for that individual before he or she gets a sunburn. If a product is applied in a smaller quantity, the actual SPF value would be lower—and likewise higher if applied in a larger quantity. Sunscreens should be applied in a smooth and uniform manner to achieve a thin film on the exposed skin.[23,51] The SPF value helps the consumer in choosing the sunscreen suited best for his or her needs (Table 5-5).

A water-resistant product maintains the SPF level after 40 minutes of water immersion and likewise a very water resistant or waterproof product is tested after 80 minutes of water immersion. The new monograph specifies an upper limit of SPF 30, which means that any product greater than 30 can be labeled only as SPF 30 plus or SPF 30+.[51]

A high SPF value gives no guarantee of protection against UVA radiation, unless the formulation is enriched with UVA absorbers (see Table 5-5). The FDA has set a SPF of 30 as the optimal value for ultrahigh protection. The calculated increase in protection with an SPF greater than 30 is negligible. A product of SPF 30 blocks 96.7% of UVR, whereas SPF 40 blocks 97.5%. A high SPF also gives a false sense of extra protection.

Sunscreens should be applied at least 30 minutes before sun exposure. This allows for the sunscreen chemical to better diffuse into the stratum corneum. Immediately after application, contact with clothing should be avoided so as not to remove the sunscreen and

Table 5-5
Sunscreen Protection Based on SPF Values

SPF Value	Protection
2 to < 4	Minimal
4 to < 8	Moderate
8 to < 12	Good or average
12 to < 16	High
16 to < 20	Very high
20 to < 30	Ultrahigh
> 30	Highest

thereby inadvertently decrease protection. For routine daily use, SPF 15 (with UVB, UVA compounds) is generally adequate, but for highest protection SPF 30 is recommended.

Women who use daily cosmetics with added sunscreens often feel protected, but generally these formulations have an SPF value less than 12. Although there is some UVR protection, it is not enough against skin hyperpigmentation and photoaging. Such formulations absolutely do not provide adequate sunburn protection, and individuals with skin types I through III must be made aware of this. One misconception that exists is that reapplication of a sunscreen can give additive value protection. For example, if a product of SPF 15 is reapplied as a second coat during sunbathing, it will not provide protection equal to an SPF value of 30.

Sun-protective clothing that can block more than 97% of harmful UVR is increasingly being used by adults and children. In the past few years tightly woven synthetic fabrics with documented SPFs greater than 15 have become more available.[23] These are especially useful for people who are increasing their outdoor leisure activities and also for those employed in outdoor jobs such as telephone linemen, construction workers, sailors, and farmers. However, the methods used to measure and test for SPF in fabrics should be standardized to provide a more consistent indication of sun protection.

Secondary Prevention

Although primary prevention involves blocking the malignancy itself, secondary prevention focuses on averting death from that malignancy. In the case of NMSC, BCC rarely metastasizes and causes death. SCC of the skin, however, can metastasize and cause death.

Screening

Protocols for High-risk Individuals

Patients who are on chronic immunosuppression—such as transplant recipient patients and the rare patient with xeroderma pigmentosum and epidermodysplasia verruciformis—are at high risk for development of AKs and aggressive SCCs.[39] Chronic immunosuppression predisposes to the development of both BCCs and SCCs. In the Dutch population, the overall incidence of SCC in the immune-suppressed patient is 250 times higher than in the general population.[39] SCC predominates over BCC by a ratio of 3.6:1, a reversal of the usual ratio. Established published protocols and guidelines for these high-risk patients do not exist but should be standardized. Generally, a whole-body examination every 3 months should provide adequate follow-up and allow early detection of neoplasia.

Management of Patients with Positive History of Skin Cancer

Patients with skin cancer are clearly at risk for the development of more skin tumors. A recent study effectively establishes the risk of developing an NMSC after having an NMSC.[1] All patients who have had a BCC should be followed for a minimum of 3 to 6 months to check for local recurrence. If there is no sign of recurrence, follow-up varies based on the patient's age, health care system, and proximity to the health care provider. Ideally, the patient should have a full skin examination every 6 months for a follow-up period of 2 to 3 years. In the case of an SCC, the patient should be followed every 3 months for the first year. The primary site and draining nodal basins should be checked. After the first year, follow-up should be at 6-month intervals. The risk of developing a second SCC within 3 years of having the first one is 18%. At these follow-up visits patients should be continually advised to restrict sun exposure; avoid noonday sun; and wear a broad hat, long sleeves, and a broad-spectrum sunscreen with an SPF of 15 or greater (Box 5-1).

BOX 5-1	"Safe Sun" Guidelines

Minimize sun exposure during the peak UVB period from 10 AM to 4 PM
Apply sunscreen of SPF 15 or more generously
Wear wide-brimmed hats, sunglasses, and additional protective clothing
Avoid deliberate tanning and tanning salons

Chemoprevention

NMSCs are the most commonly diagnosed malignancies in the United States, accounting for approximately 40% of all cancer diagnosis.[52] Skin cancer has a tremendous impact on morbidity, health, and health care economics. The development of chemopreventive strategies is a high public health priority.

Primary prevention strategies include behavior modification and use of sunscreens to minimize UVR exposure. However, secondary chemopreventive strategies are necessary, especially for individuals who are at high risk. The goal of chemoprevention is to develop oral or topical agents that will complement primary prevention of skin cancer.[52]

A few large randomized placebo-controlled phase III intervention trials of chemopreventive agents have been studied in individuals at high risk for development of NMSCs. Several laboratory results have suggested that retinoids have a chemopreventive effect. In a phase III double-blind, randomized study of retinol versus a placebo in 2297 patients with moderate to severe AKs, daily oral retinol (25,000 IU) was associated with a 32% reduction in the risk of developing SCCs of the skin.[53] No significant toxicity was noted. This study effect was especially protective in high-risk patients with eight or more freckles or moles. However, in a follow-up study of 719 patients with a prior history of four or more skin cancers who were randomized to receive oral retinol (25,000 IU), isotretinoin (5-10 mg), or a placebo,[54] neither retinol nor isotretinoin was effective in reducing or delaying the occurrence of NMSC. Retinol may be more effective in early stages of carcinogenesis. Acitretin 30 mg/day was investigated in renal transplant recipients. It was significantly more effective than a placebo in the prevention of SCC and reduced the occurrence of keratotic lesions in this group of patients.[55]

A large double-blind, multicenter, randomized, placebo-controlled phase III trial of beta carotene with or without daily application of SPF 15 sunscreen studied subjects for 4.5 years.[56] There was no significant difference between the beta carotene and placebo groups in the incidence of BCC or SCC. This result supports a previous study that showed a lack of effect of supplementary beta carotene on NMSC in participants studied for 5 years.[57] Five years may not be long enough or the dosage insufficient to study the secondary preventive effects of beta carotene on the development of skin cancer.

Considerable interest has developed in other dietary factors that modify skin carcinogenesis. Restricted-fat diets decrease the frequency of actinic keratoses and NMSC.[58] Natural factors such as green tea, caffeic acid, phenethyl ester from honey bee hives, resveratrol from grapes, silymarin from milk thistle, and ursolic acid from the rosemary plant are shown to be effective at inhibiting skin tumor formation.[23] The antioxidants vitamin C, vitamin E, and alpha-lipoic acid have been shown to have photoprotective topical effects. Long-term studies of oral regimens should be performed.[51] Precise mechanisms of inhibition and their effectiveness as chemopreventive agents for human skin cancer still must be established.

PART II: MELANOMA

INTRODUCTION

Although malignant melanoma accounts for only 8% of all skin cancers, it represents 90% of the deaths caused by skin cancer. Melanomas arise de novo from melanocytes in the skin or from preexisting moles. Moles, or nevi, are simply nests of melanocytes that reside in the dermal and epidermal layers of the skin and are for the most part benign (Figure 5-7). Melanocytes rest in the basal layer of the skin and produce melanin in response to ultraviolet light exposure. This melanin is taken up by the surrounding keratinocytes that are migrating to the superficial-most layers of the skin (Figure 5-8). This results in the familiar and highly desired "tan."

Although melanomas that arise from melanocytes or preexisting moles are generally dark in color, the melanoma lesions can be multicolored, ranging from all black, brown, white, pink, red, or any combination of these colors (Figure 5-9, A, B, and C). These colors generally represent a change in an existing mole or appearance of a new lesion and can be associated with itching, increase in size, becoming raised, developing irregular borders, or bleeding. All of these clinical changes warrant an excisional biopsy to make and appropriately microstage the diagnosis. (Microstaging is the histologic measurement of the thickness of the melanoma expressed in millimeters [Breslow level, Figure 5-10, *right*] or dermal penetration [Clark's levels, Figure 5-10, *left*]).

INCIDENCE AND MORTALITY

Melanoma is the deadliest form of skin cancer and is now occurring in 15/100,000 women and in 19/100,000 men in the United States.[59] These rates have more than doubled in the past 20 years, exceeding all other neoplasms. In fact, in Australia, the rate had been doubling

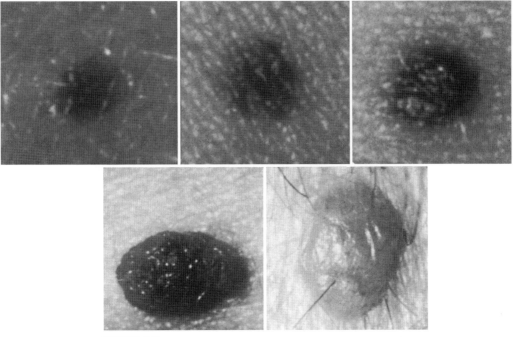

FIGURE 5-7
These photographs depict the most common flat and raised presentations of benign moles/nevi.

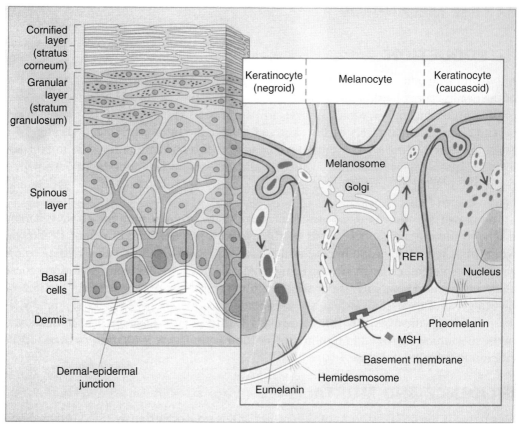

FIGURE 5-8
This diagram depicts a cross-sectional view of the skin and shows the relationship of the melanocyte to the basal cellular layer and rising keratinocytes.

every 10 years.[60] Fortunately, there is now some evidence that the current melanoma "epidemic" may be leveling off. Since 1990, the rise in the incidence has slowed and may be stabilizing for women born after 1930 and for men born after 1950.[61,62] Melanoma can occur at any age but has its peak incidence in the 40- to 50-year-old age group for both men and women. There is a second peak in both women and men in the 65- to 75-year age range. Mortality had also increased by 2% annually between 1960 and 1998, when the rate began to level off, particularly in women. This leveling has also occurred in incidence rates. It is estimated that nearly 8000 persons will die from melanoma in the United States in 2003.[59]

Although the exact etiology of melanoma is unknown, it is clear that exposure to UV light plays a critical factor in the development of this type of cancer.[63] The latitude effect demonstrates the effect of UV light on the incidence of melanoma—the farther fair-skinned people are from the north and south poles, the greater their risk for developing melanoma. Adjusted for skin type, the incidence of melanoma is highest at equatorial latitudes and falls off the farther one travels from the equator. Latitude studies of school-age children who live closer to the equator have shown significantly increased nevus and freckle counts. This phenomenon is not occurring in individuals whose skin is of darker pigmentation. The lifetime risk of developing melanoma in Caucasians is 1 in 80; it is 1 in 1100 in heavily pigmented peoples, thus suggesting that darkly pigmented and easily tanned individuals are protected.

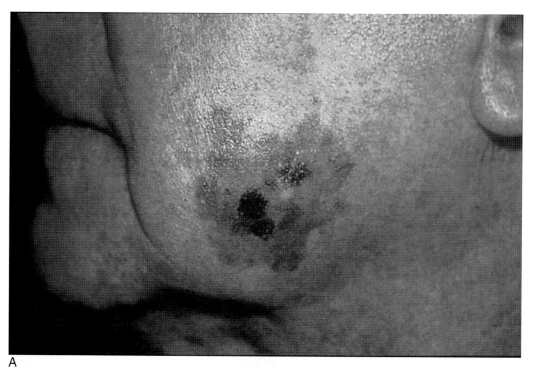

A

FIGURE 5-9

A, Characteristic presentation of the earliest form of melanoma. Lentigo maligna melanoma, pure radial growth, no vertical grown (invasion). Also called melanoma in situ.

RISK FACTORS

As previously stated, excess sun exposure, particularly a history of severe sunburn, is associated with the development of melanoma. Included in the solar risk factors are a sun-sensitive skin type, multiple common or atypical nevi, NMSCs, AK, and xeroderma pigmentosum or chronic immunosuppression. Non–solar-based risk factors include increased numbers of melanocytic nevi in children and the familial atypical mole or melanoma syndrome (FAMMS).[64-66]

Sun-sensitive skin types include persons with blond or red hair, blue or green eyes, light complexion, freckles, and inability to tan. The pattern and duration of sunlight appear to be important for the development of melanoma. In contrast to NMSCs, which are associated with cumulative sun exposure and occur most frequently in areas always exposed to the sun, melanomas are associated with intense, sporadic exposure and tend to occur in skin areas exposed to the sun sporadically.[67] In fact, sporadic exposure that results in severe burns in childhood and adolescence more than doubles the risk of developing melanoma.[68] It is possible that the first high-dose exposure of the skin to UV light causes programmed cell death of damaged keratinocytes (the cells that produce NMSCs), but melanocytes survive, probably indirectly because of the body's need for sun protection from melanin. Severely damaged melanocytes may survive for more future UV light insults, eventually undergoing some unknown mutational change to begin malignant proliferation.[69]

UVB radiation causes the majority of DNA damage. However, roughly 10 to 100 times more UVA radiation penetrates the atmosphere and is probably just as mutagenic as UVB. Animal studies have shown that UVA irradiation can cause the same DNA mutations and local skin immunosuppression as UVB, but UVA requires much longer exposure times.[63] Sunscreen

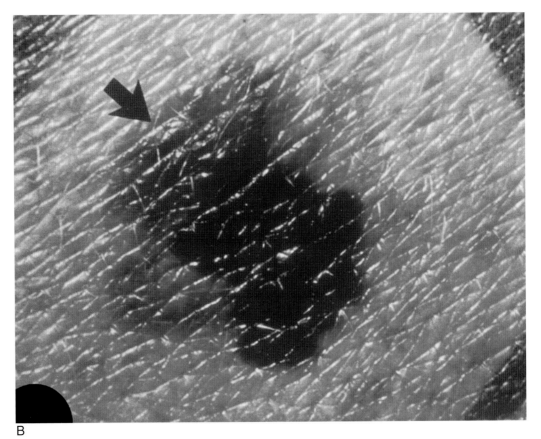

B

FIGURE 5-9, cont'd
B, Characteristic presentation of the most common form of melanoma—superficial spreading melanoma. Both radial and vertical growth.

protection, reported as an SPF number, primarily measures the protection against UVB; it does not adequately assess the photoprotective profile against UVA. There is some evidence that the UVA to UVB ratio is important because most sunscreens effectively block UVB but not UVA. This gives a false sense of protection and actually increases the nonprotected time in the sun.[70,71] It is unclear whether tanning salons, which primarily use UVA, have any impact on the development of melanoma. Controlled studies of artificial UV irradiation are difficult to interpret because people who use tanning salons also tend to purposefully tan. Although the use of tanning beds results in a slow and controlled exposure to UV light, chronic use may still result in the development of skin cancers, including melanoma. The only value to the use of tanning beds is the possible prevention of a severe burn because the skin is tanned slowly. However, no studies to date have been performed that substantiate any benefit to the use of tanning beds before any form of recreational sun exposure.

Familial history of melanoma in a first-degree relative is the greatest risk in the development of melanoma. The familial atypical mole and melanoma syndrome has been associated with mutations at chromosomes 1 and 9. These patients may have more than 100 nevi, with at least 10 that are severely clinically atypical. The incidence of melanoma in these families approaches 100%. The development of melanoma in this group appears to be independent of UV light exposure. Two genes appear to be involved: p16 or MTS1, a tumor suppressor gene that is mutated or deleted, and CDK4, an oncogene that promotes uncontrolled

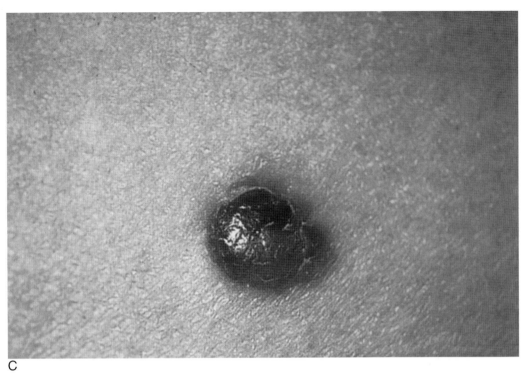

C

FIGURE 5-9, cont'd
C, Characteristic presentation of nodular melanoma—no radial growth, only vertical growth.

growth.[72,73] Both of these genetic mutations are present in most long-term cultured melanoma cell lines, uncultured melanoma cells, and the germline of melanoma families.[74] Studies of these families and of their genetic mutations have shed light on the development of sporadic melanoma. There appears to be a link between UV light irradiation and p16 expression in modulating damage induced by UVB exposure. Deletions or mutations of p16 will disable melanocytes from repairing DNA damage and allow mutations to be passed on in subsequent cell divisions.[75]

Melanoma, Pregnancy, and Exogenous Sex Hormones

The relationship between pregnancy, estrogen, and progesterone has always been entertained as a result of the clinical observations of increasing numbers of moles and melanin pigmentation (chloasma) during pregnancy. These observations suggested that melanin production can be stimulated by estrogen and therefore could cause or induce the development of melanoma. In addition, it was discovered that estrogen receptors were detected in approximately 20% to 30% of melanoma specimens.[76]

To date there is no evidence that pregnancy induces melanoma, makes melanoma more aggressive, or induces a recurrent melanoma. About 20% of women experience clinical changes in the number and color of their moles.[77] However, biopsy specimens of these moles have not shown any specific changes or activation of the melanocytes.[77,78]

All of the studies that involve melanoma and pregnancy are retrospective and show no difference in type of melanoma, site of melanoma, or aggressiveness of melanoma.[79-84] There is no evidence that the clinical course of melanoma arising or recurring during a pregnancy is adversely affected by that pregnancy. Old literature, based on very small case studies, suggested that pregnancy accelerated the process of metastasis. Since that time, in recent reviews

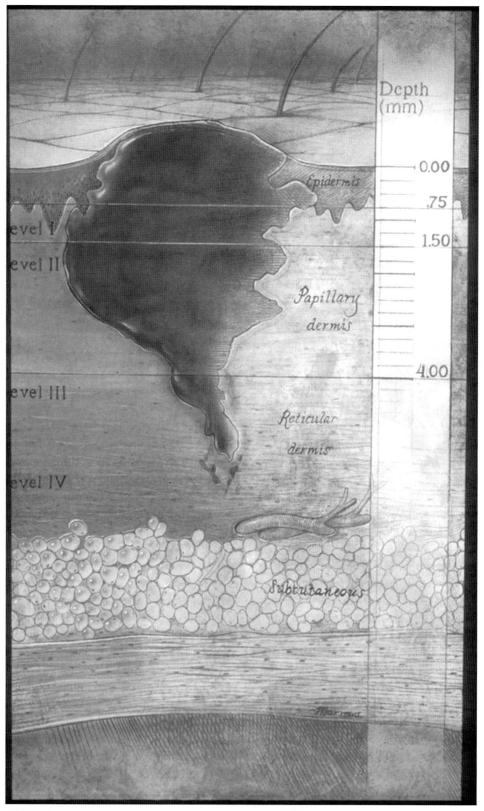

FIGURE 5-10
This figure depicts a stylized drawing of a melanoma and shows Clark's levels (I–V) on the left and Breslow depth (mm) on the right.

of larger numbers of women with early stages of melanoma diagnosed during pregnancy, the melanoma had no different clinical course than that of nonpregnant women.[79-84] In fact melanoma before, after, or during pregnancy is most probably not significantly different in its aggressiveness, compared with melanomas in nulliparous women. However, it is recommended that women wait for at least 2 years after the diagnosis of melanoma before becoming pregnant. Again, the reason for waiting is not because of the effect of pregnancy on melanoma but rather the effect of recurrent melanoma on pregnancy. Most melanomas, if they are to recur, will recur within the first 2 years of diagnosis and treatment. Therefore if a melanoma were to recur during a pregnancy, the treatment options could become severely limited. Surgical excision is almost always possible, but adjuvant therapies that use immunotherapy or chemotherapy, or both, are quite difficult and potentially lethal to the fetus. Aggressive biochemotherapy for metastatic melanoma in the face of pregnancy has not been reported and is almost certainly not indicated.[85]

Recent studies on the use of oral contraceptives before the development of melanoma have been reported from Europe and the United States.[86,87] No association with any duration of oral contraceptive use and subsequent melanoma risk was found. The use of oral contraceptives and hormone replacement therapy subsequent to a treated melanoma has not been as well studied. No large studies of the use of oral contraceptives or hormonal replacement after the diagnosis of melanoma have been conducted. There is no evidence to avoid the use of either therapy in women who have had melanoma, but the common current practice is to delay any estrogen or progesterone use for 2 years. This is the same rationale for the delay of pregnancy for 2 years after a successfully treated melanoma.[85]

PREVENTION OF MELANOMA

The primary prevention of melanoma relies on routine, frequent skin self-examination, dermatology screening, and the consistent use of sunscreens. This applies to all light-skinned individuals regardless of prior personal or family history. The only difference in high-risk individuals (prior melanoma, familial atypical mole melanoma syndrome) is the frequency of professional screening, body photographs, and mole biopsy—in general, self-examination of all body areas at least every 1 to 2 months and at least a yearly dermatologic examination. High-risk individuals should be examined every 4 to 6 months by a physician who is well versed in the diagnosis and treatment of melanoma. Total body photographs and photographs of individual moles by standard photography or digital imaging have been used primarily for people in the high-risk category but are gaining popularity for all patients with moles.

Self-examination, probably practiced by a small percentage of our population, should be carried out in a step-by-step process. A thorough examination requires the individual to undress completely, have a full-length and a hand-held mirror, a hair dryer, and excellent lighting. Using both mirrors, one can examine virtually the entire body surface. The hair dryer is used to separate the hair for a good scalp examination. For the hard-to-see areas of the scalp, back, and buttocks, it is wise to enlist the help of a family member or spouse. Educational pamphlets showing the step-by-step self-examination can be obtained from the American Academy of Dermatology, the Skin Cancer Foundation, and the American Cancer Society (Box 5-2).

All light-skinned people who live in sunny climates or whose profession requires prolonged sun exposure should seek a thorough dermatology examination at least every 6 months. This may not completely prevent all melanomas but will certainly allow for earlier diagnoses that will more likely result in cures. Any new or suspicious mole should be

---

BOX 5-2   **Resources for Patients and Providers**

American Academy of Dermatology
P.O. Box 4014
Schaumburg, IL 60168-4014
Telephone: 1-888-462-3376
www.aad.org

The Skin Cancer Foundation
245 Fifth Avenue, Suite 1403
Department SEC
New York, NY 10016
Telephone: 1-800-SKIN-490
www.skincancer.org

American Cancer Society
1599 Clifton Rd., NE
Atlanta, GA 30329
Telephone: 1-800-227-2345
www.cancer.org

---

carefully inspected under magnification and a biopsy performed if there is any clinical or historical atypia. Patients with multiple atypical moles, with or without a history of melanoma, should be photographed; photographs should incorporate the total body, body sections, and individual moles. This mole "mapping" will result in prevention and, more importantly, earlier diagnosis. Prophylactic removal of all moles does not prevent melanoma because most melanomas probably do not occur in existing moles but rather in moles or lesions yet to develop.

The most controversial method of preventing melanoma is the use of sunscreens. The best sunscreen is full clothing with all body surfaces covered, especially with clothing designed to reflect ultraviolet light. Inasmuch as this is not always practical or possible, sunscreens become our only choice. There is current evidence that sunscreens can reduce the development of moles in children, thereby possibly reducing the number of melanomas that can occur from moles destined for or capable of malignant change. However, there are still no definitive data that show that the use of sunscreens prevents melanoma. There is evidence that the improper use of sunscreen, combined with prolonged or intense sun exposure, can increase the risk of development of melanoma.[88,89] Therefore reliance on sunscreen as the sole method of sun protection is foolhardy. Avoidance of the sun; avoidance of severe, blistering sunburns; and use of protective clothing and sunscreens may all be necessary.

The types of sunscreens are divided into those that primarily block UVB irradiation and those that block both UVB (which causes the majority of DNA damage) and UVA light. It appears that it is chemically more difficult to block the longer-wavelength UVA light. Furthermore, 10 to 100 times more UVA light reaches the earth's surface than does UVB. The best UVA block is avobenzone (Parsol), followed by oxybenzone and methyl anthyranilate. The absolute best inorganic physical blocks of all UV light are titanium dioxide or zinc oxide, both of which are cosmetically and texturally unpopular. Again, as stated before, a sunscreen that can effectively block all UV light, even at high SPF levels, is not the sole answer to sun protection. Avoidance of peak sunlight hours of the day, protective clothing, wide-brimmed hats, and the proper use and reapplication of sunscreens may be the best method of melanoma prevention.

REFERENCES

1. Marcil I, Stern RS: Risk of developing a subsequent nonmelanoma skin cancer in patients with a history of nonmelanoma skin cancer: a critical review of the literature and meta-analysis. *Arch Dermatol* 2000;136:1524-1530.
2. Miller DL, Weinstock MA: Nonmelanoma skin cancer in the United States: incidence. *J Am Acad Dermatol* 1994;30:774-778.
3. Weinstock MA: Nonmelanoma skin cancer mortality in the United States, 1969 through 1988. *Arch Dermatol* 1993;129:1286-1290.
4. American Cancer Society: *Nonmelanoma skin cancer,* 2001.
5. Giles GG, Marks R, Foley P: Incidence of nonmelanocytic skin cancer treated in Australia. *Br Med J (Clin Res Ed)* 1988;296:13-17.
6. Green A, Battistutta D: Incidence and determinants of skin cancer in a high-risk Australian population. *Int J Cancer* 1990;46:356-361.
7. Marks R, Staples M, Giles GG: Trends in nonmelanocytic skin cancer treated in Australia: the second national survey. *Int J Cancer* 1993;53:585-590.
8. Glass AG, Hoover RN: The emerging epidemic of melanoma and squamous cell skin cancer [see comments]. *JAMA* 1989;262:2097-2100.
9. Gallagher RP, Hill GB, Bajdik CD, et al: Sunlight exposure, pigmentation factors, and risk of nonmelanocytic skin cancer, II: squamous cell carcinoma. *Arch Dermatol* 1995;131:164-169.
10. Gallagher RP, Hill GB, Bajdik CD, et al: Sunlight exposure, pigmentary factors, and risk of nonmelanocytic skin cancer, I: basal cell carcinoma. *Arch Dermatol* 1995;131:157-163.
11. Kricker A, Armstrong BK, English DR, et al: Pigmentary and cutaneous risk factors for nonmelanocytic skin cancer: a case-control study. *Int J Cancer* 1991;48:650-662.
12. Chuang TY, Reizner GT, Elpern DJ, et al: Nonmelanoma skin cancer in Japanese ethnic Hawaiians in Kauai, Hawaii: an incidence report. *J Am Acad Dermatol* 1995;33:422-426.
13. Vitasa BC, Taylor HR, Strickland PT, et al: Association of nonmelanoma skin cancer and actinic keratosis with cumulative solar ultraviolet exposure in Maryland watermen. *Cancer* 1990;65:2811-2817.
14. Franceschi S, Levi F, Randimbison L, et al: Site distribution of different types of skin cancer: new aetiologicalclues. *Int J Cancer* 1996;67:24-28.
15. Levi F, Franceschi S, Te VC, et al: Trends of skin cancer in the Canton of Vaud, 1976-92. *Br J Cancer* 1995;72:1047-1053.
16. Weinstock MA, Bogaars HA, Ashley M, et al: Nonmelanoma skin cancer mortality: a population-based study. *Arch Dermatol* 1991;127:1194-1197.
17. Moller R, Reymann F, Hou-Jensen K: Metastases in dermatological patients with squamous cell carcinoma. *Arch Dermatol* 1979;115:703-705.
18. Weinstock MA: Death from skin cancer among the elderly: epidemiological patterns. *Arch Dermatol* 1997;133:1207-1209.
19. Tong AKF, Fitzpatrick TB: Neoplasms of the skin. In Holland JF, Kufe DW, Pollock RE, editors: *Cancer medicine,* ed 5, Lewiston, NY, BC Decker, 2000, Section 33:1823-1848.
20. MacKie RM: *Skin cancer: An illustrated guide to the aetiology, clinical features, pathology and management of benign and malignant cutaneous tumours,* St. Louis and London, Mosby and Martin Dunitz, 1996.
21. Nomura T, Nakajima H, Hongyo T, et al: Induction of cancer, actinic keratosis, and specific p53 mutations by UVB light in human skin maintained in severe combined immunodeficient mice. *Cancer Res* 1997;57:2081-2084.
22. Ziegler A, Jonason AS, Leffell DJ, et al: Sunburn and p53 in the onset of skin cancer [see comments]. *Nature* 1994;372:773-776.
23. Freedberg IM, Fitzpatrick TB: *Fitzpatrick's dermatology in general medicine,* New York, McGraw-Hill, 1999.
24. Ren ZP, Hedrum A, Ponten F, et al: Human epidermal cancer and accompanying precursors have identical p53 mutations different from p53 mutations in adjacent areas of clonally expanded non-neoplastic keratinocytes. *Oncogene* 1996;12:765-773.
25. Coldiron BM: Thinning of the ozone layer: facts and consequences [see comments]. *J Am Acad Dermatol* 1992;27:653-662.
26. Kerr RA: Ozone hole: not over the Arctic—for now [news]. *Science* 1992;256:734.
27. Manney G, Froidevaux L, Waters J, et al: Chemical depletion of ozone in the arctic: lower stratosphere during winter 1992-93. *Nature* 1994;370:429-434.
28. Moan J, Dahlback A: The relationship between skin cancers, solar radiation and ozone depletion. *Br J Cancer* 1992;65:916-921.
29. Fears TR, Scotto J, Schneiderman MA: Mathematical models of age and ultraviolet effects on the incidence of skin cancer among whites in the United States. *Am J Epidemiol* 1977;105:420-427.
30. Okoro AN: Albinism in Nigeria. A clinical and social study. *Br J Dermatol* 1975;92:485-492.
31. Friedman RJ: *Cancer of the skin,* Philadelphia, WB Saunders, 1991.
32. Ramani ML, Bennett RG: High prevalence of skin cancer in World War II servicemen stationed in the Pacific theater. *J Am Acad Dermatol* 1993;28:733-737.
33. Stern RS, Laird N, Melski J, et al: Cutaneous squamous-cell carcinoma in patients treated with PUVA. *N Engl J Med* 1984;310:1156-1161.
34. Stern RS, Laird N: The carcinogenic risk of treatments for severe psoriasis: photochemotherapy follow-up study. *Cancer* 1994;73:2759-2764.
35. Karagas MR, Stukel TA, Greenberg ER, et al: Risk of subsequent basal cell carcinoma and squamous cell carcinoma of the skin among patients with prior skin cancer: Skin Cancer Prevention Study Group. *JAMA* 1992;267:3305-3310.
36. Smith JB, Fenske NA: Cutaneous manifestations and consequences of smoking [see comments]. *J Am Acad Dermatol* 1996;34:717-732; quiz 733-734.

37. Maize JC: Skin cancer in immunosuppressed patients [editorial]. *JAMA* 1977;237:1857-1858.

38. Lutzner MA: Skin cancer in immunosuppressed organ transplant recipients. *J Am Acad Dermatol* 1984;11:891-893.

39. Hartevelt MM, Bavinck JN, Kootte AM, et al: Incidence of skin cancer after renal transplantation in the Netherlands. *Transplantation* 1990;49:506-509.

40. Kiviat NB: Papillomaviruses in non-melanoma skin cancer: epidemiological aspects. *Semin Cancer Biol* 1999;9:397-403.

41. de Villiers EM, Lavergne D, McLaren K, et al: Prevailing papillomavirus types in non-melanoma carcinomas of the skin in renal allograft recipients. *Int J Cancer* 1997;73:356-361.

42. Guitart J, Bergfeld WF, Tuthill RJ, et al: Squamous cell carcinoma of the nail bed: a clinicopathological study of 12 cases. *Br J Dermatol* 1990;123:215-222.

43. Loescher LJ, Buller MK, Buller DB, et al: Public education projects in skin cancer: the evolution of skin cancer prevention education for children at a comprehensive cancer center. *Cancer* 1995;75:651-656.

44. Stern RS, Weinstein MC, Baker SG: Risk reduction for nonmelanoma skin cancer with childhood sunscreen use. *Arch Dermatol* 1986;122:537-545.

45. Banks BA, Silverman RA, Schwartz RH, et al: Attitudes of teenagers toward sun exposure and sunscreen use. *Pediatrics* 1992;89:40-42.

46. Crane LA, Schneider LS, Yohn JJ, et al: "Block the sun, not the fun": evaluation of a skin cancer prevention program for child care centers. *Am J Prev Med* 1999;17:31-37.

47. Dolan NC, Ng JS, Martin GJ, et al: Effectiveness of a skin cancer control educational intervention for internal medicine housestaff and attending physicians. *J Gen Intern Med* 1997;12:531-536.

48. Naylor MF, Boyd A, Smith DW, et al: High sun protection factor sunscreens in the suppression of actinic neoplasia. *Arch Dermatol* 1995;131:170-175.

49. Marks R: Non-melanoma skin cancer and solar keratoses in Australia: a review. *Eur J Epidemiol* 1985;1:319-322.

50. Fitzpatrick TB: *Dermatology in general medicine,* New York, McGraw-Hill, 1993.

51. DeBuys HV, Levy SB, Murray JC, et al: Modern approaches to photoprotection. *Dermatol Clin* 2000;18:577-590.

52. Stratton SP, Dorr RT, Alberts DS: The state-of-the-art in chemoprevention of skin cancer. *Eur J Cancer* 2000;36:1292-1297.

53. Moon TE, Levine N, Cartmel B, et al: Effect of retinol in preventing squamous cell skin cancer in moderate-risk subjects: a randomized, double-blind, controlled trial. Southwest Skin Cancer Prevention Study Group. *Cancer Epidemiol Biomarkers Prev* 1997;6:949-956.

54. Levine N, Moon TE, Cartmel B, et al: Trial of retinol and isotretinoin in skin cancer prevention: a randomized, double-blind, controlled trial. Southwest Skin Cancer Prevention Study Group. *Cancer Epidemiol Biomarkers Prev* 1997;6:957-961.

55. Bavinck JN, Tieben LM, Van der Woude FJ, et al: Prevention of skin cancer and reduction of keratotic skin lesions during acitretin therapy in renal transplant recipients: a double-blind, placebo-controlled study. *J Clin Oncol* 1995;13:1933-1938.

56. Clark LC, Combs GF Jr, Turnbull BW, et al: Effects of selenium supplementation for cancer prevention in patients with carcinoma of the skin: a randomized controlled trial, Nutritional Prevention of Cancer Study Group [see comments] [published erratum appears in *JAMA* 1997;277:1520]. *JAMA* 1996;276:1957-1963.

57. Green A, Williams G, Neale R: Does daily use of sunscreen or beta-carotene supplements prevent skin cancer in healthy adults? *West J Med* 2000;173:332.

58. Black HS, Thornby JI, Wolf JE Jr., et al: Evidence that a low-fat diet reduces the occurrence of nonmelanoma skin cancer. *Int J Cancer* 1995;62:165-169.

59. Greenlee RT, Murray T, Bolden S, et al: Cancer statistics, 2000. *CA Cancer J Clin* 2000;50:7-33.

60. Whiteman DC, Valery P, McWhirter W, et al: Risk factors for childhood melanoma in Queensland, Australia. *Int J Cancer* 1997;70:26-31.

61. Hall HI, Miller DR, Rogers JD, et al: Update on the incidence and mortality from melanoma in the United States. *J Am Acad Dermatol* 1999;40:35-42.

62. Jemal A, Devesa SS, Fears TR, et al: Cancer surveillance series: changing patterns of cutaneous malignant melanoma mortality rates among whites in the United States. *J Natl Cancer Inst* 2000;92:811-818.

63. Longstreth JD: Melanoma genesis, putative causes, and possible mechanisms. In Soong S, editor: *Cutaneous melanoma,* ed 3, St. Louis, Quality Medical, 1998.

64. Clark WH Jr, Reimer RR, Greene M, et al: Origin of familial malignant melanomas from heritable melanocytic lesions: "The B-K mole syndrome." *Arch Dermatol* 1978;114:732-738.

65. Bale SJ, Dracopoli NC, Tucker MA, et al: Mapping the gene for hereditary cutaneous malignant melanoma-dysplastic nevus to chromosome 1p. *N Engl J Med* 1989;320:1367-1372.

66. Goldstein AM, Goldin LR, Dracopoli NC, et al: Two-locus linkage analysis of cutaneous malignant melanoma/dysplastic nevi. *Am J Hum Genet* 1996;58:1050-1056.

67. Elwood JM, Gallagher RP, Hill GB, et al: Cutaneous melanoma in relation to intermittent and constant sun exposure: the Western Canada Melanoma Study. *Int J Cancer* 1985;35:427-433.

68. Weinstock MA: Controversies in the role of sunlight in the pathogenesis of cutaneous melanoma. *Photochem Photobiol* 1996;63:406-410.

69. Gilchrest BA, Eller MS, Geller AC, et al: The pathogenesis of melanoma induced by ultraviolet radiation. *N Engl J Med* 1999;340:1341-1348.

70. Gasparro FP, Mitchnick M, Nash JF: A review of sunscreen safety and efficacy. *Photochem Photobiol* 1998;68:243-256.

71. Sunscreens: are they safe and effective? *Med Lett Drugs Ther* 1999;41:43-44.

72. Kamb A, Gruis NA, Weaver-Feldhaus J, et al: A cell cycle regulator potentially involved in genesis of many tumor types. *Science* 1994;264:436-440.

73. Piepkorn M: Melanoma genetics: an update with focus on the CDKN2A(p16)/ARF tumor suppressors. *J Am Acad Dermatol* 2000;42:705-722; quiz 723-706.

74. Soufir N, Avril MF, Chompret A, et al: Prevalence of p16 and CDK4 germline mutations in 48 melanoma-prone families in France, The French Familial Melanoma Study Group. *Hum Mol Genet* 1998;7:209-216.

75. Piepkorn M: The expression of p16(INK4a), the product of a tumor suppressor gene for melanoma, is upregulated in human melanocytes by UVB irradiation. *J Am Acad Dermatol* 2000; 42:741-745.

76. Fisher RI, Neifeld JP, Lippman ME: Oestrogen receptors in human malignant melanoma. *Lancet* 1976;2:337-339.

77. Sanchez JL, Figueroa LD, Rodriguez E: Behavior of melanocytic nevi during pregnancy. *Am J Dermatopathol* 1984;6:89-91.

78. Foucar E, Bentley TJ, Laube DW, et al: A histopathologic evaluation of nevocellular nevi in pregnancy. *Arch Dermatol* 1985;121:350-354.

79. Wong JH, Sterns EE, Kopald KH, et al: Prognostic significance of pregnancy in stage I melanoma. *Arch Surg* 1989;124:1227-1230; discussion 1230-1231.

80. Reintgen DS, McCarty KS Jr, Vollmer R, et al: Malignant melanoma and pregnancy. *Cancer* 1985;55:1340-1344.

81. MacKie RM, Bufalino R, Morabito A, et al: Lack of effect of pregnancy on outcome of melanoma: for The World Health Organisation Melanoma Programme. *Lancet* 1991;337:653-655.

82. Houghton AN, Flannery J, Viola MV: Malignant melanoma of the skin occurring during pregnancy. *Cancer* 1981;48:407-410.

83. Travers RL, Sober AJ, Berwick M, et al: Increased thickness of pregnancy-associated melanoma. *Br J Dermatol* 1995;132:876-883.

84. Slingluff CL Jr, Reintgen DS, Vollmer RT, et al: Malignant melanoma arising during pregnancy: a study of 100 patients. *Ann Surg* 1990;211:552-557; discussion 558-559.

85. MacKie RM: Pregnancy and exogenous female sex hormones in melanoma. In Soong S, editor: *Cutaneous melanoma*, St. Louis, Quality Medical, 1998.

86. Holly EA, Cress RD, Ahn DK: Cutaneous melanoma in women, III: reproductive factors and oral contraceptive use. *Am J Epidemiol* 1995;141:943-950.

87. Zanetti R, Franceschi S, Rosso S, et al: Cutaneous malignant melanoma in females: the role of hormonal and reproductive factors. *Int J Epidemiol* 1990;19:522-526.

88. Bigby M: The sunscreen and melanoma controversy. *Arch Dermatol* 1999;135:1526-1527.

89. Autier P: Sunscreen and melanoma revisited. *Arch Dermatol* 2000;136:423.

chapter 6

Cervical Cancer

Alberto Manetta

INCIDENCE AND MORTALITY

The prevention of cervical cancer is one of the most successful examples of cancer control and prevention. Cervical cancer–related mortality has decreased dramatically during the last 80 years from 30/100,000 in 1930 to 3.8 per 100,000 in 2000[1] (Figure 6-1). Since 1982 cervical cancer–related mortality rates have declined 1.5% per year.[1]

There is a significant discrepancy in the incidence of cervical cancer and in cancer-related mortality among different minorities in the United States and different countries in the world. The total number of women diagnosed with cervical cancer in the United States in 1999 was 12,900, with a cancer-related mortality of 4400.[1] However, the number of women affected worldwide is approximately 471,000, with a mortality of 215,000.[2,3] In many of the developing countries, cervical cancer is the most common cause of death during the reproductive years. For instance, the incidence rate in the 35- to 64-year-old age group in Chennai, India, is 99 per 100,000, which is even higher than the rate reported from Cali, Colombia, of 77 per 100,000.[4] The success of the present cervical cancer screening program is limited to developed, Western countries.

Cervical cancer is considered a cancer of the reproductive age group but also occurs in the fifth, sixth, and seventh decades. It is common for older women not to be screened for cervical cancer. As a result, the incidence in this population is higher than expected. In the latest National Institutes of Health (NIH) Consensus Conference on cervical cancer, the higher incidence of patients older than 65 was discussed and emphasized as a public health concern.[5] The mean age for cervical cancer in this country is 52 years.[6]

In the United States, the incidence of cervical cancer is not homogeneously distributed among different ethnic groups. Statistics for most of the racial minorities show a higher incidence of disease and cancer-related deaths than for the non-Hispanic White population. Table 6-1 shows the incidence and mortality rates for U.S. Hispanics versus non-Hispanic Whites. In U.S. Hispanics, the incidence rate is 15.3 per 100,000 versus an incidence of 7.1 for non-Hispanic Whites.[7] The mortality rates parallel incidence rates with 3.4 and 2.3 cervical cancer–related deaths per 1000,000 for Hispanics and non-Hispanic Whites, respectively.[7] The incidence for African Americans is also higher than for Whites, 11.4 per 100,000.[8] The reasons for this difference in incidence are most likely related to several factors, including a higher incidence of human papillomavirus (HPV)-related premalignant lesions, cultural differences, and health care access–related issues that impede appropriate screening. The progression from dysplasia to cancer among different ethnic groups has not been appropriately studied.

HISTOLOGIC TYPES AND STAGING

Cervical carcinoma, histologically, has been divided into three main categories:
1. Squamous cell carcinoma
2. Adenocarcinoma
3. Other epithelial tumors

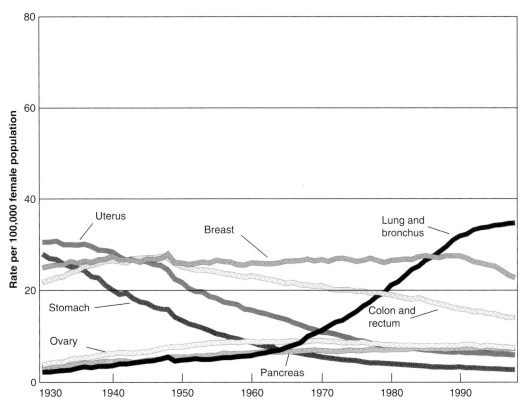

FIGURE 6-1
Cancer death rates for females in the United States, 1930-1998, per 100,000. Age adjusted to the 1970 population. (From *Cancer facts and figures 2001*. American Cancer Society, 2001. Attachment A.)

Squamous cell carcinoma represents the majority of cervical cancers, with a relative incidence of 65% to 80%.[9] The decrease in incidence of cervical cancer is mostly in squamous cell carcinoma; the incidence of adenocarcinomas remains unchanged or even shows an increase, according to some studies.[10-12] The reason for the relative increase of adenocarcinomas versus squamous cancers has not been clearly established. Although some hypotheses

Table 6-1
Hispanic and White Non-Hispanic Incidence and Mortality Rates

	INCIDENCE RATES*			MORTALITY RATES*	
	Hispanic	White Non-Hispanic		Hispanic	White Non-Hispanic
All sites combined	272.9	414.1	All sites combined	104.0	168.4
Female breast	68.9	118.7	Female breast	15.1	25.6
Colon and rectum	28.8	44.8	Colon and rectum	10.3	17.4
Lung	27.1	58.4	Lung	19.8	50.3
Prostate	101.6	149.2	Prostate	16.2	23.4
Cervix	15.3	7.1	Cervix	3.4	2.3
Stomach	10.3	5.9	Stomach	5.8	3.6
Liver	5.7	2.8	Liver	4.8	2.9

*Rates of new cases or deaths per 100,000 people in 1990-1997.
Source: Surveillance, Epidemiology and End Results Cancer Incidence CD-ROM 1990-1997, Division of Cancer Control and Population Sciences, National Cancer Institute, 1990.

Table 6-2
Carcinoma of the Cervix Uteri: FIGO Nomenclature (Montreal, 1994)

Stage 0	Carcinoma in situ, cervical intraepithelial neoplasia Grade III.
Stage I	The carcinoma is strictly confined to the cervix (extension to the corpus would be disregarded). Invasive carcinoma which can be diagnosed only by microscopy. All macroscopically visible lesions—even with superficial invasion—are allotted to Stage 1b carcinomas. Invasion is limited to a measured stromal invasion with a maximal depth of 5.0 mm and a horizontal extension of not > 7.0 mm. Depth of invasion should not be > 5.0 mm taken from the base of the epithelium of the original tissue—superficial or glandular. The involvement of vascular spaces—venous or lymphatic—should not change the stage allotment. 1a1, measured stromal invasion of not > 3.0 mm in depth and extension of not > 7.0 mm. 1a2, measured stromal invasion of > 3.0 mm and not > 5.0 mm with an extension of not > 7.00 mm. Clinically visible lesions limited to the cervix uteri or preclinical cancers greater than Stage 1a. 1b1, clinically visible lesions not > 4.0 cm. 1b2, clinically visible lesions > 4.0 cm.
Stage II	Cervical carcinoma invades beyond the uterus but not to the pelvic wall or to the lower third of the vagina. IIa, no obvious parametrial involvement. IIb, obvious parametrial involvement.
Stage III	The carcinoma has extended to the pelvic wall. On rectal examination, there is no cancer-free space between the tumor and the pelvic wall. The tumor involves the lower third of the vagina. All cases with hydronephrosis or nonfunctioning kidney are included, unless they are known to be due to other cause. IIIa, tumor involves lower-third of the vagina, with no extension to the pelvic wall. IIIb, extension to the pelvic wall and/or hydronephrosis or nonfunctioning kidney.
Stage IV	The carcinoma has extended beyond the true pelvis or has involved (biopsy-proven) the mucosa of the bladder or rectum. A bullous edema, as such, does not permit a case to be allotted to Stage IV. IVa, spread of the growth to adjacent organs. IVb, spread to distant organs.

Source: Benedet JL, Bender H, Jones H III, Ngan HY, et al: FIGO staging classifications and clinical practice guidelines in the management of gynecologic cancers. FIGO Committee on Gynecologic Oncology. *Int J Gynaecol Obstet* 2000;70:209-262.

indicate a possible carcinogenic effect of oral contraceptive pills (OCPs), differences in the effectiveness of the Papanicolaou (Pap) smear in the screening of preinvasive squamous versus glandular lesions provide a more likely explanation. The presence of adenocarcinomas in the endocervical canal instead of the outer portion of the cervix may be undetected by a Pap smear, thus leading to reports of a higher false-negative rate.

In contrast to cancer of the uterus and ovary, which are surgically staged, carcinoma of the cervix is clinically staged.[13] Table 6-2 presents the International Federation of Gynecology and Obstetrics (FIGO) staging classification of carcinoma of the cervix. The cancer-related mortality, which is between 0% and 3% for stages 0 to 1B, escalates very rapidly.

RISK FACTORS

Reproductive and Sexual Factors

For a long time it has been known that sexual behavior affects the incidence of cervical cancer. Specifically, well-controlled studies have demonstrated that age of first sexual intercourse and numbers of sexual partners have a significant influence on the incidence of cervical cancer.[14-16]

Ruth Peters investigated the risk factors associated with cervical cancer by using a case-control study. She reported that the number of sexual partners before age 20 was particularly significant.[14] The number of sexual partners seems to be a surrogate for HPV infections,[17] and the risk of cervical cancer may be directly related to the number of pregnancies and births.[15,18] This risk persisted even after adjusting for sexual and socioeconomic factors.[19] Although it would be tempting to speculate that the number of births is a surrogate for HPV infection, that does not seem to be the case. Brinton and associates demonstrated a lack of relationship between HPV types 16 and 18 infection and parity.[19]

Human Papillomavirus

During the last few decades, some sexually transmitted diseases (STDs) other than HPV have been implicated in causing cervical cancer or accelerating its progress. The etiology of cervical cancer most likely is multifactorial. However, the only STD that consistently has been associated with cervical cancer and for which a reasonable mechanism of action has been found is the HPV infection; Zur Hausen hypothesized in 1975 that HPV could be the etiologic factor for cervical cancer.[20,21]

The human papillomavirus consists of a closed-circle, double-stranded genome of approximately 8000 base pairs (Figure 6-2). The viral genome is composed of eight early expressed genes or open reading frames (E1-E8), two late-open reading frames (L1-L2), and

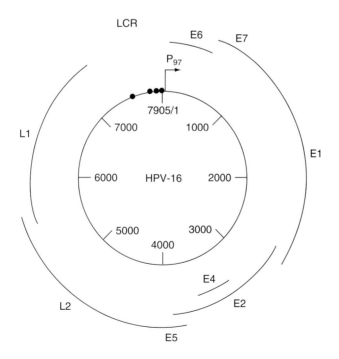

FIGURE 6-2
The genomic map of the human papillomavirus-16 (HPV-16) as deduced from the DNA sequence. (From DeVita VT, Hellman S, Rosenberg, SA: *Cancer: principles and practice of oncology,* ed 6, Philadelphia, Lippincott Williams & Wilkins, 2001.)

a long control region (LCR) or upstream regulatory control region. The role of these genes is not completely clear, but some basic functions have been established (Table 6-3). The L1 region encodes a viral structural protein, which is highly antigenic and cross-reacts with most other HPV groups. The L1 protein proved to be critical in vaccine development (see the section on vaccines).[22-25]

HPV DNA is regularly found in primary and metastatic cervical cancer as well as in premalignant lesions. Several studies have documented that HPV infection in women with normal cytology precedes cervical intraepithelial neoplasia (CIN).[26]

HPV DNA in patients with normal Pap smears is associated with an increased risk for invasive cervical cancer. The subsequent invasive cancer will be positive for the same HPV type as previously discovered in the normal Pap smear.[27] Kjaer found that the first episode of genital warts is strongly associated with cervical cancer, indicating a higher predisposition of the adolescent cervix to the development of cervical cancer when infected with HPV. Although genital warts are related to different types of HPVs than cervical cancers, it is most likely that women at risk harbored more than one HPV type or are predisposed to other types of HPV infections.[16]

Although HPV may coexist with other etiologic factors, no other STD, other than HPV, seems to have an independent association with cervical cancer. It is possible that other STDs may act as cofactors, but in general the strength of these associations decreases significantly after the data are corrected for HPV infections. HPV exposure completely explains the risk related to sexual behavior, especially the total number of sexual partners, without any need to consider other STDs.[28] In addition, the numerous HPV types that are able to cause disease in the human lack serologic tests for their detection. There are more than 75 genotypes of HPVs found to be pathogenic in the human, and many can affect the genital tract. Some of them, such as types 6 and 11, cause benign conditions such as venereal warts and some, such as 16, 18, 31, and 33, are associated with cervical cancer (Table 6-4). The association of HPV and cervical cancer is consistent not only in the United States but also around the world. In a study that included more than 1000 cervical cancer specimens from different parts of the world, HPV DNA was detected in 93% of the tumors. HPV 16 was found in 50% of the specimens and was the prevalent type in all sample countries except Indonesia, where HPV 18 was predominant.[29]

Apoptosis, or natural cell death, is what prevents cells from proliferating uncontrollably and possibly developing into cancer. Several genes are primarily responsible for apoptotic events. The tumor suppressor gene p53 and the antiapoptotic bcl-2 seem to play a significant

Table 6-3
Gene Functions of Papillomavirus

Open Reading Frame	Function
E1	Modulation, DNA replication
E2	Viral transcriptional regulation, replication
E4	Cytoplasmic protein, virus maturation, and release
E5	Affects cell cycle kinases, transformation
E6	Oncoprotein, p53 suppression, immortalizing
E7	Oncoprotein, pRb suppression, immortalizing
L1	Major capsid protein
L2	Minor capsid protein
LCR	Promoter and enhancer elements

Source: Hilleman MR: Overview of vaccinology with special reference to papillomavirus vaccines. *J Clin Virol* 2000;19:79-90.

Table 6-4
Human Papillomavirus Types

HPV Type	Location	Association
1	Cutaneous	Plantar warts
2	Cutaneous	Common warts
3	Cutaneous	Flat warts
4	Cutaneous	Common and plantar warts
5	Cutaneous	Macular lesions in EV and cancers
6	Genital tract, other mucosae	Genital warts, laryngeal papillomatosis
7	Genital tract, other mucosae	"Butcher's" warts
8	Cutaneous	Macular lesions (EV) and cancers
9	Cutaneous	Macular lesions (EV)
10	Cutaneous	Flat warts
11	Genital tract, other mucosae	Genital warts, laryngeal papillomas
12	Cutaneous	Macular lesions (EV)
13	Oral	Oral focal epithelial hyperplasia
14	Cutaneous	Macular lesions (EV) and cancers
15	Cutaneous	Macular lesions (EV)
16	Genital tract, other mucosae	Intraepithelial neoplasia and cancers
17	Cutaneous	Macular lesions (EV) and cancers
18	Genital tract, other mucosae	Intraepithelial neoplasia and cancers
19	Cutaneous	Macular lesions (EV)
20	Cutaneous	Macular lesions (EV) and cancers
21	Cutaneous	Macular lesions (EV)
22	Cutaneous	Macular lesions (EV)
23	Cutaneous	Macular lesions (EV)
24	Cutaneous	Macular lesions (EV)
25	Cutaneous	Macular lesions (EV)
26	Cutaneous	Common warts
27	Cutaneous	Common warts
28	Cutaneous	Flat warts
29	Cutaneous	Common warts
30	Genital tract, other mucosae	Intraepithelial neoplasia and cancer
31	Genital tract, other mucosae	Intraepithelial neoplasia and cancers
32	Oral	Oral focal epithelial hyperplasia, oral papillomas
33	Genital tract, other mucosae	Intraepithelial neoplasia and cancers
34	Genital tract, other mucosae	Intraepithelial neoplasia
35	Genital tract, other mucosae	Intraepithelial neoplasia and cancers
36	Cutaneous	Actinic keratosis, EV lesions
37	Cutaneous	Not yet known, isolated from a keratoacanthoma
38	Cutaneous	Not yet known, isolated from a melanoma
39	Genital tract, other mucosae	Intraepithelial neoplasia and cancers
40	Genital tract, other mucosae	Intraepithelial neoplasia
41	Cutaneous	Flat warts
42	Genital tract, other mucosae	Intraepithelial neoplasia
43	Genital tract, other mucosae	Intraepithelial neoplasia
44	Genital tract, other mucosae	Intraepithelial neoplasia
45	Genital tract, other mucosae	Intraepithelial neoplasia and cancers
46	Cutaneous	Macular lesions (EV)
47	Cutaneous	Macular lesions (EV)
48	Cutaneous	Cutaneous squamous cell carcinoma (transplant patient)

Continued

Table 6-4
Human Papillomavirus Types—cont'd

HPV Type	Location	Association
49	Cutaneous	Flat wart (immunosuppressed patient)
50	Cutaneous	Macular lesions (EV)
51	Genital tract, other mucosae	Intraepithelial neoplasia and cancers
52	Genital tract, other mucosae	Intraepithelial neoplasia and cancers
53	Genital tract, other mucosae	Intraepithelial neoplasia
54	Genital tract, other mucosae	Intraepithelial neoplasia
55	Genital tract, other mucosae	Intraepithelial neoplasia
56	Genital tract, other mucosae	Intraepithelial neoplasia and cancers
57	Oral, genital tract, other mucosae	Oral papillomas and inverted maxillary sinus papilloma
58	Genital tract, other mucosae	Intraepithelial neoplasia and cancers
59	Genital tract, other mucosae	Anogenital intraepithelial neoplasia
60	Cutaneous	Epidermoid cysts, plantar warts
61	Genital tract, other mucosae	Intraepithelial neoplasia
62	Genital tract, other mucosae	Intraepithelial neoplasia
63	Cutaneous	Isolated from a plantar wart
64	Genital tract, other mucosae	Intraepithelial neoplasia
65	Cutaneous	Isolated from a pigmented wart
66	Genital tract, other mucosae	Intraepithelial neoplasia and cancers
67	Genital tract, other mucosae	Isolated from an intraepithelial neoplasia
68	Genital tract, other mucosae	Isolated from an intraepithelial neoplasia
69	Genital tract, other mucosae	Intraepithelial neoplasia and cancers
70	Genital tract, other mucosae	Isolated from a vulvar papilloma
71	Genital tract, other mucosae	Isolated from an intraepithelial neoplasia
72	Oral	Isolated from an oral papilloma (HIV patient)
73	Oral	Isolated from an oral papilloma (HIV patient)
74	Genital tract, other mucosae	Isolated from an intraepithelial neoplasia
75	Cutaneous	Isolated from a common wart in organ allograft recipient
76	Cutaneous	Isolated from a common wart in organ allograft recipient
77	Cutaneous	Isolated from a common wart in organ allograft recipient

EV = epidermodysplasia verruciformis; HIV = human immunodeficiency virus; HPV = human papillomavirus.

Source: DeVita VT, Hellman S, Rosenberg, SA: *Cancer: principles and practice of oncology,* ed 6,. Philadelphia, Lippincott Williams & Wilkins, 2001.

role in cervical cancer. Whereas p53 is known to facilitate and perhaps initiate apoptosis, bcl-2 is known as an apoptosis inhibitor. P53 acts as a downregulator of bcl-2. Thus binding and inactivation of p53 leads to inhibition of apoptosis through the inactivity of p53 and the lack of downregulation of bcl-2. The mechanism of malignant cell conversion is most likely extremely complex. In cervical cancer, the action seems to be centered on the binding of p53 by the HPV oncoprotein E6 and the cascading events that eventually lead to the inhibition of apoptosis (Figure 6-3).[30] For an excellent analysis of the role of apoptosis in gynecologic malignancies, refer to Ellen Sheets' article.[31]

The percentage of women who are HPV-positive and have normal cervical cytology varies significantly depending on the population. In some instances the percentage is extremely high. In a recent study based on a population with a high incidence of cervical cancer in South America, a 43% incidence of HPV positivity in women with negative cervical

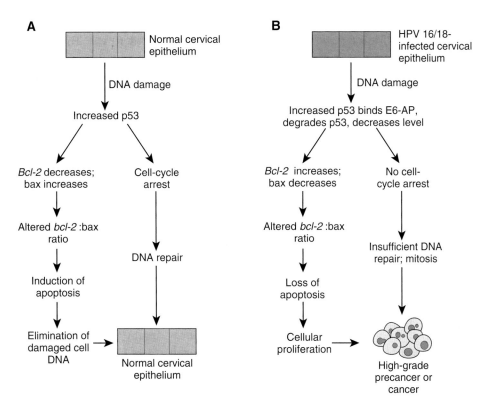

FIGURE 6-3
The interaction of HPV and p53 in normal cervical epithelium and in HPV 16/18-infected cervical epithelium. (From Scheffner M, Werness BA, Huibregtse JM, et al: *Cell* 1990;63:1129-1136.)

cytology was reported. Low-grade squamous intraepithelial lesions (LSILs), high-grade squamous intraepithelial lesions (HSILs), and invasive cancer were found to be associated with 96%, 100%, and 100% HPV positivity,[32] respectively. Most investigators would agree that if HPV is not the causative agent and primary carcinogenic factor for cervical cancer, it is certainly a required agent.[22]

Herpes Simplex Virus

Genital herpes is a common disease that has also been implicated in the development of cervical cancer. Because of the presence of multiple STDs in the same individual, it is often difficult to isolate a specific infection to establish its independent predictive value. There are two serotypes of herpes simplex, 1 and 2 (HSV-1 and HSV-2). The high seroprevalence of these infections makes investigations that rely on serologic testing difficult to interpret. Antibodies to HSV-1 can be detected in nearly 90% of adults, whereas the seroprevalence of HSV-2 is lower, with 15% of adults showing reactivity.[33-38] These rates are very dependent on the population studied and may vary significantly.

The data supporting the HSV as a risk factor are not as strong as for the HPV. It is also not clear whether these two viruses act independently or their combined effect represents a greater risk factor. Although some investigators have found no independent association between HSV-2 and cervical cancer,[39] others have determined that the association presents an increased risk for invasive and preinvasive cervical malignancies.[40,41] These differences most likely result from variations in the methodology used to detect the HSV infection and differences in the population.

Although the presence of HSV in cervical cytology indicates the presence of an active infection,[42] the implication of seropositivity is more difficult to interpret.[43] There is evidence that the true risk associated with HSV-2 is limited to HPV-negative tumors. This may indicate the existence of multiple pathways for the pathogenesis of cervical cancer and may explain the development of disease in patients with HPV-negative tumors, which account for nearly 10% of cervical cancers.[44]

Human Immunodeficiency Virus

Acquired immunodeficiency syndrome (AIDS) patients have been found to be at risk for malignancies such as Kaposi's sarcoma and B-cell non-Hodgkin's lymphoma. Additionally, human immunodeficiency virus (HIV)-infected women have been identified as being at high risk for the development of neoplastic and preneoplastic conditions of the cervix. The immunodeficiency caused by the HIV creates the opportunity for HPV infections that lead to cervical cancer. It is estimated that approximately 11 million women are infected worldwide.[45] The incidence of HIV is particularly high in developing countries where heterosexual transmission is the most common mode of infection. The largest increase in incidence is being seen in the Far East.[45]

There is a high incidence of HPV infection and CIN among HIV-seropositive women. A recent study that included 307 HIV seropositive women found an incidence of 27% and 58% for CIN and HPV infection, respectively.[46] The incidence of CIN was found to be an even higher 45% in patients with CD4 counts of less than 200 cells/mm^3.[47] In a prospective study that compares risk factors between HIV-seropositive and HIV-seronegative women, Ellerbrock found that one in five HIV-infected women will develop biopsy-confirmed CIN.[48] Cervical cytology was abnormal in 38.3% of HIV-infected women, but only 2.3% was found to be HSIL. This contrasted with 16.2% of total abnormalities and 1.2% HSIL found in a similar population of HIV-uninfected women.[49] HIV-infected women are also at higher risk for recurrence of CIN. After cone biopsy, HIV seropositive women were found to have a twofold increased risk of having a positive surgical margin.[50]

The newer treatments available in the management of HIV-positive and AIDS patients have made an enormous impact on survival. This creates even a greater need for appropriate management of HIV-positive patients affected with premalignant conditions of the cervix. All HIV-positive women should be considered at high risk for cervical cancer and counseled on the need and importance of Pap smears.

Risk factors for cervical cancer are shown in Box 6-1.

The Male Factor

The role of men's sexual behavior in the development of cervical cancer has been—and remains—a subject of controversy. Almost 25 years ago, Kessler reported on 29 "marital clusters." These clusters were composed of two women who both developed cervical cancer and were married to the same man.[51] Since then, although no definitive study has been done, several investigators have identified the male partner as a potential risk factor.[52] The prevalence of HPV DNA in penile carcinoma is very high. In a recent study 71% of patients with penile carcinoma were found to have HPV DNA, with the greatest majority being HPV 18.[53] The common origin of penile carcinoma and cervical cancer further supports the hypothesis that these diseases behave as STDs. Especially among high-risk populations, the prevalence of HPV DNA in the penises of husbands of women with cervical cancer is very high. In Cali, Colombia, it was found to be 26%. However, no statistical difference was found between men married to members of the case and control groups (26% and 19%, respectively.) The

BOX 6-1   Risk Factors for Cervical Cancer

Reproductive and Sexual Factors
Age at first sexual intercourse
Age of first pregnancy
Number of sexual partners
Number of pregnancies
Sexually transmitted diseases
• Human papillomavirus
• Herpes
• Human immunodeficiency virus (HIV)
Male factor (high-risk male)
Oral contraceptives
Socioeconomic factors
Low level of education
Low economic level
Ethnic minority
Others
Tobacco exposure
Lack of appropriate screening
Previous treatment for cervical intraepithelial neoplasia

high number of sexual partners, especially contact with prostitutes, in this very high-risk population may limit the power of this case-control study.[54]

The male factor was also investigated in Denmark. Forty-one case couples and 90 control couples participated in the study. The most significant risk factors were found to be a history of genital warts in the male and nonuse of condoms. However, only two husbands of case group members and none married to members of the control group had HPV DNA identified in the penile swabs.[16] The studied population, the test kit used, and the timing of the test may explain differences in the prevalence of HPV DNA in the men.

This is a difficult issue to discuss with patients, and most women would have limited knowledge about the sexual history of their male partners. There is a need, however, to inform women that their partners may constitute a risk for their own development of cervical cancer. The presence or history of genital warts in the male should indicate an increase in the risk. Barrier contraceptives, especially condoms, have been shown to have a protective effect.

Contraception

As expected, because of the sexually transmitted aspect of cervical cancer, barrier contraceptives overall have a negative effect and OCPs a positive one on the incidence of premalignant and malignant lesions of the cervix. However, the possibility has been raised that the effect of OCPs may be independent of other factors.

One of the few cohort studies that addressed this issue was able to demonstrate, even after standardization of rates by age, parity, smoking, social class, previous cytology, and history of sexually transmitted disease, an increase in the incidence of cervical cancer and carcinoma in situ for OCP users. This increased incidence was directly associated with increased duration of use. The risk of women who took OCPs for more than 10 years was four times greater than the risk of never-users.[55]

Some investigators were not able to demonstrate an association between the use of OCPs and cervical cancer after correcting for HPV infection. Kjellberg performed a population-based case-control study and reported a lack of association between dietary micronutrient, parity, OCP use, and cervical cancer after taking HPV infection into account.[56] A multi-institutional, case-control study was not able to demonstrate an association between OCPs and invasive adenocarcinomas, squamous cell carcinoma in situ, and invasive squamous cell carcinomas after correcting for HPV infection, sexual history, and cytologic screening. It is noteworthy that a positive association remained between current use of OCPs and cervical adenocarcinoma in situ.[57] This association may offer an explanation for the increased incidence of adenocarcinomas. Harriet Smith, using the National Cancer Institute's Surveillance, Epidemiology and End Results (SEER) program data, reported on the age-adjusted increase in incidence rates of adenocarcinomas versus squamous cell carcinomas. The age-adjusted incidence per 100,000 for all invasive cervical cancers decreased by 37% during a span of 24 years—12.35 (1973-1977) versus 7.8 (1993-1996). The age-adjusted incidence rates for squamous cell carcinoma declined by 42%—9.45 (1973-1977) versus 5.5 (1993-1996). In contrast, the age-adjusted incidence rates for adenocarcinoma increased by 29%—1.34 (1973-1977) versus 1.73 (1993-1996).[12] In addition to OCP use, this increase may be due to the relative inability of the Pap smear to detect early endocervical lesions.

Using population-based data, Brinton and associates showed a statistically significant increase in the risk of adenocarcinoma for OCP users after adjusting for Pap smear screening and sexual history.[58]

The increased incidence of cervical cancer associated with the use of OCPs may not be completely related to sexual factors but rather caused by the direct proliferative effect of these hormones on the cervical epithelium.[59] Progestins may act as a cofactor with HPV in the development of cervical cancer. Oncogenic transformation has been demonstrated in the presence of progesterone but not estrogen.[60] HPV-infected cell lines will increase their colony formation efficiency on plastic surface and soft agar when exposed to prolonged progesterone treatment. In contrast, progesterone had no effect on HPV-negative cell lines. The progesterone effect was reversed by the use of the progesterone antagonist RU 486.[61]

A comparison of women who used barrier methods with women who never used them revealed that the relative risk of invasive cervical cancer was 0.4 (95% confidence interval [CI], 0.2-0.9). Similar protection was found for premalignant cervical neoplasia, where the estimated relative risk was 0.6. The protective effect increased with duration of use.[62]

The association between contraception, as an independent risk factor, and cervical cancer is not completely resolved. Malcolm Pike and Darcy Spicer have referred to the inherent difficulties of these types of studies because of the positive association between OCP use and cervical screening and sexual risk factors. They estimated, based on the analysis of three published population-based studies, an increase of cervical cancer risk of 3.6% per year of OCP use.[59]

Should patients with CIN, especially those with persistent or of high grade CIN, be advised to discontinue the use of OCP? There is no definitive evidence in the literature to support this recommendation, and the need for contraception along with the feasibility of using other contraceptive techniques must be taken into consideration.

Dietary Factors

Several nutritional factors have been implied in the development of premalignant and malignant lesions of the cervix. Most of the research involved case-control studies that compared cervical cancer or dysplasia with the nutritional information provided by dietary intake at the time of diagnosis. In some cases the nutritional information was provided by the use of blood levels and even in fewer cases by cervical tissue levels. There are several pitfalls with this methodology. Nutritional data obtained at the time of the survey may not be representative of past dietary habits. This is especially important in a condition like CIN, in which the incubation time is unknown but is suspected to be relatively long. Most nutritional studies based on surveys rely heavily on recollection that is only relevant if women have not changed their dietary habits as a result of the diagnosis. It may be more important that most nutritional studies have not taken into account significant risk factors, especially HPV infection. This not only introduces a bias but also makes the data more difficult to interpret. There is no information concerning the effect of nutrition on the HPV infection or the effect of the HPV infection on the plasma or tissue levels of nutrients. Furthermore, disparities between tissue and plasma levels add an even a greater level of complexity.

Vitamin A

Vitamin A is one of the fat-soluble vitamins and is found in nature in two different forms: vitamin A_1, or retinol, and vitamin A_2, or retinol 2. The former, A_1, or retinol, is the most common form in mammalian tissues. The latter, A_2, or retinol 2, is found in freshwater fish. Carotenoids are common components of green and yellow vegetables. Three major groups have been defined: alpha, beta, and gamma carotene. Carotenes have no vitamin activity, but they are converted in the intestinal mucosa and the liver to vitamin A. Every molecule of beta-carotene yields two molecules of retinol, or vitamin A.

The data are contradictory, but despite the limitations related to the nutritional studies discussed above, dietary beta-carotene has been shown in several studies to protect against the development of premalignant and malignant lesions of the cervix.[63-66]

Concentrations of beta-carotene and cis-beta-carotene were found to be lower not only in the plasma but also in the cervical tissue of cancer and precancer patients in comparison with those of noncancer controls.[67] Other case-control studies failed to find an association between beta-carotene levels and cervical cancer.[68] Few investigators have taken into account HPV exposure. After adjusting for HPV positivity, Ho was not able to demonstrate a correlation between beta-carotene and CIN.[69] Others have found a decreased risk associated with high levels of alpha-carotene but not with beta.[70]

In a study involving women with high-grade CIN, a comparison of beta-carotene levels between HPV-positive and HPV-negative women failed to show a difference. This finding indicates the lack of a relationship between a HPV status and dietary beta-carotene.[71]

Vitamin E

Vitamin E or tocopherol is commonly found in plants; the most common form is alpha-tocopherol. Vitamin E is among the micronutrients found to have antioxidant activity, which is its potential benefit as a cancer protective agent. Studies focusing on the effect of vitamin E on the development of cervical cancer have yielded unclear results. Using a nested case-control study in Finland and Sweden within a joint cohort of 400,000 women followed up for an average of 4 years, investigators failed to show a statistically significant difference in the levels of unoxidized alpha-tocopherol in the blood of cervical cancer patients versus that of controls.[72] Others have reported an inverse relationship between the risk for CIN and alpha-tocopherol, thus indicating a potential protective effect.[73] Studies have shown a similar inverse correlation between plasma alpha-tocopherol and a risk of CIN (odds ratio = 0.15) result after adjusting for HPV positivity.[69,74]

Vitamin C

Vitamin C, or ascorbic acid, is one of the water-soluble vitamins and is widely distributed in plant and animal tissues. Few species, other than humans, require dietary vitamin C. Most higher animals can synthesize ascorbic acid. In general, a reverse association has been found between vitamin C intake and the risk of CIN or cervical cancer.[64,75,76] However, a few studies have been unable to show a protective effect of vitamin C.[68,77]

Folic Acid

Folic acid, or folacin, is found in vegetables. Its deficiency in humans results in anemia. Folic acid is a key component in the metabolism of amino acids, purines, and pyrimidines. Folate deficiency has been considered a risk factor for preinvasive and invasive cervical cancer. This is of particular concern because of the known negative effect of pregnancy and OCPs on folate levels. Some inverse associations have been identified between CIN and folate in both serum and diet.[75,78] However, other studies have not revealed this effect.[79] Folic acid deficiencies may act on the epithelium directly or may enhance the risk of HPV infections. Butterworth was able to show that low folate levels in red blood cells increase the effect of HPV-16 infection for cervical dysplasia. The adjusted odds ratio for women infected with HPV-16 was 1.1 and 5.1 (95% CI, 2.3 to 11) among women with folate levels above 660 mol/L or lower levels, respectively.[80]

There are no definitive studies on the risks posed by the dietary deficit of vitamins, nor has a protective effect been shown. Because of the potential benefits for cancer prevention and other conditions, eating a well-balanced diet with plenty of green and yellow vegetables is sound advice. Unless patients have a specific dietary restriction, vitamin supplements are not indicated.

Tobacco Exposure

Lung cancer is the most important cause of cancer-related mortality in the Western world; 87% is attributed to tobacco exposure mainly through cigarette smoking.[81,82] More recently, several epidemiologic studies have established a relationship between cervical cancer and cigarette smoking.[83-86] Cigarette smoking is also positively related, in a dose-dependent fashion, to intraepithelial cervical lesions.[87] Cessation of smoking decreases the risk.[88] The presence of tobacco-related carcinogens in the genital tract of smokers may explain the relationship between tobacco exposure and the development of cervical malignancies.

A potent tobacco-specific nitrosamine, NNK, has been found in the cervical mucus of smokers and nonsmokers. However, the concentration in smokers was significantly higher than in the nonsmoking group.[89]

Because of the high incidence of lung cancer and the known association with cigarette smoking, considerable attention has been focused on enzymes that toxify or detoxify carcinogens present in tobacco. Members of the gluthatione S-transferase (GST) family detoxify toxic and mutagenic compounds by conjugating them with glutathione. A deficit in this enzyme may be a risk factor for the development of tobacco-related cancers.[90]

Cytochrome P450 (CYP) enzymes are involved in the generation of active metabolites from precarcinogens found in tobacco. Polymorphisms in these enzymes have been suggested as a mechanism of carcinogenesis.[91,92] Mutations and polymorphisms that affect these enzymes may explain the difference in people's susceptibility to the development of tobacco-related cancers. Furthermore, because the distribution of these polymorphisms is ethnically based, it may also explain the ethnic differences found in the incidences of these malignancies.

An excess number of second primaries have been reported in survivors of invasive cervical cancer. These may be caused by the treatment delivered, such as radiotherapy or chemotherapy, or a common causative or promoter agent such as HPV or cigarette smoking.[93-95] It is also widely known that cervical dysplasia is associated with increased risk for invasive cervical cancer. But what is more unexpected is that it may be also be a predictor for other tobacco-related invasive neoplasms. An excess risk for tobacco-related and non-melanomatous skin cancer was found, in a population-based study, after the diagnosis of carcinoma in situ of the cervix.[96] A similar experience has been reported with other genital malignancies. Using data from nine population-based cancer registries participating in the National Cancer Institute's SEER program, Sturgeon and associates reported on an excess of second primaries after the diagnosis of vulvar or vaginal cancer. Most of the excess second cancers were smoking-related (cancers of the lung, buccal cavity, pharynx, esophagus, nasal cavity, and larynx).[97] Unpublished studies confirm these relationships.

Cigarette smoking is related to invasive and preinvasive cervical cancer. The risk, as with other tobacco-related cancers, depends on the degree of exposure. Genetic alterations on the enzymes that are responsible for the metabolism of tobacco carcinogens may increase the risk, similar to what occurs in lung cancer. Counseling of patients with CIN should include smoking cessation information. Patients with CIN should be alerted to the possibility of developing other tobacco-related malignancies.

PREVENTION

Classically, primary prevention is interpreted as any intervention that may block the development of a malignancy. Secondary prevention is defined as interventions that may lead to early diagnosis in curable patients. Tertiary prevention involves interventions that help prevent recurrences and secondary malignancies. There have been several definitions and interpretations of primary, secondary, and tertiary prevention as they apply to cancer of the cervix. Some of the confusion originates in the use of the Pap smear to detect premalignant conditions of the cervix. This could be considered a form of secondary prevention for premalignant conditions and primary prevention for invasive cervical cancer. For ease of reading—and for the purpose of this chapter—we have considered all screening methods, including HPV testing, as methods of primary prevention.

Behavioral Changes

Changes in sexual behavior may positively affect the incidence of cervical cancer. There have been very few prospective studies that demonstrate the effectiveness of behavioral changes; however, the retrospective data and population-based case-control studies overwhelmingly indicate a protective effect of some lifestyle practices and the harmful effect of others. Women who delay the onset of sexual activities and limit the number of sexual partners have a much lower incidence of cervical cancer.[69,98-103] Healthier sexual behavior in men may also decrease the incidence of cervical cancer.[104] There is no clear indication that current school-based educational programs are effective in reducing high-risk behavior,[105,106] although they may have some beneficial effects.[107] Differing school-based programs and extensive societal influences—such as media influence, peer pressure, and parental guidance—make these studies extremely difficult to carry out and control.

Use of the Pap test to screen for cervical cancer has a significant effect on the diagnosis of premalignant conditions and the subsequent decrease in the incidence of cancer. Wide discrepancies in screening percentage exist among different segments of the population in the United

States. Changes in behavior that lead to an increase in screening will positively influence cervical cancer diagnosis and prevention.

Most minorities are poorly screened,[108-110] which partially explains their higher incidence of cervical cancer. Behavioral scientists have studied the way that people change behavior and found that most people go through a series of stages and have opportunities to move forward, remain at the same stage, or even regress. One of the models that has been extensively studied and applied to intervention programs is the transtheoretical model of health behavior. Behavioral changes entail evolution through five stages (Figure 6-4): precontemplation, where there is no intention to change; contemplation, where change is expected within 6 months; preparation, where change is planned; action, where changes are being made; and maintenance, where changes are being protected.[111]

It is critical to understand how a populations fits within this model. For instance, promoting screening for cervical cancer has little chance of success if most of the population is in a precontemplation stage. Educational programs would be, under these circumstances, more effective. This model has been applied to cervical cancer screening.[112] Large percentages of minorities are in the precontemplation and contemplation stages, while nonminority women are in the action and maintenance stages. Most of the differences are attributed to

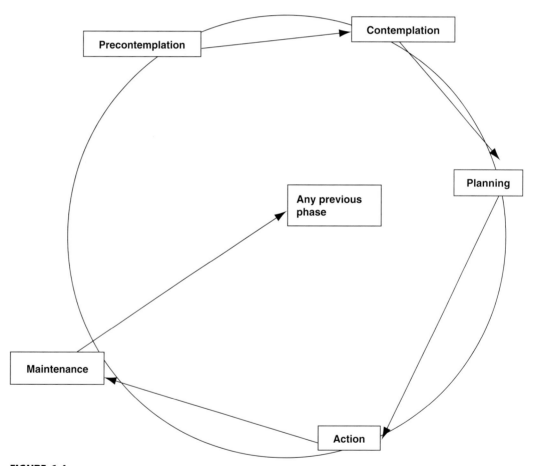

FIGURE 6-4
The transtheoretical model of health behavior, beginning with initial precontemplation stage, through contemplation, preparation, and action. The last stage, maintenance, revisits the previous stages until the behavior change is stable.

cultural or educational issues, socioeconomic status, and their repercussions in access to health care and the availability of culturally sensitive health care.[110,113-115] Fewer years of education may be one of the most important variables in explaining the higher rates of invasive cervical cancer in Hispanics.[14,17] A different value system among Hispanics, which includes a sense of fatalism, may also impede appropriate management of early cervical lesions and screening.[116] This is more pronounced in recent immigrants than in individuals with longer periods of acculturation. Even within a given minority, such as Hispanics, there are large differences among different groups. For instance, Mexican Americans and Puerto Ricans have a more fatalistic view of cancer than Cuban or Central Americans.[117]

However, there are indications that health care delivered in a culturally appropriate environment may still be successful regardless of the fatalism shown by this population. In a recent survey, more than 85% of Hispanics responded that they would believe and follow their doctor's advice (personal communication). This indicates that there is ample room for appropriate intervention in the health care of this significant minority.

Age is also an important predictor for screening. Older women are less likely to have had Pap smears.[118] In a recent consensus conference, NIH decided to target this group for screening because of its lower screening rate.[5]

Tobacco has been identified as a promoter of cervical cancer. Smoking cessation programs and the consequent decreasing number of women smokers should lessen the incidence of cervical cancer. Awareness of the relationship between tobacco exposure and cervical cancer may be an important motivator. Overall, less than half of women undergoing Pap smears know of this relationship. Health maintenance visits present an opportunity to emphasize this connection and to offer smoking cessation programs.[119]

Increasing the follow-up of women with abnormal Pap smears also would reduce the incidence of cervical cancer. The loss to follow-up after an abnormal Pap smear is extremely high. Most studies of community clinics reported losses to follow-up of 30% to 50%.[120-125] Interventions designed to increase follow-up have not been effective.[120,126] Even financial incentives, such as providing vouchers to the participants, had a modest effect.[127] Follow-up, even of high-grade lesions, remains a challenge. Less than 83% of patients with evidence of HGSIL or invasive carcinoma in Pap smears had documentation of follow-up within 6 months.[128]

Loss of follow-up of patients with abnormal Pap smears occurs for several reasons. Some are socioeconomic, cultural, and educational, all of which affect health care access. In addition, the present management of the abnormal Pap smear is a rather laborious process that includes several office visits for colposcopy, biopsies, and treatment of the dysplastic lesion. Women with poor health care access usually have transportation, communication, and child care problems and are less likely to comply. Programs that attempt to decrease the number of visits, especially programs where the initial cytology and the treatment are delivered in the same setting (single-visit programs), may decrease loss of follow-up.[129,130] However, the current screening program used in the United States may not be suitable for some of the most impoverished areas of the world, where the access to health care is far more limited than in the United States.

Prophylactic Vaccines

HPV is judged to be the main carcinogenic factor in the development of cervical cancer, and most cervical cancers are HPV-related. Vaccine use may prevent HPV infection and its associated cervical cancer.[24,25,131,132] The aim of a prophylactic or preventive vaccine is to prevent the development of HPV infections and the cascade of events that leads to cervical cancer. Strategies that use HPV-based preventive and therapeutic vaccines are presently in clinical trials. Most vaccines are based on a humoral response with a subsequent generation of neutralizing antibodies that destroy the virus before it becomes intracellular. In the same way that hepatitis B vaccination should lead to a decrease in the incidence of hepatic cancer, a preventive vaccination with HPV theoretically should lead to a decreased incidence of cervical cancer.

Several obstacles have been encountered in the development of prophylactic HPV human vaccines, including the following:

- There are more than 60 major HPV types, and many of these can cause cervical cancer.
- There is a lack of an appropriate animal model.
- HPV does not easily replicate in vitro.
- To be effective, women have to be vaccinated at an early age; it is not clear if this would be acceptable to populations at risk.

The areas of the HPV genome considered for vaccine development are the E6 and E7 early expressed oncogenic genes and the L1 and L2 viral capsid structural proteins. These proteins are antigenic, thus inducing high levels of neutralizing antibodies.[133-135] HPV 16 viral-like particle vaccines that express the virion capsule protein L1 and L2 have generated a lot of interest as possible strategies to achieve immunization against HPV 16.[136] Preclinical studies are encouraging; animals previously vaccinated with recombinant virus-like particles (VLP) respond with a substantial increase in neutralizing antibody titer.[137] What is yet to be established is whether this protection against an experimental HPV challenge will translate into a long-lasting immunity against the sexual transmission of HPV. Some of these strategies are being clinically tested in phase I and II studies.[138-141]

Although the acceptability of this approach must be confirmed in at-risk populations, preliminary reports are encouraging. In a study performed in Mexico, 84% (n = 880) of the mothers surveyed indicated they would allow their daughters to participate in clinical trials that involved HPV vaccines.[142] A study done in Finland also indicates that all prerequisites for large vaccine clinical trials have been fulfilled.[143]

The future of HPV prophylactic vaccines is very promising, but the acceptability across very heterogeneous populations with different educational levels and cultural beliefs remains questionable. In addition, the current high prevalence of HPV infections indicates that it would take several decades for even very successful immunization programs to have an impact on the incidence of cervical cancer.

Chemoprevention
Retinoids
There exists a rich background behind the rationale of using retinoids as chemopreventive agents. As discussed earlier, diets rich in carotenoids have been associated with protecting against cervical neoplasia. Also, a negative association has been found between serum retinol levels and cervical malignancies.[72,144-149] Serum retinol levels may also be a marker of progression. Women with carcinoma in situ of the cervix that progressed to invasive cancer had retinol levels 4.5 times lower than the ones that did not progress.[145] Furthermore, a decrease in the expression of nuclear retinoic acid receptor mRNA has been documented in CIN.[150] It has been hypothesized that retinoid activity may be caused by an increase in expression of p53 and the inhibition of HPV-E6/E7 transcription.[151]

The potential use of retinoids in the management of premalignant conditions of the cervix has been explored in a variety of clinical settings. Meyskens performed a study in which cervical caps with sponges containing 1.0 mL of 0.372% beta-trans-retinoic acid were used. He was able to demonstrate an increase in the complete histologic regression rate of CIN II from 27% in the placebo group to 43% in the retinoic acid treatment group (p = .041). This positive effect was limited to patients with CIN II; no difference between the two arms was found among patients with CIN III.[152] An earlier study demonstrated the potential beneficial effect of retinoic acid, documenting a reduction in size of the intraepithelial lesion by colposcopy in 6 of 18 (33%) patients and a complete resolution of the disease by cervical conization in two patients.[153] Significant side effects are associated with the use of topical retinoic acid in the vagina, thus making the clinical application questionable.

The relative lack of side effects, in contrast with topical retinoic acid, made oral beta-carotene an excellent candidate for chemoprevention. Beta-carotene does not have vitamin-like activity but is converted to vitamin A in the intestinal mucosa. The use of beta-carotene was studied in a phase II setting in patients with CIN II and I. A positive relationship between serum and tissue levels of beta-carotene was demonstrated, indicating that serum levels may be used for monitoring and that dietary supplementation would increase tissue levels. Response rates were 60%, 70%, and 33% at 3, 6, and 12 months, respectively.[154] These responses could not be confirmed in larger, phase III, placebo-controlled studies.[155]

Although initially—and on the basis of preclinical and early clinical trials—there was a high degree of enthusiasm about the use of beta-carotene, larger studies have not shown a beneficial effect of this nutrient.

All-trans-N-(4-hydroxyphenyl) retinamide (4HPR or fenretinide) is a synthetic retinoid that has been shown to induce apoptosis in cervical cancer cell lines. 4-HPR is well-tolerated and has demonstrated less toxicity than all-trans retinoic acid.[156,157] There is a high degree of enthusiasm for 4-HPR, and phase II studies are under way.[158]

Alpha-Difluoromethylornithine

Alpha-difluoromethylornithine (DFMO) is a suicide inhibitor of ornithine decarboxylase and has been studied as an antiproliferative agent in a variety of cancers.[159-161] Ornithine decarboxylase is a critical enzyme in the metabolism of polyamines. The polyamines spermidine and spermin, as well as their precursor, putrescine, are required for growth and the proliferation of all cells. A wide variation in the concentration of polyamine synthesis biomarkers between colposcopically normal and abnormal areas has been found.[162] Thirty patients with CIN III, histologically confirmed, were treated with DFMO as part of a phase I trial. The medication was well-tolerated; five patients experienced a complete response and 10 a partial response.[163] These very preliminary findings will have to be confirmed with larger, randomized studies.

The Pap Smear

In 1941 George Papanicolaou described a system based on microscopic analysis of cervical cytology for the prevention of cervical cancer. Box 6-2 shows this classification according to Pap test results. He described five different classes of abnormalities, class I to V.[164] The implementation of the Pap smear screening program was associated with a significant reduction in cervical cancer and a consequent reduction in mortality. This screening method is one of the few to have received an "A" from the U.S. Prevention Task Force, which is under the Agency for Health Care Policy and Research (AHCPR), now the Agency for Healthcare Research and Quality (AHRQ). Although the Pap smear has been determined to be cost-

BOX 6-2	Classification of Pap Test Results	
Class I	Normal	
Class II	Atypical, inflammation or uterine cells seen	
Class III	Dysplastic, mild, moderate or severe	
Class IV	Carcinoma in situ	
Class V	Suspicious for an invasive cancer	

Source: Papanicolaou GN, Traut HF: *Diagnosis of uterine cancer by the vaginal smear*, New York, The Commonwealth Fund, 1943.

effective and a valuable screening method in the United States and other countries, there has never been a randomized trial demonstrating its effectiveness in the prevention of cervical cancer.[165-168]

One of the main attributes of the Pap smear is its specificity, especially for high-grade lesions where the false-positive rate is almost negligible.[169] On the other hand, sensitivity has been the major drawback of this screening method. False-negative rates from 2% to 54% have been reported.[170-172] There is no standard definition of false-negative smears. The most reasonable approach is to consider a false-negative as any negative smear that in subsequent analysis is found to be unequivocally positive.[173] This definition eliminates all sampling errors as false-negatives, including those where the specimen may be adequate but not truly representative of the entire cervix. One possibility is to reserve the term "false-negative" for cases in which a laboratory error has caused a Pap smear to be reported as negative but subsequent review has found the test to be obviously positive. Any other disparity should be called a "discrepant smear." This term may be used for those smears in which the cytologic examination is not in agreement with the histology found at the time of cervical biopsy. This may be due to sampling error or to the intrinsic limitation of exfoliated cells to represent the true nature of the histologic abnormality. Box 6-3 lists the Pap smear inaccuracies.

Pap Smear Inaccuracies

Several decades ago Pap smears were limited to a sample of the vaginal pool without any attempt to retrieve cells from the exocervix or endocervix. These techniques have proven to be unsatisfactory. The presence of an exocervical and endocervical specimen increases the accuracy of the Pap smear. Extended-tip spatulas that reach further into the endocervix have proven to be more effective than the traditional Ayre spatula.[172] The endocervical brush is also superior to the cotton swab for the retrieval of the endocervical specimen.[174-177] The decrease in the number of unsatisfactory Pap smears has made the use of the endocervical

BOX 6-3	Pap Smear Inaccuracies

1. Sampling errors
   a. Related to technique
   b. Related to device
2. Fixation-related errors
3. Laboratory errors

brush cost-effective.[178] The best and most consistent samples are obtained with a combination of the extended-tip spatula and the endocervical brush[172] (Figure 6-5). The most common methods to fix the specimen are direct contact with 95% alcohol or the use of spray aerosol fixative. Delay or inappropriate fixation leads to air-drying, which significantly deteriorates the quality of the specimen.[179,180]

False-negatives and discrepant Pap smears have been significant sources of litigation. Patients and attorneys' lack of understanding of the limitations of the Pap smear has led to some of this litigation. Educational programs that alert women to the limitations of this test may decrease the number of legal cases. Using appropriate measures of quality control and quality assurance can minimize true laboratory errors.[181,182] One of the most important elements of the quality control programs is the rescreening of negative Pap smears. It has been determined that up to 50% of false-negative smears may be correctly diagnosed by retrospective rescreening. Most of these will be in the atypical squamous cells of undetermined significance (ASCUS) category.[183,184]

By the late 1970s and 1980s, the cytology-based screening program was indicating that the Papanicolaou classification lacked histologic correlation and was being applied inconsistently by different laboratories. These concerns about the Papanicolaou classification led the NIH to convene an expert panel in Bethesda, Maryland, in 1988. This panel developed a new classification (Box 6-4) for the interpretation of cervicovaginal cytology that has been called "the Bethesda system."[185-187]

This system addressed some of the concerns expressed earlier, especially the lack of correlation between cytologic report and histopathology. The terms LSIL and HSIL were introduced. LSIL was designated as the cytologic expression of CIN I and HSIL was reserved for CIN II and III. Changes related to HPV infection were also classified as LSIL. This decision was based on the inability of the cytopathologist to distinguish between HPV changes and

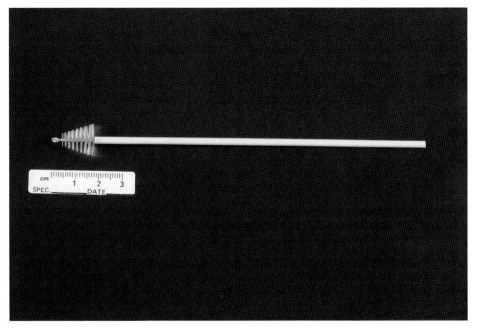

FIGURE 6-5
Endocervical brush used to retrieve the endocervical specimen. (From Martin-Hirsch P, et al: *Collection devices for obtaining cytology samples.* Cochrane Database Syst Rev 2000.)

BOX 6-4   **Bethesda System—1988**

Adequacy
- Satisfactory
- Limited
- Unsatisfactory

Descriptive
- Normal
- Benign
- Epithelial cell abnormality
  - Atypical squamous cells of unknown significance
  - Low-grade squamous intraepithelial lesion
  - High-grade squamous intraepithelial lesion
- Glandular cell abnormality
  - Atypical glandular cells
  - Adenocarcinoma

Sources: *Oncology* 1989;3:65,68; *J Reprod Med* 1989;34:779-785; Smigel K: *J Natl Cancer Inst* 1989;81:1354-1355.

LSIL. The bundling of these two entities was the subject of discussion and concern, mainly related to the possibility of overtreating HPV lesions labeled as LSIL.[188-190]

The NIH convened a second panel of experts in 1991 to address the pros and cons expressed by the scientific community about the Bethesda system. This panel revised the classification, which was made public in 1992.[191-193] This classification has become the standard for the reporting of cervical cytology in the United States and other countries.

The Bethesda classification has three major headings:

1. Adequacy of the specimen
2. General categorization
3. Descriptive diagnosis

One of the strengths of this system is that it addresses the issue of "adequacy of the cytologic specimen," which is determined by the presence of endocervical cells. Substandard specimens must be interpreted cautiously. A significant 16% of patients with inadequate specimens are subsequently found to have abnormalities.[194] There is a high level of agreement among pathologists as to what constitutes an inadequate smear.[195]

The "general categorization" class allows the pathologist to declare the smear "within normal limits" without any further explanation. Otherwise, it directs the reader of the report to the descriptive diagnosis.

Squamous cell abnormalities include ASCUS, LSIL, HSIL, and squamous cell carcinoma. The distribution of squamous cell abnormalities depends on the studied population.[196-202] For instance, there is evidence that the percentage of Pap smear abnormalities in adolescents has increased during the last decades.[203] In a recent study of more than 1100 laboratories in the United States, the following median reporting rates for epithelial cell abnormalities were reported: ASCUS 4.5%, atypical glandular cells of undetermined significance (AGUS) 0.3%, LSIL 1.6%, and HSIL 0.5%.[204] One of the most vexing issues related to screening of cervical cancer by use of the Pap smear is the significance of the low-grade abnormalities such as ASCUS and LSIL. There are approximately 60 million Pap smears performed in the United States annually. Only 8%, or 5 million, will be reported as abnormal. Of this 5 million, fewer than 20%, or one million, will have associated histologic changes. The majority of the "false-positive" smears will be in the ASCUS and LSIL categories.[205] The percentage of histologic abnormalities found in patients with ASCUS and LSIL varies considerably from study to study, but in general the percentage is low. Very few longitudinal studies with long-term follow-up have been conducted to determine the significance of these lesions. In a study limited to ASCUS in which more than 600 patients were followed for 6 years, the percentage of women found to have HSIL during the follow-up period was 9%, and none developed invasive cancer.[198] The economic impact related to the clinical management of these low-grade abnormalities is significant; most of the cost is related to the use of colposcopy and biopsies to rule out the presence of CIN. There is a great interest in designing triage protocols to minimize the number of colposcopies and biopsies.

Although the cytologic diagnosis of ASCUS is associated with a very low percentage of significant histologic lesions, that is not the case for AGUS, for which most studies have shown a high incidence of either squamous or glandular abnormalities. It has been consistently demonstrated that approximately 50% of all AGUS are associated with either squamous or glandular changes. Furthermore, 50% of these, or 25% of the total, are associated with malignant or premalignant squamous or glandular lesions.[206,207] An incidence of 0.2% of AGUS among 76,000 Pap smears studied has been reported. Forty-five percent of the patients were found to have clear histologic abnormalities, including four invasive cancers.[208]

The most common and better tested liquid-based Pap test is the Thin-Prep (Cytyc Corp.; Boxborough, MA). This test has been approved since 1996 by the Food and Drug Administration in the United States as an alternative to the conventional Pap smear. Similar technology is offered by the AutoCyte PREP system (AutoCyte, Inc.; Elon College, NC). These techniques offer the advantage of presenting to the examiner a monolayer of cells. The use of Thin-Prep (TP), compared with the conventional Pap smear, has reportedly led to an increase in the percentage of "satisfactory" examinations (91.9% TP vs. 72.2% conventional).[209-211]

A new device to retrieve the cervical sample is being used in combination with the Thin Prep (TP) test; a "brush" type of device that is designed to obtain an appropriate exocervical and endocervical sample with a single pass (Papette, Wallach Surgical Devices, Inc.; Milford, CT). It seems that this device alone is not as effective in acquiring an appropriate endocervical component as the endocervical brush.[212]

Based on a prospective study that compares TP with conventional Pap, Diaz-Rosario reported an increase in LSIL of 71.65% (from 1.58% to 2.71%) and an increase in HSIL of 102.54% (from 0.26% to 0.52%). A 40% decrease in the number of ASCUS was also reported.[211] Comparing TP with historical data, Papillo reported a 52% and 53% increase in the detection of LSIL and HSIL, respectively.[213]

Thin Prep has also been effective in detecting glandular lesions; a significant decrease in the false-negative rate was noted for biopsy-confirmed adenocarcinoma in situ (AIS) or invasive adenocarcinoma.[214]

Most studies, which use biopsy results as the gold standard, have shown an improved sensitivity of the TP in comparison with the conventional Pap smear.

The recommended frequency of Pap smears has been a subject of intense debate. The present recommendation endorsed by the American Cancer Society and the American College of Obstetrics and Gynecology states the following:

All women who are or have been sexually active, or who have reached 18 years of age, should undergo an annual Papanicolaou (Pap) test and pelvic examination. After a woman has three or more consecutive, satisfactory annual examinations with normal findings, the Pap smear may be performed less frequently at the discretion of her physician.

At the "discretion of the physician" implies that the presumed risk should determine the frequency of Pap smears. Because of the complexity of properly evaluating risk, not only of the woman but also of the male partner, and because of the difficulty encountered by many women in maintaining schedules longer than one year, this recommendation has commonly been interpreted to mean annual Pap smears. This recommendation does not exclude postmenopausal women. If the health care provider elects to decrease the frequency of Pap smears, the pelvic examination should be done annually.

Bethesda 2001 Cytology Reporting System

Because of new information from the ASCUS and low-grade triage study (ALTS), the Bethesda system was revamped in 1991. The 2001 Bethesda system terminology (Box 6-5) for the reporting of cervical cytology further refines the previous classifications (1988 and 1991).[215-218]

The 2001 system retains the statement of specimen adequacy but eliminates the use of "satisfactory but limited by." The presence or absence of endocervical cells or transformation zone component is now a qualifier under "satisfactory for evaluation." The presence of endocervical or transformation zone component can only be acknowledged if there are at least 10 endocervical or squamous metaplastic cells.

The general categorization "negative for intraepithelial lesion or malignancy" is optional in the new classification, a questionable change because this category assists clinicians with the reading of Pap smear reports.

Significant changes have been made in the "epithelial cell abnormalities" section. Atypical squamous cells (ASC) are now divided into "undetermined significance (ASC-US)" and "cannot exclude HSIL (ASC-H)." The latter is an intermediate category located between ASC and HSIL.

As in the 1991 classification the terms LSIL and HSIL are reserved for histologic changes compatible with the diagnosis of HPV infection/Cin1 and Cin2/Cin3, respectively. The term "AGUS" has also been called "AGCUS," which caused legitimate concern because AGUS and AGCUS were occasionally confused with ASCUS. AGUS has been eliminated from the current classification.

Glandular cell abnormalities in the 2001 system are classified as "atypical endocervical cells," "atypical endometrial cells," and "atypical glandular cells," the last term to be used when the origin is uncertain.

Another significant change in the 2001 system is the separation of endocervical "AIS" from "AGUS." Endocervical AIS is now listed separately.

A breach category named "atypical endocervical cells, favor neoplastic" is reserved for cases in which the cells are very suspicious but fall short of the term AIS. It is not clear if this more complex classification will be universally accepted. Even if it is commonly adopted in the United States, it is rather unlikely that countries outside the United States that have not implemented the 1991 system would agree to the 2001 classification.

Colposcopy

Colposcopy was initially introduced in Europe in the early part of the twentieth century, and Hinselmann reported on this procedure in 1925.[219] Although extensively used in Europe as a screening method, it made no impact in the United States until the 1960s. In the United States and the United Kingdom, colposcopy is seldom used as a stand-alone screening technique. It has been used as a method for the management of abnormal Pap smears and jointly with directed biopsies as an alternative to cone biopsy. Colposcopy is based on the

BOX 6-5   Bethesda System—2001

SPECIMEN TYPE: *Indicate conventional smear (Pap smear) vs. liquid-based vs. other*

SPECIMEN ADEQUACY

Satisfactory for evaluation *(describe presence or absence of endocervical/transformation zone component and any other quality indicators, e.g., partially obscuring blood, inflammation, etc.)*

Unsatisfactory for evaluation *(specify reason)*

Specimen rejected/not processed *(specify reason)*

Specimen processed and examined, but unsatisfactory for evaluation of epithelial abnormality because of *(specify reason)*

GENERAL CATEGORIZATION *(optional)*

Negative for Intraepithelial Lesion or Malignancy

Epithelial Cell Abnormality: See Interpretation/Result *(specify "squamous" or "glandular" as appropriate)*

Other: See Interpretation/Result *(e.g., endometrial cells in a woman > 40 years of age)*

AUTOMATED REVIEW

If case examined by automated device, specify device and result.

ANCILLARY TESTING

Provide a brief description of the test methods and report the result so that it is easily understood by the clinician.

INTERPRETATION/RESULT

NEGATIVE FOR INTRAEPITHELIAL LESION OR MALIGNANCY *(when there is no cellular evidence of neoplasia, state this in the General Categorization above and/or in the Interpretation/Result section of the report, regardless of whether there are organisms or other nonneoplastic findings)*

ORGANISMS:

Trichomonas vaginalis

Fungal organisms morphologically consistent with *Candida* spp.

Shift in flora suggestive of bacterial vaginosis

Bacteria morphologically consistent with *Actinomyces* spp.

Cellular changes consistent with Herpes simplex virus

OTHER NONNEOPLASTIC FINDINGS *(Optional to report; list not inclusive)*:

Reactive cellular changes associated with:

– inflammation (includes typical repair)

– radiation

– intrauterine contraceptive device (IUD)

Glandular cells status post-hysterectomy

Atrophy

OTHER

Endometrial cells *(in a woman > 40 years of age)*

   (Specify whether "negative for squamous intraepithelial lesion")

EPITHELIAL CELL ABNORMALITIES

SQUAMOUS CELL

Atypical squamous cells

– of undetermined significance (ASC-US)

– cannot exclude HSIL (ASC-H)

Low grade squamous intraepithelial lesion (LSIL) encompassing: HPV/mild dysplasia/CIN 1

High grade squamous intraepithelial lesion (HSIL) encompassing: moderate and severe dysplasia, CIS/CIN 2, and CIN 3

– with features suspicious for invasion *(if invasion is suspected)*

Squamous cell carcinoma

GLANDULAR CELL

Atypical

– endocervical cells (NOS *or specify in comments*)

– endometrial cells (NOS *or specify in comments*)

– glandular cells (NOS *or specify in comments*)

Continued

BOX 6-5	Bethesda System—2001—cont'd

Atypical
– endocervical cells, favor neoplastic
– glandular cells, favor neoplastic
Endocervical adenocarcinoma in situ
Adenocarcinoma
– endocervical
– endometrial
– extrauterine
– not otherwise specified (NOS)
OTHER MALIGNANT NEOPLASMS: (*specify*)
EDUCATIONAL NOTES AND SUGGESTIONS (*optional*)
Suggestions should be concise and consistent with clinical follow-up guidelines published by professional organizations (references to relevant publications may be included).

Source: Bethesda System 2001. 2001 Terminology. National Cancer Institute. Available at: http://bethesda2001.cancer.gov/terminology.html.

recognition of images produced by the vascularization of the abnormal epithelium. It is used to inspect the cervix and to choose the areas in which a biopsy should be performed. The reliability of colposcopy is completely dependent on the ability of the examiner. As a result, the percentage of false-negative colposcopically directed biopsies varies dramatically in different settings. It has been reported to be as high as 56%.[220] Attempts have been made to standardize colposcopy and to convert it into a more objective technique. The best-known technique is Reid's colposcopy index.[221,222]

Colposcopic images become more apparent after the application of a 4% solution of acetic acid. Abnormal epithelium becomes whiter than the surrounding area. In colposcopy terminology they are called "acetowhite" lesions. The columnar epithelium and the vasculature also become more prominent, a feature that is further accentuated by the use of a green filter. For colposcopy to be meaningful, the entire transformation zone must be visible to the examiner. When this is not the case the colposcopy is deemed to be "unsatisfactory." No judgment can be passed in unsatisfactory colposcopies because the entire area at risk cannot be properly evaluated. Colposcopic examination with endocervical curettage (ECC) has been the gold standard for the last three decades and is advocated by many colposcopists.[211-214] ECC is also used because it is possible to have a satisfactory and normal colposcopic exam in a patient who has a "skipped" lesion high in the endocervical canal. Additionally, abnormal glandular lesions may be located in the endocervix only. Some investigators have challenged the need for ECC, especially in the presence of minimally abnormal Pap smears.[223] There is less controversy in the routine use of the ECC, for the management of HSIL,[224, 225] and it is certainly mandatory for the management of patients with a diagnosis of AGUS.

HPV Testing

HPV is considered to be the major risk factor for cervical cancer and possibly the causative factor.[23,226-229] The high percentage of ASCUS and LSIL that spontaneously resolve have led investigators to the search for triage methods that would reduce the number of colposcopies and biopsies that must be performed to identify the relatively small number of patients with high-grade histologic lesions. Identification of the relatively small percentage of patients with LSIL and ASCUS that have underlying CIN should significantly reduce costs and prevent unnecessary diagnostic procedures and treatment. The use of HPV testing as a triage test is actively being studied. Most of the recent clinical studies have been performed with the Hybrid Capture II (HC2). A high degree of correlation has been reported between the Hybrid Capture (HC) and the polymerase chain reaction (PCR).[230-233] This assay, in addition to determining HPV positivity, is able to differentiate between HPV types of high- and low-risk oncogenic potential. The high-risk HPV types included in the "II" version of the assay are the following: 16, 18, 31, 33, 35, 39, 45, 51, 52, 56, 58, 59, and 68. The low risks are 6, 11, 42, 43, and 44. Some investigators have limited the use of the assay to the high-risk types, especially in clinical research.

HPV has been studied as a triage tool in the management of HSIL. Because of the high incidence of HPV positivity, it is clear that this test would not be able to discriminate between patients with serious histologic conditions, CIN II and above, and the small percentage of patients in whom there is not a clear abnormality or in whom a histologic low-grade abnormality is found. HSIL is not an indication for HPV testing. These patients should be managed with colposcopy and biopsies or loop electrosurgical excision procedure (LEEP). Approximately 80% to 90% of these lesions are HPV-positive for the high-risk viral types.[234-238]

Cytologic smears diagnosed as ASCUS and LSIL have a high percentage of spontaneous resolution and are associated with a low percentage of histologic abnormalities. Only 15% will be found to have significant histologic lesions, CIN II, or more serious conditions.[239] The work-up of ASCUS and LSIL creates an enormous financial burden with relatively small yield. As a result, HPV testing has been considered for the triage of ASCUS and LSIL. The hypothesis is that patients with ASCUS or LSIL associated with high-risk HPV types should undergo colposcopy and biopsies, and others may be ignored.

A recent multiinstitutional study has attempted to clarify the best strategy for the management of ASCUS and LSIL. One of the specific aims of this study was to test the accuracy and reliability of HPV DNA testing for the triage of patients with ASCUS or LSIL. Patients entering into this study were randomized to one of the following three arms:

1. Immediate referral for colposcopy
2. Follow-up with cytology only
3. Use of HPV DNA testing to triage to colposcopy

Preliminary data from this trial indicate that 83% of women with LSIL tested positive for HPV DNA.[240] These results suggest that positivity for HPV DNA will have limited value as a discriminant in LSIL.

This study used as a control group immediate colposcopy and biopsies. It was assumed that this control group represented the prevalence of CIN. The percentage of CIN II/III in the LSIL group was 15%, which is consistent with previous findings. In the same study, the prevalence of histologically confirmed CIN III among ASCUS patients was 5.1%.

Fifty-three percent of ASCUS patients were HPV-positive for the high-risk oncogenic potential probe. The percentage of CIN II/III in the control group (immediate colposcopy) and in the group triage with the HPV test was almost identical, approximately 15%. However, only 53% of patients in the ASCUS group were found to be HPV-positive and thus subject to colposcopy. The sensitivity to detect CIN III by testing for high-risk types HPV DNA was 96.3% (95% CI, 91.6% to 98.8%).[239]

In summary, although additional research is needed, the most important indication for HPV typing constitutes the cytologic diagnosis of ASCUS. Although only 5% to 15% of ASCUS smears will be found to have lesions compatible with a diagnosis of HSIL such as

CIN II or III, the large number of cases of ASCUS (approximately 3 million in the United States) includes a significant percentage of patients diagnosed with high-grade CIN lesions. Approximately one third of patients diagnosed with HSIL were initially identified as having ASCUS.[236]

Management of the Abnormal Pap Smear
Unsatisfactory Smear

"Unsatisfactory smear" refers to Pap smears with slides of insufficient quality for the pathologists to arrive at the proper diagnosis. The most common reason for unsatisfactory smears is the absence of endocervical cells, possibly from an inadequate sampling or related to clinical conditions that prevent the acquisition of endocervical epithelium.

Establishing better communication between clinician and pathologist may prevent many "unsatisfactory smears." Pathologists should be aware of conditions that make it difficult or impossible to find endocervical cells in the smear. Box 6-6 lists the most common conditions associated with the lack of endocervical cells in the Pap smear.

Another reason for unsatisfactory smears is the inappropriate fixation of the slide, resulting in "air-dried" slides. Slides must be fixed with the appropriate media immediately; exposure to air deteriorates the quality of the cells. Unsatisfactory or limited smears are produced in less than 0.5% of cases. A small percentage of these unsatisfactory or "limited" smears are found to have underlying SIL (9%) or carcinoma (2%).[194] In the absence of obvious reasons for the lack of endocervical cells, a second sampling should be provided.

Atypical Squamous Cell of Undetermined Significance

The expected percentage of ASCUS varies according to the characteristics of the population tested. Overall, approximately half of all abnormal Pap smears are caused by ASCUS. The age of the screened population accounts for significant differences. In a recent study, the ratio of ASCUS to SIL was 2.2 to 1. However, when women were stratified by menopausal status, there was a statistically significant difference between the groups. The ratios found were 1.9, 7.5, and 4.1 for premenopausal, perimenopausal, and postmenopausal women, respectively.[241] It is not clear why the ASCUS/SIL ratio increases with age. ASCUS possibly is overdiagnosed in perimenopausal women because of subtle atrophic artifacts.[241] Adolescents in inner city environments with a history of multiple sexual partners and STDs are at higher risk of having ASCUS Pap smears than their age-matched controls.[242]

Because only a small percentage of patients with ASCUS will eventually be found to have cervical changes that are clinically significant, it is of utmost importance to decrease the number of colposcopies and biopsies and to limit the work-up to the ones most likely to have dysplasia. Overall ASCUS is responsible for 5% to 15% of HGSIL in final biopsies.

Recent attempts have been made to further subdivide ASCUS, thus increasing the clinical significance. The terminology that has been suggested includes "favor premalignant" or "favor squamous intraepithelial lesion" (ASCUS-P, ASFS), "favor reactive" (ASCUS-R or

---

BOX 6-6	**Most Common Conditions Associated with Lack of Endocervical Cells in Pap Smear**

- Previous hysterectomy
- Elderly patients with atrophic cervix
- Patients treated with radiation therapy for cancer of the cervix, vagina, or uterus

ASFR), and "unqualified" or "not otherwise specified" (ASCUS-C, ASNOS). This subclassification has not been universally adopted. Furthermore, with the exception of ASCUS-P, it is unclear whether this further subdivision helps to identify patients with ASCUS who are in need of colposcopy and biopsies.[243,244] In the Bethesda 2001 classification a new subset of ASCUS is designated as Atypical Squamous Cell: cannot exclude high-grade SIL (ASC-H). These patients, because of the higher probability of HSIL, should be actively managed with colposcopy.

HPV testing in patients with cytologic diagnosis of ASCUS has been demonstrated to be worthwhile in identifying patients with CIN. The sensitivity to detect CIN III or more serious lesions by testing for high-risk types HPV DNA is 96%. This proved to be more sensitive than repeating the Pap smear.[239] Use of the liquid media has been adequate for HPV testing.[245] The residual volume of liquid-based media after the cytologic examination is performed may be used for HPV testing. This shifts the triage of patients with ASCUS from the health care provider's office to the laboratory and prevents unnecessary office or clinic visits.

The universal adoption of TP or similar methodology should increase the sensitivity of the Pap test, decrease the percentage of unsatisfactory or limited smears, and in conjunction with HPV testing provide a way to triage patients with ASCUS in the laboratory. The results of the ALTS trial indicate the effectiveness of using HPV for triage of patients with ASCUS.[239]

Low-Grade Squamous Intraepithelial Lesions

The management of LSIL must be guided by the clinical significance of this cytologic diagnosis. LSIL includes patients with histologic diagnosis compatible with HPV infection and CIN I. A high percentage of spontaneous regression has been documented in patients with all grades of dysplasia but particularly of CIN I. Review of the literature would indicate that the probability of regression of CIN I is 60%, persistence 30%, progression to CIN III 10%, and progression to invasion 1%.[246]

The risk of progression from CIN I to III is estimated to be approximately 1% per year.[247] Patients with a previous history of treatment for CIN are at a higher risk for progression.[248] A higher percentage of CIN (75% versus 41%) is found in patients diagnosed with LSIL by cytology and previously treated for CIN[249] A patient's age at the time of diagnosis is inversely related to the possibility of spontaneous regression. Young patients are more predisposed to progression.[250]

Because of the relatively low percentage of CIN III and the high cost of providing colposcopy services to every patient with LSIL, attention has been directed to other biomarkers. The incidence of HPV positivity in patients with LSIL was investigated as part of a large multiinstitutional study (the ALTS group). The study also attempted to determine whether HPV testing could be useful as a triage test. Through use of the Digene Hybrid Capture II (HC2), the study showed that 532 (82.9%) of 642 women (95% CI, 79.7%-85.7%) with the cytologic diagnosis of LSIL tested positive for high oncogenic potential HPV types.[239] In a subset of 210 of these patients the results of the HC2 were confirmed by use of PCR; 171 of the 2210 or 81.4% tested positive by use of both PCR and HC2.[230]

The high grade of HPV positivity makes this test ineffective for the triage of patients with cytologic diagnosis of LSIL. The management of LSIL should be guided by the reliability of the patient. Patients with a high likelihood of not returning for follow-up Pap smears should undergo colposcopy and biopsies. Reliable patients may be requested to come back for follow-up Pap smears until regression is documented by normal Pap tests. Some investigators have advocated that patients with LSIL and persistent disease ought to be actively managed for 2 years after diagnosis.[251]

Because of the lack of a test to distinguish patients with LSIL from those who may have CIN, a more conservative position must be taken than in the management of ASCUS. Patients with LSIL at high risk for CIN, such as patients previously treated for CIN, adolescents, and HIV-positive patients, should have colposcopy and biopsies as required. Patients who are unreliable or have a history of not following up with physician recommendations should be actively managed. Conservative management with repeat Pap smears taken after 3 months should be recommended to reliable patients. Although there are no strong data to support this recommendation, it is advisable that patients with persistent LSIL for 2 or more years be managed with colposcopy and biopsies.

High-grade Squamous Intraepithelial Lesion

The cytologic diagnosis of HSIL and cervical cancer are similar. This is expected because most HSIL are related to high–oncogenic-risk HPV, especially HPV 16/18. The Pap smear history of 585 women with histologically confirmed carcinoma in situ (CIN III) was reviewed by Bergeron and associates.:[252] Of the 454 patients who had one smear available for review, 9 (2%) had a negative cytologic diagnosis; 58 (13%) had LSIL; and 387 (85%) had HSIL. This study points out the significant correlation between the cytologic diagnosis of HSIL and the histologic presence of high-grade dysplasia.[252]

Because of the high degree of correlation between HSIL and high-grade CIN, all patients with HSIL should be actively managed either with colposcopy and biopsies or LEEP.

Abnormal Pap Smear in the HIV-Positive Patient

An increase in the incidence of cervical cancer and HPV has been documented in HIV-positive women. High-risk HPV types were detected in 25% and 80% of HIV seropositive patients with normal and abnormal cytology, respectively.[253] In a study involving 307 HIV-positive women, cervical disease was diagnosed in 27.0% through use of Pap smears, colposcopies, and biopsies. The presence of HPV DNA was documented by PCR in 53% of the women.[46] Goodman reported a prevalence of 37% of CIN among HIV-positive women. ASCUS diagnosis was found to be the largest contributor to false-negative Pap smears.[254] A cytologic diagnosis of ASCUS confers a significant risk for cervical dysplasia in HIV seropositive women.[255]

Since 1993 invasive cervical cancer has been designated a diagnostic criterion for AIDS in HIV-infected patients by the Centers for Disease Control and Prevention in HIV-positive women.[256]

The level of immunosuppression may be a contributory factor in the development of CIN in HIV-positive women. Patients with CIN had a lower CD4 T-lymphocyte count and higher viral loads than a control group with normal Pap smears.[257,258]

The association of premalignant and malignant conditions of the cervix has become a serious health concern as a result of the increase in HIV-positive women, the increased association of HPV infections in this population, and the greater and longer survival experienced by women with AIDS treated with modern therapy. There are little data on the effect of modern combined antiretroviral therapy on the incidence of CIN and cervical cancer in HIV-positive women. However, preliminary reports indicate an increased incidence of invasive cervical cancer in patients actively treated. This may be because of the greater survival of these patients as a result of the decreased incidence of other fatal coinfections and the opportunity for CIN to progress to invasive cancer.[259]

HIV-positive patients must adhere to a rigorous yearly screening program even in the absence of Pap smear abnormalities. Twenty percent of HIV-positive patients with no cervical abnormalities will develop dysplasia within 3 years.[48] All HIV-positive patients with Pap smear abnormalities must be actively managed with colposcopy and biopsies.

Management of Cervical Intraepithelial Neoplasia

Although recently there has been a tendency to use the cytologic descriptors LSIL and HSIL to describe histologic lesions, histologic lesions will continue to be described as CIN and the term SIL reserved for addressing cytologic abnormalities.

It is widely accepted that patients with high-grade CIN, CIN II and III, are at a very high risk for invasive cervical cancer. Because of ethical considerations, definitive observational studies have not been done using modern methodology. These patients must be treated appropriately. Nevertheless, there is an opportunity for conservative (expectant) management for patients with CIN I. Seventy percent of patients with CIN I will spontaneously reverse within a period of 9 months.[260] The term "spontaneous," within this context, must be carefully considered. To obtain the histologic diagnosis of CIN, biopsies are required. The effect that these biopsies have on the progression of CIN is unknown, especially on CIN I, where the lesions have the tendency to be small and very often are completely removed in the course of the biopsy. On the other hand, observational studies without tissue diagnosis, relying only on cytology and colposcopy, may be inaccurate and unreliable.

As previously described for LSIL, expectant management for patients with CIN I is not appropriate for unreliable individuals in whom there is a possibility of not following up with the health care provider's recommendations. In contrast, reliable patients may be followed with Pap smears and colposcopy.

The surgical management of CIN may be safely accomplished using a variety of treatment modalities. Martin-Hirsch, in a recent review that included 23 clinical trials, determined that no surgical technique is superior to others.[261] Treatment selection is usually based on personal preferences and type of training received.

Surgical techniques for the management of CIN may be divided into ablative, in which the tissue is destroyed, and excisional, in which tissue may be retained for pathologic evaluation. Ablative therapy such as cryosurgery or laser vaporization can only be employed if the complete lesion can be seen with the colposcope, there is no reason to suspect invasion, and the endocervical curettage is negative.

Cryotherapy destroys tissue by the crystallization of intracellular water. Most cryotherapy units reach the required low temperatures ($-20°$ C to $-30°$ C) necessary for the ablation of tissue by the use of carbon dioxide or nitrous oxide. This is an inexpensive and, when properly used, effective technique. The cryoprobe must accommodate the size of the lesion. Lesions larger than the largest available cryoprobe are not suitable for this treatment modality. Richart and associates reported that the cumulative risk of developing CIN after cryotherapy was 0.41% at year 5, 0.44% at year 10, and 0.44% at year 14. They found no significant differences in the risk of recurrence for CIN I, II or III.[262] Benedet and associates, reporting on a series of patients with 10 year follow-up, also found cryotherapy to be effective with no significant differences among the varying degrees of CIN.[263] Other authors have found cryotherapy not as effective when used on patients with the diagnosis of CIN III.[264] The higher failure rates reported for CIN III may be related to the selection of patients. Patients with large lesions[265] or lesions deeply penetrating the endocervical glands may have a higher failure rate.[266,267]

Laser vaporization by carbon dioxide laser offers an alternative to cryotherapy. The term "vaporization" refers to the mechanism of action. The interaction between the incident laser beam and the intracellular water results in the vaporization of the latter and subsequent cellular destruction. The patient selection criteria are the same as with other ablative techniques; namely, patients with lesions for whom invasive cancer has been ruled out by a satisfactory colposcopy with appropriate biopsies and when the ECC is negative. Compared with cryotherapy, laser vaporization offers the advantage of complete control over the depth of the tissue destruction and may be used in large lesions that may not qualify for cryotherapy treatment. This technique is efficacious and provides low failure rates. The recurrence rates, 5% to 10%, are similar to cryotherapy.[268,269] The disadvantage of this method, compared with cryotherapy, relates to the costly equipment, more demanding training, a higher opportunity for intraoperative complications, and a higher incidence of postoperative bleeding.[270] The success rate seems to be comparable regardless of the CIN degree.[270] Although more costly, this method is invaluable when the lesions are very large, the cervix is distorted because of previous surgery, or the lesions extend to the vagina.

Loop electrosurgical excision or diathermy is a surgical procedure that has not only become popular but in many centers has also become the only surgical management for CIN. This method has the advantage of being therapeutic as well as diagnostic; a specimen is obtained for pathologic evaluation. The use of electricity (i.e., electrofulguration) to destroy skin lesions has been employed for many years. The combination of high power and the use of a thin loop wire enables the surgeon to remove a portion of the cervix with relatively low thermal damage. This technique has also been called LLETZ (large loop excision of the transformation zone) or LEEP. Prendiville and associates popularized this technique using a large loop that allows the removal of the entire transformation zone with a single pass of the electrode.[271] Bigrigg reported on the safety of this method in a study that included 1000 consecutive patients; only six had to return to the clinic because of bleeding. In his study Bigrigg used what has been called the "see and treat technique."[272] Patients with abnormal Pap smears undergo the procedure without the use of colposcopically guided biopsies. Colposcopy is used only to ascertain that the complete squamous columnar junction is visible and can be excised. "See and treat" techniques are gaining in popularity, especially in Europe. Definitive studies have not been performed comparing the "usual care"—obtaining a biopsy first and confirming the diagnosis—with "see and treat." Although concerns were raised about the possibility of overtreatment by "see and treat" techniques, they are apparently unwarranted.[273] LEEP does not seem to have a negative effect on fertility.[274-277]

Cold knife cone biopsy or conization has been considered to be the "gold standard" among excisional techniques. One of the major disadvantages is that the removal of a conical area of the cervix with the scalpel usually requires general anesthesia. In general, a larger amount of healthier tissue is removed with cold knife cone than with LEEP. There is a perception that LEEP leads to a higher incidence of surgically involved margins, compared with cold knife cone. However, very often LEEP is performed in an outpatient facility with local anesthesia where retraction of the vagina and visualization of the cervix cannot be compared to the one obtained in the operating room under general anesthesia, which is the case in most cold knife cone biopsies. Furthermore, no support in the literature indicates that LEEP leads to a higher residual disease or increase in complication rate.[278-285] Excisional treatment of CIN, even CIN III, is very successful. More than 95% of patients treated will be free of disease.[286]

Mitchell and associates compared the effectiveness of cryotherapy, laser vaporization, and electrosurgical loop excision in a randomized study. The mean follow-up time was 16 months (with a 6- to 37-month range). They found a high success rate and no significant differences among the three different techniques.[287]

Aggressive treatment—LEEP, cone biopsy, or hysterectomy—is recommended for HIV-positive patients with CIN III. However, hysterectomy does not seem to decrease the recurrence rate, as judged by subsequent abnormal Pap smears, compared with cone biopsy. High recurrence rates have been found with both treatment modalities—67% for cone biopsy and 60% for hysterectomy patients.[288]

In summary, patients with CIN I who are not at high risk, are reliable, and do not indicate they will not return for follow-up may be candidates for conservative management with appropriate follow-up. Patients with CIN II and III must be treated. Cryosurgery should be used when the lesion is completely visualized and is smaller than the largest cryoprobe. This may not be an appropriate technique for CIN III. With the exception of very special cases, the use of laser therapy, either as an ablative or excisional technique, does not seem to be advantageous. LEEP offers the opportunity of definitive treatment and tissue diagnosis. It also offers the possibility of management using "see and treat" techniques. Cold knife cone, with very few exceptions, does not offer any advantages over LEEP.

Pregnancy and the Abnormal Pap Smear

In general, patients with Pap smear abnormalities during pregnancy are managed similarly to the nonpregnant patient. The biology of this condition during pregnancy is similar to the nonpregnant state.[289,290] In dependable patients with ASCUS and LSIL, after initial colposcopy and biopsies as required, patients may be managed with Pap smears and colposcopy at 8-week intervals. Any further management may be delayed until the postpartum period. Women with HSIL should undergo colposcopy and biopsies. Patients with any suspicion of microinvasive disease should undergo a cold knife or LEEP procedure. LEEP has been reported to be a safe and well-tolerated procedure during the first trimester of pregnancy.[291] The rate of progression from CIN to invasive cancer within the length of gestation seems to be very modest. In a series of 811 women referred with abnormal cervical cytology during pregnancy, Woodrow reported only a 7% progression to a higher level of dysplasia. No patient developed microinvasive or invasive cancer.[292]

There is a perception among gynecologists that vaginal deliveries, because of the possible exfoliative power, may reverse SIL. There is no evidence in the literature to support this belief.[293] All patients who carry the diagnosis of SIL or abnormal Pap smear should have a repeat Pap smear, and depending on the circumstances, colposcopy and biopsies 6 to 8 weeks postpartum.

There is evidence that the significance and management of pregnant patients with AGUS should be similar to nonpregnant patients. Patients should be actively managed, with colposcopy and LEEP or cone biopsy as indicated.[294]

REFERENCES

1. *Cancer facts and figures 2001.* Atlanta, American Cancer Society, 2001.
2. Fischer U, Raptis G, Gessner W, et al: [Epidemiology and pathogenesis of cervical cancer]. *Zentralbl Gynakol* 2001;123:198-205.
3. Pisani P, Parkin DM, Ferlay J: Estimates of the worldwide mortality from eighteen major cancers in 1985: implications for prevention and projections of future burden. *Int J Cancer* 1993;55:891-903.
4. Shanta V, Krishnamurthi S, Gajalakshmi CK, et al: Epidemiology of cancer of the cervix: global and national perspective. *J Indian Med Assoc* 2000;98:49-52.
5. Cervical cancer. *NIH Consens Statement* 1996;14:1-38; quiz 34p.
6. Hagen B, Skjeldestad FE, Halvorsen T, et al: Primary treatment of cervical carcinoma: ten years experience from one Norwegian health region. *Acta Obstet Gynecol Scand* 2000;79:1093-1099.
7. *Cancer facts and figures for Hispanics 2000-2001.* Atlanta, American Cancer Society, 2001.
8. *Cancer facts and figures 2002.* Atlanta, American Cancer Society, 2002.
9. Scully RE, Bonfiglio TA, Kurman RJ, et al: Histological typing of female genital tract tumours. *World Health Organization: international histological classification of tumours,* ed 2, New York, Springer-Verlag, 1994.
10. Parazzini F, La Vecchia C: Epidemiology of adenocarcinoma of the cervix. *Gynecol Oncol* 1990;39:40-46.
11. Zheng T, Holford TR, Ma Z, et al: The continuing increase in adenocarcinoma of the uterine cervix: a birth cohort phenomenon. *Int J Epidemiol* 1996;25:252-258.
12. Smith HO, Tiffany MF, Qualls CR, et al: The rising incidence of adenocarcinoma relative to squamous cell carcinoma of the uterine cervix in the United States: a 24-year population-based study. *Gynecol Oncol* 2000;78:97-105.
13. Benedet JL, Bender H, Jones H III, Ngan HY, et al: FIGO staging classifications and clinical practice guidelines in the management of gynecologic cancers, FIGO Committee on Gynecologic Oncology. *Int J Gynaecol Obstet* 2000;70:209-262.
14. Peters RK, Thomas D, Hagan DG, et al: Risk factors for invasive cervical cancer among Latinas and non-Latinas in Los Angeles County. *J Natl Cancer Inst* 1986;77:1063-1077.
15. Brinton LA, Hamman RF, Huggins GR, et al: Sexual and reproductive risk factors for invasive squamous cell cervical cancer. *J Natl Cancer Inst* 1987;79:23-30.
16. Kjaer SK: Risk factors for cervical neoplasia in Denmark. *APMIS Suppl* 1998;80:1-41.
17. Bosch FX, Munoz N, de Sanjose S, et al: Risk factors for cervical cancer in Colombia and Spain. *Int J Cancer* 1992;52:750-758.
18. Kjaer SK, Dahl C, Engholm G, et al: Case-control study of risk factors for cervical neoplasia in

Denmark, II: Role of sexual activity, reproductive factors, and venereal infections. *Cancer Causes Control* 1992;3:339-348.
19. Brinton LA, Reeves WC, Brenes MM, et al: Parity as a risk factor for cervical cancer. *Am J Epidemiol* 1989;130:486-496.
20. zur Hausen H, Gissmann L, Steiner W, et al: Human papilloma viruses and cancer. *Bibl Haematol* 1975;43:569-571.
21. zur Hausen H, de Villiers EM: Human papillomaviruses. *Annu Rev Microbiol* 1994;48:427-447.
22. Murakami M, Gurski KJ, Steller MA: Human papillomavirus vaccines for cervical cancer. *J Immunother* 1999;22:212-218.
23. zur Hausen H: Papillomaviruses in human cancers. *Proc Assoc Am Physicians* 1999;111:581-587.
24. Cornelison TL: Human papillomavirus genotype 16 vaccines for cervical cancer prophylaxis and treatment. *Curr Opin Oncol* 2000;12:466-473.
25. Hilleman MR: Overview of vaccinology with special reference to papillomavirus vaccines. *J Clin Virol* 2000;19:79-90.
26. Rozendaal L, Walboomers JM, van der Linden JC, et al: PCR-based high-risk HPV test in cervical cancer screening gives objective risk assessment of women with cytomorphologically normal cervical smears. *Int J Cancer* 1996;68:766-769.
27. Wallin KL, Wiklund F, Angstrom T, et al: Type-specific persistence of human papillomavirus DNA before the development of invasive cervical cancer. *N Engl J Med* 1999;341:1633-1638.
28. Kjellberg L, Wang Z, Wiklund F, et al: Sexual behaviour and papillomavirus exposure in cervical intraepithelial neoplasia: a population-based case-control study. *J Gen Virol* 1999;80:391-398.
29. Bosch FX, Manos MM, Munoz N, et al: Prevalence of human papillomavirus in cervical cancer: a worldwide perspective, International biological study on cervical cancer (IBSCC) Study Group. *J Natl Cancer Inst* 1995;87:796-802.
30. Scheffner M, Werness BA, Huibregtse JM, et al: The E6 oncoprotein encoded by human papillomavirus types 16 and 18 promotes the degradation of p53. *Cell* 1990;63:1129-1136.
31. Sheets EE, Yeh J: The role of apoptosis in gynaecological malignancies. *Ann Med* 1997;29:121-126.
32. Tonon SA, Picconi MA, Zinovich JB, et al: Human papillomavirus cervical infection and associated risk factors in a region of Argentina with a high incidence of cervical carcinoma. *Infect Dis Obstet Gynecol* 1999;7:237-243.
33. Corey L, Handsfield HH: Genital herpes and public health: addressing a global problem. *JAMA* 2000;283:791-794.
34. Janier M, Lassau F, Bloch J, et al: Seroprevalence of herpes simplex virus type 2 antibodies in an STD clinic in Paris. *Int J STD AIDS* 1999;10:522-526.
35. Oliver L, Wald A, Kim M, et al: Seroprevalence of herpes simplex virus infections in a family medicine clinic. *Arch Fam Med* 1995;4:228-232.
36. Breinig MK, Kingsley LA, Armstrong JA, et al: Epidemiology of genital herpes in Pittsburgh: sero-

logic, sexual, and racial correlates of apparent and inapparent herpes simplex infections. *J Infect Dis* 1990;162:299-305.

37. Ades AE, Peckham CS, Dale GE, et al: Prevalence of antibodies to herpes simplex virus types 1 and 2 in pregnant women, and estimated rates of infection. *J Epidemiol Community Health* 1989;43:53-60.

38. Wutzler P, Doerr HW, Farber I, et al: Seroprevalence of herpes simplex virus type 1 and type 2 in selected German populations: relevance for the incidence of genital herpes. *J Med Virol* 2000;61:201-207.

39. Murthy NS, Mathew A: Risk factors for pre-cancerous lesions of the cervix. *Eur J Cancer Prev* 2000;9:5-14.

40. Hsieh CY, You SL, Kao CL, et al: Reproductive and infectious risk factors for invasive cervical cancer in Taiwan. *Anticancer Res* 1999;19:4495-4500.

41. Viikki M, Pukkala E, Nieminen P, et al: Gynaecological infections as risk determinants of subsequent cervical neoplasia. *Acta Oncol* 2000;39:71-75.

42. Fiel-Gan MD, Villamil CF, Mandavilli SR, et al: Rapid detection of HSV from cytologic specimens collected into ThinPrep fixative. *Acta Cytol* 1999;43:1034-1038.

43. Sharma BK, Sharma R, Smith CC, et al: Prevalence of serum antibodies to LA-1 oncoprotein, herpes simplex virus type-2 glycoprotein and human papillomavirus type 16 transactivator (E2) protein among Indian women with cervical neoplasia. *Indian J Exp Biol* 1998;36:967-972.

44. Daling JR, Madeleine MM, McKnight B, et al: The relationship of human papillomavirus-related cervical tumors to cigarette smoking, oral contraceptive use, and prior herpes simplex virus type 2 infection. *Cancer Epidemiol Biomarkers Prev* 1996;5:541-548.

45. Fowler MG, Melnick SL, Mathieson BJ: Women and HIV: epidemiology and global overview. *Obstet Gynecol Clin North Am* 1997;24:705-729.

46. Heard I, Tassie JM, Schmitz V, et al: Increased risk of cervical disease among human immunodeficiency virus-infected women with severe immunosuppression and high human papillomavirus load(1). *Obstet Gynecol* 2000;96:403-409.

47. Ahr A, Scharl A, Lutke K, et al: Cervical intraepithelial neoplasia in human immunodeficiency virus-positive patients. *Cancer Detect Prev* 2000;24:179-185.

48. Ellerbrock TV, Chiasson MA, Bush TJ, et al: Incidence of cervical squamous intraepithelial lesions in HIV-infected women. *JAMA* 2000;283:1031-1037.

49. Massad LS, Riester KA, Anastos KM, et al: Prevalence and predictors of squamous cell abnormalities in Papanicolaou smears from women infected with HIV-1, Women's Interagency HIV Study Group. *J Acquir Immune Defic Syndr* 1999;21:33-41.

50. Boardman LA, Peipert JF, Cooper AS, et al: Cytologic-histologic discrepancy in human immunodeficiency virus-positive women referred to a colposcopy clinic. *Obstet Gynecol* 1994;84:1016-1020.

51. Kessler II: Venereal factors in human cervical cancer: evidence from marital clusters. *Cancer* 1977;39:1912-1919.

52. Thomas DB, Ray RM, Kuypers J, et al: Human papillomaviruses and cervical cancer in Bangkok, III: the role of husbands and commercial sex workers. *Am J Epidemiol* 2001;153:740-748.

53. Picconi MA, Eijan AM, Distefano AL, et al: Human papillomavirus (HPV) DNA in penile carcinomas in Argentina: analysis of primary tumors and lymph nodes. *J Med Virol* 2000;61:65-69.

54. Munoz N, Castellsague X, Bosch FX, et al: Difficulty in elucidating the male role in cervical cancer in Colombia, a high-risk area for the disease. *J Natl Cancer Inst* 1996;88:1068-1075.

55. Beral V, Hannaford P, Kay C: Oral contraceptive use and malignancies of the genital tract: results from the Royal College of General Practitioners' Oral Contraception Study. *Lancet* 1988;2:1331-1335.

56. Kjellberg L, Hallmans G, Ahren AM, et al: Smoking, diet, pregnancy and oral contraceptive use as risk factors for cervical intra-epithelial neoplasia in relation to human papillomavirus infection. *Br J Cancer* 2000;82:1332-1338.

57. Lacey JV Jr, Brinton LA, Abbas FM, et al: Oral contraceptives as risk factors for cervical adenocarcinomas and squamous cell carcinomas. *Cancer Epidemiol Biomarkers Prev* 1999;8:1079-1085.

58. Brinton LA, Huggins GR, Lehman HF, et al: Long-term use of oral contraceptives and risk of invasive cervical cancer. *Int J Cancer* 1986;38:399-344.

59. Pike MC, Spicer DV: Hormonal contraception and chemoprevention of female cancers. *Endocr Relat Cancer* 2000;7:73-83.

60. Pater A, Bayatpour M, Pater MM: Oncogenic transformation by human papillomavirus type 16 deoxyribonucleic acid in the presence of progesterone or progestins from oral contraceptives. *Am J Obstet Gynecol* 1990;162:1099-1103.

61. Yuan F, Auborn K, James C: Altered growth and viral gene expression in human papillomavirus type 16-containing cancer cell lines treated with progesterone. *Cancer Invest* 1999;17:19-29.

62. Parazzini F, Negri E, La Vecchia C, et al: Barrier methods of contraception and the risk of cervical neoplasia. *Contraception* 1989;40:519-530.

63. Verreault R, Chu J, Mandelson M, et al: A case-control study of diet and invasive cervical cancer. *Int J Cancer* 1989;43:1050-1054.

64. Herrero R, Potischman N, Brinton LA, et al: A case-control study of nutrient status and invasive cervical cancer, I: dietary indicators. *Am J Epidemiol* 1991;134:1335-1346.

65. Brock KE, Berry G, Mock PA, et al: Nutrients in diet and plasma and risk of in situ cervical cancer. *J Natl Cancer Inst* 1988;80:580-585.

66. La Vecchia C, Decarli A, Fasoli M, et al: Dietary vitamin A and the risk of intraepithelial and invasive cervical neoplasia. *Gynecol Oncol* 1988;30:187-195.

67. Peng YM, Peng YS, Childers JM, et al: Concentrations of carotenoids, tocopherols, and retinol in paired plasma and cervical tissue of patients with cervical cancer, precancer, and non-cancerous diseases. *Cancer Epidemiol Biomarkers Prev* 1998;7:347-350.

68. Ziegler RG, Jones CJ, Brinton LA, et al: Diet and the risk of in situ cervical cancer among white women in the United States. *Cancer Causes Control* 1991;2:17-29.

69. Ho GY, Palan PR, Basu J, et al: Viral characteristics of human papillomavirus infection and antioxidant levels as risk factors for cervical dysplasia. *Int J Cancer* 1998;78:594-599.

70. Nagata C, Shimizu H, Yoshikawa H, et al: Serum carotenoids and vitamins and risk of cervical dysplasia from a case-control study in Japan. *Br J Cancer* 1999;81:1234-1237.

71. Tabrizi SN, Fairley CK, Chen S, et al: Epidemiological characteristics of women with high grade CIN who do and do not have human papillomavirus. *Br J Obstet Gynaecol* 1999;106:252-257.

72. Lehtinen M, Luostarinen T, Youngman LD, et al: Low levels of serum vitamins A and E in blood and subsequent risk for cervical cancer: interaction with HPV seropositivity. *Nutr Cancer* 1999;34:229-234.

73. Giuliano AR, Papenfuss M, Nour M, et al: Antioxidant nutrients: associations with persistent human papillomavirus infection. *Cancer Epidemiol Biomarkers Prev* 1997;6:917-923.

74. Goodman MT, Kiviat N, McDuffie K, et al: The association of plasma micronutrients with the risk of cervical dysplasia in Hawaii. *Cancer Epidemiol Biomarkers Prev* 1998;7:537-544.

75. VanEenwyk J, Davis FG, Colman N: Folate, vitamin C, and cervical intraepithelial neoplasia. *Cancer Epidemiol Biomarkers Prev* 1992;1:119-124.

76. Slattery ML, Abbott TM, Overall JC Jr, et al: Dietary vitamins A, C, and E and selenium as risk factors for cervical cancer. *Epidemiology* 1990;1:8-15.

77. Ziegler RG, Brinton LA, Hamman RF, et al: Diet and the risk of invasive cervical cancer among white women in the United States. *Am J Epidemiol* 1990;132:432-445.

78. Kwasniewska A, Tukendorf A, Semczuk M: Folate deficiency and cervical intraepithelial neoplasia. *Eur J Gynaecol Oncol* 1997;18:526-530.

79. Potischman N, Brinton LA, Laiming VA, et al: A case-control study of serum folate levels and invasive cervical cancer. *Cancer Res* 1991;51:4785-4789.

80. Butterworth CE Jr, Hatch KD, Macaluso M, et al: Folate deficiency and cervical dysplasia. *JAMA* 1992;267:528-533.

81. Patterns of cancer in five continents. *IARC Sci Publ* 1990;102:1-159.

82. Shopland DR, Eyre HJ, Pechacek TF: Smoking-attributable cancer mortality in 1991: is lung cancer now the leading cause of death among smokers in the United States? *J Natl Cancer Inst* 1991;83:1142-1148.

83. Winkelstein W Jr, Smoking and cervical cancer—current status: a review. *Am J Epidemiol* 1990;131:945-957; discussion 958-960.

84. Baron JA, Byers T, Greenberg ER, et al: Cigarette smoking in women with cancers of the breast and reproductive organs. *J Natl Cancer Inst* 1986;77:677-680.

85. Slattery ML, Robison LM, Schuman KL, et al: Cigarette smoking and exposure to passive smoke are risk factors for cervical cancer. *JAMA* 1989;261:1593-1598.

86. La Vecchia C, Franceschi S, Decarli A, et al: Cigarette smoking and the risk of cervical neoplasia. *Am J Epidemiol* 1986;123:22-29.

87. Daly SF, Doyle M, English J, et al: Can the number of cigarettes smoked predict high-grade cervical intraepithelial neoplasia among women with mildly abnormal cervical smears? *Am J Obstet Gynecol* 1998;179:399-402.

88. Brinton LA, Schairer C, Haenszel W, et al: Cigarette smoking and invasive cervical cancer. *JAMA* 1986;255:3265-3269.

89. Prokopczyk B, Cox JE, Hoffmann D, et al: Identification of tobacco-specific carcinogen in the cervical mucus of smokers and nonsmokers. *J Natl Cancer Inst* 1997;89:868-873.

90. Seidegard J, Vorachek WR, Pero RW, et al: Hereditary differences in the expression of the human glutathione transferase active on trans-stilbene oxide are due to a gene deletion. *Proc Natl Acad Sci USA* 1988;85:7293-7297.

91. Caporaso N, Landi MT, Vineis P: Relevance of metabolic polymorphisms to human carcinogenesis: evaluation of epidemiologic evidence. *Pharmacogenetics* 1991;1:4-19.

92. Ingelman-Sundberg M, Johansson I, Persson I, et al: Genetic polymorphism of cytochromes P450: interethnic differences and relationship to incidence of lung cancer. *Pharmacogenetics* 1992;2:264-271.

93. Rabkin CS, Biggar RJ, Melbye M, et al: Second primary cancers following anal and cervical carcinoma: evidence of shared etiologic factors. *Am J Epidemiol* 1992;136:54-58.

94. Kleinerman RA, Curtis RE, Boice JD Jr, et al: Second cancers following radiotherapy for cervical cancer. *J Natl Cancer Inst* 1982;69:1027-1033.

95. Boice JD Jr, Day NE, Andersen A, et al: Second cancers following radiation treatment for cervical cancer: an international collaboration among cancer registries. *J Natl Cancer Inst* 1985;74:955-975.

96. Levi F, Randimbison L, Vecchia CL, Franceschi S: Incidence of invasive cancers following carcinoma in situ of the cervix. *Br J Cancer* 1996;74:1321-1323.

97. Sturgeon SR, Curtis RE, Johnson K, et al: Second primary cancers after vulvar and vaginal cancers. *Am J Obstet Gynecol* 1996;174:929-933.

98. Shepherd J, Weston R, Peersman G, et al: Interventions for encouraging sexual lifestyles and behaviours intended to prevent cervical cancer. *Cochrane Database Syst Rev* 2000;2:CD001035.

99. Braun V, Gavey N: Exploring the possibility of sexual-behavioural primary prevention interventions for cervical cancer. *Aust N Z J Public Health* 1998;22:353-359.

100. Sideri M, Spinaci L, Schettino F, et al: Risk factors for high-grade cervical intraepithelial neoplasia in patients with mild cytological dyskaryosis: human papillomavirus testing versus multivariate tree analysis of demographic data. *Cancer Epidemiol Biomarkers Prev* 1998;7:237-241.

101. Parazzini F, Chatenoud L, La Vecchia C, et al: Determinants of risk of invasive cervical cancer in young women. *Br J Cancer* 1998;77:838-841.

102. Chichareon S, Herrero R, Munoz N, et al: Risk factors for cervical cancer in Thailand: a case-control study. *J Natl Cancer Inst* 1998;90:50-57.

103. Morrison CS, Schwingl PJ, Cates W Jr, Sexual behavior and cancer prevention. *Cancer Causes Control* 1997;8:S21-25.

104. Giuliano AR, Papenfuss M, Schneider A, et al: Risk factors for high-risk type human papillomavirus infection among Mexican-American women. *Cancer Epidemiol Biomarkers Prev* 1999;8:615-620.

105. Moberg DP, Piper DL: The Healthy for Life project: sexual risk behavior outcomes. *AIDS Educ Prev* 1998;10:128-148.

106. Siegel DM, Aten MJ, Roghmann KJ, et al: Early effects of a school-based human immunodeficiency virus infection and sexual risk prevention intervention. *Arch Pediatr Adolesc Med* 1998;152:961-970.

107. Hawkins JD, Catalano RF, Kosterman R, et al: Preventing adolescent health-risk behaviors by strengthening protection during childhood. *Arch Pediatr Adolesc Med* 1999;153:226-234.

108. Kagawa-Singer M, Pourat N: Asian American and Pacific Islander breast and cervical carcinoma screening rates and healthy people 2000 objectives. *Cancer* 2000;89:696-705.

109. Skaer TL, Robison LM, Sclar DA, et al: Knowledge, attitudes, and patterns of cancer screening: a self-report among foreign born Hispanic women utilizing rural migrant health clinics. *J Rural Health* 1996;12:169-177.

110. Fernandez MA, Tortolero-Luna G, Gold RS: Mammography and Pap test screening among low-income foreign-born Hispanic women in USA. *Cad Saude Publica* 1998;14:133-147.

111. Prochaska JO, Redding CA, Harlow LL, et al: The transtheoretical model of change and HIV prevention: a review. *Health Educ Q* 1994;21:471-486.

112. Kelaher M, Gillespie AG, Allotey P, et al: The transtheoretical model and cervical screening: its application among culturally diverse communities in Queensland, Australia. *Ethn Health* 1999;4:259-276.

113. Buller D, Modiano MR, Guernsey de Zapien J, et al: Predictors of cervical cancer screening in Mexican American women of reproductive age. *J Health Care Poor Underserved* 1998;9:76-95.

114. Howe SL, Delfino RJ, Taylor TH, et al: The risk of invasive cervical cancer among Hispanics:

115. Lobell M, Bay RC, Rhoads KV, et al: Barriers to cancer screening in Mexican-American women [see comments]. *Mayo Clin Proc* 1998;73:301-308.

116. Brewster WR, Anton-Culver H, Ziogas A, et al: Recruitment strategies for cervical cancer prevention study. *Gynecol Oncol* 2002;85:250-254.

117. Ramirez AG, Suarez L, Laufman L, et al: Hispanic women's breast and cervical cancer knowledge, attitudes, and screening behaviors. *Am J Health Promot* 2000;14:292-300.

118. Mandelblatt JS, Gold K, O'Malley AS, et al: Breast and cervix cancer screening among multiethnic women: role of age, health, and source of care. *Prev Med* 1999;28:418-425.

119. McBride CM, Scholes D, Grothaus L, et al: Promoting smoking cessation among women who seek cervical cancer screening. *Obstet Gynecol* 1998;91:719-724.

120. Melnikow J, Chan BK, Stewart GK. Do follow-up recommendations for abnormal Papanicolaou smears influence patient adherence? *Arch Fam Med* 1999;8:510-514.

121. Alanen KW, Elit LM, Molinaro PA, et al: Assessment of cytologic follow-up as the recommended management for patients with atypical squamous cells of undetermined significance or low grade squamous intraepithelial lesions [see comments]. *Cancer* 1998;84:5-10.

122. Lavin C, Goodman E, Perlman S, et al: Follow-up of abnormal Papanicolaou smears in a hospital-based adolescent clinic. *J Pediatr Adolesc Gynecol* 1997;10:141-145.

123. Miller SM, Siejak KK, Schroeder CM, et al: Enhancing adherence following abnormal Pap smears among low-income minority women: a preventive telephone counseling strategy. *J Natl Cancer Inst* 1997;89:703-708.

124. Carey P, Gjerdingen DK: Follow-up of abnormal Papanicolaou smears among women of different races. *J Fam Pract* 1993;37:583-587.

125. Thinkhamrop J, Lumbiganon P, Jitpakdeebodin S: Loss to follow-up of patients with abnormal Pap smear: magnitude and reasons. *J Med Assoc Thai* 1998;81:862-865.

126. Kaplan CP, Bastani R, Belin TR, et al: Improving follow-up after an abnormal pap smear: results from a quasi-experimental intervention study. *J Womens Health Gend Based Med* 2000;9:779-790.

127. Marcus AC, Kaplan CP, Crane LA, et al: Reducing loss-to-follow-up among women with abnormal Pap smears: results from a randomized trial testing an intensive follow-up protocol and economic incentives. *Med Care* 1998;36:397-410.

128. Jones BA, Novis DA: Follow-up of abnormal gynecologic cytology: a college of American pathologists Q-probes study of 16132 cases from 306 laboratories. *Arch Pathol Lab Med* 2000;124:665-671.

129. Burger RA, Monk BJ, Van Nostrand KM, et al: Single-visit program for cervical cancer prevention

in a high-risk population. *Obstet Gynecol* 1995;86:491-498.

130. Holschneider CH, Felix JC, Satmary W, et al: A single-visit cervical carcinoma prevention program offered at an inner city church: a pilot project. *Cancer* 1999;86:2659-2667.

131. Da Silva DM, Eiben GL, Fausch SC, et al: Cervical cancer vaccines: emerging concepts and developments. *J Cell Physiol* 2001;186:169-182.

132. Ling M, Kanayama M, Roden R, Wu TC: Preventive and therapeutic vaccines for human papillomavirus-associated cervical cancers. *J Biomed Sci* 2000;7:341-356.

133. Evans TG, Bonnez W, Rose RC, et al: A Phase 1 study of a recombinant viruslike particle vaccine against human papillomavirus type 11 in healthy adult volunteers. *J Infect Dis* 2001;183:1485-1493.

134. Pastrana DV, Vass WC, Lowy DR, et al: NHPV16 VLP vaccine induces human antibodies that neutralize divergent variants of HPV16. *Virology* 2001;279:361-369.

135. Lowy DR, Schiller JT: Papillomaviruses: prophylactic vaccine prospects. *Biochim Biophys Acta* 1999;1423:M1-8.

136. Schiller JT, Hidesheim A: Developing HPV viruslike particle vaccines to prevent cervical cancer: a progress report. *J Clin Virol* 2000;19(1-2):67-74.

137. Breitburd F, Kirnbauer R, Hubbert NL, et al: Immunization with viruslike particles from cottontail rabbit papillomavirus (CRPV) can protect against experimental CRPV infection. *J Virol* 1995;69:3959-3963.

138. Harro CD, Pang YY, Roden RB, et al: Safety and immunogenicity trial in adult volunteers of a human papillomavirus 16 L1 virus-like particle vaccine. *J Natl Cancer Inst* 2001;93:284-292.

139. Lehtinen M, Kibur M, Luostarinen T, et al: Prospects for phase III-IV HPV vaccination trials in the Nordic countries and in Estonia. *J Clin Virol* 2000;19:113-122.

140. Muderspach L, Wilczynski S, Roman L, et al: A phase I trial of a human papillomavirus (HPV) peptide vaccine for women with high-grade cervical and vulvar intraepithelial neoplasia who are HPV 16 positive. *Clin Cancer Res* 2000;6:3406-3416.

141. van Driel WJ, Ressing ME, Kenter GG, et al: Vaccination with HPV16 peptides of patients with advanced cervical carcinoma: clinical evaluation of a phase I-II trial. *Eur J Cancer* 1999;35:946-952.

142. Lazcano-Ponce E, Rivera L, Arillo-Santillan E, et al: Acceptability of a human papillomavirus (HPV) trial vaccine among mothers of adolescents in Cuernavaca, Mexico. *Arch Med Res* 2001;32:243-247.

143. Paavonen J, Halttunen M, Hansson BG, et al: Prerequisites for human papillomavirus vaccine trial: results of feasibility studies. *J Clin Virol* 2000;19:25-30.

144. Batieha AM, Armenian HK, Norkus EP, et al: Serum micronutrients and the subsequent risk of cervical cancer in a population-based nested case-control study. *Cancer Epidemiol Biomarkers Prev* 1993;2:335-339.

145. Nagata C, Shimizu H, Higashiiwai H, et al: Serum retinol level and risk of subsequent cervical cancer in cases with cervical dysplasia. *Cancer Invest* 1999;17:253-258.

146. Kantesky PA, Gammon MD, Mandelblatt J, et al: Dietary intake and blood levels of lycopene: association with cervical dysplasia among non-Hispanic, black women. *Nutr Cancer* 1998;31:31-40.

147. Ramaswamy G, Krishnamoorthy L: Serum carotene, vitamin A, and vitamin C levels in breast cancer and cancer of the uterine cervix. *Nutr Cancer* 1996;25:173-177.

148. Potischman N, Hoover RN, Brinton LA, et al: The relations between cervical cancer and serological markers of nutritional status. *Nutr Cancer* 1994;21:193-201.

149. Bernstein A, Harris B: The relationship of dietary and serum vitamin A to the occurrence of cervical intraepithelial neoplasia in sexually active women. *Am J Obstet Gynecol* 1984;148:309-312.

150. Xu XC, Mitchell MF, Silva E, et al: Decreased expression of retinoic acid receptors, transforming growth factor beta, involucrin, and cornifin in cervical intraepithelial neoplasia. *Clin Cancer Res* 1999;5:1503-1508.

151. Narayanan BA, Holladay EB, Nixon DW, et al: The effect of all-trans and 9-cis retinoic acid on the steady state level of HPV16 E6/E7 mRNA and cell cycle in cervical carcinoma cells. *Life Sci* 1998;63:565-573.

152. Meyskens FL Jr, Surwit E, Moon TE, et al: Enhancement of regression of cervical intraepithelial neoplasia II (moderate dysplasia) with topically applied all-trans-retinoic acid: a randomized trial [see comments]. *J Natl Cancer Inst* 1994;86:539-543.

153. Surwit EA, Graham V, Droegemueller W, et al: Evaluation of topically applied trans-retinoic acid in the treatment of cervical intraepithelial lesions. *Am J Obstet Gynecol* 1982;143:821-823.

154. Manetta A, Schubbert T, Chapman J, et al: Beta-carotene treatment of cervical intraepithelial neoplasia: a phase II study [see comments]. *Cancer Epidemiol Biomarkers Prev* 1996;5:929-932.

155. Mackerras D, Irwig L, Simpson JM, et al: Randomized double-blind trial of beta-carotene and vitamin C in women with minor cervical abnormalities. *Br J Cancer* 1999;79(9-10):1448-1453.

156. Oridate N, Suzuki S, Higuchi M, et al: Involvement of reactive oxygen species in N-(4-hydroxyphenyl) retinamide-induced apoptosis in cervical carcinoma cells. *J Natl Cancer Inst* 1997;89:1191-1198.

157. Ulukaya E, Wood EJ: Fenretinide and its relation to cancer. *Cancer Treat Rev Aug* 1999;25:229-235.

158. Mitchell MF, Hittelman WN, Lotan R, et al: Chemoprevention trials in the cervix: design, feasibility, and recruitment. *J Cell Biochem Suppl* 1995;23:104-112.

159. Manni A, Wright C: Polyamines as mediators of the effect of prolactin and growth hormone on the growth of N-nitroso-N-methylurea-induced rat mammary tumor cultured in vitro in soft agar. *J Natl Cancer Inst* 1985;74:941-944.

160. Malt RA, Kingsnorth AN, Lamuraglia GM, et al: Chemoprevention and chemotherapy by inhibition of ornithine decarboxylase activity and polyamine synthesis: colonic, pancreatic, mammary, and renal carcinomas. *Adv Enzyme Regul* 1985;24:93-102.

161. Manetta A, Satyaswarcoop PG, Podczaski ES, et al: Effect of alpha-difluoromethylornithine (DFMO) on the growth of human ovarian carcinoma. *Eur J Gynaecol Oncol* 1988;9:222-227.

162. Mitchell MF, Tortolero-Luna G, Lee JJ, et al: Polyamine measurements in the uterine cervix. *J Cell Biochem Suppl* 1997;28-29:125-132.

163. Mitchell MF, Tortolero-Luna G, Lee JJ, et al: Phase I dose de-escalation trial of alpha-difluoromethylornithine in patients with grade 3 cervical intraepithelial neoplasia. *Clin Cancer Res* 1998;4:303-310.

164. Papanicolaou GN, Traut HF: *Diagnosis of uterine cancer by the vaginal smear*, New York, The Commonwealth Fund, 1943.

165. Guzick DS: Efficacy of screening for cervical cancer: a review. *Am J Public Health* 1978;68:125-134.

166. Miller AB, Lindsay J, Hill GB: Mortality from cancer of the uterus in Canada and its relationship to screening for cancer of the cervix. *Int J Cancer* 1976;17:602-612.

167. Fidler HK, Boyes DA, Worth AJ: Cervical cancer detection in British Columbia: a progress report. *J Obstet Gynaecol Br Commonw* 1968;75:392-404.

168. Matsunaga G, Tsuji I, Sato S, et al: Cost-effective analysis of mass screening for cervical cancer in Japan. *J Epidemiol* 1997;7:135-141.

169. Wilbur DC, Prey MU, Miller WM, et al: Detection of high grade squamous intraepithelial lesions and tumors using the AutoPap System: results of a primary screening clinical trial. *Cancer* 1999;87:354-358.

170. Naryshkin S: The false-negative fraction for Papanicolaou smears: how often are "abnormal" smears not detected by a "standard" screening cytologist? *Arch Pathol Lab Med* 1997;121:270-272.

171. Lazcano-Ponce EC, Alonso de Ruiz P, Lopez-Carrillo L, et al: Validity and reproducibility of cytologic diagnosis in a sample of cervical cancer screening centers in Mexico. *Acta Cytol* 1997;41:277-284.

172. Martin-Hirsch P, Jarvis G, Kitchener H, et al: Collection devices for obtaining cervical cytology samples. *Cochrane Database Syst Rev* 2000;2: CD001036.

173. Davey DD: Quality and liability issues with the Papanicolaou smear: the problem of definition of errors and false-negative smears. *Arch Pathol Lab Med* 1997;121:267-269.

174. Kohlberger PD, Stani J, Gitsch G, et al: Comparative evaluation of seven cell collection devices for cervical smears. *Acta Cytol* 1999;43:1023-1026.

175. Kavak ZN, Eren F, Pekin S, et al: A randomized comparison of the 3 Papanicolaou smear collection methods. *Aust N Z J Obstet Gynaecol* 1995;35:446-449.

176. Toffler WL, Pluedeman CK, Sinclair AE, et al: Comparative cytologic yield and quality of three Pap smear instruments. *Fam Med* 1993;25: 403-407.

177. Martin D, Umpierre SA, Villamarzo G, et al: Comparison of the endocervical brush and the endocervical curettage for the evaluation of the endocervical canal. *P R Health Sci J* 1995;14: 195-197.

178. Harrison DD, Hernandez E, Dunton CJ: Endocervical brush versus cotton swab for obtaining cervical smears at a clinic: a cost comparison. *J Reprod Med* 1993;38:285-288.

179. Schoolland M, Sterrett GF, Knowles SA, et al: The "inconclusive–possible high grade epithelial abnormality" category in Papanicolaou smear reporting. *Cancer* 1998;84:208-217.

180. Randall B, van Amerongen L: Commercial laboratory practice evaluation of air-dried/rehydrated cervicovaginal smears vs. traditionally-fixed smears. *Diagn Cytopathol* 1997;16:174-176.

181. Frable WJ, Austin RM, Greening SE, et al: Medicolegal affairs. International Academy of Cytology Task Force summary, Diagnostic Cytology Towards the 21st Century: An International Expert Conference and Tutorial. *Acta Cytol* 1998;42:76-119; discussion 120-132.

182. Greening SE: Errors in cervical smears: minimizing the risk of medicolegal consequences. *Monogr Pathol* 1997;121:16-39.

183. Wilbur DC: False negatives in focused rescreening of Papanicolaou smears: how frequently are 'abnormal' cells detected in retrospective review of smears preceding cancer or high-grade intraepithelial neoplasia? *Arch Pathol Lab Med* 1997;121:273-276.

184. Jones BA: Rescreening in gynecologic cytology. Rescreening of 8096 previous cases for current low-grade and indeterminate-grade squamous intraepithelial lesion diagnoses: a College of American Pathologists Q-Probes study of 323 laboratories. *Arch Pathol Lab Med* 1996;120:519-522.

185. New system for reporting Pap smears. *Oncology (Huntingt)* 1989;3:65, 68.

186. The 1988 Bethesda System for Reporting Cervical/Vaginal Cytologic Diagnoses. Developed and approved at a National Cancer Institute Workshop, Bethesda, Maryland, U.S.A., December 12-13, 1988. *J Reprod Med* 1989; 34: 779-785.

187. Smigel K: The Bethesda System unveiled; revamps Pap smear reporting. *J Natl Cancer Inst* 1989;81:1354-1355.

188. Herbst AL: The Bethesda System for cervical/vaginal cytologic diagnoses: a note of caution. *Obstet Gynecol* 1990;76:449-450.

189. Bottles K, Reiter RC, Steiner AL, et al: Problems encountered with the Bethesda System: the University of Iowa experience. *Obstet Gynecol* 1991;78:410-414.

190. Herbst AL: Concerns regarding the Bethesda System. *Int J Gynecol Pathol* 1991;10:326-328.

191. Sherman ME, Schiffman MH, Erozan YS, et al: The Bethesda System: a proposal for reporting abnormal cervical smears based on the reproducibility of cytopathologic diagnoses. *Arch Pathol Lab Med* 1992;116:1155-1158.

192. Luff RD: The Bethesda System for reporting cervical/vaginal cytologic diagnoses: report of the 1991 Bethesda workshop. The Bethesda System Editorial Committee. *Hum Pathol* 1992;23:719-721.

193. The revised Bethesda System for reporting cervical/vaginal cytologic diagnoses: report of the 1991 Bethesda workshop. *Acta Cytol* 1992;36:273-276.

194. Ransdell JS, Davey DD, Zaleski S: Clinicopathologic correlation of the unsatisfactory Papanicolaou smear. *Cancer* 1997;81:139-143.

195. Ciatto S, Cariaggi MP, Minuti AP, et al: Interlaboratory reproducibility in reporting inadequate cervical smears: a multicentre multinational study. *Cytopathology* 1996;7:386-390.

196. Edelman M, Fox AS, Alderman EM, et al: Cervical Papanicolaou smear abnormalities in inner city Bronx adolescents: prevalence, progression, and immune modifiers. *Cancer* 1999;87:184-189.

197. Duggan MA, Brasher PM: Accuracy of Pap tests reported as CIN I. *Diagn Cytopathol* 1999;21:129-136.

198. Raab SS, Bishop NS, Zaleski MS: Long-term outcome and relative risk in women with atypical squamous cells of undetermined significance. *Am J Clin Pathol* 1999;112:57-62.

199. Mount SL, Papillo JL: A study of 10,296 pediatric and adolescent Papanicolaou smear diagnoses in northern New England. *Pediatrics* 1999;103:539-545.

200. Utagawa ML, Pereira SM, Cavaliere MJ, et al: Cervical intraepithelial neoplasia in adolescents: study of cytological findings between 1987 and 1995 in Sao Paulo State—Brazil. *Arch Gynecol Obstet* 1998;262:59-64.

201. Shlay JC, McGill WL, Masloboeva HA, et al: Pap smear screening in an urban STD clinic. Yield of screening and predictors of abnormalities. *Sex Transm Dis* 1998;25:468-475.

202. Lawson HW, Lee NC, Thames SF, et al: Cervical cancer screening among low-income women: results of a national screening program, 1991-1995. *Obstet Gynecol* 1998;92:745-752.

203. Mangan SA, Legano LA, Rosen CM, et al: Increased prevalence of abnormal Papanicolaou smears in urban adolescents. *Arch Pediatr Adolesc Med* 1997;151:481-484.

204. Davey DD, Woodhouse S, Styer P, et al: Atypical epithelial cells and specimen adequacy: current laboratory practices of participants in the college of American pathologists interlaboratory comparison program in cervicovaginal cytology. *Arch Pathol Lab Med* 2000;124:203-211.

205. Palcic B, Garner DM, MacAulay CE: Image cytometry and chemoprevention in cervical cancer. *J Cell Biochem Suppl* 1995;23:43-54.

206. Soofer SB, Sidawy MK: Atypical glandular cells of undetermined significance: clinically significant lesions and means of patient follow-up. *Cancer* 2000;90:207-214.

207. Chhieng DC, Elgert PA, Cangiarella JF, et al: Clinical significance of atypical glandular cells of undetermined significance: a follow-up study from an academic medical center. *Acta Cytol* 2000;44:557-566.

208. Manetta A, Keefe K, Lin F, et al: Atypical glandular cells of undetermined significance in cervical cytologic findings. *Am J Obstet Gynecol* 1999;180:883-888.

209. Weintraub J, Morabia A: Efficacy of a liquid-based thin layer method for cervical cancer screening in a population with a low incidence of cervical cancer. *Diagn Cytopathol* 2000;22:52-59.

210. Guidos BJ, Selvaggi SM: Use of the ThinPrep Pap Test in clinical practice. *Diagn Cytopathol* 1999;20:70-73.

211. Diaz-Rosario LA, Kabawat SE: Performance of a fluid-based, thin-layer Papanicolaou smear method in the clinical setting of an independent laboratory and an outpatient screening population in New England. *Arch Pathol Lab Med* 1999;123:817-821.

212. Selvaggi SM, Guidos BJ: Specimen adequacy and the ThinPrep Pap Test: the endocervical component. *Diagn Cytopathol* 2000;23:23-26.

213. Papillo JL, Zarka MA, St John TL: Evaluation of the ThinPrep Pap test in clinical practice: a seven-month, 16,314-case experience in northern Vermont. *Acta Cytol* 1998;42:203-208.

214. Ashfaq R, Gibbons D, Vela C, et al: ThinPrep Pap Test: accuracy for glandular disease. *Acta Cytol* 1999;43:81-85.

215. *Bethesda System 2001. 2001 Terminology.* National Cancer Institute. Available at: http://bethesda2001.cancer.gov/terminology.html.

216. Stoler MH: New Bethesda terminology and evidence-based management guidelines for cervical cytology findings. *JAMA* 2002;287:2140-2141.

217. Solomon D, Davey D, Kurman R, et al: The 2001 Bethesda System: terminology for reporting results of cervical cytology. *JAMA* 2002;287:2114-2119.

218. Wright TC Jr, Cox JT, Massad LS, et al: 2001 Consensus Guidelines for the management of women with cervical cytological abnormalities. *JAMA* 2002;287:2120-2129.

219. Kolstad P, Stafl A: *Atlas of colposcopy*, Baltimore, University Park Press, 1972.

220. Skehan M, Soutter WP, Lim K, et al: Reliability of colposcopy and directed punch biopsy. *Br J Obstet Gynaecol* 1990;97:811-816.

221. Reid R, Stanhope CR, Herschman BR, et al: Genital warts and cervical cancer, IV: a colpo-

scopic index for differentiating subclinical papillomaviral infection from cervical intraepithelial neoplasia. *Am J Obstet Gynecol* 1984;149:815-823.

222. Reid R, Scalzi P: Genital warts and cervical cancer, VII: an improved colposcopic index for differentiating benign papillomaviral infections from high-grade cervical intraepithelial neoplasia. *Am J Obstet Gynecol* 1985;153:611-618.

223. Williams DL, Dietrich C, McBroom J: Endocervical curettage when colposcopic examination is satisfactory and normal. *Obstet Gynecol* 2000;95:801-803.

224. Ferenczy A: Management of patients with high grade squamous intraepithelial lesions. *Cancer* 1995;76:1928-1933.

225. Bornstein J, Yaakov Z, Pascal B, et al: Decision-making in the colposcopy clinic: a critical analysis. *Eur J Obstet Gynecol Reprod Biol* 1999;85:219-224.

226. Hasskarl J, Butz K, Whitaker N, et al: Differential cell cycle response of nontumorigenic and tumorigenic human papillomavirus-positive keratinocytes towards transforming growth factor-beta₁. *J Mol Med* 2000;78:94-101.

227. zur Hausen H: Papillomaviruses causing cancer: evasion from host-cell control in early events in carcinogenesis. *J Natl Cancer Inst* 2000;92:690-698.

228. Walboomers JM, Jacobs MV, Manos MM, et al: Human papillomavirus is a necessary cause of invasive cervical cancer worldwide. *J Pathol* 1999;189:12-19.

229. Beutner KR, Tyring S: Human papillomavirus and human disease. *Am J Med* 1997;102:9-15.

230. Human papillomavirus testing for triage of women with cytologic evidence of low-grade squamous intraepithelial lesions: baseline data from a randomized trial, the Atypical Squamous Cells of Undetermined Significance/Low-Grade Squamous Intraepithelial Lesions Triage Study (ALTS) Group. *J Natl Cancer Inst* 2000;92:397-402.

231. Mould TA, Singer A, Gallivan S: Quantitative detection of oncogenic HPV DNA using hybrid capture to triage borderline and mildly dyskaryotic Papanicolaou smears. *Eur J Gynaecol Oncol* 2000;21:245-248.

232. Kubota T, Ishi K, Suzuki M, et al: Usefulness of hybrid capture HPV DNA assay as a diagnostic tool for human papillomavirus infection. *Kansenshogaku Zasshi* 1998;72:1219-1224.

233. Cope JU, Hildesheim A, Schiffman MH, et al: Comparison of the hybrid capture tube test and PCR for detection of human papillomavirus DNA in cervical specimens. *J Clin Microbiol* 1997;35:2262-2265.

234. Sasagawa T, Minemoto Y, Basha W, et al: A new PCR-based assay amplifies the E6-E7 genes of most mucosal human papillomaviruses (HPV). *Virus Res* 2000;67:127-139.

235. Cavalcanti SM, Zardo LG, Passos MR, et al: Epidemiological aspects of human papillo-

mavirus infection and cervical cancer in Brazil. *J Infect* 2000;40:80-87.

236. Manos MM, Kinney WK, Hurley LB, et al: Identifying women with cervical neoplasia: using human papillomavirus DNA testing for equivocal Papanicolaou results. *JAMA* 1999;281:1605-1610.

237. Tortolero-Luna G, Mitchell MF, Swan DC, et al: A case-control study of human papillomavirus and cervical squamous intraepithelial lesions (SIL) in Harris County, Texas: differences among racial/ethnic groups. *Cad Saude Publica* 1998;14:149-159.

238. Nindl I, Zahm DM, Meijer CJ, et al: Human papillomavirus detection in high-grade squamous intraepithelial lesions: comparison of hybrid capture assay with a polymerase chain reaction system. *Diagn Microbiol Infect Dis* 1995;23:161-164.

239. Solomon D, Schiffman M, Tarone R: Comparison of three management strategies for patients with atypical squamous cells of undetermined significance: baseline results from a randomized trial. *J Natl Cancer Inst* 2001;93:293-299.

240. Schiffman M, Adrianza ME: ASCUS-LSIL Triage Study: design, methods and characteristics of trial participants. *Acta Cytol* 2000;44:726-742.

241. Keating JT, Wang HH: Significance of a diagnosis of atypical squamous cells of undetermined significance for Papanicolaou smears in perimenopausal and postmenopausal women. *Cancer* 2001;93:100-105.

242. Arora CD, Schmidt DS, Rader AE, et al: Adolescents with ASCUS: are they a high risk group? *Clin Pediatr (Phila)* 2001;40:133-138.

243. Anton RC, Ramzy I, Schwartz MR, et al: Should the cytologic diagnosis of "atypical squamous cells of undetermined significance" be qualified?: an assessment including comparison between conventional and liquid-based technologies. *Cancer* 2001;93:93-99.

244. Crum CP, Genest DR, Krane JF, et al: Subclassifying atypical squamous cells in Thin-Prep cervical cytology correlates with detection of high-risk human papillomavirus DNA. *Am J Clin Pathol* 1999;112:384-390.

245. Ferenczy A, Franco E, Arseneau J, et al: Diagnostic performance of Hybrid Capture human papillomavirus deoxyribonucleic acid assay combined with liquid-based cytologic study. *Am J Obstet Gynecol* 1996;175:651-656.

246. Ostor AG: Natural history of cervical intraepithelial neoplasia: a critical review. *Int J Gynecol Pathol* 1993;12:186-192.

247. Holowaty P, Miller AB, Rohan T, et al: Natural history of dysplasia of the uterine cervix. *J Natl Cancer Inst* 1999;91:252-258.

248. Mitchell H, Medley G, Carlin JB: Risk of subsequent cytological abnormality and cancer among women with a history of cervical intraepithelial neoplasia: a comparative study. *Cancer Causes Control* 1990;1:143-148.

249. Wright TC, Sun XW, Koulos J: Comparison of management algorithms for the evaluation of

women with low-grade cytologic abnormalities. *Obstet Gynecol* 1995;85:202-210.

250. Kataja V, Syrjanen S, Mantyjarvi R, et al: Prognostic factors in cervical human papillomavirus infections. *Sex Transm Dis* 1992;19:154-160.

251. Lee SS, Collins RJ, Pun TC, et al: Conservative treatment of low grade squamous intraepithelial lesions (LSIL) of the cervix. *Int J Gynaecol Obstet* 1998;60:35-40.

252. Bergeron C, Debaque H, Ayivi J, et al: Cervical smear histories of 585 women with biopsy-proven carcinoma in situ. *Acta Cytol* 1997;41:1676-1680.

253. Cubie HA, Seagar AL, Beattie GJ, et al: A longitudinal study of HPV detection and cervical pathology in HIV infected women. *Sex Transm Infect* 2000;76:257-261.

254. Goodman A, Chaudhuri PM, Tobin-Enos NJ, et al: The false negative rate of cervical smears in high risk HIV seropositive and seronegative women. *Int J Gynecol Cancer* 2000;10:27-32.

255. Holcomb K, Abulafia O, Matthews RP, et al: The significance of ASCUS cytology in HIV-positive women. *Gynecol Oncol* 1999;75:118-121.

256. Buehler JW, Ward JW: A new definition for AIDS surveillance. *Ann Intern Med* 1993;118:390-392.

257. Cardillo M, Hagan R, Abadi J, et al: CD4 T-cell count, viral load, and squamous intraepithelial lesions in women infected with the human immunodeficiency virus. *Cancer* 2001;93:111-114.

258. Davis AT, Chakraborty H, Flowers L, et al: Cervical dysplasia in women infected with the human immunodeficiency virus (HIV): a correlation with HIV viral load and CD4+ count. *Gynecol Oncol* 2001;80:350-354.

259. Dorrucci M, Suligoi B, Serraino D, et al: Incidence of invasive cervical cancer in a cohort of HIV-seropositive women before and after the introduction of highly active antiretroviral therapy. *J Acquir Immune Defic Syndr* 2001;26:377-380.

260. Falls RK: Spontaneous resolution rate of grade 1 cervical intraepithelial neoplasia in a private practice population. *Am J Obstet Gynecol* 1999;181:278-282.

261. Martin-Hirsch PL, Paraskevaidis E, Kitchener H: Surgery for cervical intraepithelial neoplasia. *Cochrane Database Syst Rev* 2000;2:CD001318.

262. Richart RM, Townsend DE, Crisp W, et al: An analysis of "long-term" follow-up results in patients with cervical intraepithelial neoplasia treated by cryotherapy. *Am J Obstet Gynecol* 1980;137:823-826.

263. Benedet JL, Miller DM, Nickerson KG, et al: The results of cryosurgical treatment of cervical intraepithelial neoplasia at one, five, and ten years. *Am J Obstet Gynecol* 1987;157:268-273.

264. Ostergard DR: Cryosurgical treatment of cervical intraepithelial neoplasia. *Obstet Gynecol* 1980;56:231-233.

265. Townsend DE: Cryosurgery for CIN. *Obstet Gynecol Surv* 1979;34:828.

266. Rojas I, Rodriguez T, Pierotic M, et al: [Histological evaluation of cryosurgery in high grade intraepithelial neoplasia (CIN-III)] of the uterine cervix]. *Rev Chil Obstet Ginecol* 1993;58:200-204; discussion 204-205.

267. Anderson MC, Hartley RB: Cervical crypt involvement by intraepithelial neoplasia. *Obstet Gynecol* 1980;55:546-550.

268. Kuppers V, Degen KW, Dominik S, et al: [The advantages of CO_2 laser use in treatment of cervix dysplasia]. *Geburtshilfe Frauenheilkd* 1994;54:401-405.

269. Gunasekera PC, Phipps JH, Lewis BV: Large loop excision of the transformation zone (LLETZ) compared to carbon dioxide laser in the treatment of CIN: a superior mode of treatment. *Br J Obstet Gynaecol* 1990;97:995-998.

270. Benedet JL, Miller DM, Nickerson KG: Results of conservative management of cervical intraepithelial neoplasia. *Obstet Gynecol* 1992;79:105-110.

271. Prendiville W, Cullimore J, Norman S: Large loop excision of the transformation zone (LLETZ): a new method of management for women with cervical intraepithelial neoplasia. *Br J Obstet Gynaecol* 1989;96:1054-1060.

272. Bigrigg MA, Codling BW, Pearson P, et al: Colposcopic diagnosis and treatment of cervical dysplasia at a single clinic visit: experience of low-voltage diathermy loop in 1000 patients. *Lancet* 1990;336:229-231.

273. Fung HY, Cheung LP, Rogers MS, et al: The treatment of cervical intra-epithelial neoplasia: when could we 'see and loop.' *Eur J Obstet Gynecol Reprod Biol* 1997;72:199-204.

274. Turlington WT, Wright BD, Powell JL: Impact of the loop electrosurgical excision procedure on future fertility. *J Reprod Med* 1996;41:815-818.

275. Bigrigg A, Haffenden DK, Sheehan AL, et al: Efficacy and safety of large-loop excision of the transformation zone. *Lancet* 1994;343:32-34.

276. Hallam NF, West J, Harper C, et al: Large loop excision of the transformation zone (LLETZ) as an alternative to both local ablative and cone biopsy treatment: a series of 1000 patients. *J Gynecol Surg* 1993;9:77-82.

277. Cruickshank ME, Flannelly G, Campbell DM, et al: Fertility and pregnancy outcome following large loop excision of the cervical transformation zone. *Br J Obstet Gynaecol* 1995;102:467-470.

278. Hillemanns P, Kimmig R, Dannecker C, et al: [LEEP versus cold knife conization for treatment of cervical intraepithelial neoplasias]. *Zentralbl Gynakol* 2000;122:35-42.

279. Giacalone PL, Laffargue F, Aligier N, et al: Randomized study comparing two techniques of conization: cold knife versus loop excision. *Gynecol Oncol* 1999;75:356-360.

280. Takac I, Gorisek B: Cold knife conization and loop excision for cervical intraepithelial neoplasia. *Tumori* 1999;85:243-246.

281. Huang LW, Hwang JL: A comparison between loop electrosurgical excision procedure and cold knife conization for treatment of cervical dyspla-

sia: residual disease in a subsequent hysterectomy specimen. *Gynecol Oncol* 1999;73:12-15.

282. Duggan BD, Felix JC, Muderspach LI, et al: Cold-knife conization versus conization by the loop electrosurgical excision procedure: a randomized, prospective study. *Am J Obstet Gynecol* 1999; 180:276-282.

283. Kim YT, Kim JW, Kim DK, et al: Loop diathermy and cold-knife conization in patients with cervical intraepithelial neoplasia: a comparative study. *J Korean Med Sci* 1995;10:281-286.

284. Girardi F, Heydarfadai M, Koroschetz F, et al: Cold-knife conization versus loop excision: histopathologic and clinical results of a randomized trial. *Gynecol Oncol* 1994;55:368-370.

285. Naumann RW, Bell MC, Alvarez RD, et al: LLETZ is an acceptable alternative to diagnostic cold-knife conization. *Gynecol Oncol* 1994;55:224-228.

286. Reich O, Pickel H, Lahousen M, et al: Cervical intraepithelial neoplasia III: long-term outcome after cold-knife conization with clear margins. *Obstet Gynecol* 2001;97:428-430.

287. Mitchell MF, Tortolero-Luna G, Cook E, et al: A randomized clinical trial of cryotherapy, laser vaporization, and loop electrosurgical excision for treatment of squamous intraepithelial lesions of the cervix. *Obstet Gynecol* 1998;92:737-744.

288. Williams FS, Roure RM, Till M, et al: Treatment of cervical carcinoma in situ in HIV positive women. *Int J Gynaecol Obstet* 2000;71:135-139.

289. Armbruster-Moraes E, Ioshimoto LM, Leao E, et al: Prevalence of 'high risk' human papillomavirus in the lower genital tract of Brazilian gravidas. *Int J Gynaecol Obstet* 2000;69:223-227.

290. Palle C, Bangsboll S, Andreasson B: Cervical intraepithelial neoplasia in pregnancy. *Acta Obstet Gynecol Scand* 2000;79:306-310.

291. Mitsuhashi A, Sekiya S: Loop electrosurgical excision procedure (LEEP) during first trimester of pregnancy. *Int J Gynaecol Obstet* 2000;71: 237-239.

292. Woodrow N, Permezel M, Butterfield L, et al: Abnormal cervical cytology in pregnancy: experience of 811 cases. *Aust N Z J Obstet Gynaecol* 1998;38:161-165.

293. Yost NP, Santoso JT, McIntire DD, et al: Postpartum regression rates of antepartum cervical intraepithelial neoplasia II and III lesions. *Obstet Gynecol* 1999;93:359-362.

294. Chhieng DC, Elgert P, Cangiarella JF, et al: Significance of AGUS Pap smears in pregnant and postpartum women. *Acta Cytol* 2001;45:294-299.

CHAPTER 7

Cancer of the Vagina

Alberto Manetta

INCIDENCE

The continuity of tissues between the vagina and the cervix makes the true incidence of vaginal cancer difficult to determine. The reported incidence is very low. Between 1985 and 1994, 4885 vaginal cancers were reported.[1] Twenty-one hundred cases were reported by the American Cancer Society for the year 2001; however, this number also included some other rare tumors difficult to classify in other categories.[2] By convention and according to FIGO (International Federation of Gynecology and Obstetrics), all invasive carcinomas involving the cervix and the vagina are classified as cervical.[3] In addition, the vagina is a common site of recurrence and metastatic disease from the cervix and endometrium, thus making the certainty of the primary site even more difficult. Most of the reported series indicate a vaginal cancer incidence of approximately 1% to 2% among all gynecologic cancers.[4,5] Although there are no firm data from sources outside the United States, it must be assumed that the incidence of this cancer in developing countries must be significantly higher than in the United States.

As in the cervix, the most common histologic type of vaginal cancer is the squamous or epidermoid variety, which represents approximately 95% of all vaginal malignancies. However, the vagina may also be the site of other histologic types of cancer, such as adenocarcinoma, melanoma, and sarcoma.[6]

The incidence of vaginal cancer is related to the incidence of cervical cancer.[7] This is expected because most vaginal cancers are also related to human papillomavirus (HPV). Eighty-five percent of the vaginal cancer precursor, vaginal intraepithelial neoplasia (VAIN), is associated with HPV.[8] A well-defined precancerous lesion or VAIN exists and is similar to what is found in cervical cancer. Histologically, VAIN is graded in a manner similar to that of the cervix and vulva and is divided into categories I, II, and III according to the severity of the lesion.

VAIN III is also called "carcinoma in situ" (CIS); VAIN I is mild and VAIN II is moderate.

Although invasive vaginal cancer most often occurs in older women in their 60s,[9,10] VAIN occurs earlier—from the late 20s to age 50.[11]

Similar to carcinoma of the cervix, cancer of the vagina is clinically staged. Table 7-1 contains the FIGO nomenclature in the staging of vaginal cancer.[12]

RISK FACTORS

Because of the lower incidence of vaginal cancer, in contrast to cervical cancer, it is more difficult to determine risk factors. However, HPV has been consistently identified in vaginal cancers and VAIN.[13,14] Women infected with the highly oncogenic HPV types are at higher risk for this malignancy.[15] Although not proved inconclusively with large epidemiologic studies, the risk factors for cervical and vaginal cancer are very similar and are typically related to expo-

Table 7-1
Carcinoma of the Vagina

Stage 0	Carcinoma in situ: intraepithelial neoplasia grade III (VAIN III)
Stage I	The carcinoma is limited to the vaginal wall
Stage II	The carcinoma has involved the subvaginal tissue but has not extended to the pelvic wall
Stage III	The carcinoma has extended to the pelvic wall
Stage IV	The carcinoma has extended beyond the true pelvis or has involved the mucosa of the bladder or rectum; bullous edema as such does not permit a case to be allotted to Stage IV
Stage IVA	Tumor invades bladder and/or rectal mucosa and/or direct extension beyond the true pelvis
Stage IVB	Spread to distant organs

Source: Benedet JL, Bender H, Jones H III, et al: FIGO staging classifications and clinical practice guidelines in the management of gynecologic cancers. FIGO Committee on Gynecologic Oncology. *Int J Gynaecol Obstet* 2000;70(2):209-262.

sure to HPV infections. The greatest risk factor for vaginal cancer is a previous carcinoma of the cervix or vulva, which further indicates a common cause.[6] Reporting on a series of 121 patients with VAIN, Dodge and associates found that 22% have had surgery for cervical intraepithelial neoplasia (CIN) and that 22% have had a hysterectomy.[11]

Other etiologic factors have been suggested, especially related to the chronic trauma to the vagina caused by pessaries. These studies were done long ago, without the ability to control other factors, including HPV infections.[16] There is no association between previous hysterectomy and vaginal cancer once the population is controlled for age and cervical disease.[17]

Although vaginal cancer is usually found in older women, a larger number of adenocarcinomas were diagnosed in very young women in the 1960s. These cancers histologically were adenocarcinomas, tumors rarely diagnosed in the vagina until then. Specifically these were mesonephric-like malignant tumors identified as clear cell adenocarcinomas (CCA). The first six cases of CCA were reported in 1970.[18]

In 1971 Herbst and associates described the association between intrauterine exposure to diethylstilbestrol (DES) and clear cell adenocarcinoma (CCA) of the vagina.[19] DES, a nonsteroidal synthetic estrogen, was used for the prevention of spontaneous abortion in the 1940s and 1950s. Based on the Registry for Research on Hormonal Transplacental Carcinogenesis begun by Arthur Herbst at the University of Chicago, a review done in 1987 identified 519 cases of CCA of the vagina or cervix. In 60% of these cases ingestion of DES by the patient's mother was confirmed. It is estimated that the risk of developing CCA from birth through age 34 among DES-exposed women is 1 per 1000.[19,20] The median age at diagnosis of CCA was 19.0 years. Women whose mothers were exposed to DES before the twelfth week of pregnancy were at higher risk.[21] To date, it has not been proved that daughters of DES-exposed women are at risk for any malignancy other than CCA.[22]

The possible postnatal effect of other synthetic estrogen, specifically oral contraceptives, in patients exposed in utero to DES was evaluated. In an analysis of 244 cases compared with 244 age-matched DES-exposed women, Palmer and associates were not able to find an increase in risk for CCA of the vagina among patients taking oral contraceptives.[23] It was also suggested that ionizing radiation might be an etiologic factor for vaginal cancer.[24,25] However, other studies have not confirmed this relationship.[26]

PREVENTION

As with carcinoma of the cervix, changes in sexual behavior that decrease exposure to the HPV will lead to a decrease in the incidence of vaginal carcinoma. Given the common HPV-related cause, vaginal cancer may be amenable to preventive techniques using prophylactic HPV vaccines (see Chapter 6).

Screening

The Papanicolaou (Pap) test is an effective method for the diagnosis of premalignant and malignant lesions of the vagina. The sensitivity of the Pap test in detecting VAIN in patients with previous hysterectomy is 83%.[27]

Most published series have reported that 30% to 50% of vaginal cancers are found in women who underwent hysterectomy[4,28-30] The reasons follow:

1. Most vaginal cancers occur in older women.
2. Hysterectomy is a very common surgical procedure.
3. By convention, if the cervix is involved, the malignancy will be labeled cervical in origin.

The screening of women for vaginal cancer after a hysterectomy for benign conditions has been a subject of controversy. In contrast, the consensus is that women who have had hysterectomy because of dysplastic or malignant lesions of the cervix should continue to be screened yearly. Pearce and associates reported on 9610 smears taken from women who had a hysterectomy because of benign gynecologic conditions. One hundred four of these were found to be abnormal—two with invasive cancers and six with high-grade lesions. The remainder had minor Pap smear abnormalities. Overall the possibility of patients in this group of having an abnormal Pap smear was found to be 1.1%.[31] After an extensive review of the literature, Fetters concluded that there is insufficient evidence to recommend routine vaginal smear screening for women after total hysterectomy for benign disease.[32] Other authors have arrived at similar conclusions.[33,34] However, several reports have documented cases of invasive or preinvasive vaginal cancer in patients after hysterectomy for benign conditions.[28,29,35]

The Pap smear has an appropriate sensitivity for use as a screening tool for vaginal cancer in women with previous hysterectomies. Nevertheless, because of the low incidence of this malignancy and the low prevalence of Pap smear abnormalities, it is most likely not cost-effective to do this test yearly with patients who underwent hysterectomy for benign conditions. There are no clear guidelines on how often, if any, Pap smears should be done in this population. In contrast, patients who have had hysterectomy for intraepithelial or invasive malignancies of the cervix should be examined and undergo a Pap test annually.

Daughters of women exposed to DES should be carefully examined and have Pap smears performed yearly. Four-quadrant techniques obtaining a sample of each vaginal wall are preferred in DES-exposed women. As discussed previously, these are malignancies of very young women. Because the use of DES was discontinued in the 1950s, it is unlikely that many cases of young women exposed to intrauterine DES will be seen. Nevertheless—and because the natural behavior of this condition in older women is not completely understood—patients ought be followed yearly with appropriate pelvic examinations and cytology. Because most of these tumors arise in the upper vagina, visual and digital inspection of this area is critical. A biopsy should be performed on any suspicious lesions. A large percentage of these patients will have adenosis, which is the presence of nonneoplastic endocervical epithelium, primarily in the upper vagina. There is no evidence in the literature to support the treatment of adenosis.

Management of Vaginal Intraepithelial Neoplasia

Prevention of vaginal cancer includes the appropriate diagnosis and treatment of the premalignant lesion or VAIN. Patients with abnormal Pap smears should have, in addition to a careful assessment of the cervix and the vulva, a thorough inspection of the vagina. Synchronous dysplastic lesions of the cervix, vulva, and the vagina are not uncommon. As in the cervix, dysplastic lesions of the vagina turn white in the presence of 4% acetic acid. Any suspicious lesions should be carefully examined with the colposcope, and a biopsy should be performed. Occasionally the abnormality may be in the vagina only, with the cervix being completely normal. Any woman who has an abnormal Pap smear that cannot be explained by the presence of a cervical lesion should have a colposcopic assessment of the vagina.

VAIN is primarily found in the upper vagina, but it is very often a multifocal disease.[36-38] In fact, more than 50% of VAIN cases will present as a multifocal disease.[39] As a result, careful examination of the entire vagina cannot be overemphasized.

Because there is no clear consensus as to what constitutes the best treatment for this condition, the treatment must be individualized.

As in the treatment of CIN, VAIN may be treated using excisional or ablative techniques.

The role of surgery in the treatment of VAIN is rather limited for patients with widespread disease who are sexually active. Large vaginal excisions may lead to sexual dysfunction. The use of skin grafts to replace the vaginal mucosa adds significant morbidity to the procedure and is not favored by most surgeons. In contrast, small lesions or lesions confined to the vaginal apex may be treated with wide local excision or upper vaginectomy. The main advantage of this approach is the availability of a specimen that allows the surgeon to categorically exclude the possibility of invasion. Some have recommended against ablative techniques for VAIN III because of the possibility of missing a focus of invasion.[40] Excisional treatment has been reported to be associated with cure rates of 69%.[36] However, "cure rates" vary widely depending on the population and the duration of follow-up.[41]

CO_2 laser vaporization is a common ablative modality of treatment for VAIN. The treatment is well localized, with little damage to surrounding tissues. Laser ablation is well tolerated and few complications have been reported.[42-45]

One of the advantages of this modality is the ability to treat large lesions without significantly harming sexual function.[46,47] One of the shortcomings of laser therapy is that lesions must be well exposed to apply the laser beam. Areas in the vaginal apex adjacent to or in the surgical scar formed after a hysterectomy may be difficult to expose and may go untreated.[48] The use of submucosal injections of saline, skin hooks, and small dental mirrors can prevent some of these obstacles.[49] Twenty percent to 25% of patients will require more than one laser treatment.[47]

Topical 5-fluorouracil (5-FU) is well suited for effectively treating widespread VAIN. As with any other ablative modality, the presence of invasive cancer is first ruled out. Then 5-FU is used as a 5% ointment. Various schedules have been proposed. One of the recommended schedules is a daily application of 1 g of 5% cream inserted in the vagina nightly to for 1 week; this is to be repeated after a 2-week rest. Another schedule involves the weekly application of a 1.5 g of 5-FU for 10 weeks. Both schedules have been shown to be equally effective.[50] Leakage of the cream and the subsequent skin irritation of the vulva is the most common complication. The skin of the vulva and perineum should be protected with petrolatum or zinc oxide to minimize the possibility of this complication.

Radiation therapy has occasionally been used in the management of VAIN in postmenopausal patients. This rarely used treatment is an alternative to vaginectomy.

Radiotherapy is usually delivered as brachytherapy. More recently, the use of high-dose-rate delivery systems has made these treatments more convenient for the patients. Nevertheless this is a last resort type of treatment.[51,52] Table 7-2 shows the treatment of VAIN according to clinical presentation.[53]

Table 7-2
Treatment of Vaginal Intraepithelial Neoplasia (VAIN)

	Clinical Presentation	Treatment
1	Single lesion	Wide local excision or laser
2	Several lesions in upper vagina	Upper vaginectomy or laser
3	Widespread lesions beyond upper vagina	5% fluorouracil cream or laser
4	Extreme circumstances, repeated failure after other treatments in young patients	Total vaginectomy with split-skin graft
5	Extreme circumstances, repeated failure after other treatments in postmenopausal, sexually inactive patients	Radiation therapy or total vaginectomy

REFERENCES

1. Creasman WT, Phillips JL, Menck HR: The National Cancer Data Base report on cancer of the vagina. *Cancer* 1998;83:1033-1040.
2. American Cancer Society: *Cancer facts & figures 2001*. Atlanta, American Cancer Society, 2001.
3. Benedet JL, Bender H, Jones H III, et al: FIGO staging classifications and clinical practice guidelines in the management of gynecologic cancers, FIGO Committee on Gynecologic Oncology. *Int J Gynaecol Obstet* 2000;70:209-262.
4. Manetta A, Pinto JL, Larson JE, et al: Primary invasive carcinoma of the vagina. *Obstet Gynecol* 1988;72:77-81.
5. Gallup DG, Talledo OE, Shah KJ, et al: Invasive squamous cell carcinoma of the vagina: a 14-year study. *Obstet Gynecol* 1987;69:782-785.
6. Cotran RS, Kumar V, Collins T, et al: *Robbins pathologic basis of disease*, Philadelphia, WB Saunders, 1999.
7. Senkus E, Konefka T, Nowaczyk M, et al: Second lower genital tract squamous cell carcinoma following cervical cancer: a clinical study of 46 patients. *Acta Obstet Gynecol Scand* 2000;79:765-770.
8. Minucci D, Cinel A, Insacco E, et al: Epidemiological aspects of vaginal intraepithelial neoplasia (VAIN). *Clin Exp Obstet Gynecol* 1995;22:36-42.
9. Tewari KS, Cappuccini F, Puthawala AA, et al: Primary invasive carcinoma of the vagina: treat-

ment with interstitial brachytherapy. *Cancer* 2001;91:758-770.
10. Bouma J, Burger MP, Krans M, et al: Squamous cell carcinoma of the vagina: a report of 32 cases. *Int J Gynecol Cancer* 1994;4:389-394.
11. Dodge JA, Eltabbakh GH, Mount SL, et al: Clinical features and risk of recurrence among patients with vaginal intraepithelial neoplasia. *Gynecol Oncol* 2001;83:363-369.
12. Shepherd JH, Sideri M, Benedet JL, et al: *FIGO Staging of Gynecologic Cancer: Carcinoma of the vagina*, The International Federation of Gynecology and Obstetrics (FIGO). Available at: *http://www.figo.org*.
13. van Beurden M, ten Kate FW, Tjong AHSP, et al: Human papillomavirus DNA in multicentric vulvar intraepithelial neoplasia. *Int J Gynecol Pathol* 1998;17:12-16.
14. Merino MJ: Vaginal cancer: the role of infectious and environmental factors. *Am J Obstet Gynecol* 1991;165:1255-1262.
15. Bjorge T, Dillner J, Anttila T, et al: Prospective seroepidemiological study of role of human papillomavirus in non-cervical anogenital cancers. *BMJ* 1997;315:646-649.
16. Rutledge F: Cancer of the vagina. *Am J Obstet Gynecol* 1967;97:635-655.
17. Herman JM, Homesley HD, Dignan MB: Is hysterectomy a risk factor for vaginal cancer? *JAMA* 1986;256:601-603.

18. Herbst AL, Scully RE: Adenocarcinoma of the vagina in adolescence: a report of 7 cases including 6 clear-cell carcinomas (so-called mesonephromas). *Cancer* 1970;25:745-757.

19. Herbst AL, Ulfelder H, Poskanzer DC: Adenocarcinoma of the vagina: association of maternal stilbestrol therapy with tumor appearance in young women. *N Engl J Med* 1971;284:878-881.

20. Melnick S, Cole P, Anderson D, et al: Rates and risks of diethylstilbestrol-related clear-cell adenocarcinoma of the vagina and cervix: an update. *N Engl J Med* 1987;316:514-516.

21. Herbst AL, Anderson S, Hubby MM, et al: Risk factors for the development of diethylstilbestrol-associated clear cell adenocarcinoma: a case-control study. *Am J Obstet Gynecol* 1986;154:814-822.

22. Hatch EE, Palmer JR, Titus-Ernstoff L, et al: Cancer risk in women exposed to diethylstilbestrol in utero. *JAMA* 1998;280:630-634.

23. Palmer JR, Anderson D, Helmrich SP, et al: Risk factors for diethylstilbestrol-associated clear cell adenocarcinoma. *Obstet Gynecol* 2000;95:814-820.

24. Pride GL, Schultz AE, Chuprevich TW, et al: Primary invasive squamous carcinoma of the vagina. *Obstet Gynecol* 1979;53:218-225.

25. Boice JD Jr, Engholm G, Kleinerman RA, et al: Radiation dose and second cancer risk in patients treated for cancer of the cervix. *Radiat Res* 1988;116:3-55.

26. Lee JY, Perez CA, Ettinger N, et al: The risk of second primaries subsequent to irradiation for cervix cancer. *Int J Radiat Oncol Biol Phys* 1982;8:207-211.

27. Davila RM, Miranda MC: Vaginal intraepithelial neoplasia and the Pap smear. *Acta Cytol* 2000;44:137-140.

28. Bell J, Sevin BU, Averette H, et al: Vaginal cancer after hysterectomy for benign disease: value of cytologic screening. *Obstet Gynecol* 1984;64:699-702.

29. Benedet JL, Murphy KJ, Fairey RN, et al: Primary invasive carcinoma of the vagina. *Obstet Gynecol* 1983;62:715-719.

30. Manetta A, Gutrecht EL, Berman ML, et al: Primary invasive carcinoma of the vagina. *Obstet Gynecol* 1990;76:639-642.

31. Pearce KF, Haefner HK, Sarwar SF, et al: Cytopathological findings on vaginal Papanicolaou smears after hysterectomy for benign gynecologic disease. *N Engl J Med* 1996;335:1559-1562.

32. Fetters MD, Fischer G, Reed BD: Effectiveness of vaginal Papanicolaou smear screening after total hysterectomy for benign disease. *JAMA* 1996;275:940-947.

33. Piscitelli JT, Bastian LA, Wilkes A, et al: Cytologic screening after hysterectomy for benign disease. *Am J Obstet Gynecol* 1995;173:424-430; discussion 430-422.

34. Miller JM, Chambers DC: The need for Pap tests after hysterectomy for benign disease: results of a study of black patients. *Postgrad Med* 1987;82: 200-202, 205.

35. Ruiz-Moreno JA, Garcia-Gomez R, Vargas-Solano A, et al: Vaginal intraepithelial neoplasia: report of 14 cases. *Int J Gynaecol Obstet* 1987;25: 359-362.

36. Rome RM, England PG: Management of vaginal intraepithelial neoplasia: a series of 132 cases with long-term follow-up. *Int J Gynecol Cancer* 2000; 10:382-390.

37. Audet-Lapointe P, Body G, Vauclair R, et al: Vaginal intraepithelial neoplasia. *Gynecol Oncol* 1990; 36:232-239.

38. Kalogirou D, Antoniou G, Karakitsos P, et al: Vaginal intraepithelial neoplasia (VAIN) following hysterectomy in patients treated for carcinoma in situ of the cervix. *Eur J Gynaecol Oncol* 1997; 18:188-191.

39. Aho M, Vesterinen E, Meyer B, et al: Natural history of vaginal intraepithelial neoplasia. *Cancer* 1991;68:195-197.

40. Cheng D, Ng TY, Ngan HY, et al: Wide local excision (WLE) for vaginal intraepithelial neoplasia (VAIN). *Acta Obstet Gynecol Scand* 1999;78: 648-652.

41. Curtis P, Shepherd JH, Lowe DG, et al: The role of partial colpectomy in the management of persistent vaginal neoplasia after primary treatment. *Br J Obstet Gynaecol* 1992;99:587-589.

42. Townsend DE, Levine RU, Crum CP, et al: Treatment of vaginal carcinoma in situ with the carbon dioxide laser. *Am J Obstet Gynecol* 1982;143:565-568.

43. Capen CV, Masterson BJ, Magrina JF, et al: Laser therapy of vaginal intraepithelial neoplasia. *Am J Obstet Gynecol* 1982;142:973-976.

44. Curtin JP, Twiggs LB, Julian TM: Treatment of vaginal intraepithelial neoplasia with the CO_2 laser. *J Reprod Med* 1985;30:942-944.

45. Jobson VW, Campion MJ: Vaginal laser surgery. *Obstet Gynecol Clin North Am* 1991;18:511-524.

46. Sopracordevole F, Parin A, Scarabelli C, et al: [Laser surgery in the conservative management of vaginal intraepithelial neoplasms]. *Minerva Ginecol* 1998;50:507-512.

47. Campagnutta E, Parin A, De Piero G, et al: Treatment of vaginal intraepithelial neoplasia (VAIN) with the carbon dioxide laser. *Clin Exp Obstet Gynecol* 1999;26:127-130.

48. Hoffman MS, Roberts WS, LaPolla JP, et al: Laser vaporization of grade 3 vaginal intraepithelial neoplasia. *Am J Obstet Gynecol* 1991;165: 1342-1344.

49. Sherman AI: Laser therapy for vaginal intraepithelial neoplasia after hysterectomy. *J Reprod Med* 1990;35:941-944.

50. Krebs HB: Treatment of vaginal intraepithelial neoplasia with laser and topical 5-fluorouracil. *Obstet Gynecol* 1989;73:657-660.

51. MacLeod C, Fowler A, Dalrymple C, et al: High-dose-rate brachytherapy in the management of high-grade intraepithelial neoplasia of the vagina. *Gynecol Oncol* 1997;65:74-77.

52. Ogino I, Kitamura T, Okajima H, et al: High-dose-rate intracavitary brachytherapy in the management of cervical and vaginal intraepithelial neoplasia. *Int J Radiat Oncol Biol Phys* 1998;40: 881-887.

53. National Cancer Institute: *Vaginal cancer (PDQ): Treatment.* National Cancer Institute. January, 2002. Available at: *http://www.cancer.gov/cancer_information/*

Cancer of the Vulva

Krishnansu Sujata Tewari

INTRODUCTION

In 1769, John Baptist Morgagni first described vulvar cancer in *The Seats and Causes of Diseases Investigated by Anatomy*.[1] He stated that he had "seen many cancers of the genital parts of women, but as yet I have never had any opportunity of dissecting them." A depiction of vulvar anatomy appears in Figure 8-1. Previously, lack of vulvar hygiene; the accidental application of toxic substances, including arsenic compounds given for vulvar pruritus; and bituminous oils and dyes found in cotton spinning areas and dye works had been implicated as etiologic agents. In recent decades, however, infection by oncogenic strains of the human papillomavirus (HPV) has been considered the etiologic agent. A classic epidermoid vulvar cancer is presented in Figure 8-2.

The lymphatics of the vulva were first investigated by Philibert Constant Sappey in 1874.[2] In 1912, the French gynecologist A. Basset demonstrated the importance of lymphatic drainage in vulvar cancer and developed the forerunner to the modern radical vulvectomy; interestingly, Basset believed that the cancer began as a primary epithelioma of the clitoris.[3] In Basset's operation, the vulva was first excised through a *horseshoe incision*, and then 2 weeks later the inguinal, iliac, and hypogastric glands were removed by using an extraperitoneal approach.

In the 1940s, the American gynecologist Frederick J. Taussig adopted the Basset procedure and popularized vulvar surgery in the English-speaking world, reporting a 5-year survival rate of 52.6% when the inguinal but not the pelvic lymph nodes were involved.[4,5] In 1930, Walter Stoeckel introduced the method of removal of the lymph nodes at the time of radical vulvectomy through a *butterfly incision*.[6] The most serious complication of en bloc resection of the vulva and bilateral inguinofemoral lymph nodes was wound sepsis. Philip John DiSaia first described the method of the *triple incision technique* to minimize postsurgical morbidity.[7]

Additional modifications in treatment have evolved. The Gynecologic Oncology Group demonstrated that radical vulvectomy with bilateral groin node dissection followed by tailored inguinofemoral and pelvic irradiation, when indicated, was superior to radical vulvectomy with bilateral groin and pelvic lymphadenectomy. In addition, modifications of the radical vulvectomy procedure have become popular, with only one half or one quarter of the organ being resected during primary surgery. The possibility of sentinel node identification through isosulfan blue dye injection and lymphoscintigraphy is currently being investigated by the Gynecologic Oncology Group. It is anticipated that the number of groin node dissections and hence chronic lower extremity lymphedema will be decreased, similar to what has been done for the other cutaneous (i.e., external genital) malignancy, specifically breast cancer.[8] Finally, in an effort to avoid primary exenterative surgery (i.e., ultraradical surgery involving resection of the vulva with the vagina, pubic bone, bladder, or rectum) for locally advanced lesions, the effectiveness of neoadjuvant chemoradiation before surgery and interstitial brachytherapy is currently being studied.[9]

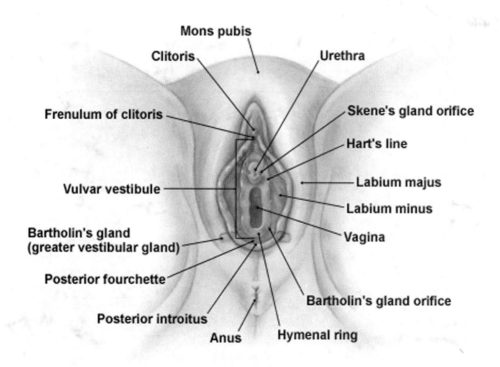

FIGURE 8-1
Normal vulvar anatomy.

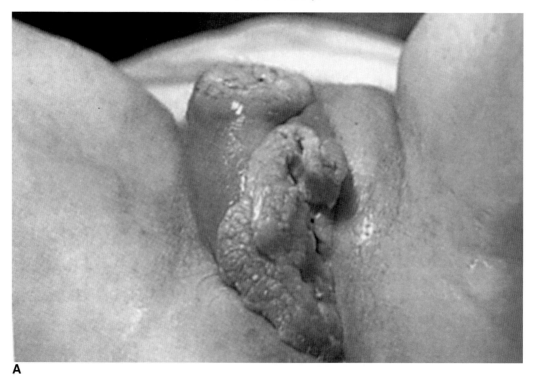

A

FIGURE 8-2
Squamous cell carcinoma of the vulva. **A,** Typical appearance of vulvar carcinoma, showing an ulcerating mass with rolled edges.

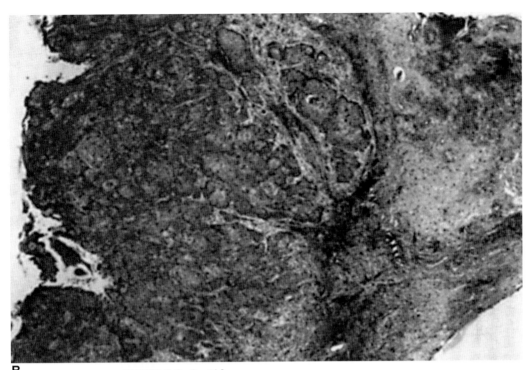

FIGURE 8-2, Cont'd
B, Histologic section of squamous cell carcinoma of the vulva.

The pathogenesis of vulvar cancer is most likely different than the other reproductive tract cancers (Table 8-1). Mitotically active centers are present in the cervix, uterus, and ovary, where it is believed that errors in DNA repair or influence by viruses or exogenous or endogenous hormones may play a role in resulting malignant transformation. Specifically, most cervical carcinomas arise in the squamocolumnar junction or transformation zone of the uterine cervix where active squamous metaplasia occurs. Similarly, the endometrial lining undergoes numerous cycles of proliferation and desquamation during the phases of each menstrual cycle, and it is this circuitry through which unopposed estrogens may affect the development of some uterine corpus carcinomas. Finally, ovulation itself disrupts the surface coelomic epithelium of the ovary, which needs to be repaired each month after an ovulatory cycle. No such mitotically active region of the vulva exists, which perhaps explains why cancer of this organ is less common than malignancies arising from the others.[10]

In the 1960s, Richart coined the term "cervical intraepithelial neoplasia" (CIN) and designed a grading system based on the percentage of cells from the basement membrane to the surface that were undifferentiated.[11] The term "vulvar intraepithelial neoplasia" (VIN) was introduced in the early 1980s and originally used to designate severe squamous epithelial atypia (i.e., severe dysplasia) and squamous cell carcinoma in situ of the vulva.[12-15] This concept was later expanded to encompass the entire spectrum of morphologic changes that carried a potential for malignant transformation.[16] Pathologically, VIN indicates a squamous epithelial lesion characterized by disordered maturation and nuclear abnormalities, such as loss of polarity, pleomorphism, coarsening of nuclear chromatin, irregularities of the nuclear membrane, and mitotic figures, including atypical forms, at various levels in the epithelium.[17] When one third or less of the distance from the basement membrane to the surface is

Table 8-1

Reproductive Tract Site	New Cases per Year (U.S.)	Precursor	Cellular Activity	Oncogenic Theory	Early Detection	Effect of Surgery on Fertility
Ovary	38,300	None	Ovulation	Incessant ovulation	No	Compro-mised
Uterine corpus	23,400	Complex hyperplasia with atypia	Menstruation	Unopposed estrogen	Post-menopausal vaginal bleeding	Compro-mised
Uterine cervix	12,800	Cervical dysplasia	Metaplasia at the squamo-columnar junction	Oncogenic strains of HPV	Papanicoloau test	Compro-mised
Vulva	3,200	Vulvar intraepithelial neoplasia	No specific site	HPV?	Examination & symptom-atology	Not com-promised

involved, the lesions are called VIN 1 or grade I.[18-20] When more than one third but less than or equal to two thirds is involved, the lesions are called VIN 2 or grade II.[18-20] Finally, when more than two thirds is involved or there is full-thickness involvement (i.e., carcinoma in situ or CIS), the term VIN 3 is used.[18-20]

The VIN terminology was adopted by the International Society for the Study of Vulvar Disease in 1986 to present a scheme that would be accepted by gynecologists, pathologists, and dematologists.[21] In its latest classification of gynecologic tumors in 1994, the World Health Organization and the International Society of Gynecological Pathologists incorporated the VIN terminology.[17] Indeed, the VIN terminology is appealing because previously confusing diagnostic terms such as "Bowen's disease," erythroplasia of Queyrat," simplex carcinoma in situ," and "atypia" have been deleted.[22] Furthermore, standardization and comparability of vulvar pathology is desirable not only on an interdisciplinary basis but also internationally. Perhaps most importantly, nonneoplastic vulvar disorders such as lichen sclerosis, other dermatoses, and squamous cell hyperplasia (formerly called "hyperplastic dystrophy") are not included in the VIN terminology.[23] Mixed disorders that can occur if either squamous cell hyperplasia or lichen sclerosis is associated with VIN should be reported as VIN.[24]

Vulvar cancer is an uncommon tumor, accounting for only 3% to 5% of genital tract malignancies.[25,26] Vulvar carcinoma is amenable to early diagnosis because of readily apparent symptomatic lesions.[25] Asymptomatic vulvar lesions may be detected during a thorough pelvic examination performed as part of an annual comprehensive physical examination. For this reason, the vulva is an organ that is ideally situated for early detection of disease and cancer prevention.

VIN may represent a precursor to invasive vulvar cancer.[27] It is likely that the lesions of VIN are subject to regression, just as the lesions associated with CIN may spontaneously regress. Not all VIN lesions progress to invasive cancer as is indicated by the manifestation of vulvar carcinomas as solitary lesions, whereas VIN is typically multifocal.[28]

Paget's disease, first identified in the breast and associated with an underlying breast adenocarcinoma in 100% of cases, may also develop in other sites of the body. The extramammary form of Paget's disease that occurs in the vulva is uncommonly associated with underlying adenocarcinoma. In addition, malignant melanoma of the vulva has also been reported and represents the second most common histologic type of vulvar cancer after squamous cell carcinomas—an unusual circumstances because the vulva is not typically a sun-exposed cutaneous region. Both extramammary Paget's disease of the vulva and malignant melanoma of the vulva will be discussed later in this chapter.

INCIDENCE OF VULVAR INTRAEPITHELIAL NEOPLASIA AND INVASIVE CANCER

Although the incidence of VIN in the United States has increased from 1.2 to 2.1 per 100,000 women in the last two decades,[29] the actual incidence is difficult to calculate because many cases are asymptomatic. In the United States, the Surveillance, Epidemiology and End Results (SEER) data from 1973 to 1976 and 1985 to 1987 were drawn from a sample of approximately 10% of the country's population and were noteworthy for indicating an increase in the incidence of in situ lesions but not invasive cancers. Epidemiologists have been unable to determine whether this increase was caused by more frequent use of health services by women, heightened awareness, or changes in sexual behavior, the latter behavior supporting the argument that there may be two distinct etiologies for VIN and invasive vulvar cancer.[29]

The increase in the incidence of VIN is a phenomenon that has also been observed in Norway and in New Zealand. The Norwegian data are derived from the national cancer registry and encompass the years 1973-1992,[30] and the New Zealand data are taken from a regional gynecologic oncology unit and include patients diagnosed from 1961 to 1992.[31] With an average annual age-adjusted incidence of 1.6 per 100,000 women in the United States, vulvar cancer accounts for 1% of all malignancies in women and approximately 3% to 5% of all female genital tract cancers.[32,33] An association between poorly developed countries and the incidence in vulvar cancer is evident in worldwide distributions.[34] The incidence rates are highest in Latin America and Asia and lowest in Japan and China.[25] Parenthetically, the low risk in Asian populations has been confirmed in Asian women who have migrated to Australia and continue to be at significantly lower risk for this genital tract malignancy.[35] Worldwide, the incidence increases with age, and more than 50% of patients are 70 years of age or older.[36]

STAGING OF INVASIVE VULVAR CANCER

Regional spread occurs in the inguinal and femoral lymph node, and the status of the groin lymph nodes remains the most significant prognosticator of vulvar cancer.[37,38] Before 1988, vulvar cancer was clinically staged and required comprehensive physical examination, chest and bone radiographs, cystoscopy, and proctoscopy. Clinical staging depended on the surgeon's ability to determine inguinofemoral lymph nodal status by direct palpation. Unfortunately, an unacceptably large discrepancy between clinical assessment and surgical-pathologic examination of the groin contents was indicated in a report submitted by Iverson from the Norwegian Radium Hospital; 15% of 258 patients were overdiagnosed (i.e., clinically suspicious nodes but negative pathologically). Furthermore, 36% of the pathologically documented inguinal nodal metastases diagnosed in 100 women were missed upon palpation.[39]

In 1988 the International Federation of Gynecology and Obstetrics (FIGO) agreed to adopt a new surgical staging system.[40] FIGO stage can only be assigned after a rigorous histopathologic evaluation of the operative specimens (i.e., vulva and inguinofemoral lymph nodes). This staging system is based on the TNM (tumor, nodes, metastases) classification. FIGO stage I lesions are less than or equal to 2 cm in size and are confined to the vulva without regional or distant spread; it should be noted that FIGO stage I has been subdivided into IA and IB categories, with the former denoting a superficially invasive lesion 2 cm or less in greatest diameter but with 1.0 mm or less of stromal invasion. FIGO stage II indicates lesions greater than 2 cm confined to the vulva, whereas a lesion of any size with unilateral groin node involvement is designated stage III. Bilateral groin node involvement; urethral, pelvic bone, or bladder or rectal mucosal involvement; or both are categorized as FIGO IVA disease, whereas pelvic nodal or other distant metastases are designated FIGO IVB.

SURVIVAL FIGURES

The FIGO Annual Reports dating from 1978 contain the only readily available published material relating to vulvar cancer survival worldwide.[41] In the 24th volume, 50 centers contributed worldwide. Of these, only 23 have treated more than 20 patients in the 3-year period that the current report encompasses. Those 23 centers supplied data on 80% of the 1034 patients in the annual report. The following discussion highlights important findings contained in the 24th volume.[41]

The age distribution showed that 75% of patients were diagnosed at 60 years of age or older, with a peak in the eighth decade of life. Squamous cell carcinomas represent 70% of cases. Thirty percent of patients were diagnosed with FIGO stage 0 to II disease.[41]

Age, tumor size, number of inguinofemoral lymph nodes that test positive, and FIGO stage were accurate predictors of overall survival. For the 715 women with squamous cell carcinomas, overall survival at 5 years for women diagnosed between 30 to 69 years of age, 70 to 79 years of age, and older than 80 years of age was 69.6% to 75%, 57.1%, and 38.7%, respectively.[41]

Overall survivorship at 5 years for tumor sizes smaller than 2 cm in maximal diameter was 86.2%. For lesions whose maximal diameter ranged from 2 cm to 5 cm, the overall 5-year survival fell to 66%. Women with tumors 6 cm or larger experienced a disappointing 5-year survival rate of 41.5% to 45.7%.[41]

Overall survival at 5 years decreases from 81.1% to 49.7% when one positive inguinofemoral lymph node is discovered. Metastases to two nodes were found to decrease overall 5-year survival to 37%. Fewer than one third of patients with four or more positive nodes were alive at 5 years.[41] Overall survivorship was carefully examined based on FIGO stage. For stage I lesions, the 2-, 3-, and 5-year survivorships were 90.7%, 88.1%, and 86.5%, respectively. The stage II tumors exhibited a 2-, 3-, and 5-year overall survival rate of 77.2%, 72.9%, and 67.7%, respectively. Women diagnosed with stage III disease survived 2 years in 57% of cases, 3 years in 49.5% of cases, and 5 years in 40.3% of cases. Finally, women with advanced FIGO stage IV vulvar cancers had very poor survivorship—33.7% at 2 years, 31.4% at 3 years, and an abysmal 21.7% at 5 years of follow-up. The survival distribution by FIGO stage appears in Figure 8-3.[41]

Disease-free survival was also stratified by FIGO stage. Although 89.4% of women with stage I disease did not experience recurrence at 1 year of follow-up, recurrence rates at 1 year of 15.5%, 31.4%, and 46.5% were observed for stage II, III, and IV lesions, respectively. At 2 years of follow-up, there were recurrences of 20.9%, 32.7%, 48.9%, and 58.4% of stage I, II, III and IV tumors, respectively. By 5 years of follow-up, only 71.7% of women diagnosed with stage I disease were relapse-free. For stage II disease, 41.6% of women were disease-free

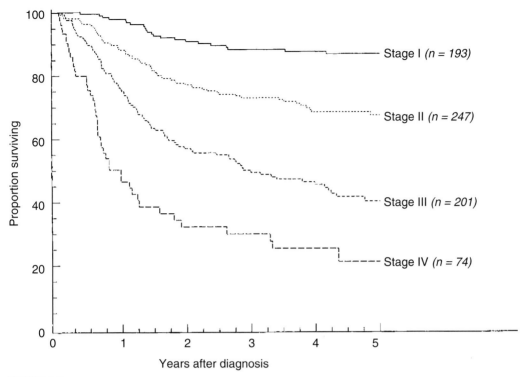

FIGURE 8-3
Carcinoma of the vulva: patients treated in 1993-95. Survival by FIGO stage (epidermoid invasive cancer only), n = 715.

at 5 years and for stage III cancers, only 35.7% of patients had not experienced recurrence at 5 years. Finally, it was noted that only 14.6% of women with stage IV vulvar cancer were disease-free at 5 years of follow-up.[41]

RISK FACTORS

There has been no etiologic agent identified that causes invasive vulvar cancer, although race, education, income, diet, total body mass, smoking, multiple sexual partners, abnormal cervical Papanicolaou (Pap) test, diabetes, hypertension, young age at first birth, high coffee consumption, working in laundry cleaning or garment industries, a history of venereal and chronic nonspecific disease, inflammation, and vulvar dystrophy have all been implicated.[25] Some of these risk factors are surrogates for cervical cancer risk and for this reason some investigators have postulated that there may be two distinct forms of vulvar cancer, specifically an HPV-related warty vulvar carcinoma and a non–HPV-related keratinizing squamous cell vulvar cancer.

Human Papillomavirus and Vulvar Cancer

The HPV is a double-stranded DNA virus, and oncogenic strains are now believed to be responsible for the development of CIN and invasive cervical carcinoma. During the early 1980s, Rastkar and associates[42] and Pilotti and associates[43] were among the first groups to identify HPV viral associations in vulvar carcinoma specimens through immunohistochemistry and electron microscopy. The ensuing 10 years bore witness to the accumulation of a body of work in which HPV nucleic acids were identified through in situ hybridization and polymerase chain reaction (PCR) in several laboratories where vulvar cancer and intraepithelial neoplastic tissues were under investigation.[26,44-64]

Noteworthy results from more recent studies include the population-based analysis conducted by Madeleine and associates from the Fred Hutchinson Cancer Research Center in Seattle, in which the risk for invasive vulvar cancer was calculated based upon exposure to HPV, cigarette smoking, or the herpes simplex virus 2.[65] They examined 400 incident cases of carcinoma in situ and 110 squamous cell carcinomas and estimated the relative risks through adjusted odds ratios of developing in situ and invasive disease to be 3.6 and 2.8, respectively, with HPV 16 seropositivity; 6.4 and 3.0, respectively, with current cigarette smoking; and 1.9 and 1.5, respectively, with HSV 2 seropositivity. The relative risk was as high as 18.8 among current smokers who were HPV 16 seropositive in comparison with never-smokers who were HPV 16 seronegative.[65] Hildesheim's team from the National Cancer Institute at Bethesda studied 142 histologically confirmed cases of vulvar intraepithelial neoplasia (VIN) grade 3 and invasive vulvar cancer and 126 community controls. Subjects testing positive for HPV 16 antibodies were at a 5.3-fold increased risk of vulvar neoplasia. In concordance with Madeleine's observations, the risk associated with HPV 16 seropositivity was higher among smokers than among nonsmokers.[66] In addition to the observational data relating high-risk sexual behavior (and hence, HPV infection) to vulvar cancer, the laboratory evidence linking HPV infection to vulvar dysplasia and invasive vulvar carcinoma is striking. Junge and colleagues from the University of Copenhagen studied the surgical specimens from 62 women with vulvar dysplasia and carcinoma in situ.[67] HPV DNA was detected by PCR in 51 of 58 cases (88% had oncogenic HPV subtype 16) and was evenly distributed in all age groups. In situ hybridization studies detected oncogenic HPV 16 and 33 predominantly in warty carcinomas. The investigators concluded that oncogenic strains of HPV were associated with dysplasia and carcinoma in situ of the vulva. Kagie's group from Leiden University Medical Center in the Netherlands employed consensus primer-PCR to study HPV infection in 66 patients with vulvar carcinoma. Patients with HPV-positive carcinomas were younger, presented in lower stages, and had high-grade VIN more often than those with HPV-negative carcinomas.[68]

Sun and co-workers from the Johns Hopkins medical institutions in Baltimore studied the HPV-specific serologic response in VIN, warty (i.e., HPV-related) squamous cell carcinoma of the vulva, and keratinizing (i.e., non–HPV-related) squamous cell carcinoma of the vulva. The presence of HPV-specific antibodies in sera was established by enzyme-linked immunosorbent assay (ELISA) and in radioimmunoprecipitation assays and was found to be significantly higher in HPV-associated VIN and warty squamous cell carcinoma than in keratinizing squamous cell vulvar cancers.[69]

At the University of California, Irvine, the prognostic significance of HPV DNA in 55 newly diagnosed primary invasive vulvar cancers was studied. Thirty-three (60%) tumors contained HPV DNA. Patients younger than 70 years of age or who smoked were more likely to have HPV-positive vulvar cancers. Using life-table analysis, the absence of HPV DNA and the presence of regional nodal metastases were predictive of recurrence and death from vulvar cancer. After investigators controlled for lesion size, age, tumor grade, and nodal metastasis by using the Cox proportional hazards model, only HPV status remained an independent prognostic factor. It was concluded that HPV DNA is more common in vulvar cancers of young women who smoke than in older nonsmokers and that women with HPV-negative tumors are at an increased risk of recurrence and death from vulvar cancer.[70] The study of HPV nucleic acids has become increasingly sophisticated during the last 5 years, as researchers continue to discern the molecular circuitry through which the virus infects and transforms normal vulvar epithelium.[71-77]

Geographic Distribution

Unfortunately, it is difficult to describe the global incidence and mortality of vulvar cancer because in national tumor registries it falls under the heading of *cancer of other genital sites,* which also includes vaginal and fallopian tube cancers. There is an association between poorly developed countries and the incidence of vulvar cancer, with the highest rates reported in Latin America and Asia.[78] During the period from 1978 to 1982, Costa Rica, Puerto Rico, and Colombia had the highest incidences,[79] whereas the lowest incidence rates of 0.3 to 0.4 per 100,000 were observed in Japan and China. Although mortality rates have not increased during the past 20 years, as discussed previously, the incidences of both VIN and vulvar CIS have increased.

Anastasiadis and colleagues performed a 13-year retrospective analysis of preinvasive and invasive vulvar cancer in Thrace, Greece, and identified data in support of the hypothesis that different epidemiologic characteristics are present in women with invasive and in situ vulvar lesions.[80] Aynaud and co-workers examined 423 cases of intraepithelial carcinoma and invasive carcinoma of the vulva, vagina, and penis in Ile-de-France.[81] They noted a correlation in younger age clusters for preinvasive disease (25-45 years) and more advanced ages (59-68 years) for the development of invasive disease, leading them to postulate a common etiologic factor for the development of the disease in both sexes.

Additional information concerning the geographic distributions of VIN may be found in the report prepared by Tidy and associates from the United Kingdom in which the investigators studied the referral patterns not only for VIN but also for lichen sclerosus and Paget's disease of the vulva.[82] The extreme heterogeneity of VIN lesions was verified by the Italian Study Group on Vulvar Disease after an examination of the clinicopathologic features of 370 cases.[83] Bjørge and associates summarized the 1970 to 1992 Norwegian experience, in which women carrying a diagnosis of carcinoma in situ of the uterine cervix were followed and evaluated for the development of a second primary cancer.[84] Among 37,001 women followed, there were 1037 second primary cancers in 989 individuals, with cancers of the esophagus, nose, nasal cavities, trachea, bronchus, lung, bladder, skin, vagina, and vulva occurring most frequently, thus suggesting that populations at risk for vulvar cancer include those in which there is a high density of cervical neoplasia.

OTHER RISK FACTORS

Several attempts to characterize epidemiologic factors of invasive vulvar cancer and VIN appeared in the 1980s,[85-88] but it was not until the 1990s that sufficient numbers had been accumulated by various academics to permit a careful analysis of emerging trends and associations.[89-93]

Diet

Sturgeon and colleagues noted a moderately increased age-adjusted risk of vulvar cancer in a case-control study of 543 subjects who had decreased intake of dark yellow–orange vegetables.[94] This suggested that lack of alpha-carotene may predispose women to the development of vulvar neoplasia. Coffee consumption was also associated with an increase in risk, but alcohol consumption, intake of dark green vegetables, citrus fruits, legumes, vitamins A and C, and folate were unrelated to the risk of vulvar cancer.[94]

Parazzini's team examined 125 women with histologically confirmed invasive vulvar cancer in Milan and compared their eating habits to 541 control subjects.[95] They found that the risk of vulvar cancer was inversely related to green vegetable and carrot consumption. No consistent association emerged between milk, meat, liver, alcohol, and coffee consumption and risk of vulvar cancer. The authors concluded that the risk of vulvar cancer is related to a number of nutritional and dietary factors.[95]

Obesity

Andreasson and associates first suggested that obesity may be a risk factor for vulvar cancer in 1982.[96] Mabuchi and colleagues were unable to detect a relationship between body weight and vulvar cancer in a case-control study from 1985.[97] Brinton's group did observe a relative risk of 1.3 among obese women for the development of vulvar cancer in 1990, but this did not reach statistical significance.[33] Similarly, Parazzini's team in Milan noted an association between body mass index (BMI) above 30 and vulvar cancer that was not statistically significant.[98] Finally, Kirschner and colleagues retrospectively examined 136 women with invasive squamous cell carcinoma of the vulva and found no negative impact of the BMI on either the development or survival of invasive vulvar cancer; specifically, 52.9% of patients had a normal BMI, 29.4% were moderately obese, and 13.2% were severely obese.[99]

Race

In a presentation of 249 vulvar cancer patients from the M.D. Anderson Hospital and Tumor Institute in Houston, Franklin and Rutledge considered the possibility of different pathogenic mechanisms among black and white populations.[100] Henson and Tarone contributed to the Third National Cancer Survey in the United States in which cases of invasive and in situ carcinoma of the lower female genital tract were examined, paying close attention paid to age, race, and geographic distribution.[101] No difference in the rates of vulvar carcinoma in situ between White and Black women was found, and although there was a slightly higher incidence of invasive vulvar cancer for Black women, the difference was not statistically significant.

Kosary evaluated the prognostic impact of FIGO stage, histology, histologic grade, age, and race by using cases obtained from the National Cancer Institute's SEER program that were diagnosed between 1973 and 1987.[102] An analysis of 2575 cases of vulvar cancer indicated that FIGO stage, histology, histologic grade, age, and race were all prognostically significant; however, the investigator suggested that the interaction of factors may be more predictive of outcome than any one factor separately.[102] With respect to racial incidences, Sturgeon noted that the overall incidence of CIS from 1973 to 1976 was 1.6 per 100,000 for Black women, compared with 1.1 per 100,000 for White women.[29] From 1985 to 1987, Black women again had a higher incidence of vulvar CIS, compared with that of White women (2.3 and 2.1 per 100,000, respectively).[29] The incidence of invasive vulvar cancer was not significant between Black and White populations (1.7 and 1.3 per 100,000, respectively) from 1973 to 1976 and (1.2 and 1.1 per 100,000 respectively) from 1985 to 1987.[29] Although these data may be interpreted as indicating a slightly higher risk for in situ and invasive disease to Black women, confounding factors such as socioeconomic status, barriers to health care access, and education levels must be considered.

Socioeconomic Factors

Both the 1972 Franklin and Rutledge paper[100] and the 1977 Henson and Tarone paper[101] would suggest that low socioeconomic status is linked to an increased risk of developing invasive vulvar cancer. In a case-control study that included only 37 women with CIS and 22 with invasive cancer, Newcomb and associates reported an inverse association between education level and vulvar CIS but not invasive cancer.[88] Parazzini and colleagues also performed a case-control study with 73 Italian subjects and concluded that the risk of vulvar cancer was inversely correlated with education level, which is a surrogate for socioeconomic status.[98] Specifically, women with 7 to 11 years of education had a 0.6 per 100,000 risk for developing vulvar cancer, compared with the risk of women with less than 7 years of education; for women with 12 or more years of education, the risk was decreased to 0.4 per 100,000, compared with women with less than 7 years of education.[98] Just as with race, socioeconomic status is very difficult to measure and may be a confounder of important risks such as lifestyle issues, personal hygiene, and barriers to health care.[25]

Sexuality

Interestingly, there has been no association between sexual behavior and the risk of vulvar cancer. For example, age at first intercourse and number of sexual partners, which serve as surrogates for cervical cancer risk by virtue of HPV infection, have not been implicated in the development of vulvar cancer. Perhaps those women caught in the surges of the sexual revolution have not had sufficient time for the HPV epidemic to manifest. It is possible that in upcoming years we will be able to use sexual history to target populations at high risk for developing vulvar cancer.[33,97,98]

Reproductive History

The papers by Andreasson and associates[96] and by Newcomb and associates[88] from the early 1980s suggested that early menarche, nulliparity, and early menopause are risk factors for vulvar cancer. These claims, however, have been refuted by case-control studies prepared by Ansink and associates[32] and by Mabuchi and associates.[97]

Genital Tract Infections Other than HPV

As discussed earlier, virology studies have detected HPV nucleic acids in up to 60% of invasive vulvar cancers,[57,103,104] with the oncogenic strain HPV subtype 16 found in 70% of VIN III and CIS of the vulva.[88,105] In addition to the HPV, sexually transmitted pathogens such as *Treponema pallidum* (the etiologic agent for syphilis), *Chlamydia trachomatis*, and the herpes simplex virus have been implicated.[88,96] A history of genital warts (cervical, vaginal, vulvar) also places a woman at risk for the development of vulvar cancer;[33] conversely, women with vulvar cancer are felt to be at risk for the development of cervical cancer because they may be infected with oncogenic HPV.

Tobacco

Brinton and associates identified a 34% increased risk for vulvar cancer among women who ever smoked.[33] In women who also had a history of genital warts, the relative risk was significantly increased. Newcomb and associates reported a relative risk for the development of invasive cancer of 2.2 for current smokers.[88] Interestingly, the relative risk for vulvar CIS was even higher among smokers, at 4.4. The study by Parazzini and associates in 1993, however, detected an overall risk of 0.9 among smokers for the development of vulvar cancer in Italian women.[98]

Oral Contraceptive Use

The studies carried out by Newcomb and associates,[88] Parazzini and associates,[98] and Brinton and associates[33] are inconclusive when it comes to describing the risk of vulvar cancer among oral contraceptive users, with the latter two papers finding no association.

Newcomb's analysis identified an association between oral contraceptive use and the development of CIS, but not for invasive disease.[88] This is surprising, because the use of birth control pills often is accompanied by a lack of use of barrier methods in contraception; hence, one would anticipate a greater opportunity for HPV transmission as has been observed among women with invasive cervical cancer. At one time it was believed that the oral contraceptive agents themselves had some type of direct transforming effect, but further study has shown that lack of concomitant use of barrier methods with oral contraceptives permits ready access of the HPV to its target, the cervical transformation zone. The higher incidence of vulvar CIS in oral contraceptive users also suggests that vulvar CIS and invasive vulvar cancer may have two different causes or that there may be a form of invasive vulvar cancer for which vulvar CIS is a precursor. What is needed is a description of the risk associated with oral contraceptives, stratified by the warty (i.e., HPV-associated) and nonwarty types of invasive vulvar cancer.

Immunosuppressive Disease

During the last three decades it has become clear that immunologic dysfunction is important in cancer. Carter and associates[106] and Franklin and Rutledge[100] have considered immunosuppressive conditions to be risk factors for invasive vulvar cancer, especially when the disease develops in women during the second and third decades of life. Specific disease states would include diabetes mellitus, pregnancy, systemic lupus erythematosus, and organ transplant recipients.[107-109] Thus far, none of these conditions has been independently and conclusively associated with an increase in the risk of vulvar cancer. Perhaps the most important observation has come from studying that population of women infected with the human immunodeficiency virus (HIV), for whom invasive cervical cancer has now become an acquired immunodeficiency syndrome (AIDS)–defining illness.[110,111] Accordingly, VIN has been reported to occur more frequently in HIV-infected women than in control groups of self-identified non–HIV-infected women.[112-114] Because women with HIV are now living longer, they face an increased probability of contracting oncogenic HPVs and are ultimately at increased risk for the long-term sequelae of malignant transformation. Wright and associates have discovered two cases of invasive vulvar cancer in HIV-infected women previously diagnosed with VIN.[115]

Papanicoloau Testing Frequency

The data by Brinton and associates indicate that women who have never been screened for cervical cancer have a relative risk of 2.46 for the development of vulvar cancer.[33] Additionally, the presence of an abnormal Pap test increased the risk for vulvar CIS (relative risk, 1.92) and for invasive vulvar cancer (relative risk, 1.41).[33] These findings suggest that the performance of a Pap test lowers the risk of vulvar cancer through concomitant external genital examination through which precursor vulvar lesions may be identified. This has been substantiated by the work of Franklin and Rutledge,[100] Newcomb and associates,[88] and Parazzini and associates,[98] the latter group reporting a relative risk of 0.3 for vulvar cancer among women who have had at least two Pap tests in their lives.

Risk Factors—Summary

Age, HPV infection, and smoking are established risk factors. Obesity may make examination of the external genitalia difficult and thereby increase the risk for premalignant lesions to go undetected. Finally, routine Pap screening can decrease the risk by leading to early diagnosis of premalignant conditions.

EARLY DIAGNOSIS

The clinical presentation of VIN may be variable. Lesions may be multifocal or solitary. In addition, they may be pigmented or pale, with irregular borders or raised, or both. Oftentimes, multiple lesions may manifest, all of which appear different and unrelated. Some examples are presented in Figures 8-4 and 8-5.

Most women will report a history of vulvar itching and irritation. The duration of symptoms is often for 6 months or longer. A clinical conundrum arises because there are infections (e.g., monilial vulvovaginitis) and many vulvar dystrophies (e.g., lichen sclerosis) that may simulate the clinical symptoms complex of VIN.[116-119] Interestingly, some investigators have reported squamous cell carcinomas arising within a bed of lichen sclerosis.[120,121] When Buscema and associates reviewed 98 consecutive cases of invasive disease, they noted that less than 20% demonstrated classic in situ neoplasia in the adjacent areas, whereas more than 50% revealed patterns suggestive of the vulvar dystrophies.[122] Although the dystrophies are not necessarily the precursory lesions, they did represent probable long-term irritation, which is significant in the development of vulvar cancer.

The clinician must be vigilant and ready to perform a biopsy of any suspicious lesion, especially because VIN is being diagnosed with increasing frequency among younger subjects. The biopsy should be mandatory in those patients treated for dystrophies and infectious processes, if satisfactory resolution of physical examination findings and symptoms has not occurred after a sufficient period of time. A long delay in diagnosis of premalignant change is common in many VIN cases because the primary treating clinician repeatedly prescribes ineffective topical and oral remedies for persistent inflammation.[123] However, it is unlikely for VIN to present without a lesion in patients with vulvodynia.[124] Furthermore, it is uncommon for vulvar vestibulitis to be mistaken for VIN because the characteristic blocked and inflamed gland duct openings are practically pathognomonic for the glandular condition.[125] Finally, Edwards and colleagues reiterate the importance of obtaining that crucial biopsy to determine whether an underlying neoplasm is present in cases of persistent vulvar condyloma after treatment with Condylox or laser vaporization or excisional therapy.[25]

As noted previously, lesions may be varied in appearance and texture. With the aid of acetic acid staining, acetowhite changes may be observed with or without punctuation; leukoplakia; velvety, erythematous, ulcerated, umbilicated, or pigmented lesions; or a combination of these changes.[126] Lesions therefore may be any shade of brown, a dull red, white, gray, or even rosette. Some cases resemble condyloma acuminata, whereas others are similar to condylomata lata, nevi, lentigo, or seborrheic keratoses.

The multifocal nature of VIN must always be kept in mind and therefore entire vulva, including the clitoris, must be inspected. Most women with VIN will have disease restricted to the labium minorum, although the labium majorum may become overgrown by extensive lesions. Perianal involvement occurs in 40% of cases. Occasionally, the lesions may be observed at the labiocrural fold or even on the mons pubis. The vagina may be a target for a preneoplastic process and therefore inspection and palpation of the vaginal cylinder is essential. Finally, if the cervix has remained in situ, a careful examination of this structure must be accomplished with the aid of Pap testing. Edwards and colleagues have indicated that perhaps the most common clinical presentation of VIN occurs in a woman who has previously been treated for CIN, cervical CIS, vaginal intraepithelial neoplasia, or occasionally invasive carcinoma of the cervix uteri or for a combination of these conditions.[25]

The apparent lack of homogeneity and highly variable nature of the disease may prove frustrating. Fortunately, there are certain clinical hallmarks of VIN, the most notable being

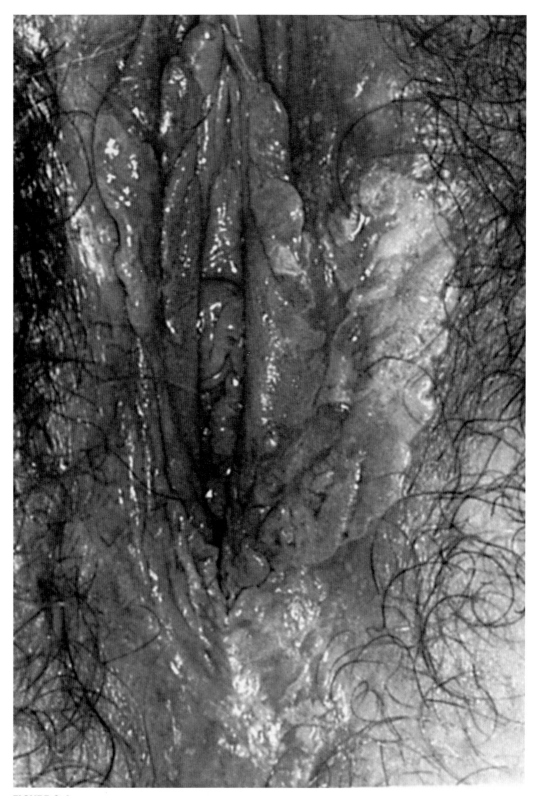

FIGURE 8-4
Solitary left labial plaque demonstrating vulvar intraepithelial neoplasia (VIN) grade III on biopsy. The plaque was excised under general anesthesia, and the surrounding skin was laser ablated to second and third surgical planes (see discourse in text on laser surgery for VIN).

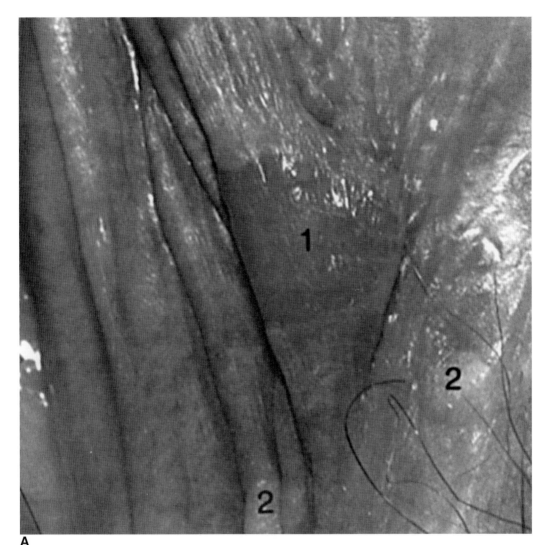

FIGURE 8-5
Multifocal vulvar intraepithelial neoplasia (VIN) lesions of variegated appearance. **A,** The midvulvar red lesion *(1)* is raised and resembles red velvet. There are elevated white patches *(2)*. Biopsies were performed on all these variations in clinical pattern to produce a comprehensive record of the status of this patient's vulva. The red lesion was confirmed as VIN, as were the white lesions.

that cases of vulvar CIS are papular or raised above the level of the surrounding skin and have a somewhat roughened edge in nearly all cases. In the 1980 study by Friedrich and colleagues, 90% of lesions exhibited this characteristic.[127]

Of course, when the lesions are very small, the degree of rise above the skin surface may be very difficult to appreciate. For this reason, the experienced vulvologist has a hand-held 2 × or 4 × magnification reading glass available in his or her examination room to study the vulvar skin and any associated abnormalities in detail. A colposcope may also be used for this purpose (if a hand-held lens is not available) but may be cumbersome.[128] It is uncertain whether the higher magnification afforded by the colposcope adds any information beneficial to clinical evaluation.

Under normal circumstances, the squamous keratinocyte is converted to keratin above the granular zone and the nucleus is lost; therefore surface nuclei are not present on normal

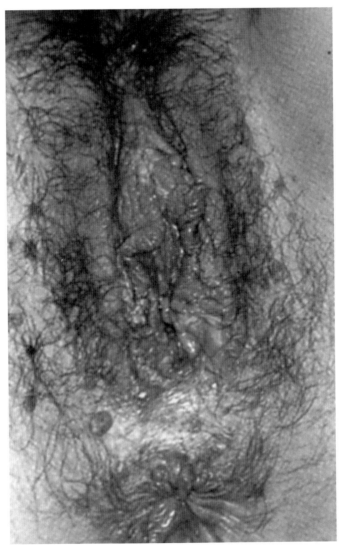

B

FIGURE 8-5, Cont'd
B, VIN manifest as brown papules.

vulvar skin. When nuclear chromatin material is retained in the acellular keratin layer of the epithelium, the phenomenon is called parakeratosis and is a manifestation of abnormal maturation, resulting in the presence of nuclear chromatin overlying areas of vulvar CIS.[129] Collins reported the use of a 1% aqueous solution of toluidine blue dye as a nuclear stain that becomes fixed to areas of superficial nuclei.[130] After a minute of fixation, 1% acetic acid is used to decolorize the area, indicating regions of parakeratosis that have acquired a faint bluish tinge by retaining the dye.[130] The clinician may expect invasive lesions to become intensely blue. A depiction of the effects of acetic acid and the toluidine blue dye staining appears in Figure 8-6.

Additional vulvar evaluation will indicate two additional hallmarks of the disease. First, many lesions are papular, if only slightly, with a smooth surface. Second, the rapid rate of cell division in vulvar CIS causes nearby melanocytes to become stimulated and increase pigment production, leading to spillage into the underlying dermis and resultant pigmentation. Parakeratosis, papule formation, and so-called "pigment incontinence" are clinical

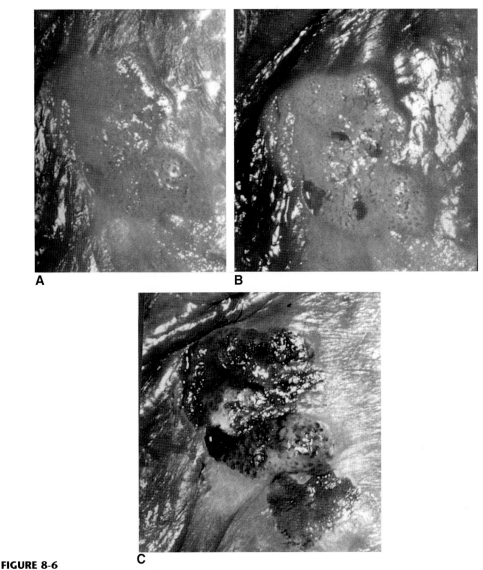

FIGURE 8-6
The appearance of vulvar intraepithelial neoplasia before, **A,** and after application of acetic acid, **B,** and toluidine blue, **C.**

earmarks of vulvar CIS, and one of these three features typically will be present in patients with severe VIN.[129,131,132]

Because VIN has a multifocal nature, nearly 75% of cases exhibit classic lesions separated by bands of normal tissue. Contiguous involvement of adjacent structures may occur with anal lesions, glans clitoris, distal vagina, and urethral meatus. Of these, anal involvement will most likely be missed unless anoscopy is performed. Whereas careful anoscopy is probably not necessary for all cases of VIN, anoscopy should be performed in the presence of pre-treated vulvar CIS because isolated foci of disease have been detected within the squamous portion of the anal canal below the dentate line, even when the external anal skin appeared normal. For this reason, Franklin and Rutledge have emphasized the concept of the "anogenital unit" when evaluating the external genitalia.[100] Disease restricted to the anus has been given the term "anal intraepithelial neoplasia" (AIN).[133-135]

Evaluation for VIN must be performed in good light, and as stated previously, the entire perineum should be examined. Shaving the vulva may be helpful in certain situations.

Equivocal lesions may be stained for approximately 2 minutes with acetic acid, and a biopsy should be performed on any acetowhite epithelium. CIS or invasive carcinoma should be suspected in lesions that are erythematous, ulcerated, and thickened, and these lesions should be sampled in several areas to detect invasive disease and to determine its extent for subsequent treatment planning.

Accordingly, definitive diagnosis can only be accomplished through a vulvar biopsy. This is a simple and rapid office procedure that can be performed with the dermatologic Keyes skin biopsy punch and a pair of short scissors and small forceps. Following infiltration of 1% lidocaine without epinephrine, a circular 5-mm plug of skin is drilled out in a manner similar to that of a small cork borer (Figure 8-7). The defect may be easily reapproximated with a single stitch of absorbable suture material. The specimen should be placed epidermal side upwards on a small piece of absorbent cardboard tissue, allowing the tissue fluids to seep out of the cut dermis and adhere to the cardboard surface. The entire unit is inverted to float upon the surface of the fixative solution, thus permitting the necessary orientation for the pathologist to exact tissue sections perpendicular to the surface. It is important to avoid the creation of tangential sections that can easily misrepresent the epithelial thickness and cellular populations. Because of the multicentricity of VIN, it is important to sample widely.

A comprehensive evaluation for VIN should also include a Pap specimen retrieved from the uterine cervix (if still present) or the vagina. The performance of cervical or vaginal colposcopy or biopsies, or any combination of these, is guided by what is observed grossly and by cytologic results.

HISTOLOGY

Under the light microscope, VIN 3 may be described as warty, basaloid, and differentiated.[13,19,22] The warty or condylomatous lesion has an undulating and spiked surface with

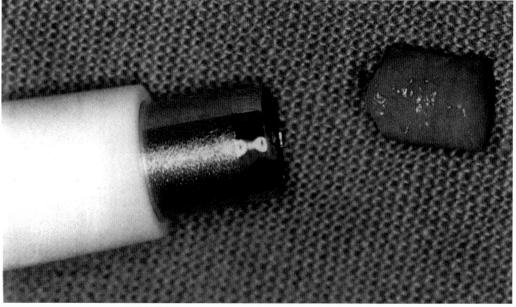

FIGURE 8-7
Vulvar disposable biopsy punch (5 to 6 mm in diameter).

large cells, nuclear pleomorphism, abundant mitoses, and surface keratinocytes containing koilocytotic features and multinucleation (Figure 8-8, A).[13,22] The basaloid subtype of VIN 3 is also considered the usual type and appears flat with atypical immature parabasal-type cells with abundant mitotic figures (Figure 8-8, B).[19,22] Finally, the differentiated or simplex subtype of VIN 3 exhibits an eosinophilic cytoplasm, large nuclei, and prominent nucleoli in basal or parabasal cells (Figure 8-8, C).[13,22]

In vulvar CIS, the epithelial architecture of the vulva is destroyed, and a desynchronous pattern replaces the orderly maturation of squamous cells as they reach the surface (Figure 8-8, D).[20] What results is a histologic appearance similar to cervical carcinoma in situ. Rete ridges may coalesce or become attenuated, with a prevalence of acanthosis.[20] Among the nuclear abnormalities are include pyknosis, chromatin clumping, multiple nucleoli, binucleation, and as mentioned previously, higher orders of multinucleation. Round bodies composed of densely pyknotic nuclei surrounded by clear halos of pale, vacuolated cytoplasm result in corps ronds formation. Mitotic aberrations occur through errors in cell division and result in tripolar mitoses, nuclear grains, and bilobed and folded nuclei. Those lesions with surface keratinization contain a granular zone beneath the keratin layer that may appear normal even though the keratin is thickened. Another constant feature is an underlying dermal connective tissue—inflammatory cell infiltrate. An ominous finding is the rare occurrence of intraepithelial pearl formation at the tip of the rete ridges because such lesions may be associated with foci of early stromal invasion.[20]

According to the 1984 Proposal by the International Society for the Study of Vulvar Diseases, superficially invasive or early invasive squamous cell carcinoma of the vulva (i.e., FIGO stage

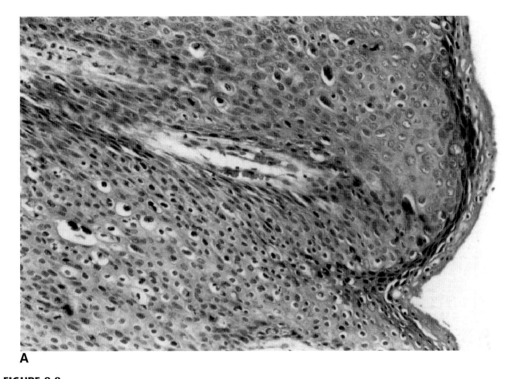

A

FIGURE 8-8
Histologic appearances of vulvar intraepithelial neoplasia (VIN). **A,** *Warty type,* in which the superficial keratinocytes have enlarged hyperchromatic nuclei with multinucleation and koilocytosis. Parakeratosis is present. The epithelium has disorganized epithelial cell growth with lack of evidence of cellular maturation involving nearly the full thickness. The deeper rete ridges have a well-defined epidermal-dermal junction with a mild chronic inflammatory infiltrate in the superficial dermis.

Continued

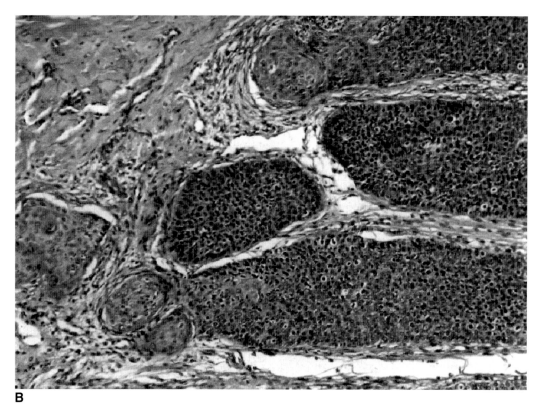

B

FIGURE 8-8, cont'd
B, *Basaloid type,* with associated squamous cell carcinoma antigen seen at the deep rete tips and in the dermis.

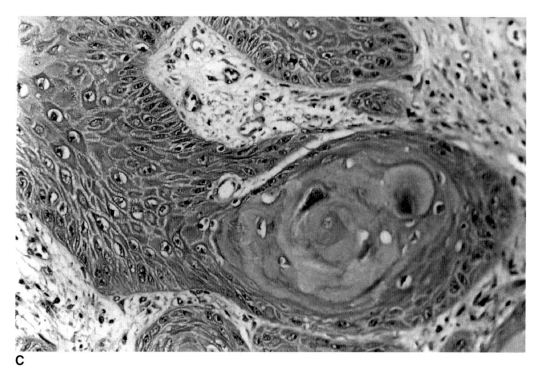

C

FIGURE 8-8
C, *Differentiated type* VIN: Within the tip of a rete rige, keratinocytes with increased eosinophilic cytoplasm, dyskeratosis, and nuclear pleomorphism with prominent nucleoli are present within the parabasalar area.

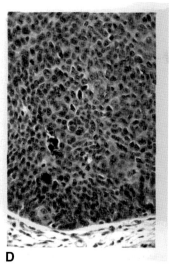

FIGURE 8-8, cont'd
D, Histologic section revealing a carcinoma in situ.

IA) is defined by a single lesion that measures 2 cm or less in diameter, with a depth of stromal invasion of 1 mm or less (Figure 8-9).[40] The depth of invasion is measured from the epithelial-stromal junction of the most superficial adjacent dermal papilla to the deepest point of invasion (Figure 8-10). In contrast, tumor thickness may be measured from the tumor surface or from the granular layer when keratinization is present (Figure 8-10). Finally, tumor diameter must be confirmed histologically, with any regions of adjacent intraepithelial neoplasia excluded from the measurement. It is important to note that patients harboring lesions with more than one site of invasion cannot be classified as FIGO stage IA.

The majority of squamous cell carcinomas of the vulva are well-differentiated lesions with numerous foci of keratinization and well-developed intercellular bridges.[34,136,137] Clitoral and vestibular lesions tend to be less differentiated and harbor lymphatic channel and perineural invasion. The tumor-stromal interface may have prognostic importance, with relatively better survival rates afforded lesions containing pushing borders and heavy lymphoplasmacytic infiltrates rather than infiltrating margins and fibroblastic reaction.[34,136] Infrequently, the origin of a vulvar squamous cell carcinoma may be traced to the squamous epithelium lining the outer portion of the excretory duct of a Bartholin's gland.

It is imperative that the clinician and pathologist record the microscopic appearance of the overlying skin and that adjacent to the lesion in an effort to deepen our understanding of the pathogenic relationship between invasive carcinoma and conditions such as atrophy, lichen sclerosis, hyperplastic dystrophia, atypia, intraepithelial neoplasia, granuloma inguinale, and lymphogranuloma venereum.

The responsibility rests with the astute pathologist, who remains aware that many conditions may mimic carcinoma in situ of the vulva—including condylomata acuminata, hyperplastic dystrophy, condylomata lata, seborrheic keratoses, acanthosis nigricans, lentigo, and, of course, nevi.

NATURAL HISTORY

What is the natural history of VIN?[24] Spontaneous regression has been documented in squamous cell carcinoma in situ lesions of the vulva, just as it has in cases of CIN. The first

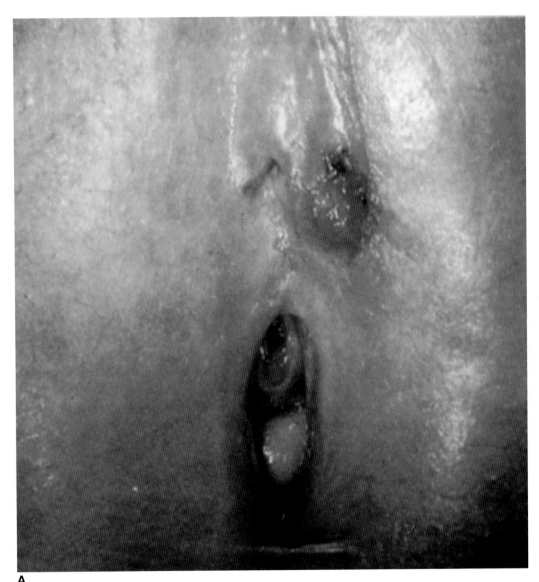

A
FIGURE 8-9
Superficially invasive vulvar carcinoma. **A,** Superficially invasive vulvar cancer arising in a bed of lichen sclerosus.

occurrence of this phenomenon was reported by Friedrich in 1972 and described as a "reversible vulvar atypia."[138] Since then, several additional cases of spontaneous regression have been documented by vulvologists, notably Skinner and colleagues,[139] Gardner (as discussed by Dean and associates),[140] and Berger and Hori,[141] who have each identified one patient for whom spontaneous regression of vulvar carcinoma in situ has occurred; Buscema and associates,[142] Friedrich and associates,[127] and Jones and Rowan[143] have reported an additional 21 cases.

The series by Friedrich and colleagues is notable for including five patients for whom complete regression of the intraepithelial lesion was confirmed by a follow-up vulvar biopsy.[142] These five women were among a case series of 50 patients, and for this reason, the authors have calculated the spontaneous regression rate in the population studied at 10%. In these cases, regression occurred at 4 months to 2 years from initial diagnosis, with the initial lesions exhibiting aneuploidy by DNA photometric analysis and the follow-up tissue

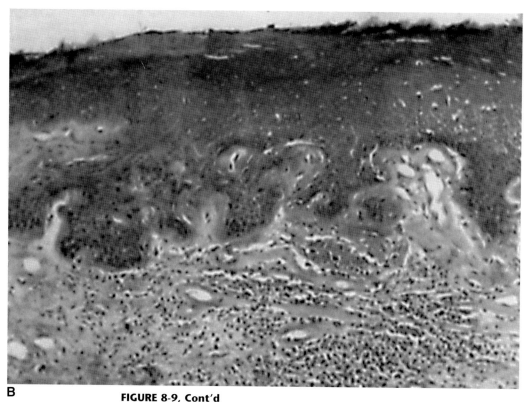

B

FIGURE 8-9, Cont'd
B, Histologic section with less than 1 mm of stromal invasion.

from photographically documented vulvar sites being uniformly euploid. All five of these women have had extended follow-up and no recurrences. Several examples of spontaneous regression recorded in the medical literature are included in Table 8-2.[137-143]

Very few cases in which the progression rates for histologically documented vulvar carcinoma in situ have occurred with certainty have been reported; Table 8-3 includes information about some of these cases.[15,141,142,144-158] Gardiner and associates irradiated two women with in situ lesions; after long-term observation, invasive vulvar cancer was detected.[144] Collins found a single case of an invasive recurrence after a vulvectomy,[145] and Jones and Buntine describe a 72-year-old woman for whom a vulvar carcinoma in situ progressed to invasion over an 8-year period.[146] Buscema and co-workers summarized the Baltimore experience of 102 cases of vulvar carcinoma in situ: There were two cases of documented invasion subsequent to surgical resection of vulvar carcinoma in situ in women aged 75 years and 83 years, and two others in which invasive carcinoma at the anal orifice occurred in women who were immunosuppressed.[142] Similarly, Friedrich and colleagues cared for a severely immunosuppressed woman with vulvar carcinoma in situ for whom progression to invasive disease occurred within 1 year.[127] A final example appears in Jones' and McLean's report of five women with untreated VIN for whom follow-ups from 2 to 8 years were recorded. During this time all five patients developed invasive vulvar cancer (they were between the ages of 40 years and 60 years when the condition was diagnosed).[147]

Additional knowledge can be gathered from those cases in which occult invasion has been found in a bed of VIN. Such findings are not infrequent, and examples may be found in the reports by Buscema and associates,[142] Friedrich and associates,[127] Woodruff and associates,[159] and Forney and associates.[160] Table 8-4 records these and several additional

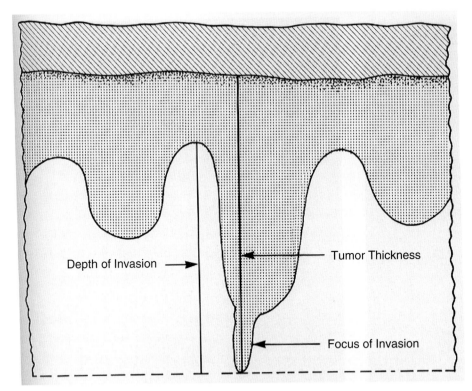

FIGURE 8-10
Measurements for the depth of invasion and tumor thickness for squamous cell carcinoma of the vulva. The depth of invasion is measured from the epithelial dermal junction to the adjacent dermal papillae to the deepest point of invasion. The tumor thickness is measured from the bottom of the granular zone to the deepest point of invasion or, if the epithelium is not keratinized, from the surface to the deepest point of invasion.

noteworthy cases.[127,142,159-169] Because of the lack of standardized nomenclature and the anecdotal and retrospective nature of many of the studies, the denominators remain obscure; it is therefore not feasible to calculate with any certainty the rates of spontaneous regression, progression to invasion, and presence of concomitant invasion. Tables 8-2, 8-3, and 8-4 provide further detail from individual studies.

It is not known whether a preclinical phase of vulvar cancer exists that would lend itself to early detection via screening. Whether all invasive squamous cell carcinomas of the vulva begins with an in situ or an intraepithelial lesion is controversial. Most invasive lesions arise in older women, are solitary and well circumscribed, and are not usually associated with the HPV, whereas VIN lesions are multifocal, associated with the HPV, and manifest in younger women. Perhaps most or all lesions are destined to regression, leaving behind that occasional "dominant" lesion with a tendency for malignant progression (i.e., invasion). The question that must be asked is what percentage of elderly women with invasive carcinomas carry with them a gynecologic lexicon containing a history of pathologically documented VIN. As indicated by previous discussion, the available literature is sparse on this topic.

The possibility exists that there may be two types of invasive vulvar cancer, one that is associated with the HPV and one that is not linked with HPV infection.[105] Edwards and colleagues state in their survey that because most invasive cancers begin as stage I, well-circumscribed lesions with a low association for lymph node metastases and 5-year survivorship of 90% to 95%, patients would benefit from early detection even if a preinvasive phase does not exist.[25]

Table 8-2

Year	Author	Number of Cases
1972	Friedrich et al[137]	1
1973	Skinner et al[138]	1
1974	Gardner (as discussed by Dean)[139]	2
1978	Berger and Hori[140]	1
1979	Buscema et al[141]	2
1980	Friedrich et al[142]	5
2000	Jones & Rowan[143]	14

Specifically, the natural history of early or microinvasive vulvar cancer must be examined. The association with nodal spread remains the single most important prognosticator. Kneale, Elliot, and McDonald surveyed the published experiences and found 20 cases of 7.8% inguinofemoral or pelvic lymph node involvement, or both, among 257 cases that would meet the definition of FIGO Stage IA.[170] It should be noted, however, that lymphadenectomies were not performed in all 257 cases. Because the size of the primary invasive lesion is predictive of nodal spread, by definition FIGO stage I (and hence FIGO stage IA) carries a low risk of nodal metastases by virtue of size alone, with several small series noting 1% to 4% positive nodes when the lesions are less than 1 cm in maximal diameter. Similarly, site of disease on the vulva is not predictive of lymph node metastases because tumors in the labia majora, clitoris, fourchette, and urethra as well as the labia minora all drain to regional lymph nodes. Other pathologic factors that will require further study as investigators accumulate additional cases of FIGO stage IA include the significance of angiolymphatic permeation, anaplastic tumors, and microscopic confluence and their effect on the biologic and clinical behavior of the superficially invasive vulvar neoplasm.

Table 8-3

Year	Author	Number of Cases
1953	Gardiner et al[144]	2
1968	Jones and Buntine[146]	1
1970	Collins et al[145]	1
1979	Buscema et al[141]	4
1980	Friedrich et al[142]	1
1982	Friedman et al[156]	1
1982	Caglar et al[158]	5
1982	Ulbright et al[157]	1
1984	Buckley et al[154]	2
1984	Östör et al[155]	1
1984	Crum et al[14]	5
1986	Jones and McLean[147]	6
1987	Ragnarsson et al[153]	3
1990	Van Sickle et al[152]	3
1995	Bakri and Dimitrievich[149]	2
1995	Sadler and Jones[150]	2
1995	Hørding et al[151]	12
1996	Herod et al[148]	9

Table 8-4

Year	Author	Number of Cases
1973	Woodruff et al[159]	3
1977	Forney et al[160]	2
1979	Buscema et al[141]	2
1980	Friedrich et al[142]	3
1982	Zaino et al[169]	2
1986	Powell et al[168]	4
1989	Pickel[167]	33*
1995	Haefner et al[166]	15
1996	Herod et al[165]	26
1998	Modesitt et al[164]	16
1999	Husseinzadeh and Recinto[162]	16
1999	Rettenmaier[163]	1
2001	Rouzier et al[161]	25

*Among a total of 305 vulvectomy/vulvar biopsy specimens (i.e., number of patients not specified).

TREATMENT OF VULVAR INTRAEPITHELIAL NEOPLASIA

The treatment of VIN is somewhat controversial.[171-174] A primary surgical approach ranging from wide local excision to simple vulvectomy is often advocated. If the disease focus is small, a wide local excision may be expected to produce excellent results. In cases of extensive or multifocal disease, a skinning vulvectomy with skin grafting may be the optimal surgical approach, and although this is less morbid than a simple (i.e., conventional) vulvectomy, the cosmetic and functional end results have continued to be poor for many patients. For these reasons, the treatment of choice for VIN in women under the age of 40, for whom invasion has been adequately ruled out, is carbon dioxide (CO_2) laser vaporization. The CO_2 laser may also be employed in cases where multifocal disease is present and the suspicion for invasion is low (Figure 8-11).[175-182]

To exploit the full potential of the sophisticated laser instrument, it is important that there is accurate delineation of the disease and use of optimum power densities; in addition, the surgeon must be able to exercise precise control over the depth of ablation. In an effort to avoid surgical misadventure, superficial laser vulvectomy using the CO_2 laser should be performed by expert physicians. For example, it may be tempting to direct the laser on a patch of VIN, but poor control of depth can lead to full-thickness epithelial destruction and the resulting cosmesis will be similar to a third-degree burn. Thus, to avoid delayed healing and scar formation, the clinician must learn to recognize the four surgical planes as outlined by Reid and associates in 1985.[182]

The target tissues at the first and second surgical planes are the surface epithelium and the dermal papillae.[182] The target tissues at the third and fourth surgical planes are the pilosebaceous ducts and pilosebaceous glands.[182] For the first and second surgical planes, the zones of vaporization are the proliferating layer of the surface epithelium and the superficial papillary dermis. The corresponding zones of vaporization for the third and fourth surgical planes are the upper and midreticular dermis, respectively. Finally, the zones of necrosis for surgical planes 1 through 4 include the basement membrane, deep papillary dermis, and midreticular and deep reticular dermises.

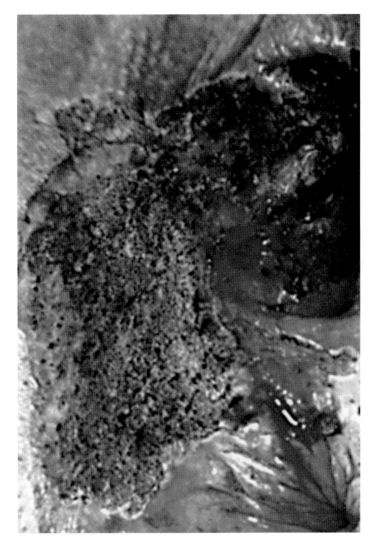

FIGURE 8-11
CO_2 laser vaporization to the second surgical plane for vulvar intraepithelial neoplasia. The exposed papillary dermis has been gently relased, sufficient to scorch (but not cut) the dermal surface.

Because many cases of VIN are multicentric (especially in young women) and are often surrounded by pockets of subclinical HPV infection, regional or general anesthesia is required before the laser can be applied. The perineum is shaved carefully after anesthesia is induced. Antiseptic solutions should not be used because they impair the response of the tissues to acetic acid application; furthermore, antiseptic prophylaxis is unnecessary because the high temperatures at the laser site will kill any unruly microorganisms. The vulva, perineum, and anus should be soaked with acetic acid for 3 minutes and then carefully examined with the colposcope. Before the acetic acid reaction fades, the borders of the VIN and outer margins along the perimeter of subclinical papillomavirus infection must be outlined clearly. Wet towels should be placed around the surgical field to prevent the drapes from igniting, and protective eyewear should be worn by everyone in the operating room.

The laser is first used to expose the proliferating zone of the epidermis by brushing the skin surface with a layer of laser energy. A moistened gauze swab can be used to gently wipe the epidermal debris from the operative field. This move then reveals the smooth pink-white basement membrane overlying the anatomically intact papillary dermis.

Moving the laser beam quickly across the exposed dermal surface will allow the laser to scorch to the second plane rather than crater the area. In contrast, lasing to the third plane must be done slowly with careful deliberate movements and hand-eye coordination to control the depth of penetration. The third surgical plane is appropriate for VIN not involving the pilosebaceous glands; however, if the pilosebaceous glands are involved, lasing to the fourth surgical plane will be required.

Postoperative care is aimed at counteracting the inflammation and edema caused by mild thermal injury to the underlying tissues. The vulva should be liberally dressed with 0.1% triamcinolone cream while the patient is still in the lithotomy position. The postoperative regimen involves soaking the surgical area for 30 minutes every 4 hours in a bath of reconstituted sea water (Instant Ocean) or hypertonic Epsom salt solution (1 cup per gallon). The vulva should then be dried with a hair dryer adjusted to a cool setting and dressed with a thin application of neomycin-bacitracin ointment. When used correctly, the CO_2 laser permits the vulva to be treated with little scarring and no disfigurement. Prescriptions for a stool softener and 2% lidocaine gel should be provided because the surgical site may be painful during the postoperative period. Patients should be seen weekly for the first 3 weeks. Recurrences occur in 10% to 20% of cases and are highly associated with continued tobacco use.

Ferenczy and colleagues compared CO_2 laser vaporization to the loop electrosurgical excision and fulguration procedure (LEEP) in 28 women with VIN.[183] To avoid selection bias, they treated half of the lesional area with laser vaporization, and they electro-excised the other half.[183] Although the overall operating time when controlled for lesional size was twice as fast for the laser (mean, 8 minutes), compared with the LEEP (mean, 20 minutes), at a mean follow-up of 12 months (range, 9 months to 26 months), there was no significant difference between the laser- or LEEP-treated areas with respect to disease recurrence, healing time (mean, 18 days), postoperative discomfort, and complications.[182] These results should be verified in a larger clinical trial before a recommendation can be made to perform LEEP instead of laser vaporization or wide local excision with a scalpel.

For women older than 40 to 45 years of age or in those for whom there is any suspicion of invasion, the treatment of choice for VIN I to VIN III (excluding those cases of VIN III in which there is full-thickness involvement of the epithelium) is wide local excision (i.e., partial simple vulvectomy).[184,185] After careful pathologic analysis of the surgical specimen to rule out invasive disease, patients may expect a 75% cure rate. A management algorithm for VIN appears in Figure 8-12.

For cases of squamous cell carcinoma in situ (i.e., VIN 3), the original treatment proposed by Knight had been wide local excision (Figure 8-13).[186] This method has been sanctioned by dermatologists for Bowen's disease elsewhere on the body, but because of fears that vulvar CIS is preinvasive, many clinicians advocate a simple vulvectomy as the treatment of choice. Those who have routinely employed total vulvectomy have reported recurrence rates of less than 10%; however, this approach is not without risk. Two cases of fatal pulmonary embolism have been recorded, and anorgasmia usually results from removal of the clitoris. Scarring around the urethral meatus may divert the urinary stream. Friedrich suggests that perhaps the greatest consequence is emotional, because many women view the surgery as similar to mastectomy.[127] Once their relief at "escape from cancer" subsides, they regret the loss of the vulva and consider themselves permanently disfigured. Because many cases of VIN 3 that are found pathologically to contain a focus of invasion have occurred in the

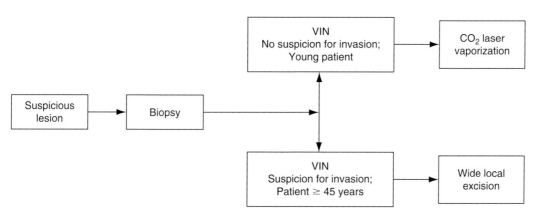

FIGURE 8-12
Management algorithm for the diagnosis and treatment of vulvar intraepithelial neoplasia.

immunosuppressed or elderly patient, the risk of malignant progression is insufficient in younger, healthier women to justify a mutilating surgical procedure.

Rutledge and Sinclair promoted the less drastic procedure of partial amputation of the clitoris in selected patients.[187] Following the skinning vulvectomy, a split-thickness skin graft to the vulva from a donor site on the medial thigh was applied (Figure 8-14). Patients were pleased with the initial cosmetic result; however, the additional scar at the donor site from which the graft had been procured was a disadvantage. Prolonged hospitalization for bed rest in a special bed, along with antibiotic prophylaxis that employs chloramphenicol, is required to ensure that the graft takes to the perineum.[188,189] Kaplan and associates noted that when the disease extended to the anal canal, the skinning vulvectomy and split-thickness skin graft were effectively employed in clearing the neoplasia; however, failure to recognize anal extension resulted in persistent disease following surgical therapy.[190] There has been increasing interest in treating vulvar carcinoma in situ with wide local excision. Forney treated 11 women and noted one case of persistent disease.[160] Woodruff found two recurrences among 17 women treated by wide local excision.[159] The two recurrences discovered by Dean and colleagues in their series of 16 cases were successfully managed by repeat excision.[140] Finally, Friedrich and associates treated 17 women with vulvar carcinoma in situ by using wide local excision and observed three recurrences.[127] Thus the documented recurrence rate following wide local excision for vulvar CIS is less than 20%, ranging from 9% to 17%.[127,140,159,160]

If the status of the surgical margins of the wide local excision specimen is taken into consideration, Friedrich correctly observed that a somewhat different picture emerges. In the Milwaukee study, 31 of 37 women treated by primary surgery had specimens with clear margins, and only three patients (i.e., 10%) developed a late recurrence; in contrast, 50% of the six women with positive surgical margins experienced recurrence.[127] Thus the likelihood of recurrence of vulvar CIS depends more upon the histologic quality of the surgical margins than on the extent of the procedure. It should also be noted that the recurrence of an in situ disease does not carry with it the ominous implications of recurrence of an invasive cancer, and therefore a repeat excision may be expected to provide successful therapy.[191] The ideal surgical approach would be a wide local excision to encompass all visible lesions with a 8-mm to 10-mm surgical margin, sparing those areas of the vulva that are not involved. If the clitoral glans is unaffected, it should be spared, and if it is involved, careful and controlled CO_2 laser vaporization rather than amputation should be the rule.

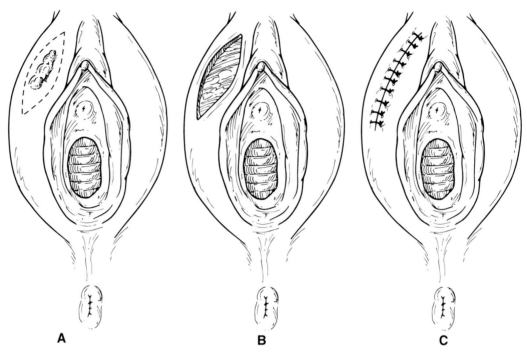

A	**B**	**C**

FIGURE 8-13

A, Vulva lesion with intended path of wide local excision. **B,** Wide local excision for vulvar intraepithelial neoplasia. **C,** Closure of wide local excision. An epithelial section of the vulva is removed. The defect is enclosed with interrupted sutures of biodegradable material.

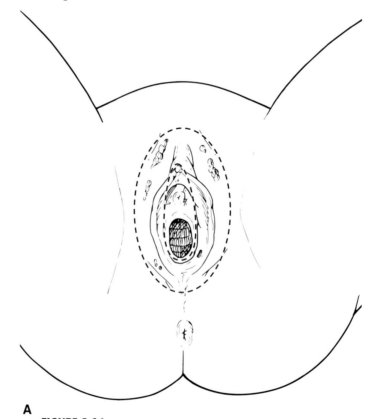

A

FIGURE 8-14

A, Multifocal vulva lesion with intended path for skinning vulvectomy.

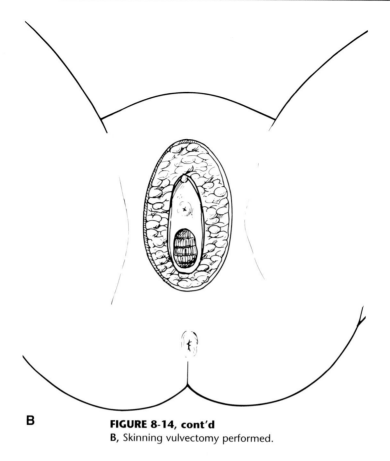

B

FIGURE 8-14, cont'd
B, Skinning vulvectomy performed.

Even with a wide local excision, depending on the extent, the vulva may still be disfigured. However, in most cases, the surgical bed may be reapproximated longitudinally along the anterior-posterior creases of the labia by using 2-0 vicryl suture material. The skin should be closed first by placing a stitch midway, thus bisecting the defect. The next two stitches should be placed midway between the first stitch and the top of the defect and between the first stitch and the inferior aspect of the defect. Several additional interrupted stitches may then be placed to reapproximate the skin. It is important that the repair be done without tension so that the suture material will not tear through the vulva. Furthermore, it is paramount that the urethra not deviate because of undue traction on a suture. Following excisional therapy, appropriate attention must be directed towards the potential long-term cosmetic and functional morbidities, including sexual function and somatopsychic reactions.[192,193] Occasionally, swinging a flap over the surgical bed is an effective strategy for minimizing sexual morbidity associated with the surgical management of VIN.[194]

In addition to CO_2 laser vaporization, nonsurgical approaches to the treatment of VIN include the use of topical 5-fluorouracil (5-FU), cryosurgery, dinitrochlorobenzene (DNCB)-induced hypersensitivity, photodynamic therapy, antiviral agents, interferon gel, and chemopreventive agents such as retinyl acetate gel (Box 8-1). 5-FU is an antineoplastic agent that blocks the methylation of deoxyuridylic acid to thymidylic acid, effectively inhibiting DNA synthesis.[195-200] When 5-FU is applied at a concentration of 5% in a cream base, the pooled experience in treating vulvar CIS is a noteworthy 47% response rate. The cream is applied twice daily for 6 consecutive weeks, and patients may note an erythema and irritation at 2 weeks with ulceration and sloughing beginning at 4 weeks. Although pain may be intense

Continued

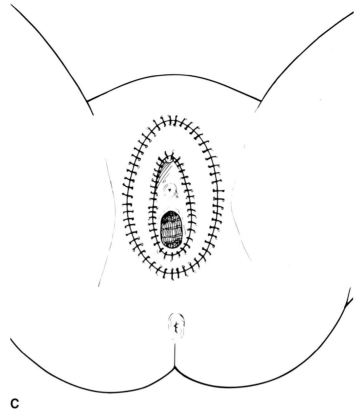

C

FIGURE 8-14, cont'd
C, Schematic representation of skinning vulvectomy with split-thickness skin graft for the treatment of extensive vulvar intraepithelial neoplasia.

and the discomfort significant during the healing period, the end results leave a healed vulva free from scarring, functional impairment, or both. Contact dermatitis and delayed hypersensitivity may be associated with the use of 5-FU.

Cryotherapy may be effectively used to treat vulvar, vaginal, and cervical condylomas.[201] When it has been used in patients with vulvar CIS, the results have been mixed. Forney and associates found four cases of small, unifocal lesions that were receptive to cryosurgery.[167] But when the entire vulva was deeply frozen under a pudendal block, a total slough was

---

BOX 8-1

Nonsurgical Methods
CO_2 laser vaporization
Antineoplastic agents (5-fluorouracil)
Cryotherapy
Induced hypersensitivity (2,4-dinitrochlorobenzene)
Immunotherapy (alpha-interferon)
Photodynamic therapy (5-aminolevulinic acid)
Chemopreventive agents (retinyl acetate)
Antiviral agents (cidofovir)

produced with resultant protracted, painful healing. The use of cryotherapy for extensive VIN is not recommended.

A novel method of treating vulvar CIS was introduced by Weintraub and Lagasse when they sensitized two patients to DNCB by applying 2 mg of DNCB dissolved in 0.1 mL acetone to the skin of an upper extremity.[202] After 2 weeks, a 0.1% DNCB cream was applied to the vulvar lesions, which then ulcerated and sloughed. Another approach has been to use the immunostimulant alpha-interferon (alpha-IFN) in gel form to treat VIN. In a prospective trial of topical alpha-IFN, Spirtos and colleagues instructed 18 patients to apply the gel to affected areas every 8 hours and to present to the cancer clinic for an evaluation for response biweekly.[203] Overall, 14 of 18 (78%) patients demonstrated some response to alpha-IFN applied topically. Their data support the observations of other investigators that alpha-IFN is an active agent in the treatment of VIN III.

Topical 5-aminolevulinic acid (5-ALA)–based photodynamic therapy (PDT) has produced complete response rates in more than 90% of nonmelanoma skin carcinomas, most of which are HPV negative. Employing a similar treatment procedure, Abdel-Hady and associates observed a short-term response in only 10 of 32 women with VIN 2-3 lesions.[204] The investigators found that unifocal lesions were more responsive than multifocal and pigmented lesions. They concluded that high-risk HPV infection and lack of cell-mediated immunity might play a role in the observed poor response of lower genital lesions to topical PDT. These observations were supported by Hillemanns and associates' study in which 24 women with 111 lesions of VIN 1-3 were topically sensitized with 10 mL of a 20% solution of 5-ALA and treated with 57 cycles of laser light at 635 nm (100 J/cm^2).[205] A complete response was achieved in 13 patients (52%) with 27 lesions. All patients with VIN 1 and monofocal and bifocal VIN 2-3 showed complete clearance. However, a complete response could be achieved in only 4 (27%) of 15 women with multifocal VIN 2-3. No response was seen in two women with multifocal VIN 3. The investigators concluded that PDT with 5-ALA is easy to perform and has the advantages of minimal tissue destruction, few side effects, and excellent cosmetic results; however, multifocal VIN with pigmented lesions remains difficult to treat.

The clinical trial by Fehr and associates sought to compare the results of topically applied 5-ALA for photosensitization with those of laser vaporization and local excision.[206] Fifteen women with VIN 3 had 10 grams of 10% ALA gel applied to the entire vulva; 2 to 3 hours later the vulva was irradiated with 120 J/cm^2 laser light at a wavelength of 635 nm. In most women, the procedure was performed without anesthesia. Thirty women with VIN 3 were treated with light-based therapy and 27 patients by surgical excision. At 8 weeks of followup, 11 of 15 women's biopsies were proved free of VIN 3 after photodynamic therapy. Excellent tissue preservation was achieved, and no ulcers or scarring occurred. There were three recurrences following PDT at 5, 6, and 7 months after therapy. At 1 year of follow-up, there was no statistically significant difference in disease-free status between patients treated with PDT and patients treated with conventional treatment modalities. The authors concluded that although the effectiveness of PDT for VIN 3 is similar to that of conventional treatment modalities, unique advantages offered by PDT include shorter healing time, excellent preservation of vulvar appearance, and the ability to render therapy without regional or general anesthesia. Kurwa and associates[207] and Lobraico and Grossweiner[208] have also reported on the successful use of PDT in cases of VIN refractory to traditional therapy.

Perhaps most exciting is the use of chemopreventive agents such as retinoids in the form of a retinyl acetate gel.[209] Retinoids may induce or accelerate the process of spontaneous regression, thereby reversing the precancerous changes. Thus transformed tissue may return to normal. The use of chemoprevention on the vulva is based on those studies in which retinoids were used on the uterine cervix and reversal has been successfully documented.

Finally, the antiviral agent cidofovir prevents replication of HPV by targeting viral DNA polymerase and preventing transcription. Koonsaeng and associates have recently demonstrated the therapeutic effectiveness of cidofovir in recurrent VIN that is resistant to interferon and retinoids.[210]

MOLECULAR RISK ASSESSMENT

It is anticipated that molecular markers may be able to determine which asymptomatic patients with a normal-appearing vulva are at risk for the development of VIN and vulvar cancer. With respect to VIN, *markers of differentiation* that have been studied involve keratin expression, specifically AE1, AE2, AE3, and CAM-5.2 antikeratin monoclonal antibodies.[25] Keratin expression[211] as well as Ki67[212] and markers for angiogenesis[213;214] may also prove to be useful. The role of HPV typing as a predictor of lesion behavior has been debated.[215] Certainly the risk of progression to invasive disease is minimal mainly in younger patients with HPV-positive, multifocal lesions.[216] Conversely, HPV-negative lesions are typically found in older women and exhibit a greater risk for progression to invasion.[217]

Clinical evaluation of visible lesions remains the cornerstone of diagnosis. Edwards and colleagues feel that because vulvar lesions may be easily visualized and accessible for biopsy, it is unlikely that research will be able to identify useful biomarkers that may be used.[25]

With respect to *general genomic markers* for invasive vulvar cancer, alterations in DNA ploidy and cytogenetics have been described, with aneuploidy being a common occurrence.[218-221] Specific genetic aberrations include HPV nucleic acids, given the hypothesis that VIN consists of two distinct entities (HPV-positive and HPV-negative lesions).[215-217] HPV DNA was more often found in vulvar cancers with adjacent foci of severe vulvar dysplasia, in younger patients, and in those with multifocal disease.[222] Nevertheless, the precise role of HPV as a cofactor in the etiology of vulvar cancer continues to be elusive. Because the presence of two viral oncogenes (E6 and E7) can result in the degradation of cellular tumor suppressor gene products (p53 and pRb, respectively), it is possible that they may serve as specific genetic markers through molecular staging.[223,224]

Markers of proliferation for invasive vulvar cancer include the S-phase fraction whereas those *markers of differentiation* include the extracellular and investigational glycoprotein tenacin.[25] Laminin expression as well as transforming growth factor (TGF)-alpha (a ligand for the epidermal growth factor receptor [EGF-R]) may also prove to be of use in the future.[225,226] *Tumor markers*, although sounding attractive, have not yet been shown to aid in the utility of facilitating the diagnosis of recurrent or metastatic disease. As an example, the serum squamous cell carcinoma (SCC) antigen levels were studied in 34 women with primary or recurrent vulvar cancer; of the 27 cases with primary disease, the SCC antigen level was elevated in only four cases, but all 27 had clinical evidence of advanced disease.[227] SCC levels might be of benefit in the rare patient who failed at distant sites without manifesting a locoregional recurrence. Plasminogen activators[228] have also been studied through use of invasive vulvar tissues, and lectins have been investigated in normal vulvar epithelium as well as in intraepithelial and invasive lesions.[229,230]

MALIGNANT MELANOMA

Cutaneous malignant melanoma accounts for 3% of all skin cancers but is responsible for two thirds of skin cancer–associated deaths. The disease derives from the basal layer of the epidermis, where neural crest cells give rise to melanocytes. These neuroectodermal tumors may also originate from junctional nevi or from compound nevi. The worldwide incidence of this aggressive lesion has been doubling every two decades.[231,232] Although only 1% to 2% of the body's surface area comprises the skin of the vulva, 3% to 7% of cutaneous melanomas arise there.[231] This may be attributed to the more complex cutaneous and mucosal surfaces that occur in the vulva, which may make this cutaneous organ more susceptible to the development of malignant melanoma. Overall, vulvar cancer accounts for approximately 8% of all gynecologic malignancies, and malignant melanoma of the vulva represent approximately 8% to 10% of all vulvar malignancies, occurring less often only than squamous cell carcinomas.[232] The disease was first described by Hewett in 1861.[233]

Three distinct histologic types of vulvar melanoma have been described. The *superficial spreading melanoma* occurs when the radial growth of the melanoma involves four or more adjacent rete ridges.[234] *Nodular melanoma* has no adjacent radial growth phase, and the *acral lentiginous melanoma* is restricted to the vestibule and displays both vertical and radial growth phases.[234] When the diagnosis of a malignant melanoma of the vulva is the subject of debate among pathologists, immunohistochemical staining is mandatory and should include a panel of melanoma markers (e.g., S-100 protein or Melanoma Specific Antigen [HMB45]) and epithelial, hematopoietic, histiocytic, neural, and neuroendocrine antibodies.

Although a surgical FIGO stage for vulvar cancer may be assigned to a vulvar melanoma, progress in understanding and managing this disease has occurred through the development of prognosticating microstaging systems. In 1969 Clark and colleagues defined five levels of tumor invasion in cutaneous melanoma of nongenital origin, the concept of which was useful for future determination of staging, prognostication, and treatment.[235] Clark's level I contains neoplastic cells confined to the epithelium, whereas a lesion that penetrates the basement membrane and extends into the loose papillary dermis is designated Clark's level II. The reticular dermis is invaded in Clark's levels III and IV, and the subcutaneous adipose tissue is violated in Clark's level V.

In 1970, Breslow and co-workers advanced the concept that tumor thickness was paramount.[236] Tumor thickness may be measured with an ocular micrometer. Breslow levels 1 through 5 progress with increments of 0.75 mm, with a Breslow Level 5 lesion being thicker than 3.0 mm. During the subsequent two decades, many reports commented on the usefulness of the Clark and Breslow microstaging systems. Unfortunately, the Clark's system would ultimately prove to be too subjective. For this reason Chung and colleagues designed a new microstaging system specifically for the staging of vulvar melanoma.[237] The Chung system is a modification of the Clark's microstaging system. Clark's levels I and V correspond to Chung's levels I and V; however, the remaining Chung's levels are differentiated by including measurements from the granular layer of vulvar skin or the outermost epithelial layer of the squamous mucosa, with Chung's level II attained at 1 mm of invasion, Chung's level III at 1 to 2 mm of invasion, and Chung's level IV at greater than 2mm of invasion but not into the underlying adipose tissue.

The Chung and Breslow microstaging recommendations are most frequently used in the staging of vulvar melanoma and can be used to estimate the risk of regional and distant metastases. Recently, however, the American Joint Committee on Cancer (AJCC) has formally approved the final version of a revised melanoma staging system that was constructed along the tumor-node-metastasis (TNM) classification scheme.[238] The T classification is stratified by tumor thickness and ulceration status; the N classification is determined by the number of nodal metastases and whether the nodes are microscopically or macroscopically involved; the M classification is based on site of distant dissemination and whether the serum lactate dehydrogenase is normal or elevated. The microstaging systems of Clark, Chung, and Breslow are outlined in Table 8-5; please refer to the AJCC's 2001 consensus statement for more information about the new but complex TNM classification scheme.[238]

The apparent "natural history" of vulvar melanoma underscores the importance of early detection. Most series have attributed a poor prognosis to the tendencies for local recurrence and for the melanocytes to establish distant metastases. Some investigators have speculated, however, that the aggressive behavior is the clinical manifestation of the advanced disease that is usually present upon discovery because the vulva has a low level of accessibility and visibility, compared with other cutaneous sites.

Ragnarsson-Olding and colleagues from the Radiumhemmet in Stockholm conducted a 25-year nationwide study of 219 Swedish women diagnosed with a new vulvar melanoma. The study results were recorded in the Swedish National Cancer Registry from 1960 through 1984. A complete follow-up of survival until 1994 was legally mandated.[239,240] This nation-wide Cancer Registry has been calculated to represent 99% of all cancer patients in Sweden and is linked to the National Causes of Death Registry by means of an individual 10-digit identification code. With permission from the Swedish National Data Inspection Authority and the Human Ethical Committee at the Karolinska Institute, the investigators broke the codes, reviewed all clinical records, and concluded that the historically cited poorer prognosis for patients with vulvar melanoma, compared with other cutaneous melanomas, was supported by their 5-year relative survival rate of 47%. The corresponding survival rate for patients of both genders with cutaneous melanoma has improved from roughly 50% in 1960 to 80% in the 1990s.[240] The Swedish investigators suggested that this difference was to a large extent due to the earlier detection of other cutaneous melanomas. The high recurrence rate and low survival rates are similar to those observed with truncal melanomas rather than the somewhat more favorable extremity melanomas.

There are important epidemiologic considerations when comparing vulvar mela-noma with other cutaneous melanomas. First, the mean age at diagnosis of cutaneous

Table 8-5

Microstaging Level	Clark et al[255]	Breslow et al[256]	Chung et al[257]
Level I	All tumor cells above basement membrane (in situ)	<0.75 mm depth of invasion	Intraepithelial
Level II	Tumor extends to papillary dermis	0.76 – 1.5 mm depth of invasion	< 1mm invasion into dermis or lamina propria
Level III	Tumor extends to interface between papillary and reticular dermis	1.51-2.25 mm depth of invasion	1 to 2 mm invasion into subepithelial tissue
Level IV	Tumor extends between bundles of collagen of reticular dermis	2.26-3.0 mm depth of invasion	> 2 mm invasion into fibrous or fibromuscular tissue
Level V	Tumor invasion of subcutaneous tissue	> 3 mm depth of invasion	Extension into subcutaneous fat[*]

melanoma is 30 to 40 years, with one third of patients diagnosed before the age of 45 years.[234] In contrast, most series have noted a mean age of older than 60 years for vulvar melanomas; it is rarely diagnosed in young women or teenagers. In the Swedish study, only 11 of 219 subjects were diagnosed with malignant melanoma of the vulva before the age of 45 years. Demographic factors such as birthing numbers, hereditary influences, and hormonal exposure may be unrelated to the development of vulvar melanoma.[239]

Melanoma typically manifests in skin with low levels of pigmentation and is known to occur with greater frequency among white women than in African Americans and Asians. Although an association between the development of malignant melanoma and ultraviolet radiation exposure has been known for some time, this does little to explain the etiology of vulvar melanoma, which does not lend itself easily to ultraviolet irradiation by virtue of its specific location.

The most common presenting symptom in women with vulvar melanoma is the discovery of a lump.[237] Bleeding and pruritus may also occur, but ulceration, discharge, and dysuria are only occasionally reported. Systemic manifestations include nocturia, weight loss, headaches, and emesis. The primary anatomic site of origin is often either a labium majorum, labium minorum, or the clitoris (Figures 8-15, A and B). According to the 1999 Swedish study, the labia majora were involved in 27.3% of cases, the labia minora in 19.2% of subjects, and the clitoral area in 30.8% of cases.[239] The investigators also examined the histologic localization and reported that in 45.5% of cases, the lesions occurred in glabrous skin; malignant melanoma was found at the junctional area in 34.8% of subjects and in the hairy skin of 11.6% of cases.

Many women will not always recognize a preexisting nevus, but when one is known to be present, it may be the *change* in a mole that is the presenting symptom in a woman for whom a diagnosis of vulvar melanoma is imminent. Tissue sampling is imperative to establish a diagnosis and the biopsies must extend into the subcutaneous tissue to allow pathologic evaluation of the thickness of the lesion.

Although the pathogenesis of vulvar melanoma has not been developed sufficiently to allow the application of good preventative measures, some considerations are intuitive. Specifically, fair-skinned women are at risk and therefore a high index of suspicion should be employed when examining the vulva, and an immediate biopsy must be performed on any new lesion or change in a preexisting nevus. Although a premalignant phase has yet to be identified, early diagnosis may translate to enhanced survival, similar to what is currently observed for persons afflicted with a cutaneous melanoma.

Quality of life may be considered as important as absolute survival.[241-243] Hence early detection of vulvar melanoma allows for more conservative vulvar surgery to preserve psychosexual self-image and enhance cosmesis. Furthermore, sentinel lymph node identification that employs lymphoscintigraphy and isosulfan blue dye may also be applicable to early vulvar melanomas, thus preventing the need for a formal inguinofemoral lymphadenectomy when the sentinel is negative and thereby preserving lower extremity lymphatic drainage.[244-248] These methods of treating the primary lesion with less radical surgery and limiting the groin dissection follow the same arguments set forth previously for SCCs of the vulva.

EXTRAMAMMARY PAGET'S DISEASE OF THE VULVA

The clinician-pathologist Sir James Paget published the first description of Paget's disease from St. Bartholomew's Hospital in London in 1874.[249] In the original series, the disease was

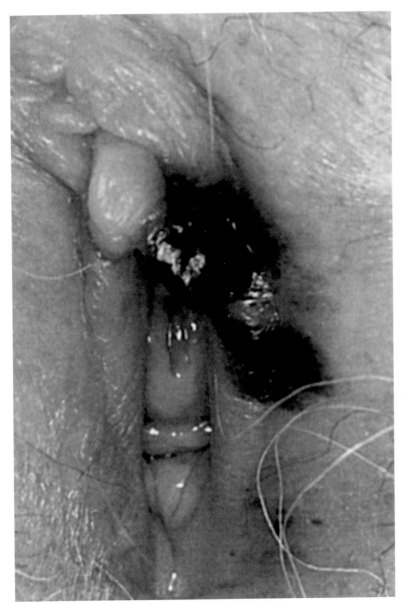

A
FIGURE 8-15
Malignant melanoma of the vulva. **A,** Note the dark hue and irregular borders.

detected on the nipple and areola and was associated with an underlying adenocarcinoma of the breast. The series that have since followed are notable for a 100% association with underlying breast malignancy. Paget's disease may also occur at sites distant from the breast ("extramammary Paget's disease" {EMPD}), in which case the association with underlying adenocarcinoma is variable.

EMPD of the vulva was first described by Dubrewilh in 1901 as a variant of mammary Paget's carcinoma.[250] By 1955, Woodruff contributed two of his own cases to the existing world literature, bringing the total number of reported cases to 23.[251] From his detailed analysis Woodruff concluded that wide local excision was the treatment of choice, provided that the underlying tissue could be removed deeply enough to include the skin appendages. By the end of the century, nearly 250 cases of EMPD of the vulva had been reported.[252-259]

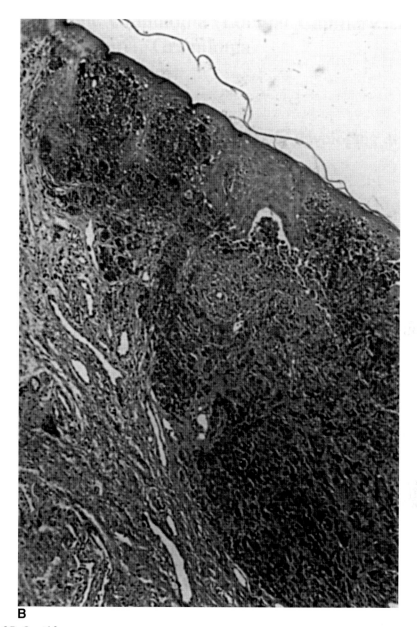

B

FIGURE 8-15, Cont'd
B, Superficial spreading malignant melanoma with vertical (invasive) growth. The superficial spreading component is present adjacent to the invasive melanoma. Melanin pigment is present in the superficial spreading and invasive components. The tumor has eroded the overlying epithelium.

The EMPD of the vulva is a lesion found most commonly in postmenopausal Caucasian women, with the mean age at diagnosis approximately 65 years.[252] When EMPD of the vulva is associated with an underlying adenocarcinoma (0%-25% of cases), it is very aggressive, with metastases to the lymph nodes and other sites. The natural history of the intraepithelial disease involves multiple local recurrences over a period of many years, often requiring numerous surgical procedures.[260]

The clinical manifestations of EMPD are varied and lack an observed pattern of progression. This has led some investigators to speculate that a disease spectrum exists involving several separate pathologic entities.[261-268] EMPD may be confined to the epidermis (noninvasive Paget's disease), or it may be associated with a contiguous invasive adenocarcinoma considered to have a cutaneous adnexal gland nature (i.e., invasive Paget's disease).[267] A third category of patients with EMPD has been reported and shows a variety of types of carcinomas arising in nearby internal as well as distant organs (e.g., rectum, prostate, bladder, bile duct).[267,268] Cases in this third category of EMPD with noncutaneous, noncontiguous "underlying carcinomas" are somewhat heterogeneous, with invasive malignancies sometimes only tenuously associated with the cutaneous Paget's disease phenomenon.

Aside from age and ethnicity, there are no known risk factors; for this reason a high index of suspicion must be maintained by the clinician when examining any red lesion of the vulva. Paget's disease of the vulva may manifest with an isolated flat reddish lesion or may be composed of a bright reddish base upon which are scattered islands of white epithelium or bridges of hyperkeratotic skin (Figure 8-16, A). The trap lies in dismissing the lesion as simple eczema or monilia candidiasis, and it is only after an extraordinary delay in diagnosis during which time topical remedies have failed that the physician is usually prompted to perform a biopsy. The blame does not always lie with the gynecologist because although most series contain reports of pruritus, pain, and burning upon presentation, there are many cases underscored by considerable patient delay.

The disease begins on the hair-bearing portions of the vulva, within the genital folds, or in the perianal region, thus being limited at the onset to the apocrine gland–bearing regions. The umbilicus, axilla, and external ear canal represent additional extramammary sites where Paget's disease has been found in association with apocrine glands. The innate pathologic

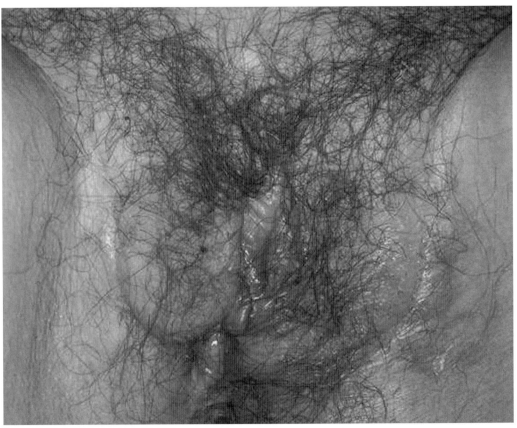

A

FIGURE 8-16
Extramammary Paget's disease of the vulva. **A,** Typical clinical appearance.

intuition for clinical detective work led many to surmise that because mammary Paget's disease is always associated with underlying malignancy, the presence of Paget's cells involving another organ signals a similar apocrine malignancy in the underlying glands.[252]

Clearly the most striking feature that distinguishes Paget's disease of the vulva from Paget's disease in other sites is the low association with underlying adenocarcinoma. Indeed, an adenocarcinoma is present in the majority of cases of nonvulvar Paget's disease. As stated previously, this association approaches 100% when the disease arises in the breast, whereas the incidence of underlying adenocarcinoma is significantly lower among the 250 cases of vulvar EMPD described in the literature.[252-259]

In addition to an associated underlying adenocarcinoma, the development of Paget's disease in the vulva may signify a malignancy at a separate site.[268] For example, Breen and colleagues surveyed the English-language medical literature and pooled 98 recorded cases of EMPD of the vulva, in which the association with a noncontiguous carcinoma reached

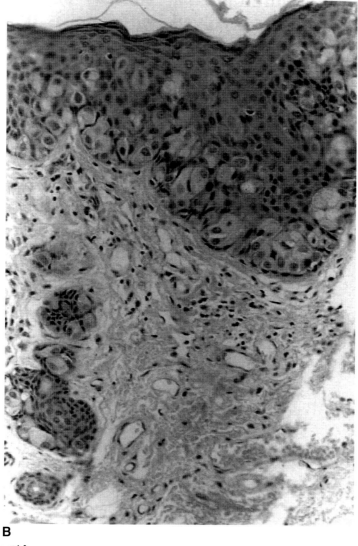

B

FIGURE 8-16, cont'd
B, Histologic section demonstrating Paget cells with prominent clear cytoplasm throughout the epithelium.

25%.[253] Breast cancer occurred most frequently, followed by SCCs of the vulva, uterine cervix, and vagina.[253] The investigators found several cases of EMPD of the vulva associated with several noncontiguous malignancies—specifically, three basal cell carcinomas of the skin, two of the urinary bladder, and two gallbladder carcinomas.[253] An unknown carcinogenic stimulus that could affect the epidermis of the vulva, the uterine cervix, and other structures in the pelvis, independently and concomitantly, may exist and account for multiple malignancies in one patient. Thus the woman with EMPD of the vulva presents a means of cancer prevention and early detection. A thorough and comprehensive physical examination including a solid pelvic examination and computed tomography or magnetic resonance imaging is essential to exclude the presence of other malignancies nearby.

Histologically, the Paget's cell occurs in nests clustered close to the basal layer or in a file along the basement membrane within the epidermal adnexae.[257] Paget's cells may be detected in hair follicles, apocrine and eccrine ducts, secretory apparatus, and even in sebaceous glands.[257] When they occur within the epidermis with epithelial maturation, the Paget's cells occur at progressively higher levels, eventually being shed at the surface along with keratinized squames where they can be identified in cytologic preparations from contact smears (e.g., a vulvar Pap).[257] The cells are large, with abundant cytoplasm that stain faintly with hematoxylin and eosin (Figure 8-16, B). The nuclei appear folded and the chromatin is finely dispersed, with rare mitotic figures. The Paget's cells stain strongly with periodic acid-Schiff (PAS), and in many cases organelle populations similar to those of apocrine and eccrine secretory cells have been observed, whereas in those cases of Paget's disease in which the cells lack secretory structure, they are possessed by tonofilaments and desmosomes characteristic of keratinocytes.[257]

Woodruff's and Pauerstein's concept of histogenesis of the Paget's cell reconciles many of the microscopic and clinical observations.[269] An aberration of differentiation of an epidermal stem cell, the Paget's cell may arise in situ from a primitive precursor cell in the epidermis and adnexal structures. Thus when Paget's disease arises from stem cells in the apocrine apparatus, the Paget cells contain secretory organelles, but when it arises from squamous basal cells, the Paget cells lack a Golgi complex and are rich in desmosomes. Thus one can follow the concept of histogenesis from a basic stem cell capable of multiple lines of differentiation. However, regardless of their local origin, Paget cells may migrate within the epithelium both horizontally and vertically, thus accounting for the multiple recurrences that often develop in patients and occasionally invest in an autologous orthotopic skin graft.

Bergen and co-workers reported on 14 cases of EMPD of the vulva and concluded that it is almost always a noninvasive intraepithelial lesion similar in behavior to SCC in situ of the vulva and can be managed conservatively without loss of sexual function and cosmesis.[256] Initial treatment is surgical and may consist of wide local excision or, in selected cases, of a skinning vulvectomy with split-thickness skin grafting as described by Rutledge and Sinclair.[185]

Whereas a mandatory intraoperative frozen section analysis of proposed surgical margins is important to ensure resection of all clinically involved areas, it may not be as significant as was once believed because local recurrences are common despite negative margins of resection. This is due to the multifocal nature of the disease. An extremely uncommon occurrence is the finding of relapsing disease in the skin graft, which typically has been taken as a dermatome from the medial thigh.[263] Perhaps there is an underlying subcutaneous substance that is able to transform the overlying epidermis regardless of whether it is primary or orthotopic. Another explanation for such clinical behavior may be attributed to "retrodissemination," a migratory behavior of Paget's cells into the skin graft from a peripheral occult metastatic site.[263]

Recurrence should be addressed from a philosophical angle. Recurrent Paget's disease of the vulva does not pose the threat carried by the original presentation of the disease because a subjacent carcinoma will have been excluded during the initial operation. Although there have been a few cases of Paget's disease "progressing" to invasive Paget's disease over time,[264-267] the de novo development of an underlying adenocarcinoma with a recurrence has not yet been reported. For this reason, recurrent areas should be considered confined to the epidermis and adnexal structures. Although reexcision still remains the treatment of choice, topical therapy employing 5-FU or laser treatment may be considered.

The disease without underlying adenocarcinoma remains, for the most part, an intraepithelial lesion and has only occasionally been reported to become invasive and metastasize. Patients with vulvar Paget's disease are at risk for the development of multiple local recurrences, metastatic disease, and second primary tumors. The occurrence of EMPD on the vulva may be regarded as a cutaneous signal that invasive carcinoma may exist elsewhere in the body, with an estimated rate of up to 25%. The breasts and axilla should be examined carefully by palpation and screening mammography, and the vulva, perineum, vagina, and uterine cervix should be screened both by colposcopy and by cytologic preparations. If an underlying or associated carcinoma cannot be found in the breasts, external genitalia, vagina, or uterine cervix, then other areas should be searched. In every patient, close follow-up is prudent and all symptoms should be thoroughly investigated.

CONCLUSION

Writing from the Gynaecological Oncology Unit of the Royal Hospital for Women in New South Wales, Grant conceded to Giles and Kneale[93] that vulvar cancer appears to be the Cinderella of oncology and stated that it frequently goes unrecognized for long periods, is often poorly treated by those who should know better, and, just as one slipper does not fit all feet, one method of therapy does not treat all vulvar neoplasms.[270] Prevention is the cornerstone of effective therapy, and careful periodic examinations conducted by a sophisticated gynecologist should detect the vast majority of (if not all) intraepithelial lesions. In addition, with the breast paradigm as a template, women should be encouraged to self-examine.[271] Finally, although no chemopreventive agents are available for women with VIN and invasive vulvar cancer, several HPV vaccine strategies are being investigated and appear to be promising.[272,273]

REFERENCES

1. Morgagni G, Alexander B: *The seats and causes of diseases investigated by anatomy; in five books, containing a great variety of dissections, with remarks. To which are added . . . copious indexes.* London, A. Millar; and T. Cadell, his successor [etc.]; 1769.

2. Sappey PC: *Traite d'anatomie, physiologie et pathologie des vaisseaux lymphatiques, considerés chez l'homme et les vertebres.* Paris, Adrien Delahaye, 1876.

3. Basset A: *L'epithelioma primitif du clitoris: son retentissment ganglionaire et son traitment operatoire.* Paris, G. Steinheil, 1912.

4. Taussig FJ: Cancer of the vulva: analysis of 155 cases, 1911-40. *Am J Obstet Gynecol* 1940;40:764.

5. Taussig FJ: Results in treatment of lymph node metastasis in cancer of the cervix and the vulva. *Am J Roent* 1941;45:813.

6. Way SA: *Malignant disease of the female genital tract.* Philadelphia, Blakiston, 1951.

7. DiSaia PJ, Creasman WT, Rich WM: An alternate approach to early cancer of the vulva. *Am J Obstet Gynecol* 1979;133(7):825-832.

8. De Cicco C, Sideri M, Bartolomei M, et al: Sentinel node biopsy in early vulvar cancer. *Br J Cancer* 2000;82(2):295-299.

9. Moore DH, Thomas GM, Montana GS, et al: Preoperative chemoradiation for advanced vulvar cancer: a phase II study of the Gynecologic Oncology Group. *Int J Radiat Oncol Biol Phys* 1998;42(1):79-85.

10. Garsia S, Origoni M, Sideri M, et al: Preneoplastic lesions of the vulva. *Eur J Gynaecol Oncol* 1988;9(4):342-345.

11. Richart RM: Clinical and laboratory studies of cervical dysplasia. *Trans N Engl Obstet Gynecol Soc* 1964;18:105-111.

12. Crum CP, Braun LA, Shah KV, et al: Vulvar intraepithelial neoplasia: correlation of nuclear DNA content and the presence of a human papilloma virus (HPV) structural antigen. *Cancer* 1982;49(3):468-471.

13. Crum CP, Fu YS, Levine RU, et al: Intraepithelial squamous lesions of the vulva: biologic and histologic criteria for the distinction of condylomas from vulvar intraepithelial neoplasia. *Am J Obstet Gynecol* 1982;144(1):77-83.

14. Crum CP: Vulvar intraepithelial neoplasia: the concept and its application. *Hum Pathol* 1982;13(3):187-189.

15. Crum CP, Liskow A, Petras P, et al: Vulvar intraepithelial neoplasia (severe atypia and carcinoma in situ): a clinicopathologic analysis of 41 cases. *Cancer* 1984;54(7):1429-1434.

16. Kiryu H, Ackerman AB: A critique of current classifications of vulvar diseases. *Am J Dermatopathol* 1990;12(4):377-392.

17. Scully RE, Boniglio TA, Kurman RJ, et al: *Histological typing of female genital tract tumours,* ed 2. New York, Springer-Verlag, 1994.

18. Edwards L: Desquamative vulvitis. *Dermatol Clin* 1992;10(2):325-337.

19. Shatz P, Bergeron C, Wilkinson EJ, et al: Vulvar intraepithelial neoplasia and skin appendage involvement. *Obstet Gynecol* 1989;74(5):769-774.

20. Baggish MS, Sze EH, Adelson MD, et al: Quantitative evaluation of the skin and accessory appendages in vulvar carcinoma in situ. *Obstet Gynecol* 1989;74(2):169-174.

21. Wilkinson EJ, Kneale BL, Lynch PJ: Report of the ISSVD terminology committee. *J Reprod Med* 1986;31(10):973-974.

22. Lininger RA, Tavassoli FA: The pathology of vulvar neoplasia. *Curr Opin Obstet Gynecol* 1996;8(1):63-68.

23. Wright VC, Chapman W: Intraepithelial neoplasia of the lower female genital tract: etiology, investigation, and management. *Semin Surg Oncol* 1992;8(4):180-190.

24. Jones RW: The natural history of vulvar intraepithelial neoplasia. *Br J Obstet Gynaecol* 1995;102(10):764-766.

25. Edwards CL, Tortolero-Luna G, Linares AC, et al: Vulvar intraepithelial neoplasia and vulvar cancer. *Obstet Gynecol Clin North Am* 1996;23(2):295-324.

26. Beckmann AM, Acker R, Christiansen AE, et al: Human papillomavirus infection in women with multicentric squamous cell neoplasia. *Am J Obstet Gynecol* 1991;165(5 Pt 1):1431-1437.

27. Scully RE: Definition of precursors in gynecologic cancer. *Cancer* 1981;48(2 Suppl):531-537.

28. Hewitt H: Pre-neoplastic lesions of the vulva. *Eur J Gynaecol Oncol* 1988;9(5):377-380.

29. Sturgeon SR, Brinton LA, Devesa SS, et al: In situ and invasive vulvar cancer incidence trends (1973 to 1987). *Am J Obstet Gynecol* 1992;166(5):1482-1485.

30. Iversen T, Tretli S: Intraepithelial and invasive squamous cell neoplasia of the vulva: trends in incidence, recurrence, and survival rate in Norway. *Obstet Gynecol* 1998;91(6):969-972.

31. Jones RW, Rowan DM: Vulvar intraepithelial neoplasia III: a clinical study of the outcome in 113 cases with relation to the later development of invasive vulvar carcinoma. *Obstet Gynecol* 1994;84(5):741-745.

32. Ansink AC, Heintz AP: Epidemiology and etiology of squamous cell carcinoma of the vulva. *Eur J Obstet Gynecol Reprod Biol* 1993;48(2):111-115.

33. Brinton LA, Nasca PC, Mallin K, et al: Case-control study of cancer of the vulva. *Obstet Gynecol* 1990;75(5):859-866.

34. Campion MJ, Hacker NF: Vulvar intraepithelial neoplasia and carcinoma. *Semin Cutan Med Surg* 1998;17(3):205-212.

35. Giles G, Farrugia H, Silver B: Cancer registration in Victoria, Australia, 1982-1987. *Eur J Cancer* 1991;27(5):659-662.

36. Woodruff JD: Carcinoma in situ of the vulva. *Clin Obstet Gynecol* 1991;34(3):669-676.

37. Hart WR: Vulvar intraepithelial neoplasia: historical aspects and current status. *Int J Gynecol Pathol* 2001;20(1):16-30.

38. Jebakumar S, Woolley PD, Bhattacharyya MN: Vulval intraepithelial neoplasia. *Int J STD AIDS* 1996;7(1):10-13.

39. Iversen T: The value of groin palpation in epidermoid carcinoma of the vulva. *Gynecol Oncol* 1981;12(3):291-295.

40. Shepherd JH: Revised FIGO staging for gynaecological cancer. *Br J Obstet Gynaecol* 1989;96(8): 889-892.

41. Beller U, Sideri M, Maisonneuve P, et al: Carcinoma of the vulva. *J Epidemiol Biostat* 2001;6(1):155-173.

42. Rastkar G, Okagaki T, Twiggs LB, et al: Early invasive and in situ warty carcinoma of the vulva: clinical, histologic, and electron microscopic study with particular reference to viral association. *Am J Obstet Gynecol* 1982;143(7):814-820.

43. Pilotti S, Rilke F, Shah KV, et al: Immunohistochemical and ultrastructural evidence of papilloma virus infection associated with in situ and microinvasive squamous cell carcinoma of the vulva. *Am J Surg Pathol* 1984;8(10):751-761.

44. Gupta J, Pilotti S, Shah KV, et al: Human papillomavirus-associated early vulvar neoplasia investigated by in situ hybridization. *Am J Surg Pathol* 1987;11(6):430-434.

45. Beckmann AM, Kiviat NB, Daling JR, et al: Human papillomavirus type 16 in multifocal neoplasia of the female genital tract. *Int J Gynecol Pathol* 1988;7(1):39-47.

46. Mitrani-Rosenbaum S, Gal D, Friedman M, et al: Papillomaviruses in lesions of the lower genital tract in Israeli patients. *Eur J Cancer Clin Oncol* 1988;24(4):725-731.

47. Kaufman RH, Bornstein J, Adam E, et al: Human papillomavirus and herpes simplex virus in vulvar squamous cell carcinoma in situ. *Am J Obstet Gynecol* 1988;158(4):862-871.

48. Downey GO, Okagaki T, Ostrow RS, et al: Condylomatous carcinoma of the vulva with special reference to human papillomavirus DNA. *Obstet Gynecol* 1988;72(1):68-73.

49. Carson LF, Twiggs LB, Okagaki T, et al: Human papillomavirus DNA in adenosquamous carcinoma and squamous cell carcinoma of the vulva. *Obstet Gynecol* 1988;72(1):63-67.

50. Bornstein J, Kaufman RH, Adam E, et al: Multicentric intraepithelial neoplasia involving the vulva: clinical features and association with human papillomavirus and herpes simplex virus. *Cancer* 1988;62(8):1601-1604.

51. Bistoletti P, Zellbi A, Moreno-Lopez J, et al: Genital papillomavirus infection after treatment for cervical intraepithelial neoplasia (CIN) III. *Cancer* 1988;62(9):2056-2059.

52. Husseinzadeh N, Newman NJ, Wesseler TA: Vulvar intraepithelial neoplasia: a clinicopathological study of carcinoma in situ of the vulva. *Gynecol Oncol* 1989;33(2):157-163.

53. Pilotti S, Rotola A, D'Amato L, et al: Vulvar carcinomas: search for sequences homologous to human papillomavirus and herpes simplex virus DNA. *Mod Pathol* 1990;3(4):442-448.

54. Milde-Langosch K, Becker G, Loning T: Human papillomavirus and c-myc/c-erbB2 in uterine and vulvar lesions. *Virchows Arch A Pathol Anat Histopathol* 1991;419(6):479-485.

55. Toki T, Kurman RJ, Park JS, et al: Probable nonpapillomavirus etiology of squamous cell carcinoma of the vulva in older women: a clinicopathologic study using in situ hybridization and polymerase chain reaction. *Int J Gynecol Pathol* 1991;10(2):107-125.

56. Schneider A, Meinhardt G, Kirchmayr R, et al: Prevalence of human papillomavirus genomes in tissues from the lower genital tract as detected by molecular in situ hybridization. *Int J Gynecol Pathol* 1991;10(1):1-14.

57. Rusk D, Sutton GP, Look KY, et al: Analysis of invasive squamous cell carcinoma of the vulva and vulvar intraepithelial neoplasia for the presence of human papillomavirus DNA. *Obstet Gynecol* 1991;77(6):918-922.

58. Andersen WA, Franquemont DW, Williams J, et al: Vulvar squamous cell carcinoma and papillomaviruses: two separate entities? *Am J Obstet Gynecol* 1991;165(2):329-335; discussion 335-326.

59. Park JS, Rader JS, Wu TC, et al: HPV-16 viral transcripts in vulvar neoplasia: preliminary studies. *Gynecol Oncol* 1991;42(3):250-255.

60. Brandenberger AW, Rudlinger R, Hanggi W, et al: Detection of human papillomavirus in vulvar carcinoma: a study by in situ hybridisation. *Arch Gynecol Obstet* 1992;252(1):31-35.

61. Della Torre G, Donghi R, Longoni A, et al: HPV DNA in intraepithelial neoplasia and carcinoma of the vulva and penis. *Diagn Mol Pathol* 1992;1(1): 25-30.

62. Vuopala S, Pollanen R, Kauppila A, et al: Detection and typing of human papillomavirus infection affecting the cervix, vagina, and vulva: comparison of DNA hybridization with cytological, colposcopic and histological examinations. *Arch Gynecol Obstet* 1993;253(2):75-83.

63. Mitchell MF, Prasad CJ, Silva EG, et al: Second genital primary squamous neoplasms in vulvar carcinoma: viral and histopathologic correlates. *Obstet Gynecol* 1993;81(1):13-18.

64. Fang BS, Guedes AC, Munoz LC, et al: Human papillomavirus type 16 variants isolated from vulvar Bowenoid papulosis. *J Med Virol* 1993;41(1): 49-54.

65. Madeleine MM, Daling JR, Carter JJ, et al: Cofactors with human papillomavirus in a population-based study of vulvar cancer. *J Natl Cancer Inst* 1997;89(20):1516-1523.

66. Hildesheim A, Han CL, Brinton LA, et al: Human papillomavirus type 16 and risk of preinvasive and invasive vulvar cancer: results from a seroepidemiological case-control study. *Obstet Gynecol* 1997;90(5):748-754.

67. Junge J, Poulsen H, Horn T, et al: Human papillomavirus (HPV) in vulvar dysplasia and carcinoma in situ. *APMIS* 1995;103(7-8):501-510.

68. Kagie MJ, Kenter GG, Zomerdijk-Nooijen Y, et al: Human papillomavirus infection in squamous cell carcinoma of the vulva, in various synchronous epithelial changes and in normal vulvar skin. *Gynecol Oncol* 1997;67(2):178-183.

69. Sun Y, Hildesheim A, Brinton LA, et al: Human papillomavirus-specific serologic response in vulvar neoplasia. *Gynecol Oncol* 1996;63(2):200-203.

70. Monk BJ, Burger RA, Lin F, et al: Prognostic significance of human papillomavirus DNA in vulvar carcinoma. *Obstet Gynecol* 1995;85(5 Pt 1):709-715.

71. Frisch M, Goodman MT: Human papillomavirus-associated carcinomas in Hawaii and the mainland U.S. *Cancer* 2000;88(6):1464-1469.

72. van Beurden M, ten Kate FW, Tjong AHSP, et al: Human papillomavirus DNA in multicentric vulvar intraepithelial neoplasia. *Int J Gynecol Pathol* 1998;17(1):12-16.

73. Flowers LC, Wistuba, II, Scurry J, et al: Genetic changes during the multistage pathogenesis of human papillomavirus positive and negative vulvar carcinomas. *J Soc Gynecol Investig* 1999;6(4):213-221.

74. Trimble CL, Hildesheim A, Brinton LA, et al: Heterogeneous etiology of squamous carcinoma of the vulva. *Obstet Gynecol* 1996;87(1):59-64.

75. Sagerman PM, Choi YJ, Hu Y, et al: Human papilloma virus, vulvar dystrophy, and vulvar carcinoma: differential expression of human papillomavirus and vulvar dystrophy in the presence and absence of squamous cell carcinoma of the vulva. *Gynecol Oncol* 1996;61(3):328-332.

76. Pilotti S, D'Amato L, Della Torre G, et al: Papillomavirus, p53 alteration, and primary carcinoma of the vulva. *Diagn Mol Pathol* 1995;4(4):239-248.

77. van Beurden M, ten Kate FJ, Smits HL, et al: Multifocal vulvar intraepithelial neoplasia grade III and multicentric lower genital tract neoplasia is associated with transcriptionally active human papillomavirus. *Cancer* 1995;75(12):2879-2884.

78. Reagan JW: Vaginal and vulvar disease. In Wied GL, Keebler CM, Koss LG, editors: *Compendium of diagnostic cytology.* Chicago, International Academy of Cytology, 1988.

79. Muir C, Waterhouse J, Mack T: Cancer incidence in five continents. Volume V. *IARC Sci Publ* 1987;V(88):1-970.

80. Anastasiadis P, Skaphida P, Koutlaki N, et al: Trends in epidemiology of preinvasive and invasive vulvar neoplasias: 13 year retrospective analysis in Thrace, Greece. *Arch Gynecol Obstet* 2000;264(2):74-79.

81. Aynaud O, Asselain B, Bergeron C, et al: [Intraepithelial carcinoma and invasive carcinoma of the vulva, vagina and penis in Ile-de-france. Enquete PETRI on 423 cases]. *Ann Dermatol Venereol* 2000;127(5):479-483.

82. Tidy JA, Soutter WP, Luesley DM, et al: Management of lichen sclerosus and intraepithelial neoplasia of the vulva in the UK. *J R Soc Med* 1996;89(12):699-701.

83. Clinicopathologic analysis of 370 cases of vulvar intraepithelial neoplasia. Italian Study Group on Vulvar Disease. *J Reprod Med* 1996;41(9):665-670.

84. Bjorge T, Hennig EM, Skare GB, et al: Second primary cancers in patients with carcinoma in situ of the uterine cervix: the Norwegian experience 1970-1992. *Int J Cancer* 1995;62(1):29-33.

85. Sherman KJ, Daling JR, Chu J, et al: Multiple primary tumours in women with vulvar neoplasms: a case-control study. *Br J Cancer* 1988;57(4):423-427.

86. Bernstein SG, Kovacs BR, Townsend DE, et al: Vulvar carcinoma in situ. *Obstet Gynecol* 1983;61(3):304-307.

87. Iversen T, Abeler V, Kolstad P: Squamous cell carcinoma in situ of the vulva: a clinical and histopathological study. *Gynecol Oncol* 1981;11(2):224-229.

88. Newcomb PA, Weiss NS, Daling JR: Incidence of vulvar carcinoma in relation to menstrual, reproductive, and medical factors. *J Natl Cancer Inst* 1984;73(2):391-396.

89. Joura EA, Losch A, Haider-Angeler MG, et al: Trends in vulvar neoplasia: increasing incidence of vulvar intraepithelial neoplasia and squamous cell carcinoma of the vulva in young women. *J Reprod Med* 2000;45(8):613-615.

90. Basta A, Adamek K, Pitynski K: Intraepithelial neoplasia and early stage vulvar cancer: epidemiological, clinical, and virological observations. *Eur J Gynaecol Oncol* 1999;20(2):111-114.

91. Jones RW, Baranyai J, Stables S: Trends in squamous cell carcinoma of the vulva: the influence of vulvar intraepithelial neoplasia. *Obstet Gynecol* 1997;90(3):448-452.

92. Kuppers V, Stiller M, Somville T, et al: Risk factors for recurrent VIN: role of multifocality and grade of disease. *J Reprod Med* 1997;42(3):140-144.

93. Giles GG, Kneale BL: Vulvar cancer: the Cinderella of gynaecological oncology. *Aust N Z J Obstet Gynaecol* 1995;35(1):71-75.

94. Sturgeon SR, Ziegler RG, Brinton LA, et al: Diet and the risk of vulvar cancer. *Ann Epidemiol* 1991;1(5):427-437.

95. Parazzini F, Moroni S, Negri E, et al: Selected food intake and risk of vulvar cancer. *Cancer* 1995;76(11):2291-2296.

96. Andreasson B, Bock JE, Weberg E: Invasive cancer in the vulvar region. *Acta Obstet Gynecol Scand* 1982;61(2):113-119.

97. Mabuchi K, Bross DS, Kessler II: Epidemiology of cancer of the vulva: a case-control study. *Cancer* 1985;55(8):1843-1848.

98. Parazzini F, La Vecchia C, Garsia S, et al: Determinants of invasive vulvar cancer risk: an Italian case-control study. *Gynecol Oncol* 1993;48(1):50-55.

99. Kirschner CV, Yordan EL, De Geest K, et al: Smoking, obesity, and survival in squamous cell carcinoma of the vulva. *Gynecol Oncol* 1995;56(1):79-84.

100. Franklin EW III, Rutledge FD: Epidemiology of epidermoid carcinoma of the vulva. *Obstet Gynecol* 1972;39(2):165-172.

101. Henson D, Tarone R: An epidemiologic study of cancer of the cervix, vagina, and vulva based on the Third National Cancer Survey in the United States. *Am J Obstet Gynecol* 1977;129(5):525-532.

102. Kosary CL: FIGO stage, histology, histologic grade, age and race as prognostic factors in determining survival for cancers of the female gynecological system: an analysis of 1973-87 SEER cases of cancers of the endometrium, cervix, ovary, vulva, and vagina. *Semin Surg Oncol* 1994;10(1):31-46.

103. Bloss JD, Liao SY, Wilczynski SP, et al: Clinical and histologic features of vulvar carcinomas analyzed for human papillomavirus status: evidence that squamous cell carcinoma of the vulva has more than one etiology. *Hum Pathol* 1991;22(7):711-718.

104. Husseinzadeh N, DeEulis T, Newman N, et al: HPV changes and their significance in patients with invasive squamous cell carcinoma of the vulva: a clinicopathologic study. *Gynecol Oncol* 1991;43(3):237-241.

105. Hording U, Junge J, Daugaard S, et al: Vulvar squamous cell carcinoma and papillomaviruses: indications for two different etiologies. *Gynecol Oncol* 1994;52(2):241-246.

106. Carter J, Carlson J, Fowler J, et al: Invasive vulvar tumors in young women: a disease of the immunosuppressed? *Gynecol Oncol* 1993;51(3):307-310.

107. Moscicki AB, Hills N, Shiboski S, et al: Risks for incident human papillomavirus infection and low-grade squamous intraepithelial lesion development in young females. *JAMA* 2001;285(23):2995-3002.

108. Blohme I: Carcinoma of the vulva in renal transplant patients. *Transplant Sci* 1994;4(1):6-7; discussion 7-8.

109. Penn I: Cancers of the anogenital region in renal transplant recipients: analysis of 65 cases. *Cancer* 1986;58(3):611-616.

110. Rose PG, Fraire AE: Multiple primary gynecologic neoplasms in a young HIV-positive patient. *J Surg Oncol* 1993;53(4):269-272.

111. Spitzer M: Lower genital tract intraepithelial neoplasia in HIV-infected women: guidelines for evaluation and management. *Obstet Gynecol Surv* 1999;54(2):131-137.

112. Chiasson MA, Ellerbrock TV, Bush TJ, et al: Increased prevalence of vulvovaginal condyloma and vulvar intraepithelial neoplasia in women infected with the human immunodeficiency virus. *Obstet Gynecol* 1997;89(5 Pt 1):690-694.

113. Korn AP, Abercrombie PD, Foster A: Vulvar intraepithelial neoplasia in women infected with human immunodeficiency virus-1. *Gynecol Oncol* 1996;61(3):384-386.

114. Abercrombie PD, Korn AP: Vulvar intraepithelial neoplasia in women with HIV. *AIDS Patient Care STDS* 1998;12(4):251-254.

115. Wright TC, Koulos JP, Liu P, et al: Invasive vulvar carcinoma in two women infected with human immunodeficiency virus. *Gynecol Oncol* 1996;60(3):500-503.

116. Scurry JP, Vanin K: Vulvar squamous cell carcinoma and lichen sclerosus. *Australas J Dermatol* 1997;38(Suppl 1):S20-25.

117. Carlson JA, Ambros R, Malfetano J, et al: Vulvar lichen sclerosus and squamous cell carcinoma: a cohort, case control, and investigational study with historical perspective; implications for chronic inflammation and sclerosis in the development of neoplasia. *Hum Pathol* 1998;29(9):932-948.

118. Joura EA, Zeisler H, Losch A, et al: Differentiating vulvar intraepithelial neoplasia from nonneoplastic epithelial disorders: the toluidine blue test. *J Reprod Med* 1998;43(8):671-674.

119. Carli P, Cattaneo A, De Magnis A, et al: Squamous cell carcinoma arising in vulval lichen sclerosus: a longitudinal cohort study. *Eur J Cancer Prev* 1995;4(6):491-495.

120. Franck JM, Young AW Jr: Squamous cell carcinoma in situ arising within lichen planus of the vulva. *Dermatol Surg* 1995;21(10):890-894.

121. Di Paola GR, Leverone NG, Belardi MG: Recurrent vulvar malignancies in an 11-year prospectively followed vulvar dystrophy: a gynecologist's permanent concern. *Gynecol Oncol* 1983;15(1):120-121.

122. Buscema J, Stern J, Woodruff JD: The significance of the histologic alterations adjacent to invasive vulvar carcinoma. *Am J Obstet Gynecol* 1980;137(8):902-909.

123. Jones RW, Joura EA: Analyzing prior clinical events at presentation in 102 women with vulvar carcinoma: evidence of diagnostic delays. *J Reprod Med* 1999;44(9):766-768.

124. Fischer G, Spurrett B, Fischer A: The chronically symptomatic vulva: aetiology and management. *Br J Obstet Gynaecol* 1995;102(10):773-779.

125. Apgar BS, Cox JT: Differentiating normal and abnormal findings of the vulva. *Am Fam Physician* 1996;53(4):1171-1180.

126. Wright VC, Chapman WB: Colposcopy of intraepithelial neoplasia of the vulva and adjacent sites. *Obstet Gynecol Clin North Am* 1993;20(1):231-255.

127. Friedrich EG Jr, Wilkinson EJ, Fu YS: Carcinoma in situ of the vulva: a continuing challenge. *Am J Obstet Gynecol* 1980;136(7):830-843.

128. Stefanon B, De Palo G: Is vulvoscopy a reliable diagnostic technique for high grade vulvar intraepithelial neoplasia? *Eur J Gynaecol Oncol* 1997;18(3):211.

129. Benedet JL, Wilson PS, Matisic J: Epidermal thickness and skin appendage involvement in vulvar intraepithelial neoplasia. *J Reprod Med* 1991;36(8):608-612.

130. Collins CG, Kushner J, Lewis GN, et al: Noninvasive malignancy of the vulva: program for management. *Obstet Gynecol* 1955;6:339-346.

131. Kashimura M, Matsuura Y, Kawagoe T, et al: Cytology of vulvar squamous neoplasia. *Acta Cytol* 1993;37(6):871-875.

132. MacCormac L, Lew W, King G, et al: Gynaecological cytology screening in South Australia: a 23-year experience. *Med J Aust* 1988;149(10):530-536.

133. Fenger C, Nielsen VT: Intraepithelial neoplasia in the anal canal: the appearance and relation to genital neoplasia. *Acta Pathol Microbiol Immunol Scand [A]* 1986;94(5):343-349.

134. Scholefield JH, Hickson WG, Smith JH, et al: Anal intraepithelial neoplasia: part of a multifocal disease process. *Lancet* 1992;340(8830):1271-1273.

135. Ogunbiyi OA, Scholefield JH, Robertson G, et al: Anal human papillomavirus infection and squamous neoplasia in patients with invasive vulvar cancer. *Obstet Gynecol* 1994;83(2):212-216.

136. Kaufman RH: Intraepithelial neoplasia of the vulva. *Gynecol Oncol* 1995;56(1):8-21.

137. Prat J: Pathology of vulvar intraepithelial lesions and early invasive carcinoma. *Hum Pathol* 1991;22(9):877-883.

138. Friedrich EG Jr: Reversible vulvar atypia: a case report. *Obstet Gynecol* 1972;39(2):173-181.

139. Skinner MS, Sternberg WH, Ichinose H, et al: Spontaneous regression of Bowenoid atypia of the vulva. *Obstet Gynecol* 1973;42(1):40-46.

140. Dean RE, Taylor ES, Weisbrod DM, et al: The treatment of premalignant and malignant lesions of the vulva. *Am J Obstet Gynecol* 1974;119(1):59-68.

141. Berger BW, Hori Y: Multicentric Bowen's disease of the genitalia: spontaneous regression of lesions. *Arch Dermatol* 1978;114(11):1698-1699.

142. Buscema J, Woodruff JD, Parmley TH, et al: Carcinoma in situ of the vulva. *Obstet Gynecol* 1980;55(2):225-230.

143. Jones RW, Rowan DM: Spontaneous regression of vulvar intraepithelial neoplasia 2-3. *Obstet Gynecol* 2000;96(3):470-472.

144. Gardiner SH, Stout FE, Arbogast JL, et al: Intraepithelial carcinoma of the vulva. *Am J Obstet Gynecol* 1953;65:539-549.

145. Collins CG, Roman-Lopez JJ, Lee FY: Intraepithelial carcinoma of the vulva. *Am J Obstet Gynecol* 1970;108(8):1187-1191.

146. Jones I, Buntine D: Progression of vulval carcinoma-in-situ. *Aust N Z J Obstet Gynaecol* 1978;18(4):274-276.

147. Jones RW, McLean MR: Carcinoma in situ of the vulva: a review of 31 treated and five untreated cases. *Obstet Gynecol* 1986;68(4):499-503.

148. Herod JJ, Shafi MI, Rollason TP, et al: Vulvar intraepithelial neoplasia: long term follow up of treated and untreated women. *Br J Obstet Gynaecol* 1996;103(5):446-452.

149. Bakri Y, Dimitrievich E: Vulvar intraepithelial neoplasia III: a clinical study of the outcome in 113 cases with relation to the later development of invasive vulvar carcinoma. *Obstet Gynecol* 1995;85(3):481-482.

150. Sadler LC, Jones RW: The progression of noncontiguous intra-epithelial neoplasia in the lower urinary and genital tracts to invasive carcinoma. *Br J Obstet Gynaecol* 1995;102(2):162.

151. Hording U, Junge J, Poulsen H, et al: Vulvar intraepithelial neoplasia III: a viral disease of undetermined progressive potential. *Gynecol Oncol* 1995;56(2):276-279.

152. Van Sickle M, Kaufman RH, Adam E, et al: Detection of human papillomavirus DNA before and after development of invasive vulvar cancer. *Obstet Gynecol* 1990;76(3 Pt 2):540-542.

153. Ragnarsson B, Raabe N, Willems J, et al: Carcinoma in situ of the vulva: long term prognosis. *Acta Oncol* 1987;26(4):277-280.

154. Buckley CH, Butler EB, Fox H: Vulvar intraepithelial neoplasia and microinvasive carcinoma of the vulva. *J Clin Pathol* 1984;37(11):1201-1211.

155. Ostor AG, Sfameni SF, Kneale BL, et al: Progression of squamous carcinoma in situ of the vulva to invasive carcinoma after systemic bleomycin therapy. *Aust N Z J Obstet Gynaecol* 1984;24(1):55-58.

156. Friedman M, White RG, Moar JJ, et al: Progression of vulval carcinoma in situ: a case report. *S Afr Med J* 1983;64(19):748-749.

157. Ulbright TM, Stehman FB, Roth LM, et al: Bowenoid dysplasia of the vulva. *Cancer* 1982;50(12):2910-2919.

158. Caglar H, Tamer S, Hreshchyshyn MM: Vulvar intraepithelial neoplasia. *Obstet Gynecol* 1982;60(3):346-349.

159. Woodruff JD, Julian C, Puray T, et al: The contemporary challenge of carcinoma in situ of the vulva. *Am J Obstet Gynecol* 1973;115(5):677-686.

160. Forney JP, Morrow CP, Townsend DE, et al: Management of carcinoma in situ of the vulva. *Am J Obstet Gynecol* 1977;127(8):801-806.

161. Rouzier R, Morice P, Haie-Meder C, et al: Prognostic significance of epithelial disorders adjacent to invasive vulvar carcinomas. *Gynecol Oncol* 2001;81(3):414-419.

162. Husseinzadeh N, Recinto C: Frequency of invasive cancer in surgically excised vulvar lesions with intraepithelial neoplasia (VIN 3). *Gynecol Oncol* 1999;73(1):119-120.

163. Rettenmaier MA: Vulvar intraepithelial neoplasia III: occult cancer and the impact of margin status on recurrence. *Obstet Gynecol* 1999;93(4):633-634.

164. Modesitt SC, Waters AB, Walton L, et al: Vulvar intraepithelial neoplasia III: occult cancer and the impact of margin status on recurrence. *Obstet Gynecol* 1998;92(6):962-966.

165. Herod JJ, Shafi MI, Rollason TP, et al: Vulvar intraepithelial neoplasia with superficially invasive carcinoma of the vulva. *Br J Obstet Gynaecol* 1996;103(5):453-456.

166. Haefner HK, Tate JE, McLachlin CM, et al: Vulvar intraepithelial neoplasia: age, morphological phenotype, papillomavirus DNA, and coexisting invasive carcinoma. *Hum Pathol* 1995;26(2):147-154.

167. Pickel H: Early stromal invasion of the vulva. *Eur J Gynaecol Oncol* 1989;10(2):97-101.

168. Powell LC Jr, Dinh TV, Rajaraman S, et al: Carcinoma in situ of the vulva: a clinicopathologic study of 50 cases. *J Reprod Med* 1986; 31(9):808-814.

169. Zaino RJ, Husseinzadeh N, Nahhas W, et al: Epithelial alterations in proximity to invasive squamous carcinoma of the vulva. *Int J Gynecol Pathol* 1982;1(2):173-184.

170. Kneale BLG, Elliot PM, McDonald IA: Microinvasive carcinoma of the vulva. In Coppleson M, Monaghan JM, Morrow CP, editors: *Gynecologic oncology: fundamental principles and clinical practice*, ed 2. Edinburgh, New York, Churchill Livingstone, 1992, 320-328.

171. Andreasson B, Bock JE: Intraepithelial neoplasia in the vulvar region. *Gynecol Oncol* 1985; 21(3):300-305.

172. Reid R: The management of genital condylomas, intraepithelial neoplasia, and vulvodynia. *Obstet Gynecol Clin North Am* 1996;23(4):917-991.

173. Basta A: Diagnostic and therapeutic procedures in the vulvar intraepithelial neoplasia (VIN) and early invasive cancer of the vulva. *Eur J Gynaecol Oncol* 1989;10(1):55-59.

174. Fiorica JV, Cavanagh D, Marsden DE, et al: Carcinoma in situ of the vulva: 24 years' experience in southwest Florida. *South Med J* 1988; 81(5):589-593.

175. Bornstein J, Kaufman RH: Combination of surgical excision and carbon dioxide laser vaporization for multifocal vulvar intraepithelial neoplasia. *Am J Obstet Gynecol* 1988;158(3 Pt 1): 459-464.

176. Baggish MS, Dorsey JH: CO2 laser for the treatment of vulvar carcinoma in situ. *Obstet Gynecol* 1981;57(3):371-375.

177. Leuchter RS, Townsend DE, Hacker NF, et al: Treatment of vulvar carcinoma in situ with the CO2 laser. *Gynecol Oncol* 1984;19(3):314-322.

178. Stein S: CO2 laser surgery of the cervix, vagina, and vulva. *Surg Clin North Am* 1984;64(5):885-897.

179. Simonsen EF: CO2 laser used for cancer in situ/Bowen's disease (VIN) and lichen sclerosus in the vulvar region. *Acta Obstet Gynecol Scand* 1989;68(6):551-553.

180. Sporri S, Frenz M, Altermatt HJ, et al: Treatment of human papillomavirus-associated vulvar disease with the CO2-laser: physical and histological aspects with use of a new scanning device, the SwiftLase. *Arch Gynecol Obstet* 1996;259(1):25-35.

181. Sideri M, Spinaci L, Spolti N, et al: Evaluation of CO(2) laser excision or vaporization for the treatment of vulvar intraepithelial neoplasia. *Gynecol Oncol* 1999;75(2):277-281.

182. Reid R, Elfont EA, Zirkin RM, et al: Superficial laser vulvectomy. II: the anatomic and biophysical principles permitting accurate control over the depth of dermal destruction with the carbon dioxide laser. *Am J Obstet Gynecol* 1985;152(3): 261-271.

183. Ferenczy A, Wright TC, Richart RM: Comparison of CO2 laser surgery and loop electrosurgical excision/fulguration procedure (LEEP) for the treatment of vulvar intraepithelial neoplasia (VIN). *Int J Gynecol Cancer* 1994;4(1):22-28.

184. DiSaia PJ, Rich WM: Surgical approach to multifocal carcinoma in situ of the vulva. *Am J Obstet Gynecol* 1981;140(2):136-145.

185. Wolcott HD, Gallup DG: Wide local excision in the treatment of vulvar carcinoma in situ: a reappraisal. *Am J Obstet Gynecol* 1984;150(6):695-698.

186. Knight RVD: Bowen's disease of the vulva. *Am J Obstet Gynecol* 1943;46:514-524.

187. Rutledge F, Sinclair M: Treatment of intraepithelial carcinoma of the vulva by skin excision and graft. *Am J Obstet Gynecol* 1968;102(6):807-818.

188. Caglar H, Delgado G, Hreshchyshyn MM: Partial and total skinning vulvectomy in treatment of carcinoma in situ of the vulva. *Obstet Gynecol* 1986;68(4):504-507.

189. Ayhan A, Tuncer ZS, Dogan L, et al: Skinning vulvectomy for the treatment of vulvar intraepithelial neoplasia 2-3: a study of 21 cases. *Eur J Gynaecol Oncol* 1998;19(5):508-510.

190. Kaplan AL, Kaufman RH, Birken RA, et al: Intraepithelial carcinoma of the vulva with extension to the anal canal. *Obstet Gynecol* 1981; 58(3):368-371.

191. Wharton JT, Gallager S, Rutledge FN: Microinvasive carcinoma of the vulva. *Am J Obstet Gynecol* 1974;118(2):159-162.

192. Thuesen B, Andreasson B, Bock JE: [Assessment of sex life and psychological reactions after local excision of vulvar carcinoma in situ]. *Ugeskr Laeger* 1993;155(15):1129-1131.

193. Thuesen B, Andreasson B, Bock JE: Sexual function and somatopsychic reactions after local excision of vulvar intra-epithelial neoplasia. *Acta Obstet Gynecol Scand* 1992;71(2):126-128.

194. Narayansingh GV, Cumming GP, Parkin DP, et al: Flap repair: an effective strategy for minimising sexual morbidity associated with the surgical management of vulval intra epithelial neoplasia. *J R Coll Surg Edinb* 2000;45(2):81-84.

195. Jansen GT, Dillaha CJ, Honeycutt WM: Bowenoid conditions of the skin: treatment with topical 5-fluorouracil. *South Med J* 1967;60(2):185-188.

196. Limmer BL: Bowen's disease: Treatment with topical 5-fluorouracil. *Cutis* 1975;16:660-663.

197. Carson TE, Hoskins WJ, Wurzel JF: Topical 5-fluorouracil in the treatment of carcinoma in situ of the vulva. *Obstet Gynecol* 1976;47(1):59S-62S.

198. Krupp PJ, Bohm JW: 5-fluorouracil topical treatment of in situ vulvar cancer: a preliminary report. *Obstet Gynecol* 1978;51(6):702-706.

199. Lifshitz S, Roberts JA: Treatment of carcinoma in situ of the vulva with topical 5-fluorouracil. *Obstet Gynecol* 1980;56(2):242-244.

200. Sillman FH, Sedlis A, Boyce JG: A review of lower genital intraepithelial neoplasia and the use of topical 5-fluorouracil. *Obstet Gynecol Surv* 1985;40(4):190-220.

201. Townsend DE, Marks EJ: Cryosurgery and the CO2 laser. *Cancer* 1981;48(2 Suppl):632-637.

202. Weintraub I, Lagasse LD: Reversibility of vulvar atypia by DNCB-induced delayed hypersensitivity. *Obstet Gynecol* 1973;41(2):195-199.

203. Spirtos NM, Smith LH, Teng NN: Prospective randomized trial of topical alpha-interferon (alpha-interferon gels) for the treatment of vulvar intraepithelial neoplasia III. *Gynecol Oncol* 1990;37(1):34-38.

204. Abdel-Hady ES, Martin-Hirsch P, Duggan-Keen M, et al: Immunological and viral factors associated with the response of vulval intraepithelial neoplasia to photodynamic therapy. *Cancer Res* 2001;61(1):192-196.

205. Hillemanns P, Untch M, Dannecker C, et al: Photodynamic therapy of vulvar intraepithelial neoplasia using 5-aminolevulinic acid. *Int J Cancer* 2000;85(5):649-653.

206. Fehr MK, Hornung R, Schwarz VA, et al: Photodynamic therapy of vulvar intraepithelial neoplasia III using topically applied 5-aminolevulinic acid. *Gynecol Oncol* 2001;80(1):62-66.

207. Kurwa HA, Barlow RJ, Neill S: Single-episode photodynamic therapy and vulval intraepithelial neoplasia type III resistant to conventional therapy. *Br J Dermatol* 2000;143(5):1040-1042.

208. Lobraico RV, Grossweiner LI: Clinical experiences with photodynamic therapy for recurrent malignancies of the lower female genital tract. *J Gynecol Surg* 1993;9(1):29-34.

209. Del Priore G, Herron MM: Retinoids for vulvar dysplasia in the HIV-infected patient. *Int J Gynaecol Obstet* 1996;55(1):77-78.

210. Koonsaeng S, Verschraegen C, Freedman R, et al: Successful treatment of recurrent vulvar intraepithelial neoplasia resistant to interferon and isotretinoin with cidofovir. *J Med Virol* 2001; 64(2):195-198.

211. Esquius J, Brisigotti M, Matias-Guiu X, et al: Keratin expression in normal vulva, non-neoplastic epithelial disorders, vulvar intraepithelial neoplasia, and invasive squamous cell carcinoma. *Int J Gynecol Pathol* 1991;10(4):341-355.

212. Modesitt SC, Groben PA, Walton LA, et al: Expression of Ki-67 in vulvar carcinoma and vulvar intraepithelial neoplasia III: correlation with clinical prognostic factors. *Gynecol Oncol* 2000;76(1):51-55.

213. MacLean AB, Reid WM, Rolfe KJ, et al: Role of angiogenesis in benign, premalignant and malignant vulvar lesions. *J Reprod Med* 2000;45(8): 609-612.

214. Bancher-Todesca D, Obermair A, Bilgi S, et al: Angiogenesis in vulvar intraepithelial neoplasia. *Gynecol Oncol* 1997;64(3):496-500.

215. Korhonen MO, Kaufman RH, Roberts D, et al: Carcinoma in situ of the vulva: the search for viral particles. *J Reprod Med* 1982;27(12):746-748.

216. Yang B, Hart WR: Vulvar intraepithelial neoplasia of the simplex (differentiated) type: a clinicopathologic study including analysis of HPV and p53 expression. *Am J Surg Pathol* 2000;24(3): 429-441.

217. Kim YT, Thomas NF, Kessis TD, et al: p53 mutations and clonality in vulvar carcinomas and squamous hyperplasias: evidence suggesting that squamous hyperplasias do not serve as direct precursors of human papillomavirus-negative vulvar carcinomas. *Hum Pathol* 1996;27(4):389-395.

218. Pinto AP, Lin MC, Sheets EE, et al: Allelic imbalance in lichen sclerosus, hyperplasia, and intraepithelial neoplasia of the vulva. *Gynecol Oncol* 2000;77(1):171-176.

219. Holway AH, Rieger-Christ KM, Miner WR, et al: Somatic mutation of PTEN in vulvar cancer. *Clin Cancer Res* 2000;6(8):3228-3235.

220. Lin MC, Mutter GL, Trivijisilp P, et al: Patterns of allelic loss (LOH) in vulvar squamous carcinomas and adjacent noninvasive epithelia. *Am J Pathol* 1998;152(5):1313-1318.

221. Tate JE, Mutter GL, Boynton KA, et al: Monoclonal origin of vulvar intraepithelial neoplasia and some vulvar hyperplasias. *Am J Pathol* 1997;150(1):315-322.

222. Wilkinson EJ, Friedrich EG Jr, Fu YS: Multicentric nature of vulvar carcinoma in situ. *Obstet Gynecol* 1981;58(1):69-74.

223. Kohlberger PD, Kirnbauer R, Bancher D, et al: Absence of p53 protein overexpression in precancerous lesions of the vulva. *Cancer* 1998;82(2):323-327.

224. Rosenthal AN, Ryan A, Hopster D, et al: p53 codon 72 polymorphism in vulval cancer and vulval intraepithelial neoplasia. *Br J Cancer* 2000;83(10):1287-1290.

225. Ehrmann RL, Dwyer IM, Yavner D, et al: An immunoperoxidase study of laminin and type IV collagen distribution in carcinoma of the cervix and vulva. *Obstet Gynecol* 1988; 72(2):257-262.

226. Berchuck A, Rodriguez G, Kamel A, et al: Expression of epidermal growth factor receptor and HER-2/neu in normal and neoplastic cervix, vulva, and vagina. *Obstet Gynecol* 1990;76(3 Pt 1): 381-387.

227. Hefler L, Obermair A, Tempfer C, et al: Serum concentrations of squamous cell carcinoma antigen in patients with vulvar intraepithelial neoplasia and vulvar cancer. *Int J Cancer* 1999; 84(3):299-303.

228. Parolini S, Rosa D, Flagiello D, et al: Immunocytochemical localization of plasminogen activators in carcinomas in the cervix and vulva. *Int J Tissue React* 1994;16(5-6):251-258.

229. Naik R, Cross P, de Barros Lopes A, et al: Lectins in the vulva. I: normal vulvar epithelium and epithelium adjacent to vulvar intraepithelial neoplasia and squamous cell carcinoma. *Int J Gynecol Pathol* 1998;17(2):154-161.

230. Naik R, Cross P, de Barros Lopes A, et al: Lectins in the vulva. II: vulvar intraepithelial neoplasia and squamous cell carcinoma. *Int J Gynecol Pathol* 1998;17(2):162-170.

231. Raspagliesi F, Ditto A, Paladini D, et al: Prognostic indicators in melanoma of the vulva. *Ann Surg Oncol* 2000;7(10):738-742.

232. Dunton CJ, Berd D: Vulvar melanoma, biologically different from other cutaneous melanomas. *Lancet* 1999;354(9195):2013-2014.

233. Hewett P: Sequel to a case of recurrent melanosis of both groins and back; the disease reappearing in the brain, heart, pancreas, liver, and other organs. *Lancet* 1861:263-264.

234. Dunton CJ, Kautzky M, Hanau C: Malignant melanoma of the vulva: a review. *Obstet Gynecol Surv* 1995;50(10):739-746.

235. Clark WH Jr, From L, Bernardino EA, et al: The histogenesis and biologic behavior of primary human malignant melanomas of the skin. *Cancer Res* 1969;29(3):705-727.

236. Breslow A: Thickness, cross-sectional areas and depth of invasion in the prognosis of cutaneous melanoma. *Ann Surg* 1970;172(5):902-908.

237. Chung AF, Woodruff JM, Lewis JL Jr: Malignant melanoma of the vulva: a report of 44 cases. *Obstet Gynecol* 1975;45(6):638-646.

238. Balch CM, Buzaid AC, Soong SJ, et al: Final version of the American Joint Committee on Cancer staging system for cutaneous melanoma. *J Clin Oncol* 2001;19(16):3635-3648.

239. Ragnarsson-Olding BK, Kanter-Lewensohn LR, Lagerlof B, et al: Malignant melanoma of the vulva in a nationwide, 25-year study of 219 Swedish females: clinical observations and histopathologic features. *Cancer* 1999; 86(7): 1273-1284.

240. Ragnarsson-Olding BK, Nilsson BR, Kanter-Lewensohn LR, et al: Malignant melanoma of the vulva in a nationwide, 25-year study of 219 Swedish females: predictors of survival. *Cancer* 1999;86(7):1285-1293.

241. Piura B, Rabinovich A, Dgani R, et al: Malignant melanoma of the vulva: report of six cases and review of the literature. *Eur J Gynaecol Oncol* 1999;20(3):182-186.

242. Raber G, Mempel V, Jackisch C, et al: Malignant melanoma of the vulva: report of 89 patients. *Cancer* 1996;78(11):2353-2358.

243. Scheistroen M, Trope C, Koern J, et al: Malignant melanoma of the vulva. Evaluation of prognostic factors with emphasis on DNA ploidy in 75 patients. *Cancer* 1995;75(1):72-80.

244. Levenback C, Burke TW, Gershenson DM, et al: Intraoperative lymphatic mapping for vulvar cancer. *Obstet Gynecol* 1994;84(2):163-167.

245. Valdes Olmos RA, Hoefnagel CA, Nieweg OE, et al: Lymphoscintigraphy in oncology: a rediscovered challenge. *Eur J Nucl Med* 1999;26(4 Suppl):S2-S10.

246. Leong SP: The role of sentinel lymph nodes in malignant melanoma. *Surg Clin North Am* 2000;80(6):1741-1757.

247. Wong JH: A historical perspective on the development of intraoperative lymphatic mapping and selective lymphadenectomy. *Surg Clin North Am* 2000;80(6):1675-1682.

248. Clary BM, Brady MS, Lewis JJ, et al: Sentinel lymph node biopsy in the management of patients with primary cutaneous melanoma: review of a large single-institutional experience with an emphasis on recurrence. *Ann Surg* 2001;233(2):250-258.

249. Paget JS: *On a form of chronic inflammation of bones (osteitis deformans) ... Additional cases of osteitis deformans ... On disease of the mammary areola preceding cancer of the mammary gland.* Baltimore, Williams & Wilkins, 1936.

250. Dubrewilh W: Paget's disease of the vulva. *Br J Dermatol* 1901;13:407-416.

251. Woodruff JD, Hildebrandt EE: Carcinoma in situ of the vulva. *Obstetrics and Gynecology* 1958;12:414-424.

252. Urabe A, Matsukuma A, Shimizu N, et al: Extramammary Paget's disease: comparative histopathologic studies of intraductal carcinoma of the breast and apocrine adenocarcinoma. *J Cutan Pathol* 1990;17(5):257-265.

253. Gregori CA, Smith CI, Breen JL: Extramammary Paget's disease. *Clin Obstet Gynecol* 1978;21(4):1107-1115.

254. Friedrich EG Jr, Wilkinson EJ, Steingraeber PH, et al: Paget's disease of the vulva and carcinoma of the breast. *Obstet Gynecol* 1975;46(2):130-134.

255. Curtin JP, Rubin SC, Jones WB, et al: Paget's disease of the vulva. *Gynecol Oncol* 1990;39(3):374-377.

256. Bergen S, DiSaia PJ, Liao SY, et al: Conservative management of extramammary Paget's disease of the vulva. *Gynecol Oncol* 1989;33(2):151-156.

257. Parker LP, Parker JR, Bodurka-Bevers D, et al: Paget's disease of the vulva: pathology, pattern of involvement, and prognosis. *Gynecol Oncol* 2000;77(1):183-189.

258. Crawford D, Nimmo M, Clement PB, et al: Prognostic factors in Paget's disease of the vulva: a study of 21 cases. *Int J Gynecol Pathol* 1999;18(4):351-359.

259. Lee SC, Roth LM, Ehrlich C, et al: Extramammary Paget's disease of the vulva: a clinicopathologic study of 13 cases. *Cancer* 1977;39(6):2540-2549.

260. Fanning J, Lambert HC, Hale TM, et al: Paget's disease of the vulva: prevalence of associated vulvar adenocarcinoma, invasive Paget's disease, and recurrence after surgical excision. *Am J Obstet Gynecol* 1999;180(1 Pt 1):24-27.

261. Kodama S, Kaneko T, Saito M, et al: A clinicopathologic study of 30 patients with Paget's disease of the vulva. *Gynecol Oncol* 1995;56(1):63-70.

262. Ganjei P, Giraldo KA, Lampe B, et al: Vulvar Paget's disease: is immunocytochemistry helpful in assessing the surgical margins? *J Reprod Med* 1990;35(11):1002-1004.

263. DiSaia PJ, Dorion GE, Cappuccini F, et al: A report of two cases of recurrent Paget's disease of the vulva in a split-thickness graft and its possible pathogenesis-labeled "retrodissemination." *Gynecol Oncol* 1995;57(1):109-112.

264. Parmley TH, Woodruff JD, Julian CG: Invasive vulvar Paget's disease. *Obstet Gynecol* 1975; 46(3):341-346.

265. Hart WR, Millman JB: Progression of intraepithelial Paget's disease of the vulva to invasive carcinoma. *Cancer* 1977;40(5):2333-2337.

266. Fine BA, Fowler LJ, Valente PT, et al: Minimally invasive Paget's disease of the vulva with extensive lymph node metastases. *Gynecol Oncol* 1995;57(2):262-265.

267. Cappuccini F, Tewari K, Rogers LW, et al: Extramammary Paget's disease of the vulva: metastases to the bone marrow in the absence of an underlying adenocarcinoma: case report and literature review. *Gynecol Oncol* 1997;66(1):146-150.

268. Degefu S, O'Quinn AG, Dhurandhar HN: Paget's disease of the vulva and urogenital malignancies: a case report and review of the literature. *Gynecol Oncol* 1986;25(3):347-354.

269. Woodruff JD, Pauerstein CJ: Differential metabolic activity in Paget's cells and associated epithelia of the vulva. *Obstet Gynecol* 1966;28(5):663-669.

270. Grant PT: Vulvar cancer. *Aust N Z J Obstet Gynaecol* 1995;35(1):70.

271. Lawhead RA Jr, Majmudar B: Early diagnosis of vulvar neoplasia as a result of vulvar self-examination. *J Reprod Med* 1990;35(12):1134-1137.

272. Stern PL, Brown M, Stacey SN, et al: Natural HPV immunity and vaccination strategies. *J Clin Virol* 2000;19(1-2):57-66.

273. Muderspach L, Wilczynski S, Roman L, et al: A phase I trial of a human papillomavirus (HPV) peptide vaccine for women with high-grade cervical and vulvar intraepithelial neoplasia who are HPV 16 positive. *Clin Cancer Res* 2000;6(9): 3406-3416.

CHAPTER 9

Prevention and Early Diagnosis of Ovarian Cancer

Mark S. Shahin
Joel I. Sorosky

EPIDEMIOLOGY

Epithelial ovarian carcinoma is the leading cause of death from gynecologic cancer in the United States. In 2001 there were an estimated 23,400 new cases (3.75% of all cancer diagnoses), and approximately 13,900 women will die of this disease each year.[1] Ovarian cancer is the fourth most frequent cause of cancer death in women and accounts for 5.2% of all cancer deaths. The incidence of ovarian cancer increases with age and peaks in the eighth decade. Based upon cancer registry data from the Surveillance, Epidemiology, and End Results Program (SEER) of the National Cancer Institute (NCI), epithelial ovarian cancer is infrequent in women younger than age 40.[2] The rate of epithelial ovarian cancer increases from 15 to 16 per 100,000 in women aged 40 to 44 to a peak of 57 per 100,000 in women aged 70 to 74. The median age of diagnosis is 63, and 48% of patients are 65 years or older.

The risk for ovarian cancer among African-American women is significantly lower than in Caucasian women (odds ratio 0.7, 95% confidence interval [CI] 0.5 to 0.9). This difference persisted after adjusting for the most common and well-known risk factors (odds ratio 0.8, 95% CI 0.6 to 1.0).[3]

From 1973 to 1994 the overall incidence of ovarian cancer remained relatively unchanged, with a declining incidence for younger women but an increasing incidence for older women.[4] During the same time period, other studies have found an increasing ovarian cancer mortality rate in older women and a decreasing mortality rate in younger women.[5] The increasing use of oral contraceptives may contribute to the decreasing incidences in mortality rates among younger women in the United States. Younger women have their cancers diagnosed typically at an earlier stage, and several studies suggest that older patients are often administered less aggressive treatment. Although the NCI reports indicate that there is a slight decline in age-adjusted ovarian mortality rate, other epidemiologic databases do not demonstrate a reduction in overall mortality.[4]

Although some improvement has been made in the overall survival of ovarian cancer patients, the 5-year survival for advanced-stage disease remains a low 25% to 30%.[6] Specific ovarian cancer death rates adjusted for stage and age are higher for African-American patients than for Caucasian; rates were 1.20 to 1.32.[7] The offspring of some Asian immigrants retain a partial protection against ovarian cancer.[8]

The incidence of ovarian cancer varies in different geographic locations throughout the world. Western countries, including the United States and the United Kingdom, have an incidence of ovarian cancer that is three to seven times greater than in Japan, where epithelial ovarian cancers are considered rare. However, the incidence of epithelial ovarian cancers among Japanese immigrants and their descendants in the United States has increased significantly, approaching that of Caucasian women from the United States. It has been suggested that this increased incidence may be related to change in dietary habits.[9]

STAGING

Cancer of the ovary is surgically staged. The International Federation of Gynecology and Obstetrics (FIGO) stages are shown in Table 9-1.[10]

RISK FACTORS

The cause of ovarian cancer is currently unknown. There has been speculation that an etiologic agent or a potentiator of oncogenesis enters the peritoneal cavity through the lower genital tract and spreads to the uterus and the fallopian tubes. Possible carcinogens, such as infectious agents, have been studied, and although case-control studies have failed to document a specific agent, some studies have linked environmental exposure to talc with the development of epithelial tumors.

Table 9-1
Carcinoma of the Ovary (FIGO Nomenclature)

Stage I	Growth limited to the ovaries
Ia	Growth limited to one ovary; no ascites that contain malignant cells present. No tumor on the external surface; capsule intact
Ib	Growth limited to both ovaries; no ascites that contain malignant cells present. No tumor on the external surfaces; capsules intact
Ic*	Tumor either stage Ia or Ib but with tumor on surface of one or both ovaries or with capsule ruptured or with ascites present that contain malignant cells, or with positive peritoneal washings
Stage II	Growth involving one or both ovaries with pelvic extension
IIa	Extension or metastases to the uterus, tubes, or both
IIb	Extension to other pelvic tissues
IIc*	Tumor either stage IIa or IIb, but with tumor on surface of one or both ovaries or with capsule(s) ruptured or with ascites present that contain malignant cells or with positive peritoneal washings
Stage III	Tumor involving one or both ovaries with histologically confirmed peritoneal implants outside the pelvis or positive retroperitoneal or linguinal nodes. Superficial liver metastases equals stage III. Tumor is limited to the true pelvis but with histologically proven malignant extension to small bowel or omentum
IIIa	Tumor grossly limited to the true pelvis, with negative nodes, but with histologically confirmed microscopic seeding of abdominal peritoneal surfaces or histologically proven extension to small bowel or mesentery
IIIb	Tumor of one or both ovaries with histologically confirmed implants, peritoneal metastasis of abdominal peritoneal surfaces, none exceeding 2 cm in diameter; nodes are negative
IIIc	Peritoneal metastasis beyond the pelvis > 2 cm in diameter and/or positive retroperitoneal or inguinal nodes
Stage IV	Growth involving one or both ovaries with distant metastases. If pleural effusion is present, there must be positive cytology to allot a case to stage IV. Parenchymal liver metastasis equals stage IV

*To evaluate the impact on prognosis of the different criteria for allotting cases to stage Ic or IIc, it would be of value to know whether rupture of the capsule was spontaneous or caused by the surgeon and whether peritoneal washings or ascites were the source of detected malignant cells.
Source: Staging announcement: FIGO Cancer Committee. *Gynecol Oncol* 1986;25:383.

Reproductive Factors

Prior reproductive history and duration of the reproductive interval have the greatest impact on the disease, with low-parity infertility, early menarche, and late menopause increasing the risk for development of ovarian cancer. The increased incidence of ovarian cancer in single women, nuns, and nulliparous women suggests that continued ovulation, uninterrupted by pregnancy, may predispose women to develop this malignancy.[11,12] This relationship of parity to the risk of ovarian cancer has led to the hypothesis that suppression of ovulation may be an important factor. According to this hypothesis, ovarian cancer develops from an aberrant repair process of the surface epithelium, which is ruptured and repaired during each ovulatory cycle. The probability that ovarian cancer would develop is therefore a function of the total number of ovulatory cycles, together with a genetic predisposition and other, as yet other undefined, environmental factors. Theoretically, the surface epithelium undergoes repetitive disruption and repair. This process may eventually lead to a higher probability of spontaneous mutations, which may subsequently unmask a germline mutation or otherwise directly lead to an oncogenetic phenotype.

Multiple pregnancies exert an increasingly protective effect on the risk for development of ovarian cancer. Compared with nulliparity, one to two pregnancies result in a relative risk (RR) of 0.49 to 0.97. Women with greater than three pregnancies have a decreased risk of 0.35 to 0.76, compared with the control population.[12] Another factor that also reduces the risk is a history of breast-feeding, although no consistent relationship has been established between breast-feeding duration and decreased risk.

Hormonal Factors

The protective effects of parity, multiple births, history of breast-feeding, and oral contraceptive use support the incessant ovulation hypothesis for the cause of ovarian cancer. Case-control studies have consistently demonstrated that the users of oral contraceptives have a 30% to 60% lower chance of developing ovarian cancer than women without a history of oral contraceptive use.[13,14] The World Health Organization investigated the relationship between the use of combined oral contraceptives and the risk of epithelial ovarian cancer in 368 women, compared with 2398 matched controls. The relative risk for women who have ever used oral contraceptives was 0.75. The risk of ovarian cancer decreased with increasing time since the cessation of use, and in contrast to other studies, the risk decreased with a longer duration of use. The decreased risk was substantially greater in nulliparous women compared with parous women, 0.16 versus 0.85, respectively.[15] Cramer and associates have estimated that oral contraceptives have resulted in the prevention of 1700 cases of ovarian cancer in the United States per year.[13]

The use of low-dose oral contraceptive pills has been questioned in regard to the effect on ovarian cancer risk reduction. However, Ness and associates have reported that the use of low-estrogen/low-progestin pills afforded an estimated risk reduction (RR 0.5, CI 0.2-0.6) that was identical to that for high-estrogen/high-progestin pills (RR 0.5, CI 0.3-0.7).[16]

Evidence in the literature supports an increased risk of ovarian cancer in women with a prior history of breast cancer. Furthermore, women with a history of ovarian cancer have a twofold to fourfold increased risk of breast cancer, which supports the significance of the altered hormonal environment in the etiology of ovarian cancer.[12,17] Individual studies have not established a direct association between ovarian cancer risk and use of hormone replacement therapy.[18] However, a metaanalysis of 21 studies did show a small increase in the overall RR, 1.15.[19] Rodriguez and associates have recently reported that in a large prospective study of 211,581 postmenopausal women who used postmenopausal estrogen for 10 or more years, there was an increased risk of ovarian cancer mortality (RR 1.51, CI 1.16-1.96) that persisted up to 29 years after cessation of estrogen replacement therapy.[20]

Under the influence of numerous hormonal effects through systemic and paracrine mechanisms, the surface epithelium of the ovaries undergoes changes. Excessive gonadotropin secretion has been also hypothesized to play a role in ovarian oncogenesis. Under excessive gonadotropin stimulation and resulting estrogen stimulation, the surface epithelium of the ovary may develop an inclusion cyst that may proliferate and ultimately undergo malignant transformation. Additional epidemiologic and experimental data suggest that hormones, including androgens and progesterone, might also have an etiologic influence.[17] Increasing data also support a sequential transition from simple endometriosis to atypical endometriosis and eventually to endometrioid and clear cell neoplasms of the ovary.[21]

Elevations in ovarian cancer risks have been related to a prior use of infertility drugs, particularly those stimulating ovulation.[22,23] Although results from these studies must be cautiously interpreted because of limitations in sample size, the association is of interest given that incessant ovulation has been proposed as a possible mechanism underlying the occurrence of ovarian cancer. An extensive review of the literature by Ness and associates concluded that infertility itself, but not fertility drugs, increases the risk for ovarian cancer.[24]

Dietary Factors

Availability of data that correlate per capita fat availability with the increases in ovarian cancer among Japanese immigrants to the United States has stimulated interest in dietary factors.[25] Most of the attention has been focused on the effects of dietary fat and has yielded mixed results from epidemiologic studies. Bosetti and associates and others have reported significantly elevated risks of ovarian cancer among Italian women who reported frequent consumption of red meat. Inverse associations were found for fish and vegetable consumption.[26] A study in China reported a significant dose-response relationship between intake of fat from animal sources and increased risk of ovarian cancer.[27]

Cramer and others found a higher risk of ovarian cancer associated with consumption of yogurt, cottage cheese, and other lactose-rich dairy products. This association was restricted to women with low levels of galactose-1-phosphate uridyl transferase activity, and enzyme linked with hypergonadotropic hypogonadism. These findings led to speculation that lactose consumption may be an environmental risk factor and transferase activity a genetic risk factor for ovarian cancer. One recent study found lactose and cholesterol levels to be predictive of subsequent ovarian cancer risk, but several other case-control studies have found no association of ovarian cancer risk with either lactose consumption or transferase activity.[28,29]

Genetic Factors

The majority of epithelial ovarian cancers are sporadic; familial or hereditary patterns account for only 5% to 10%. Family history remains an important factor in assigning an individual woman's probability of developing epithelial ovarian cancer.[30] The baseline lifetime risk of ovarian cancer for the general population is 1.6%. However, if a woman has a single family member affected by ovarian cancer, this risk increases to 4% to 5%.[31-34] In cases where there are two relatives with ovarian cancer, a woman's risk increases to

7%. Women with hereditary ovarian cancer syndromes, defined as at least two first-degree relatives with ovarian cancer, may have a lifetime probability of developing ovarian cancer as high as 25% to 50%.[18] It is noteworthy that only 7% of all ovarian cancer patients will report a first-degree relative with ovarian cancer.[35] The precise incidence of familial ovarian cancer remains to be determined, despite multiple ovarian cancer registries similar to that in place at the Roswell Park Memorial Institute in Buffalo, New York.[36] Despite the low incidence of hereditary ovarian cancer, compared with the vastly more common sporadic form, the offspring of the ovarian cancer, patients are the focus of intense research efforts because three genes carrying a genetic predisposition to ovarian cancer have already been identified (BRCA1, BRCA2, and mismatch repair genes).[37]

As previously indicated, it has been estimated that approximately 10% of all ovarian cancers result from a hereditary predisposition. Germline inheritance of a mutant gene transmitted in an autosomal dominant manner leads to increased susceptibility to ovarian cancer with variable penetrance. Two distinct clinical syndromes associated with hereditary ovarian cancer have been described. The most common of these is termed hereditary breast/ovarian cancer (HBOC), which accounts for 85% to 90% of all hereditary cancers identified. The vast majority of these cases are associated with mutations of the BRCA1 locus, which is located on chromosome 17 (17q21). More than 100 mutations in this gene have been identified. BRCA1 consists of 22 coding exons and encodes for a protein of 1863 amino acids. BRCA1 is a tumor-suppressor gene that acts as a negative regulator of tumor growth. Typically, the inheritance of a cancer-predisposing mutant allele of BRCA1 is followed by the loss of inactivation of the wild-type allele, thus resulting in nonregulation of cell growth and progression toward malignancy. BRCA1 function appears to have a role in regulation of differentiation and cell proliferation. It is also involved in the repair of damaged DNA and maintenance of genomic stability. Mutations of BRCA1 occur throughout the gene, and 80% of these mutations result in loss of function. Epidemiologic studies of genetic mutations have identified the existence of specific mutations in women of Ashkenazi-Jewish descent; 185DelAG and 5382insC on BRCA1 are present in approximately 1% and 0.1%, respectively, of the Ashkenazi-Jewish population.[37]

A second breast/ovarian cancer susceptibility gene, BRCA2, is localized to chromosome 13 (13q12).[38] The expression of BRCA2 is similar to that of the BRCA1 gene, and the two appear to share structural and functional similarities. Both genes apparently are involved in the regulated coordination of gene expression during cell cycle progression and cell differentiation. Numerous mutations of BRCA2 have been identified; specifically 6174delT on BRCA2 has been identified in approximately 1.4% of Ashkenazi-Jewish population.[39] It appears that a large fraction of all ovarian cancers in Ashkenazi-Jewish women may be associated with germline mutations in either BRCA1 or BRCA2 genes. Somatic mutations of BRCA1 and BRCA2 locus are rare in sporadic ovarian cancers.[40] Initial data from families with evidence of linkage to BRCA1 suggest that a lifetime risk of ovarian cancer is as high as 63% in women carrying BRCA1 mutations. However, further extensive studies have indicated that this risk appears to be between 28% and 44% among women with BRCA1 mutations and 27% among those with BRCA2 mutations.[41] Other studies of Ashkenazi-Jewish women with founder mutations of BRCA1 and BRCA2 who were selected for family history suggested a lifetime ovarian risk of 16% in carriers of these three founder mutations.[42] In addition to well-established HBOC syndromes, there has been a hypothesis regarding a site-specific form of ovarian cancer based on family pedigrees that reveal multiple cases of ovarian cancer without any apparent increase in breast cancer. However, linkage studies have not identified any locus other than BRCA1 and BRCA2, which suggests that site-specific manifestation is not a distinct hereditary syndrome but rather represents ovarian manifestation of HBOC in which early-onset breast cancer is infrequent.[30,39]

Hereditary nonpolyposis colorectal cancer (HNPCC) syndrome (Lynch syndrome) includes multiple adenocarcinomas involving a combination of familial colon cancer (known as the Lynch I syndrome) with a high rate of ovarian, endometrial, and breast cancers and other malignancies of the gastrointestinal and genitourinary systems.[30] Mutations of genes MSH-2, MLH-1, PMS-1, and PMS-2 have been associated with this syndrome. These mutations account for 2.9% of genetic abnormalities associated with hereditary ovarian cancer syndromes. Mutations in DNA mismatch repair genes listed earlier were related to HNPCC. Ovarian cancer occurs in approximately 5% to 10% of HNPCC patients with one of four described germline mutations. Mutations in hMSH-2 are associated with marked excessive carcinomas of the endometrium and ovary.

Ovarian cancers with germline BRCA1 mutations appear to have distinct clinical and pathologic features. Rubin and colleagues identified 53 patients with germline mutations of BRCA1 and compared their characteristics with those of controls. The patients with cancers associated with BRCA1 mutations had a significantly more favorable course and an earlier age of diagnosis, and a significant majority of these cancers were serous adenocarcinomas. The Gynecologic Oncology Group is performing a prospective study of the clinical course of ovarian cancer patients with BRCA1 mutation, compared with the more common sporadic form of the disease.

Other ovarian tumors, few of which are epithelial, have been associated with other genetic disorders as well. Peutz-Jeghers syndrome (mucocutaneous pigmentation and intestinal polyps) is associated with an increased risk for ovarian tumor of sex cord stromal origin (sex cord tumor with annular tubules) and very rarely with mucinous tumors. Patients with mixed gonadal dysgenesis (46XY genotype or mosaic) can develop gonadoblastoma, another type of sex cord stromal tumor.

Environmental Factors

The industrialized Western countries with the exception of Japan have the highest incidence of epithelial ovarian cancers. The risk for Japanese immigrants to the United States and to their offspring increases but does not reach the level observed in the Caucasian population. It has been suggested that a diet high in meat and animal fat characteristic of industrialized nations is associated with an increased risk of ovarian cancer.[12] A later study performed in Utah, however, failed to demonstrate that calories, fat, protein, fiber, or vitamin A or C appreciably affects the risk of ovarian carcinoma. Other dietary risk factors have been investigated.[12] An Italian case-control study, conducted between 1992 and 1999, involving 1031 women failed to prove an association between the intake of tobacco or coffee and the incidence of epithelial ovarian cancer.[43] Evidence in the literature suggests a protective effect from mumps infection on subsequent development of ovarian cancer,[43] but this finding has been not been confirmed in recent studies.

Current epidemiologic studies do not suggest any definite association with industrial exposure to carcinogens or to diagnostic or therapeutic radiation.[12] However, there have been conflicting reports regarding the association of the use of talcum powder, which in the past has been shown to contain asbestos, with the development of ovarian cancer.[44] It has been postulated that the exposure to asbestos and talc particulates in the form of dusting powders could lead to passage of such materials through the vaginal canal and tract to the ovaries.[45]

Gertig and associates, using data from the Nurses' Health Study, did a prospective analysis of the use of perineal talc and the risk of ovarian cancer and found no substantial association. However, they found a very modest increase limited to serous tumors (RR 1.40, 95% CI 1.02-1.91).[44] Other investigators have not been able to demonstrate an association between talcum powder use and the risk of ovarian cancer.[46,47]

GYNECOLOGIC SURGERY

Numerous studies have noted a reduced risk of ovarian cancer associated with either hysterectomy or tubal ligation.[12,15,23,48-50] This apparent protective effect has ranged from 30% to 40%. This association does not appear to be secondary to a screening bias via better visualization and removal of abnormal ovaries during surgery. This effect may reflect that these operations result in compromised ovarian blood supply or discontinuation of the passage of carcinogens from the vagina to the peritoneal cavity.

Narod and associates studied the protective effect of tubal ligation in carriers of BRCA1 or BRCA2 mutations. After adjusting for other factors such as oral contraceptive use, ethnicity, parity, and history of breast cancer, they found that tubal ligation reduces the risk of ovarian cancer in the population but that this protective effect is limited to carriers of BRCA1 mutations (odds ratio = 0.28). No effect was seen in carriers of BRCA2 mutations.[51]

PREVENTION

Prevention is the ideal method of cancer control. Cancer prevention research seeks to identify the preventable causes of cancer and to reduce cancer incidence by effective application of prevention strategies to target populations. Efforts leading to cancer prevention currently exist via three different routes. Primary prevention is the identification and elimination of cancer-causing agents; reduction to exposure to carcinogens in tobacco smoke is an example of an effective prevention strategy based on exposure and elimination. Unfortunately, for the majority of cancers, including the gynecologic epithelial cancers, a single physical or chemical etiologic factor has not been identified, thereby limiting the application of exposure-based prevention strategies. Secondary prevention consists of screening individuals so that early detection and treatment will improve survival. The third mechanism (tertiary) is the lifetime surveillance of women who have been diagnosed and successfully treated for cancer.

Primary Prevention

Three processes probably contribute to carcinogenesis: abnormal genes acquired through heredity; exogenous mutagens; and uninterrupted exposure to gonadotropins. These three factors lead to a hyperproliferative state of the germinal epithelium, where acquired genetic damage occurs more readily and transformation subsequently occurs.

Pedigrees in all women with a clinical or family history of ovarian or breast cancer should be constructed. In addition, information regarding the incidence of prostate cancer in male relatives should also be carefully documented because there is an association with this hormone-dependent cancer.[37] Once the risk of ovarian cancer development in a patient is assessed and determined to be above baseline, preventive strategies are recommended. Many studies have reported a decrease in the incidence of ovarian cancer risk in women who take oral contraceptive pills. This reduction in risk increases with the duration of usage, approaching 40% to 50% after 5 years of use. More importantly, this effect appears to occur regardless of the parity of the woman. More recent data indicate that this protective effect results from the use of low-dose oral contraceptives as well.[52] Narod and colleagues[53] studied the effect of oral contraceptive pills on patients with BRCA1 or BRCA2 mutations. A total of 271 women were reviewed, and 161 of their sisters were used in the case-controlled study. The adjusted odds ratio for ovarian cancer associated with any past use of oral contraceptives was .5, and the risk decreased with prolonged duration of use. This study strongly argues for oral contraceptive use for carriers of BRCA1 and BRCA2 mutations. Similar evidence with regard to the use of tamoxifen, however, is lacking in the literature. Similar current studies report that tubal ligation reduces the risk of ovarian cancer; the Nurses' Health Study demonstrated a 33% decrease in the risk of ovarian cancer development among women who underwent tubal sterilization.[54] Most importantly, in a preliminary analysis of a 5-year fenretinide (4-HPR) prevention trial in women with T1-T2 breast cancer, DePalo and colleagues reported six cases of ovarian cancer in the placebo-treated group and no cases of ovarian cancer observed in the 4-HPR group ($p = .01$). This study strongly argues that 4-HPR may protect against the development of ovarian cancer, even though this finding was not an objective of the trial. In preclinical studies, fenretinide demonstrates a marked dose-dependent gross inhibition and change that is typical of apoptosis in cell lines that cause human ovarian cancer.[55,56] The Gynecologic Oncology Group has reviewed these data and is currently planning to conduct a trial for ovarian cancer protection using fenretinide in women after prophylactic oophorectomy.

There is considerable interest in hormonal effects on the development of ovarian carcinoma. Rodriguez and others reported on the results of a randomized study that compare the effects of ethinyl estradiol, the oral contraceptive Triphasil (ethinyl estradiol plus levonorgestrel), levonorgestrel, or a placebo on the ovarian epithelium of macaque monkeys.[57] In the progesterone (levonorgestrel)-treated group a significant degree of apoptosis was noted (sixfold increase), whereas a lesser effect was seen in the oral contraceptive–treated group. No changes, however, were seen from the baseline in the control or estrogen-treated group. If these results are verified in extensive human trials, development of safe chemopreventive agents for patients at high risk for ovarian cancer will be possible. Currently, the best known and established chemoprevention modality for ovarian cancer has been the use of oral contraceptives, which decreases the relative risk of dying from ovarian cancer to 0.2.[58,59] Some researchers have recently voiced some concern about the potential deleterious effects of oral contraceptives on the development of breast cancer in BRCA gene mutation carriers.[60] Although the risk reduction for death from ovarian cancer with oral contraceptive use has been well established, there is concern that oral contraceptives may increase the risk of breast cancer.

Prophylactic oophorectomy is currently the only option other than use of oral contraceptives for preventing ovarian cancer. Indications for prophylactic oophorectomy either as a primary procedure or as secondary to abdominal surgery vary according to the estimated risk. The risk of subsequent ovarian cancer has been compared in women at high risk of developing ovarian cancer who are undergoing prophylactic oophorectomy and in women at similar risk who did not undergo surgery. Overall, a reduction by 46% in the risk of ovarian cancer has been observed.[61] Prophylactic oophorectomy should be accompanied at the time of surgery by careful inspection and cytology of the peritoneal cavity because of the risk of microscopic ovarian cancer or primary peritoneal carcinomatosis. One of the most important issues to consider is the morbidity associated with the procedure chosen for prophylactic oophorectomy. Laparoscopy can be effectively used for prophylactic oophorectomy, similar to its widespread application in the diagnosis and treatment of benign adnexal masses. A recent prospective study reported an adnexal surgery complication rate of approximately 10%, regardless of whether laparotomy or laparoscopy was performed, although the only cases of major complications were associated with laparoscopy.[62] None of the patients suffered long-term side effects. Ureteral complications have not been observed during prophylactic oophorectomies.[63] Bilateral salpingo-oophorectomy appears to be the treatment of choice for prophylaxis because it reduces the risk of ovarian remnants. It is the responsibility of the primary surgeon performing bilateral salpingo-oophorectomy in a prophylactic setting to communicate an indication for surgery with the primary pathologists in charge of examining the specimen because these specimens must be sectioned at more frequent intervals (of 2 mm). The fallopian tube must also be similarly evaluated because there have been recent reports of occult fallopian tube cancers in the carriers of BRCA1 and BRCA2 mutations who are undergoing prophylactic oophorectomy. Based upon our current knowledge, prophylactic hysterectomy in conjunction with prophylactic oophorectomy cannot be justified on the basis of increased cancer risks, although some would argue that a portion of the fallopian tube within the myometrium is tissue at risk for development of occult fallopian tube cancer. However, concurrent hysterectomy is beneficial in certain circumstances. A subset of patients with HNPCC related to mismatched repair genes, alluded to earlier, are at an increased risk not only for colorectal and ovarian cancer but also for endometrial cancers. These individuals would clearly benefit from a hysterectomy at the time of oophorectomy. One should also consider that some of the patients referred for prophylactic oophorectomy have been previously treated with tamoxifen, either as the primary chemoprevention for breast cancer or to reduce the risk of developing contralateral breast cancer. Because of the mildly increased risk of endometrial cancer and hyperplasia with tamoxifen treatments, these patients might also benefit from prophylactic hysterectomy at the time of prophylactic oophorectomy.

The decision to remove apparently normal ovaries at the time of unrelated pelvic or abdominal surgery will also be influenced by the primary reason for the surgery, the age of the patient, and the patient's risk of developing ovarian cancer. Approximately one of two patients will undergo bilateral prophylactic oophorectomy at the time of hysterectomy.[64] There is no apparent advantage to performing only a unilateral oophorectomy because it does not appear to reduce the risk of ovarian cancer development. In addition, approximately one third of patients undergoing hysterectomy with preservation of one ovary developed menopausal symptoms within 1 to 2 years after surgery, and another group had significantly lower bone density despite conservation of both ovaries at the time of surgery.[65,66]

A review of cases from 1950 to 1990 from various institutions reveals that almost 8.4% of patients who were diagnosed with ovarian cancer had undergone previous pelvic surgery, and in 5% of all women undergoing pelvic surgery, prophylactic oophorectomy would have prevented the development of ovarian cancer. Applying this decrease nationally would represent a decrease of 1000 ovarian cancer cases annually.[67,68] A U.S. national survey performed in the mid-1980s indicated that 18.2% of patients diagnosed with ovarian cancer reported previous hysterectomy with ovarian conservation, and more than half of the hysterectomies were performed after the age of 40.[69] In a prospective Danish cohort of 22,135 women who had undergone hysterectomy for a benign indication with conservation of at least one ovary, compared with Danish women who had not undergone hysterectomy and had a follow-up of 12½ years, the extrapolated lifetime risk of developing ovarian cancer was 2.1% after hysterectomy and 2.7% in the general population.[70] It should be noted that the prognosis of ovarian cancer in the residual ovaries appears to be similar to that in patients with no previous surgery.[68,71,72-74] It is generally agreed that oophorectomy is an integral part of surgery performed for endometrial cancer because of the risk of ovarian metastasis and also because hormone production by the ovary might be detrimental.

Oophorectomy is clearly indicated during colorectal surgery in the context of HNPCC or in the presence of gross disease on the ovary. More voices are being raised to support the addition of oophorectomy as routine in both postmenopausal and perimenopausal patients undergoing abdominal surgery for bowel cancer.[73-75] In this context, oophorectomy could enable resection of microscopic metastasis; prevention of future metastasis to the ovary, which has been reported in 2% to 8% of the cases; and prevention of primary ovarian pathology. It has been demonstrated that prophylactic oophorectomy reduces the risk of breast cancer by more than half and also confers a survival benefit for patients suffering from breast cancer.[76,77]

Extensive counseling is needed, taking into account the patient's age in relation to menopause and the possible risk of ovarian cancer. The mean age of ovarian cancer onset in the general population is 59. In hereditary ovarian cancer, the disease will occur at a younger age: 45 years in families suffering from HNPCC, 52 years in patients carrying one of the founder mutations in BRCA1, and 59 years in patients carrying founder mutations in BRCA2.[78] The age of onset among affected family members is crucial because there is a significant correlation between the ages of death among sisters in familial ovarian cancer syndromes. Based on decision analysis, oophorectomy may be delayed until the age of 40 with little loss of life expectancy, while allowing the patient to complete childbearing.[79,80]

Prophylactic oophorectomy has facilitated investigation for the presence of hypothetical ovarian cancer precursor lesions. Some investigators have described histologic abnormalities in the surface epithelium, such as inclusions, clefts and fissures, ovarian epithelial metaplasia, or papillae in greater frequency than that found in supposedly normal ovaries.[81] Other authors have described the same abnormalities in prophylactically removed ovaries but found no difference between ovaries of patients at high risk because of BRCA1 mutations and patients without these risk factors.[82]

Recent attention has been focused on peritoneal serous papillary carcinoma and its development after prophylactic oophorectomy. Peritoneal serous papillary carcinoma is histologically indistinguishable from ovarian cancer, yet it arises in the epithelial lining of the perineum, which is of the same embryologic origin as the epithelium of the ovary. Peritoneal serous papillary carcinoma appears to be multifocal in origin, based on differing patterns of gene mutations and expression at various metastatic sites. As contrasted with ovarian cancer, which has been shown to be monoclonal,[83,84] recent publications on genetic analysis of peritoneal serous papillary carcinoma of the perineum reveal that peritoneal serous papillary carcinoma is part of the malignant phenotype associated with hereditary ovarian cancer.[85,86] Several studies have reported the occurrence of tumors arising from the peritoneal surface in women after prophylactic oophorectomy.[60,83,86] Karlan and associates reported that 7 of 8 invasive cancers diagnosed in 1261 participants in the Gilda Radner Ovarian Detection Program were actually peritoneal serous papillary cancers.[61,84,87] This finding argues against the benefits of prophylactic oophorectomy in high-risk populations. It is also of further concern that present screening strategies do not allow detection of peritoneal serous papillary carcinomatosis before advanced stage disease.

Secondary Prevention

In recent years a great deal of attention has been placed on programs for early detection of ovarian cancer. Most of the programs have used different combinations of physical examination, ultrasound with and without color, Doppler analysis, and biologic markers.[88] The predictive value of early detection programs has varied significantly with the population examined and the screening tests used. A recent review evaluated 25 separate studies of ovarian cancer screening performed on approximately 90,000 women.[89] Jacobs reported results from one of the few prospective randomized studies that used multiple modalities of screening tests. The control group consisted of 10,958 women who were followed with no screening test; 10,997 women underwent CA125 (three annual tests). Women in the screening arm with raised CA125 values underwent ultrasound testing and were referred for surgery if this test was abnormal. In the screening group, 468 women underwent 781 ultrasound scans because of raised CA125, and 29 women underwent surgery. Of these 29 women, six were found to have ovarian cancer and 23 had false-positive results because of benign ovarian tumors. The overall positive predictive value of screening was 20.7%. In addition to these six index cancers, ovarian cancer was diagnosed in another 10 women within the screening group during the subsequent 8 years of follow-up. A total of 20 women were identified with ovarian cancer in the control group.[90]

Women in the screening arm survived an average of 73 months after diagnosis, whereas unscreened patients in the control group survived 42 months ($p = 0.01$). Neither the number of deaths due to ovarian cancer nor the number of stage I or stage II cancers between the two groups was statistically significant. The results of this ovarian cancer screening approach that used multiple modalities seems to be encouraging because it shows a significant difference in survival among women in the screening group.[90]

Clearly a high number of unnecessary surgeries were performed on otherwise healthy women in the aforementioned studies. Early detection programs can also cause additional distress and anxiety in many women who do not have cancer. Therefore randomized control trials have been initiated to test the effectiveness of early detection programs and to evaluate their impact on these programs, survival, and the quality of life. Early detection may be more advantageous for individuals at increased risk for developing ovarian cancer because fewer women will need to be screened for each case detected. It remains to be demonstrated whether treating cancers detected earlier by screening improves overall survival or only gives the patient a false sense of security. In 1999 Jacobs and colleagues made the first step toward addressing these questions by publishing the data from a pilot randomized control trial.[90] The screening protocol adopted in that study included three annual measurements of CA125 and pelvic ultrasonography if the CA125 level was elevated. During the 7 years of follow-up in this study, improved median survival was observed in this screened group: 16 patients had median survival of 72.9 months, compared with the control group (20 patients) with a median survival of 41.8 months ($p = .01$); nine deaths occurred in the screened group, compared with 18 deaths in the control group. In this study 23 otherwise healthy women without cancer underwent surgery, and 10 patients who developed cancer were missed during screening.[90] Although the performance of this screening strategy is encouraging, no recommendations can be made until there is confirmation of these results in larger prospective studies expected to be completed by 2004. It remains controversial whether patients who have had ovulation induction are at sufficient increased risk to warrant earlier screening, as epidemiologic studies have previously suggested. Recent data, however, suggest that if such a risk exists, it appears to be very small.[91-93]

The detection of an asymptomatic pelvic mass during routine physical examination may identify an ovarian carcinoma before abdominal dissemination occurs, but no data related to the frequency at which ovarian cancer is detected exist based on an annual pelvic examination in these asymptomatic women. Furthermore, there is little evidence that the detection of ovarian cancer based on an abnormal pelvic examination alters morbidity and mortality in asymptomatic women. Although frequent pelvic examination continues to be a common recommendation for women older than 40 years of age, its benefits as a screening procedure for ovarian cancer have not been established.

The use of ultrasonography as a screening procedure for ovarian cancer has been the subject of intense research. It has been proposed that transvaginal ultrasound is a more specific alternative to abdominal sonography; additionally transvaginal ultrasound does not require any patient preparation.[94-96] At the University of Kentucky 3220 asymptomatic postmenopausal women were screened using transvaginal ultrasound. Surgery was performed in 44 women with ovarian abnormalities and the following findings were noted: two stage I ovarian cancers (one granulosa cell, one epithelial carcinoma); one stage IIIB cancer; and 41 benign pathologies, including 21 serous cystadenomas. In this study the sensitivity was 100%, the specificity 98.7%, and the positive predictive value 6.7%. These investigators reported that removal of cystadenomas may also decrease the risk of ovarian cancers because, based on their histologic review, such tumors may be precursors of invasive epithelial ovarian cancers.[95] Adding color-flow imaging with transvaginal ultrasound may further improve the accuracy of sonography and reduce the unacceptably high rate of false-positive results that currently have been reported with ultrasound alone.[97] Neovascularization and the alterations in blood flow may be useful in discriminating benign from malignant ovarian tumors. Initial results have demonstrated no abnormalities of neovascularization in morphologically normal ovaries. Nonmalignant masses also showed no signs of neovascularization and had a pulsatility index markedly different from invasive ovarian cancer. Kurjak and associates studied a spectrum of ultrasound systems (two-dimensional transvaginal, transvaginal color Doppler, three-dimensional transvaginal, three-dimensional color Doppler, and contrast-enhanced three-dimensional power Doppler) on 251 preoperative patients diagnosed with adnexal masses. Pathologically, the sensitivity and specificity of all these techniques ranged from 80% to 100% and 95% to 99%, respectively (Table 9-2).[97] Thirty of

Table 9-2
Sensitivity and Specificity As a Result of Ultrasound Techniques on Preoperative Patients Diagnosed with Adnexal Masses

Technique	Sensitivity, %	Specificity, %	PPV, %	CI	NPV, %	CI
2DS/TVCDS	80	95	71	0.0-1.0	97	0.0-1.0
3DS	87	96	74	0.649-1.0	98	0.716-1.0
2DS	89	98	86	0.122-1.0	99	0.758-1.0
3Ds/3DPDS	97	99	97	0.607-1.0	99	0.823-1.0
Contrast-enhanced 3DPDS	100	99	93	0.453-1.0	100	1.0-1.0

CI = 95% confidence interval; 3DS = three-dimensional sonography; 2DS = two-dimensional sonography; 3DPDS = three-dimensional power Doppler sonography; PPV = positive predictive value; NPV = negative predictive value; TVCDS = transvaginal color Doppler sonography.
Source: Kurjak A, Kupesic S, Sparac V, et al: *J Ultrasound Med* 2001; 20:829-840.

these patients were found to have ovarian malignancies, and 221 were diagnosed with benign processes.

The finding that approximately 50% of women with stage I/II ovarian cancers have serum CA125 levels greater than 65 U/mL suggests that serum CA125 levels are sufficiently sensitive to identify patients with early-stage disease.[98] When CA125 levels were tested in 915 Roman Catholic nuns, only 0.5% of women older than 50 years of age had elevated test results.[99] As previously noted, false-positive test results have been reported in a number of nonmalignant gynecologic conditions such as peritonitis, pancreatitis, renal and heart failure, and hepatitis.[98] Because of the high false-positive rates and relatively low incidence of epithelial ovarian cancers, the single CA125 assay is not useful in detecting early-stage cancer. In a large study from Sweden, serum CA125 levels were measured annually in approximately 6000 women older than 40 years of age.[100] In women who had CA125 levels greater than 30, surveillance was undertaken with sequential CA125 levels every 3 months; pelvic examinations and transabdominal ultrasounds were performed every 6 months. If the CA125 level doubled or was greater than 95 at the time of screening or if an adnexal mass was detected by either ultrasound or pelvic examination, the patients underwent a laparotomy. One hundred seventy-five patients were found to have elevated CA125 levels, and six ovarian cancers were detected. Three women with normal CA125 levels developed ovarian cancers. For women younger than 50 years of age, a CA125 value above 35 had a specificity of 97%, compared with 99% for women older than 50 years of age. The specificity was increased to 99.8% for both groups if this serum CA125 level was set at 95 U/mL.

Macrophage colony-stimulating factor (MCS-F) is a growth factor that has been detected in epithelial ovarian cancers and may have a role in both screening and monitoring responses to treatment. It is secreted by ovarian cancer cell lines in vitro and acts as a chemoattractant for monocytes.[101] Elevated serum MCS-F levels have been found in 70% of the serum or ascites of patients with epithelial ovarian cancer.[101] Measurement of serum MCS-F levels together with CA125 levels may be more predictive of disease status than CA125 levels alone.[101]

Lysophosphatidic acid (LPA) has been reported in a preliminary study to be a predictive biomarker for ovarian cancer.[102] LPA is present in malignant ascites and was shown to stimulate proliferation of ovarian cancer cells in vitro. In a preliminary study, elevated LPA levels were found in 9 of 10 patients with early-stage ovarian cancer. Additional studies of specificity and sensitivity are in progress, including an assessment of LPA levels together with a determination of serum CA125.

Multimodal screening preliminary studies using serum CA125 levels, pelvic examinations, and ultrasonography have demonstrated that ovarian cancer can be detected in asymptomatic women. However, as noted, these procedures are associated with a significant false-positive rate and an unacceptably large number of negative laparotomies. Because a laparotomy is required to diagnose ovarian cancer, there is a defined morbidity and mortality associated with this screening. When the positive predictive value is below 10%, more harm (complications of unnecessary laparotomy) than good (diagnosing early-stage ovarian cancer) may come to a screened population.[34] Furthermore, in a recent review of uncontrolled trials of ovarian cancer screening in 36,208 women, 29 cases of ovarian cancers were identified, with only 12 or 41% at stage I. Survival is unlikely to be significantly affected by an earlier diagnosis of an advanced stage disease. Based on these considerations, the National Institutes of Health Consensus Conference on Ovarian Cancer in 1994 did not recommend screening for ovarian cancer in the general population without any increased risk factors.

Even in women with positive family history, there is no evidence that screening can affect mortality from this disease. In 1500 asymptomatic women who had at least one close relative with ovarian cancer and who were screened by transvaginal ultrasound, seven ovarian cancers were found, three of which were borderline in nature.[103] Even in women who have first-degree relatives with ovarian cancer or who are carriers of the BRCA1 or BRCA2 gene, the ability of screening tests to detect earlier stage ovarian cancer has not been established. However, it seems prudent to couple pelvic and ultrasound examination with monitoring of serum CA125 levels on a regular basis after these women reach 30 to 35 years of age and also to consider prophylactic oophorectomy in this high-risk group of patients. However, as mentioned earlier, the role of prophylactic oophorectomy in such patient populations continues to be controversial (Figure 9-1).

CONCLUSION

There is no currently reliable procedure for detection of early ovarian cancer. Available potential screening techniques have included pelvic examination, ovarian ultrasound, examination via transvaginal route, and monitoring of CA125 and other tumor markers combined with the ultrasound approaches. At the current time there are no recommended guidelines for screening of the general population. Depending on age and desire to maintain fertility in women at high risk for ovarian cancer, one may consider the use of oral contraceptive pills in combination with periodic CA125 level measurement and pelvic ultrasound

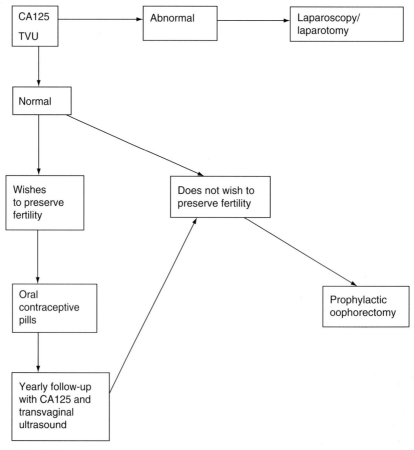

FIGURE 9-1
Screening and management of women at high risk for epithelial ovarian cancer.

or prophylactic oophorectomy. The patients must be counseled at length about the risk of each procedure and must also be advised of possible increased risks of breast cancer and future development of peritoneal carcinoma. Several national early detection and prevention programs are currently in place, and patients at high risk for development of ovarian cancer should be channeled into these programs so that understanding of the development of this disease and consideration of guidelines for prevention and early detection continues to improve.

REFERENCES

1. Greenlee RT, Hill-Harmon MB, Murray T, at al: Cancer statistics, 2001. *CA Cancer J Clin* 2001;51(1):15-36.
2. Yancik R, Ries LG, Yates JW: Ovarian cancer in the elderly: an analysis of surveillance, epidemiology, and end results program data. *Am J Obstet Gynecol* 1986;154(3):639-647.
3. Ness RB, Grisso JA, Klapper J, et al: Racial differences in ovarian cancer risks. *J Natl Med Assoc* 2000;92(4):176-182.
4. Ries LAG, Kosary CL, Hankey BF, et al: *SEER Cancer Statistics Review, 1973-1994.* Bethesda, MD, National Cancer Institute, 1997.
5. Oriel KA, Hartenbach EM, Remington PL: Trends in United States ovarian cancer mortality, 1979-1995. *Obstet Gynecol* 1999;93(1):30-33.
6. Memarzadeh S, Berek JS: Advances in the management of epithelial ovarian cancer. *J Reprod Med* 2001;46(7):621-629; discussion 629-630.
7. McGuire V, Herrinton L, Whittemore AS: Race, epithelial ovarian cancer survival, and membership in a large health maintenance organization. *Epidemiology* 2002;13(2):231-234.
8. Herrinton LJ, Stanford JL, Schwartz SM, et al: Ovarian cancer incidence among Asian migrants to the United States and their descendants. *J Natl Cancer Inst* 1994;86(17):1336-1339.
9. Kato I, Tominaga S, Kuroishi T: Relationship between westernization of dietary habits and mortality from breast and ovarian cancers in Japan. *Jpn J Cancer Res* 1987;78(4):349-357.
10. Heintz AP, Odicino F, Maisonneuve P, et al: Carcinoma of the ovary. *J Epidemiol Biostat* 2001;6(1):107-138.
11. Fathalla MF: Incessant ovulation: a factor in ovarian neoplasia? *Lancet* 1971;2(7716):163.
12. Greene MH, Clark JW, Blayney DW: The epidemiology of ovarian cancer. *Semin Oncol* 1984;11(3):209-226.
13. Cramer DW, Hutchison GB, Welch WR: Factors affecting the association of oral contraceptives and ovarian cancer. *N Engl J Med* 1982;307(17):1047-1051.
14. Epithelial ovarian cancer and combined oral contraceptives: the WHO Collaborative Study of Neoplasia and Steroid Contraceptives. *Int J Epidemiol* 1989;18(3):538-545.
15. Rosenblatt KA, Thomas DB: Reduced risk of ovarian cancer in women with a tubal ligation or hysterectomy: the World Health Organization Collaborative Study of Neoplasia and Steroid Contraceptives. *Cancer Epidemiol Biomarkers Prev* 1996;5(11):933-935.
16. Ness RB, Grisso JA, Klapper J, et al: Risk of ovarian cancer in relation to estrogen and progestin dose and use characteristics of oral contraceptives: SHARE study group, steroid hormones and reproductions. *Am J Epidemiol* 2000;152(3):233-241.
17. Risch HA: Hormonal etiology of epithelial ovarian cancer, with a hypothesis concerning the role of androgens and progesterone. *J Natl Cancer Inst* 1998;90(23):1774-1786.
18. Daly M, Obrams GI: Epidemiology and risk assessment for ovarian cancer. *Semin Oncol* 1998;25(3):255-264.
19. Garg PP, Kerlikowske K, Subak L, et al: Hormone replacement therapy and the risk of epithelial ovarian carcinoma: a meta-analysis. *Obstet Gynecol* 1998;92(3):472-479.
20. Rodriguez C, Patel AV, Calle EE, et al: Estrogen replacement therapy and ovarian cancer mortality in a large prospective study of US women. *JAMA* 2001;285(11):1460-1465.
21. Ness RB, Cottreau C: Possible role of ovarian epithelial inflammation in ovarian cancer. *J Natl Cancer Inst* 1999;91(17):1459-1467.
22. Rossing MA, Daling JR, Weiss NS: Ovarian tumors in a cohort of infertile women. *N Engl J Med* 1994;331(12):771-776.
23. Whittemore AS, Harris R, Itnyre J: Characteristics relating to ovarian cancer risk: collaborative analysis of 12 US case-control studies, II: invasive epithelial ovarian cancers in white women, Collaborative Ovarian Cancer Group. *Am J Epidemiol* 1992;136(10):1184-1203.
24. Ness RB, Cramer DW, Goodman MT, et al: Infertility, fertility drugs, and ovarian cancer: a pooled analysis of case-control studies. *Am J Epidemiol* 2002;155(3):217-224.
25. Armstrong B, Doll R: Environmental factors and cancer incidence and mortality in different countries, with special reference to dietary practices. *Int J Cancer* 1975;15(4):617-631.
26. Bosetti C, Negri E, Franceschi S, et al: Diet and ovarian cancer risk: a case-control study in Italy. *Int J Cancer* 2001;93(6):911-915.
27. Shu XO, Gao YT, Yuan JM, et al: Dietary factors and epithelial ovarian cancer. *Br J Cancer* 1989;59(1):92-96.
28. Cramer DW, Greenberg ER, Titus-Ernstoff L, et al: A case-control study of galactose consumption and metabolism in relation to ovarian cancer. *Cancer Epidemiol Biomarkers Prev* 2000;9(1):95-101.

29. Cramer DW, Muto MG, Reichardt JK, et al: Characteristics of women with a family history of ovarian cancer, I: galactose consumption and metabolism. *Cancer* 1994;74(4):1309-1317.

30. Lynch HT, Bewtra C, Lynch JF: Familial ovarian carcinoma: clinical nuances. *Am J Med* 1986; 81(6):1073-1076.

31. Casagrande JT, Louie EW, Pike MC, et al: "Incessant ovulation" and ovarian cancer. *Lancet* 1979;2(8135):170-173.

32. Kerlikowske K, Brown JS, Grady DG: Should women with familial ovarian cancer undergo prophylactic oophorectomy? *Obstet Gynecol* 1992; 80(4):700-707.

33. Schildkraut JM, Thompson WD: Familial ovarian cancer: a population-based case-control study. *Am J Epidemiol* 1988;128(3):456-466.

34. National Institutes of Health Consensus Development Conference Statement. Ovarian cancer: screening, treatment, and follow-up. *Gynecol Oncol* 1994;55(3 Pt 2):S4-14.

35. Whittemore AS: Characteristics relating to ovarian cancer risk: implications for prevention and detection. *Gynecol Oncol* 1994;55(3 Pt 2):S15-19.

36. Piver MS, Baker TR, Piedmonte M, et al: Epidemiology and etiology of ovarian cancer. *Semin Oncol* 1991;18(3):177-185.

37. Lynch HT, Casey MJ, Lynch J, et al: Genetics and ovarian carcinoma. *Semin Oncol* 1998;25(3):265-280.

38. Wooster R, Neuhausen SL, Mangion J, et al: Localization of a breast cancer susceptibility gene, BRCA2, to chromosome 13q12-13. *Science* 1994;265(5181):2088-2090.

39. Boyd J: Molecular genetics of hereditary ovarian cancer. *Oncology (Huntingt)* 1998;12(3):399-406; discussion 409-410, 413.

40. Lynch HT, Lynch JF, Casey MJ: Genetics and gynecologic cancer. In Young RC, editor: *Principles and practice of gynecological oncology*, 3rd ed. Philadelphia, Lippincott-Raven; 1997.

41. Frank TS: Testing for hereditary risk of ovarian cancer. *Cancer Control* 1999;6(4):327-334.

42. Struewing JP, Hartge P, Wacholder S, et al: The risk of cancer associated with specific mutations of BRCA1 and BRCA2 among Ashkenazi Jews. *N Engl J Med* 1997;336:1401-1408.

43. Menczer J, Modan M, Ranon L, et al: Possible role of mumps virus in the etiology of ovarian cancer. *Cancer* 1979;43(4):1375-1379.

44. Gertig DM, Hunter DJ, Cramer DW, et al: Prospective study of talc use and ovarian cancer. *J Natl Cancer Inst* 2000;92(3):249-252.

45. Cramer DW, Welch WR, Scully RE, et al: Ovarian cancer and talc: a case-control study. *Cancer* 1982;50(2):372-376.

46. Wong C, Hempling RE, Piver MS, et al: Perineal talc exposure and subsequent epithelial ovarian cancer: a case-control study. *Obstet Gynecol* 1999;93(3):372-376.

47. Whysner J, Mohan M: Perineal application of talc and cornstarch powders: evaluation of ovarian cancer risk. *Am J Obstet Gynecol* 2000;182(3):720-724.

48. Booth M, Beral V, Smith P: Risk factors for ovarian cancer: a case-control study. *Br J Cancer* 1989; 60(4):592-598.

49. Kreiger N, Sloan M, Cotterchio M, et al: Surgical procedures associated with risk of ovarian cancer. *Int J Epidemiol* 1997;26(4):710-715.

50. Miracle-McMahill HL, Calle EE, Kosinski AS, et al: Tubal ligation and fatal ovarian cancer in a large prospective cohort study. *Am J Epidemiol* 1997; 145(4):349-357.

51. Narod SA, Sun P, Ghadirian P, et al: Tubal ligation and risk of ovarian cancer in carriers of BRCA1 or BRCA2 mutations: a case-control study. *Lancet* 2001;357(9267):1467-1470.

52. Rosenblatt KA, Thomas DB, Noonan EA: High-dose and low-dose combined oral contraceptives: protection against epithelial ovarian cancer and the length of the protective effect, The WHO Collaborative Study of Neoplasia and Steroid Contraceptives. *Eur J Cancer* 1992;28A(11):1872-1876.

53. Narod SA, Risch H, Moslehi R, et al: Oral contraceptives and the risk of hereditary ovarian cancer, Hereditary Ovarian Cancer Clinical Study Group. *N Engl J Med* 1998;339(7):424-428.

54. Hankinson SE, Colditz GA, Hunter DJ, et al: A quantitative assessment of oral contraceptive use and risk of ovarian cancer. *Obstet Gynecol* 1992;80(4):708-714.

55. De Palo G, Veronesi U, Camerini T, et al: Can fenretinide protect women against ovarian cancer? *J Natl Cancer Inst* 1995;87(2):146-147.

56. Supino R, Crosti M, Clerici M, et al: Induction of apoptosis by fenretinide (4HPR) in human ovarian carcinoma cells and its association with retinoic acid receptor expression. *Int J Cancer* 1996;65(4):491-497.

57. Rodriguez GC, Walmer DK, Cline M, et al: Effect of progestin on the ovarian epithelium of macaques: cancer prevention through apoptosis? *J Soc Gynecol Investig* 1998;5(5):271-276.

58. Beral V, Hermon C, Kay C, et al: Mortality associated with oral contraceptive use: 25 year follow up of cohort of 46,000 women from Royal College of General Practitioners' oral contraception study. *BMJ* 1999;318(7176):96-100.

59. Whiting JR, Billoski TV, Jones VR: Herding instincts of cretaceous duck-billed dinosaurs. *Journal of Paleontology* 1987;75:112-132.

60. Ursin G, Henderson BE, Haile RW, et al: Does oral contraceptive use increase the risk of breast cancer in women with BRCA1/BRCA2 mutations more than in other women? *Cancer Res* 1997; 57(17):3678-3681.

61. Struewing JP, Watson P, Easton DF, et al: Prophylactic oophorectomy in inherited breast/

ovarian cancer families. *J Natl Cancer Inst Monogr* 1995(17):33-35.

62. Meltomaa SS, Taalikka MO, Helenius HY, et al: Complications and long-term outcomes after adnexal surgery by laparotomy and laparoscopy. *J Am Assoc Gynecol Laparosc* 1999;6(4):463-469.

63. Tamussino KF, Lang PF, Breinl E: Ureteral complications with operative gynecologic laparoscopy. *Am J Obstet Gynecol* 1998;178(5):967-970.

64. Averette HE, Nguyen HN: The role of prophylactic oophorectomy in cancer prevention. *Gynecol Oncol* 1994;55(3 Pt 2):S38-41.

65. Siddle N, Sarrel P, Whitehead M: The effect of hysterectomy on the age at ovarian failure: identification of a subgroup of women with premature loss of ovarian function and literature review. *Fertil Steril* 1987;47(1):94-100.

66. Watson NR, Studd JW, Garnett T, et al: Bone loss after hysterectomy with ovarian conservation. *Obstet Gynecol* 1995;86(1):72-77.

67. Shoham Z: Should prophylactic oophorectomy be performed on post-menopausal women undergoing laparotomy or laparoscopy for non-gynaecological indications? *Hum Reprod* 1997;12(2):201-202.

68. Sightler SE, Boike GM, Estape RE, et al: Ovarian cancer in women with prior hysterectomy: a 14-year experience at the University of Miami. *Obstet Gynecol* 1991;78(4):681-684.

69. Averette HE, Hoskins W, Nguyen HN, et al: National survey of ovarian carcinoma, I: a patient care evaluation study of the American College of Surgeons. *Cancer* 1993;71(4 Suppl):1629-1638.

70. Loft A, Lidegaard O, Tabor A: Incidence of ovarian cancer after hysterectomy: a nationwide controlled follow up. *Br J Obstet Gynaecol* 1997;104(11):1296-1301.

71. Fine BA, Yazigi R, Risser R: Prognosis of ovarian cancer developing in the residual ovary. *Gynecol Oncol* 1991;43(2):164-166.

72. Yaegashi N, Sato S, Yajima A: Incidence of ovarian cancer in women with prior hysterectomy in Japan. *Gynecol Oncol* 1998;68(3):244-246.

73. Koves I, Vamosi-Nagy I, Besznyak I: Ovarian metastases of colorectal tumours. *Eur J Surg Oncol* 1993;19(6):633-635.

74. Schutt U, Wedell J, Koppen P, et al: (Preventive ovariectomy in colorectal cancer.) *Chirurg* 1993;64(12):1040-1043.

75. Gemos K, Rizzotti L, Tsardis P, et al: (Indications for prophylactic ovariectomy in patients with colorectal carcinoma.) *Minerva Chir* 1995;50(1-2):89-92.

76. Rebbeck TR, Levin AM, Eisen A, et al: Breast cancer risk after bilateral prophylactic oophorectomy in BRCA1 mutation carriers. *J Natl Cancer Inst* 1999;91(17):1475-1479.

77. Meijer WJ, van Lindert AC: Prophylactic oophorectomy. *Eur J Obstet Gynecol Reprod Biol* 1992;47(1):59-65.

78. Gotlieb WH, Friedman E, Bar-Sade RB, et al: Rates of Jewish ancestral mutations in BRCA1 and BRCA2 in borderline ovarian tumors. *J Natl Cancer Inst* 1998;90(13):995-1000.

79. Houlston RS, Hampson J, Collins WP, et al: Correlation in ages at death from familial ovarian cancer among sisters. *Gynecol Oncol* 1992;47(2):253-254.

80. Grann VR, Whang W, Jacobson JS, et al: Benefits and costs of screening Ashkenazi Jewish women for BRCA1 and BRCA2. *J Clin Oncol* 1999;17(2):494-500.

81. Salazar H, Godwin AK, Daly MB, et al: Microscopic benign and invasive malignant neoplasms and a cancer-prone phenotype in prophylactic oophorectomies. *J Natl Cancer Inst* 1996;88(24):1810-1820.

82. Tonin P, Weber B, Offit K, et al: Frequency of recurrent BRCA1 and BRCA2 mutations in Ashkenazi Jewish breast cancer families. *Nat Med* 1996;2(11):1179-1183.

83. Muto MG, Welch WR, Mok SC, et al: Evidence for a multifocal origin of papillary serous carcinoma of the peritoneum. *Cancer Res* 1995;55(3):490-492.

84. Karlan BY, Baldwin RL, Lopez-Luevanos E, et al: Peritoneal serous papillary carcinoma, a phenotypic variant of familial ovarian cancer: implications for ovarian cancer screening. *Am J Obstet Gynecol* 1999;180(4):917-928.

85. Bandera CA, Muto MG, Schorge JO, et al: BRCA1 gene mutations in women with papillary serous carcinoma of the peritoneum. *Obstet Gynecol* 1998;92(4 Pt 1):596-600.

86. Schorge JO, Muto MG, Welch WR, et al: Molecular evidence for multifocal papillary serous carcinoma of the peritoneum in patients with germline BRCA1 mutations. *J Natl Cancer Inst* 1998;90(11):841-845.

87. Piver MS, Baker TR, Jishi MF, et al: Familial ovarian cancer: a report of 658 families from the Gilda Radner Familial Ovarian Cancer Registry 1981-1991. *Cancer* 1993;71(2 Suppl):582-588.

88. Gotlieb WH, Berek JS: (The proper application of biological markers.) In Guastala JP, editor: *Cancer de l'ovaire.* Paris, Arnette Blackwell, 1996.

89. Bell R, Petticrew M, Sheldon T: The performance of screening tests for ovarian cancer: results of a systematic review. *Br J Obstet Gynaecol* 1998;105(11):1136-1147.

90. Jacobs IJ, Skates SJ, MacDonald N, et al: Screening for ovarian cancer: a pilot randomised controlled trial. *Lancet* 1999;353(9160):1207-1210.

91. Gotlieb WH, Flikker S, Davidson B, et al: Borderline tumors of the ovary: fertility treatment, conservative management, and pregnancy outcome. *Cancer* 1998;82(1):141-146.

92. Venn A, Watson L, Bruinsma F, et al: Risk of cancer after use of fertility drugs with in-vitro fertilisation. *Lancet* 1999;354(9190):1586-1590.

93. Potashnik G, Lerner-Geva L, Genkin L, et al: Fertility drugs and the risk of breast and ovarian cancers: results of a long-term follow-up study. *Fertil Steril* 1999;71(5):853-859.

94. DePriest PD, van Nagell JR, Jr., Gallion HH, et al: Ovarian cancer screening in asymptomatic post-menopausal women. *Gynecol Oncol* 1993;51(2): 205-209.

95. van Nagell JR, Jr., Higgins RV, Donaldson ES, et al: Transvaginal sonography as a screening method for ovarian cancer: a report of the first 1000 cases screened. *Cancer* 1990;65(3): 573-577.

96. van Nagell JR, Jr., DePriest PD, Puls LE, et al: Ovarian cancer screening in asymptomatic post-menopausal women by transvaginal sonography. *Cancer* 1991;68(3):458-462.

97. Kurjak A, Kupesic S, Sparac V, et al: Preoperative evaluation of pelvic tumors by Doppler and three-dimensional sonography. *J Ultrasound Med* 2001;20(8):829-840.

98. Olt GJ, Berchuck A, Bast RC, Jr, Gynecologic tumor markers. *Semin Surg Oncol* 1990;6(6):305-313.

99. Zurawski VR Jr, Broderick SF, Pickens P, et al: Serum CA 125 levels in a group of nonhospitalized women: relevance for the early detection of ovarian cancer. *Obstet Gynecol* 1987;69(4):606-611.

100. Einhorn N, Sjovall K, Knapp RC, et al: Prospective evaluation of serum CA 125 levels for early detection of ovarian cancer. *Obstet Gynecol* 1992;80(1): 14-18.

101. Elg SA, Yu Y, Carson LF, et al: Serum levels of macrophage colony-stimulating factor in patients with ovarian cancer undergoing second-look laparotomy. *Am J Obstet Gynecol* 1992;166(1 Pt 1):134-7.

102. Xu Y, Shen Z, Wiper DW, et al: Lysophosphatidic acid as a potential biomarker for ovarian and other gynecologic cancers. *JAMA* 1998;280(8): 719-723

103. Bourne TH, Campbell S, Reynolds K, et al: The potential role of serum CA 125 in an ultrasound-based screening program for familial ovarian cancer. *Gynecol Oncol* 1994;52(3): 379-385.

CHAPTER 10

Cancer of the Uterine Corpus

Howard D. Homesley
Alberto Manetta

Endometrial carcinoma is a highly curable disease when diagnosed and treated in its earliest stages. A summary of current information on incidence, risk factors, prevention, diagnosis, and characteristics of special histologic types related to cancer of the uterine corpus follows.

INCIDENCE AND MORTALITY

Endometrial carcinoma accounts for 6% of all cancers in women. It is the most common gynecologic malignancy in the United States, with 39,300 new cases and 6600 deaths estimated for 2002.[1] If adjusted to account for women who have undergone hysterectomy, incidence rates would be higher.[2] There are no simple screening tests for cancer of the uterine corpus, but abnormal vaginal bleeding occurs early in the disease process. When treated in the early stages, endometrial carcinoma is highly curable.

If abnormal bleeding is ignored, the outcome for women diagnosed with advanced-stage disease remains poor. Mortality associated with cancer of the uterine corpus accounts for 2% of cancer deaths in women.[1] Among cases retrospectively reviewed at one institution for the period 1976 through 1992, median survival was 12 months in women with surgical stage IV endometrial carcinoma.[3] The National Cancer Institute (NCI) Surveillance, Epidemiology, and End Results (SEER) survival data for 1992-1997 by stage of disease and race are summarized in Table 10-1.[4] The three SEER stages are broadly inclusive of the surgical staging categories adopted by the International Federation of Gynecology and Obstetrics (FIGO).[5] Histopathologic types and grades for cancer of the corpus uteri are listed in Box 10-1. The FIGO surgical staging categories are summarized in Table 10-2.

Endometrial carcinoma incidence and mortality rates, age-adjusted to the 1970 U.S. standard population, increase with advancing age in most racial or ethnic groups.[4] For Chinese-American and Filipino-American women however, the incidence is highest between 55 and 69 years of age.[6] Incidence and mortality rates per 100,000 women younger and older than 50 years of age are shown in Figure 10-1. At age 65 years and older, the incidence rate is 97.3, and the mortality rate is 22.2 per 100,000, with age-specific incidence highest between 75 and 79 years of age (109.1 per 100,000).[4]

Mundt and associates[7] reviewed studies in which age was shown to influence recurrence and survival as well as studies in which age did not affect outcomes. Differences were noted in adjustments for pathologic factors among subjects in the various studies. In their cohort study of three pathologically comparable groups (<60, n = 156; 60-69, n = 147; ≥70, n = 152), the authors found that 5-year disease-free survivals were not significantly different

Table 10-1
SEER Endometrial Cancer Survival Data, 1992-1997, by Stage of Disease and Race*⁺

Stage of Disease	ALL RACES (N = 16,472)		WHITE FEMALES (N = 14,369)		BLACK FEMALES (N = 1019)	
	% of Cases	5-Year Relative Survival (%)	% of Cases	5-Year Relative Survival (%)	% of Cases	5-Year Relative Survival (%)
All stages	100	84.0	100	85.8	100	58.9
Carcinoma limited to the corpus uteri	73	96.1	75	96.9	52	82.9
Regional involvement	14	62.7	18	65.1	22	42.7
Presence of distant metastases	8	25.8	13	27.7	18	13.1
Unstaged disease	5	49.1	4	47.6	9	48.9

*SEER Program population-based registry data, 9 regions.
⁺Includes cancers of the uterus, corpus, and not otherwise specified (NOS).
Data Source: National Cancer Institute SEER Cancer Statistics Review, 1973-1998.

BOX 10-1 Corpus Uteri Carcinoma Histopathologic Types and Grades

Histopathologic Types
- Endometrioid carcinoma (75%-80%)
  - Ciliated adenocarcinoma
  - Secretory adenocarcinoma
  - Papillary or villoglandular
  - Adenocarcinoma with squamous differentiation
    - Adenocanthoma
    - Adenosquamous
- Uterine papillary serous (<10%)
- Mucinous (1%)
- Clear cell (4%)
- Squamous cell (<1%)
- Mixed carcinoma (10%)
- Undifferentiated

Histopathologic Grades
- Gx—Grade cannot be assessed
- G1—Well differentiated; 5% or less of a nonsquamous or nonmorular solid growth pattern
- G2—Moderately differentiated; 6% to 50% of a nonsquamous or nonmorular solid growth pattern
- G3—Poorly or undifferentiated; more than 50% of a nonsquamous or nonmorular solid growth pattern

Sources: International Federation of Gynecology and Obstetrics (*www.figo.org*) and National Cancer Institute, Endometrial Cancer (PDQ): Treatment (*www.cancer.gov*)

among the groups. When the two younger groups were combined and compared with the older group, there was a significant difference in disease-free survival ($p = .03$). Multivariate analysis, however, confirmed that race, stage, grade, and lymphovascular invasion were significant predictors of recurrence, but age was not significant when the other pathologic factors were included in the analysis.

Non-Hispanic White females have the highest incidence of endometrial carcinoma (22.9 per 100,000 population, age-adjusted, 1992-1998). Incidence rates for Black,

Table 10-2
FIGO Surgical Staging for Carcinoma of the Corpus Uteri

Stage*	Description of Stage
IA	Tumor limited to the endometrium
IB	Invasion to less than half of the myometrium
IC	Invasion equal to or more than half of the myometrium
IIA	Endocervical glandular involvement only
IIB	Cervical stromal invasion
IIIA	Tumor invades the serosa of the corpus uteri and/or adnexae and/or positive cytologic findings
IIIB	Vaginal metastases
IIIC	Metastases to pelvic and/or paraaortic lymph nodes
IVA	Tumor invasion of bladder and/or bowel mucosa
IVB	Distant metastases, including intraabdominal metastasis and/or inguinal lymph nodes

*In each stage, histopathologic grades of G1, G2, or G3 are assigned (see Box 10-1).
Source: International Federation of Gynecology and Obstetrics (*www.figo.org*)

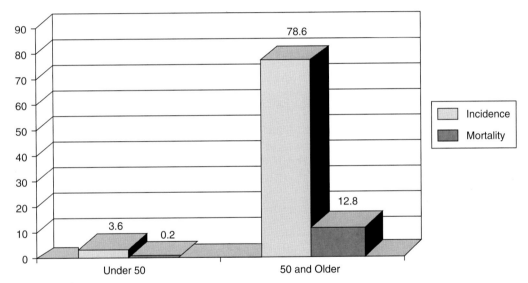

FIGURE 10-1
Incidence and mortality rates per 100,000 for cancer of the uterus and corpus (includes cancers of the uterus, corpus, and not otherwise specified [NOS]). *(From National Cancer Institute SEER Cancer Statistics Review, 1973-1998.)*

Hispanic, and Asian/Pacific Islander females range from 15.3 to 13.2 per 100,000 population. Native Americans/Alaskan Natives have the lowest incidence of endometrial carcinoma at 8.8 per 100,000 population.[8] Mortality rates among Hispanics, Native American/Alaskan Natives, and Asian/non-Hawaiian Pacific Islanders are lower than those for non-Hispanic White females, ranging from 2.5 to 1.8 per 100,000 population.[9]

Black women have an age-adjusted mortality rate approaching twice that of White women (5.7 vs. 3.1 per 100,000 population; see Table 10-1).[9] In a retrospective cohort analysis of 12,079 incident cases, Black women had a 40% lower risk of developing endometrial carcinoma but a 54% greater chance of mortality if they developed cancer of the uterine corpus.[10] A retrospective analysis of medical records for 401 women with a mean age of 63.7 years (±11.6 years) diagnosed with endometrial carcinoma between 1982 and 1995 identified an association between race and pathologic characteristics. Of the patients in the sample, 59.5% (n = 229) were Black, and 40.1% (n = 153) were non-Blacks. The carcinomas were primarily endometrioid (n = 346; 86.3%), of which 79% were stage I or II. Of the 42 (10.5%) papillary serous carcinomas, only 26% were stage I or II. The remaining 13 (3.2%) were clear cell carcinomas, of which 58% were stage I or II. The majority of papillary serous (88%) and clear cell (77%) carcinomas occurred in Black women, who had a poorer 5-year survival (56%) than non-Black women (71%). Multivariate analysis of age, stage, race, and histology found only stage and histology to be independent risk factors for survival.[11]

Reasons for racial differences in endometrial cancer mortality have been the subject of epidemiologic and genetic studies. A review of California Cancer Registry data from 1988 to 1994 using age-adjusted data showed that Black women (n = 423) had the same risk of developing high-risk endometrial cancer as did White women (n = 11,674) but had a significantly lower chance of developing low-risk tumors. Grade 1 and 2 endometrioid adenocarcinomas were considered low-risk lesions. High-risk lesions included endometrioid adenocarcinoma greater than grade 2 and papillary serous, clear cell, and adenosquamous cell types.[12] A Duke University study of 164 women with stage I endometrial adenocarcinomas identified racial disparities in overexpression of the p53 tumor suppressor gene and associated poor outcomes. Overexpression of p53 protein occurred in 28 (17%) cases and was associated with poor histologic grade and nonendometrioid appearance of tumor cells. Black women (15 of 44; 34%) were significantly more likely to exhibit overexpression of p53 than were White women (13 of 117, 11%; p = .003). Disease recurred twice as frequently when p53 overexpression was present.[13] Mutation of the *PTEN* tumor suppressor gene, associated with a more favorable prognosis, was present in significantly more White women (17 of 78; 22%) than Black women (3 of 62; 5%) in a sample of 140 females with stage III or IV endometrial carcinomas. Lower mutation rates of the *PTEN* tumor suppressor gene in Black women may contribute to racial differences in survival. Microsatellite instability was not significantly different between the two racial groups.[14]

RISK FACTORS

The risk of developing cancer of the uterine corpus has been related to reproductive, endocrine, lifestyle, and genetic factors. The Harvard Cancer Risk Index listing of *definite, probable, and possible* exposures related to developing endometrial carcinoma and the relative risk of the exposure are presented in Table 10-3. Both positively and negatively correlated factors appear. Estrogen replacement for more than 10 years is the exposure with the strongest relative risk (RR) relationship.[15] Endometrial cancer risk associated with presence of the hereditary nonpolyposis colorectal cancer (HNPCC) gene is not included in the list but is important in this subset of women.[16]

Reproductive Risk

Nulliparity has been shown to independently increase the risk of endometrial carcinoma and may be related to the higher incidence of anovulation among nulliparous women. Absence of a term birth increased the RR of developing endometrial cancer in an NCI case-control study of 405 women with endometrial carcinoma and 297 population controls (RR 2.8, 95% confidence interval [CI] 1.7-4.6). Spontaneous and induced abortions and age at first birth were unrelated to risk.[17] A total of 24,848 postmenopausal women aged 55 to 69 years were enrolled in the Iowa Women's Health Study in 1986. Of these, 167 developed endometrial carcinoma. The mean number of births was significantly lower in women who developed endometrial carcinoma (2.6 vs. 3.5, p <.0001). Ages at first and last birth were not significant when results were adjusted for number of births.[18] In a prospective study of

Table 10-3
Harvard Cancer Risk Index Exposures and Strength of Association for Endometrial Carcinoma: Definite, Probable, and Possible Associations

DEFINITE ASSOCIATION[a]			PROBABLE ASSOCIATION[b]			POSSIBLE ASSOCIATION[c]		
Exposure	Relative Risk		Exposure	Relative Risk		Exposure	Relative Risk	
Obesity (body mass index >27 vs. <21)	2.0	++	Smoke (≥25 cigarettes/ day vs. 0)	0.7	–	Vegetables[d]	0.7	–
Nulliparous (0 vs. ≥1 child)	1.2	+	Family history (first-degree relative)	1.5	++	Fruits[d]	0.8	–
Age menopause (5-yr increment)	1.2	+	Diabetes type II (yes vs. no)	1.5	++	Saturated fat[d]	1.4	+
Oral contraceptive use (≥5 years vs. none)	0.5	—				Age at first period (≥15 vs. ≤11)	0.9	–
Estrogen replacement (≥10 years vs. none)	4.0	++						

[a]An association has been established between the exposure and outcome, in which chance, bias, and confounding can be ruled out with reasonable confidence.
[b]An association has been observed between the exposure and the outcome but chance, bias, and confounding cannot be ruled out with reasonable confidence.
[c]The available studies are of insufficient quality, consistency, or statistical power to permit a conclusion of probable or definite association between the exposure and outcome.
[d]Upper quartile (25%) vs. lower quartile (25%).
Source: Colditz GA, Atwood KA, Emmons A, et al: Harvard report on cancer prevention, vol 4, Harvard Cancer Risk Index. *Cancer Causes Control* 2000;11:477-488.

765,756 Norwegian women, the decrease in risk of endometrial carcinoma with increasing parity ($p < .001$) was greatest with the first full-term pregnancy. RR, however, increased as time since last birth increased (RR = 1.20; 95% CI 1.08-1.34 per 5-year interval), reducing the parity risk benefit between parous and nulliparous women. Risk benefit of increasing age at first and last birth was not significant after adjusting for time since last birth.[19] In contrast, analysis of data on 40,951 women in Sweden from 1955 to 1995 demonstrated that increasing age at first birth increased the relative risk of endometrial carcinoma. Multiple births also increased the relative risk in this cohort.[20]

The influence of nulliparity on survival varies across studies. A study of 431,604 Norwegian women aged 45 to 74 found an age-adjusted decrease in mortality of 9.2% (95% CI 5.2-13.0) for each birth. Age of 35 years or older at first birth was associated with an RR of 0.53 (95% CI 0.34-0.83). There was no significant effect of age at last birth.[21] In a study of 316 women diagnosed with endometrial carcinoma between 1981 and 1990 in Norway, nulliparous women had a poorer 5-year survival rate than women with parity of one or more (57% vs. 81%, $p = .0001$). The nulliparous women were older and had more advanced disease. After adjustments were made for other risk factors, nulliparous women had a hazard ratio of 2.81 (95% CI 1.55-5.06), when compared with parous women.[22] A retrospective study of 328 Japanese women with endometrial cancer was reviewed to evaluate the effects of nulliparity on survival in relation to age. Individuals younger than 50 years of age were compared with those age 50 years and older. There was no effect of nulliparity on survival in the younger group or in the older group with stage I and II tumors. Ten-year survival rates were significantly worse for nulliparous women, compared with women with parity one or two and women with parity of three or more (p = .03). Delay in diagnosis was also significantly associated with survival rates of 57.1% for delay of 6 months or less and 16.6% for delays of 7 months or more (p = .02). When the data were adjusted for delay in diagnosis, there was no longer an effect from parity.[23] Delay in diagnosis among nulliparous women has been mentioned in other studies as a potential contributor to poorer prognosis.[22]

Endocrine Risk

The major risk factor for endometrial carcinoma is thought to be endogenous or exogenous estrogen exposure unopposed by progesterone or synthetic progestins. The unopposed estrogen theory suggests that there is a resultant increase in mitotic activity of endometrial cells, DNA replication errors, and somatic mutations causing endometrial hyperplasia and malignancy, or type I endometrial carcinoma. Type II endometrial carcinoma is likely unrelated to estrogen exposure and results from atrophic rather than hyperplastic epithelium.[24-28] Known risk factors were compared in 48 women with atrophy-associated carcinoma and 28 women with hyperplasia-associated carcinoma. Women in the hyperplasia-associated group were younger, weighed more, did not smoke, and experienced menarche earlier than women in the atrophy-associated group. The hyperplasia-associated risks support the unopposed estrogen theory for that group and a separate pathway for atrophy-related carcinomas.[28] Because the two types differ in histopathologic appearance and biologic behavior, differences may be associated with distinct molecular genetic alterations.[29]

In a case-control study of premenopausal and postmenopausal women, risk of developing endometrial carcinoma was related to levels of circulating steroid hormones and sex hormone–binding globulin (SHBG). High estrone levels were related to increased risk (odds ratio [OR] 2.2; 95% CI 1.2-4.4 after adjustment for body mass index). High circulating levels of androstenedione were related to a 3.6-fold increase in endometrial carcinoma risk in premenopausal women and a 2.8-fold increase in postmenopausal women. Among postmenopausal women, high SHBG levels were associated with reduced risk (OR 0.51; 95% CI 0.27-0.95). Risks associated with obesity and fat distribution in both premenopausal and postmenopausal women were not affected by adjustments for hormone levels.[30] Researchers suggest that a common biologic pathway proposed for type I endometrial carcinoma may not fully account for the independent effects of all hormone influences and other risk factors[30,31] but that several of the risk factors for endometrial cancer are mediated, in part, through increased endogenous hormone levels.[32]

Endogenous risk factors that are known to increase the risk of developing endometrial carcinoma include obesity, menstruation span, anovulation, diabetes, and other endocrinopathies. Exogenous factors include estrogen replacement therapy (ERT), oral contraceptive use, and tamoxifen adjuvant therapy.

Obesity

In postmenopausal women, conversion of androstenedione to estrone in adipose tissue is postulated as a mechanism for increased risk of endometrial cancer associated with obesity. In premenopausal obese women, progesterone insufficiency and increased anovulatory cycles are hypothesized as a mechanism.[27,30]

The NCI case-control study findings indicated an RR of 7.2 (95% CI 3.9-13.3) for weight greater than 200 pounds, compared with weight less than 125 pounds.[17] Further analysis indicated that women whose weight exceeded 172 pounds were 2.3 times as likely to develop endometrial carcinoma than women weighing 128 pounds or less (95% CI 1.4 to 3.7).

Upper-body obesity, determined by the waist-to-thigh circumference ratio, was an independent risk factor with risks of 1.0, 1.5, 1.8, and 2.6 related to increasing quartiles.[33] A nested case-control study within the Iowa Women's Health Study was conducted to determine whether additional risk was associated with abdominal adiposity beyond that ascribed to obesity. The 63 women with endometrial carcinoma had higher age-adjusted mean values of upper body adiposity higher than the 1274 controls, but differences in waist-to-hip and trunk-to-limb circumference ratios were not associated with incidence when adjusted for body mass index (BMI). A BMI increase of 5 kg/m^2 was associated with an RR of 1.80 (95% CI 1.46-2.22).[34]

A retrospective review of data was undertaken on 95 women younger than 40 years of age (age range 24 to 40 years) whose BMI ranged from 17.5 to 63.6 and who had endometrial carcinoma. Of these, 48 were not obese (BMI < 30). Women with a BMI < 25 had more advanced disease (p = .04) and high-risk histology (p = .04). All but four patients had endometrioid cancer, but all four patients with clear cell or serous papillary histology had a BMI < 25. Further investigation of a separate mechanism for disease in slender women is proposed.[35]

Elevated insulin levels have been proposed as a possible explanation for the relationship of obesity to increased risk of endometrial carcinoma. This relationship was not found in a sample of 165 women with endometrial carcinoma and 180 controls. There was a strong relationship between BMI and endometrial risk in the cohort, but it was not affected to any great extent by adjustment for C-peptide. Conversely, associations observed between C-peptide and risk of endometrial carcinoma were eliminated when adjustments were made for BMI and other risk factors.[36]

Menstruation Span

It is theorized that both early menarche age and older age at menopause increase uterine exposure to estrogens, thereby increasing risk of developing endometrial carcinoma. Data from the Iowa Women's Health Study showed that, in addition to number of pregnancies, early age at menarche, late age at natural menopause, and total length of ovulation span were associated with occurrence.[18] The prospective study of 62,079 women in Norway also found significant risk associated with early menarche and late menopause.[37] In an early case-control study of 167 cases and 903 controls in Connecticut between 1977 and 1979, older age at menopause was associated with increased risk.[38] A case-control study of 254 women with endometrial carcinoma and 254 age-matched controls found associations with late menopause as well as nulliparity. In women older than 69 years, however, neither variable discriminated between groups. When parity, age at menarche, and age at menopause were combined into a measure of unopposed estrogen exposure (menstruation span), women with endometrial carcinoma had a significantly longer menstruation span than controls (33.6 vs. 31.2 years; p < .001).[39] Menarche before age 12 was associated with an RR of 2.4, compared with menarche at 15 years of age or older in the NCI case-control study; no relationship was found with late age at menopause.[17]

Diabetes

In a population-based case-control study of Wisconsin women (cases, n = 723; controls, n = 2291), women with diabetes had an adjusted OR of 1.86 (95% CI 1.37-2.52) for developing endometrial carcinoma. The association was influenced and modified by BMI. Comparisons between diabetic and nondiabetic patients based on three weight categories indicated that nonoverweight and overweight diabetic women did not have an increased risk of developing endometrial cancer. When obese (BMI > 31.9), diabetic women had an elevated risk (OR 2.95, CI 1.60-5.46).[40]

Estrogen Replacement Therapy

Parallel increases in the incidence of endometrial carcinoma and use of ERT in the mid 1970s focused attention on the role of estrogen in risk for cancer of the uterine corpus. A metaanalysis of 30 studies with risk estimates and use of appropriate controls confirmed an RR of 2.3 (95% CI 2.1-2.5) for women taking estrogen, compared with those not taking estrogen. Among women taking estrogen for 10 years or longer, the RR was 9.5. The RR remained elevated at 2.3 for 5 years after discontinuation of unopposed estrogen.[41]

Progestins appear to antagonize the effects of estrogen on the endometrium and prevent or reverse endometrial hyperplasia.[26] The Postmenopausal Estrogen/Progestin Interventions (PEPI) trial evaluated the endometrial histologic findings from 596 postmenopausal women aged 45 through 64 years who were randomly assigned to placebo, estrogen-only, or one of three estrogen-plus-progestin regimens. The estrogen-only group had rates of hyperplasia significantly higher than those of the placebo group ($p \leq .001$) for all types of hyperplasia (simple/cystic, 27.7% vs. 0.8%; complex/adenomatous, 22.7% vs. 0.8%; or atypical, 11.8% vs. 0%). Women in the three estrogen-plus-progestin regimens had rates of hyperplasia similar to those of women in the placebo group. Biopsy results from 34 of 36 (94%) of women with hyperplasia returned to normal after progestin therapy.[42]

The Menopause Study Group trial evaluated the preventive potential of four combinations of estrogen and medroxyprogesterone acetate (MPA) in a double-blind study of 1724 postmenopausal women. The control group received only conjugated estrogens. Endometrial hyperplasia developed in 20% of the control group and in less than 1% of any of the estrogen-MPA dosage groups.[43] Retrospective analysis identified that they also had more bleeding days than women without hyperplasia ($p > .001$).[44]

Incidence of endometrial cancer decreased concurrently among participants in a prepaid health plan from 1991 to 1993 with increases in prescriptions for opposed conjugated estrogens, providing additional support for the probable affect of progestins in protecting the endometrium.[45] Continuous combined estrogen-progestin therapy has been found superior to estrogen and progestin given sequentially because of bleeding and other adverse affects associated with sequential therapy. Individualization of protocols to best fit patients is recommended to increase adherence.[46]

The use of ERT after primary treatment for endometrial cancer is a matter of debate. Although hormone replacement therapy modifies the menopausal symptoms, is helpful in preventing osteoporosis, and may have cardiopreventive effects; the theoretical possibility of a hormonal role in recurrence limits use. To evaluate the risk of recurrence and death from ERT after primary treatment, a retrospective analysis of women with surgical stage I, II, and III endometrial cancer was undertaken. A total of 130 women received estrogen; 49% also received progesterone. Comparison of 75 matched control pairs among hormone and nonhormone users identified that hormone users had a significantly longer disease-free interval than those not receiving ERT (p = .006). There were two recurrences (1%) in the estrogen group, including those with and without added progestins, and 11 recurrences (14%) in the nonhormone user group.[47] Other researchers have reported similar findings.[48] After reviewing current studies on the effects of hormone replacement therapy in cancer survivors, including those with endometrial carcinoma, DiSaia concluded that categorical prohibition of replacement therapy is not warranted. He suggests the benefits of hormone replacement therapy as well as potential risks should be considered and discussed with patients.[49,50] The preventive effects of ERT have recently been questioned primarily because of the results of the Women's Health Initiative, an NIH-sponsored study of more than 16,000 postemenopausal women. This study, which was limited to the use of a combination (E-P) of estrogen (conjugated equine estrogens) and progesterone (medroxyprogesterone acetate) versus placebo, concluded that overall the health risks exceeded the benefits of the E-P treatment. The study, which was prematurely stopped after 5.2 years in May 2002, revealed an increase incidence of strokes, breast cancer, and coronary heart disease with a decrease in the incidence of endometrial cancer, colorectal cancer, and hip fractures. It is noteworthy that these findings were in women taking the combination of estrogen and progesterone and not estrogen alone, which makes the applicability of this data to endometrial cancer survivors conjectural.[51]

Oral Contraceptives

Oral contraceptives have been shown to reduce the incidence of endometrial carcinoma as well as epithelial ovarian cancer.[52] The relationship between oral contraceptive use and endometrial carcinoma was evaluated as part of the Cancer and Steroid Hormone Study (CASH) of the Centers for Disease Control. A total of 433 women aged 20 to 54 years with endometrial carcinoma were compared with 3191 women randomly selected from the same areas of the country. In the CASH study, women who used combination oral contraceptives for at least 12 months had a reduced risk of developing endometrial carcinoma, compared with women who never used oral contraceptives (age-adjusted risk = 0.6; 95% CI 0.3-0.9). The protective effect was present up to 15 years after women stopped taking oral contraceptives.[53] Findings from the Oxford Family Planning Association contraceptive study indicate an RR for developing endometrial carcinoma of 0.1 (95% CI 0.0-0.7) for women who took oral contraceptives at any time, compared with those who did not.[54] In a study that compared 405 women who had invasive epithelial endometrial cancer with 297 population controls, combination-type oral contraceptive use resulted in an adjusted OR of 0.4 (95% CI 0.3-0.7) for women who used oral contraceptives at any time, compared with nonusers. The reduced risk was evident even in the presence of other risk factors, including age, menopausal status, parity, obesity, ERT, smoking history, or history of infertility. Reduced risk was present even in women who had discontinued use of oral contraceptives up to 20 years earlier (OR 0.7). In nulliparous women and women who were on ERT for 3 years or more, the negative association was present, but the magnitude of the association was diminished.[55]

Tamoxifen

Tamoxifen belongs to a group of drugs known as selective estrogen receptor modulators (SERMs) that produce varied effects in different body organs.[56] Tamoxifen increases survival from breast cancer by inhibiting estrogen-receptor positive cells, but incidence rates for endometrial cancer are increased somewhat in patients who take the drug, either because of coincident risk of developing endometrial carcinoma or direct and indirect estrogen-like effects on the endometrium. Whether tamoxifen promotes growth of preexisting, clinically occult endometrial carcinomas or is etiologic for the development of new cancers is unknown.[57] Assiskis and Jordan reviewed more than 250 studies on the relationship of tamoxifen to increased incidence of endometrial carcinoma. They observed that 80% of the cases are stage I disease, which is similar to the proportion of stage I disease (74%) in the SEER data. They conclude that tamoxifen therapy does not foster late-stage endometrial cancer out of proportion to early-stage cancers. The risk of developing endometrial carcinoma while on tamoxifen was calculated from previous studies to be 2 to 3 per 1000 women per year, as opposed to 1 per 1000 women per year who are not taking tamoxifen. The authors suggest that the low incidence rate does not warrant aggressive detection strategies before starting tamoxifen and that patient education be used to alert women to symptoms of disease.[58]

Tamoxifen benefits in the treatment of breast cancer outweigh the risk of developing endometrial carcinoma because most tamoxifen-related endometrial cancers are detected early and are highly curable at early stages.[2,59] Raloxifene, another SERM, is under investigation as an alternative to tamoxifen because it appears to be less likely to cause endometrial stimulation.[56]

Anovulation and Other Endocrinopathies

Among cases and controls in the CASH study, women with infertility diagnosed by a physician and of at least 2 years' duration had an OR, adjusted for age, of 1.7 (95% CI 1.1-2.6) for endometrial cancer. The researchers suggest that much of the increased risk for endometrial carcinoma associated with infertility may be explained by anovulation.[60] This would also explain the increased in risk in nulliparous women.

Polycystic ovary syndrome (PCOS) is characterized by anovulation, hyperandrogenism, and menstrual dysfunction and affects between 4% and 7% of women of reproductive age. Other endocrinopathies associated with PCOS include hyperinsulinemia, luteinizing hormone hypersecretion, elevated testosterone levels, and acyclic estrogen production. Obesity and hyperlipidemia are associated with PCOS. Insulin resistance increases risks for type II diabetes mellitus and cardiaovascular disease. Chronic anovulation associated with PCOS increases risks for endometrial carcinoma caused by unopposed estrogen. The increased risk persists after risk associated with obesity is controlled.[61-63] Hyperandrogenocity and hyperinsulinism may act independently or interdependently with unopposed estrogen in PCOS to contribute to increased risk of endometrial carcinoma.[64]

Lifestyle-Related Risk

Smoking and dietary habits have been shown to be related to the risk of developing endometrial carcinoma. Effects of smoking differ in premenopausal and postmenopausal women.

Smoking

Several case-control studies have shown a reduced risk of endometrial carcinoma in cigarette smokers. In a study that compared 405 individuals who had epithelial endometrial carcinoma with 297 controls, cigarette smokers had an RR of developing endometrial carcinoma of 0.6 (95% CI 0.2-0.7), when compared with nonsmokers. The effect was seen primarily in postmenopausal women, and current postmenopausal smokers had the greatest reduction in risk (RR 0.4; 95% CI 0.2-0.7). An extraovarian endogenous hormonal mechanism is postulated.[65] Multivariate analysis of data from 740 Wisconsin women with endometrial carcinoma and 2372 controls identified a reduced risk in current smokers, compared with those who never smoked (RR 0.8, 95% CI 0.6-1.0). Risk reduction was greatest in women who are obese or who use postmenopausal hormones.[66]

Smoking, however, was associated with advanced-stage and higher tumor grade in 157 women who underwent hysterectomy for endometrial carcinoma. Multivariate analysis of smokers compared with nonsmokers indicated that those with stage II-IV disease were more likely to be smokers than women with stage 0-I disease. Smokers accounted for 12 of 30 women (40%) with stage II-IV disease and 14 of 127 women (11%) with stage 0-I disease, resulting in an OR of 5.38 (CI 2.23-11.31).[67]

Dietary Factors

In addition to the role they play in obesity, specific dietary factors have been linked to increased and decreased risk of endometrial carcinoma. In a case-control study that compared 399 women who had endometrial carcinoma with 296 controls, caloric intake was associated with a slightly increased risk when the lowest and highest quartiles of intake were compared (OR 1.5, 95% CI 0.9-2.5). Dietary inclusion of complex carbohydrates such as breads and cereals was associated with reduced risk (OR 0.6, CI 0.4-1.1), whereas higher levels of animal fat were associated with higher risk (OR 1.5). Associations related to complex carbohydrates and animal fat were independent.[68]

Analysis of endometrial cancer risk associated with diet was undertaken in the Western New York Diet Study (1986-1991) and compared 232 women who had endometrial cancer with 639 controls. Researchers identified decreased risks for women with highest quartiles of protein intake (OR 0.4, 95% CI 0.2-0.9) and dietary fiber (OR 0.5, 95% CI 0.3-1.0). Reduced risks of OR ≤ 0.6 (range, OR 0.3 to 0.6) were found with phytosterols, vitamin C, folate, alpha-carotene, beta-carotene, lycopene, lutein with zeaxanthin, and vegetables, thus pointing to reduced risks associated with diets high in plant foods. An OR of 1.6 (95% CI 0.7-3.4) was related to fat intake.[69]

Risks of developing endometrial cancer were related to percent energy from fat among participants in a case-control study of 679 women with endometrial carcinoma diagnosed between 1985 and 1991, compared with 944 population-based controls. Comparisons of highest and lowest quartiles of energy from fat with adjustments for age, county, energy intake, hormone use, smoking, and separately for BMI resulted in an OR of 1.8 (95% CI 1.3-2.6) Comparisons of highest and lowest quartiles identified reduced risks with diets high in fruits (OR 0.65, 95% CI 0.46-0.93) and vegetables (OR 0.61, 95% CI 0.43-0.88).[70]

Iowa Women's Health Study participants who were "never users" of hormone replacement therapy and were in the highest quartile of grain intake, compared with those in the lowest quartile had a reduced risk of endometrial carcinoma (RR 0.63, 95% CI 0.39-1.01). There was no association between whole grain intake and risk of endometrial carcinoma among women who had taken hormone replacement therapy.[71]

Genetic Risks

Family history of cancer or the presence of HNPCC has associated risks for the development of endometrial carcinoma. The role of alterations in oncogenes and tumor suppressor genes in the genesis of cancer of the uterine corpus and the molecular pathogenesis of endometrial carcinoma is of increasing interest.

Family History

Family history of cancer has been shown to be an independent risk factor for endometrial carcinoma in some but not all studies. The Cancer and Steroid Hormone Study Group (CSHSG) population-based study of 455 women with primary epithelial endometrial carcinoma and 3216 community-residing controls found that the risk of endometrial cancer was substantially increased (OR 2.8, 95% CI 1.9-4.2) in women who had a first-degree female relative with endometrial carcinoma.[72] A family history of colorectal cancer was also associated with increased risk of endometrial carcinoma in the CSHSG study (OR 1.9; 95% CI 1.1-3.3).[72] The 1977-1979 Connecticut study also found increased risk in women when a mother or sister had either endometrial or ovarian carcinoma.[38]

In the prospective Iowa study, 322 of 24,848 postmenopausal women aged 55 to 69 years developed endometrial carcinoma over a 10-year period. Positive family history of cancer at any site did not increase risk for endometrial carcinoma in these women, and controlling for possible confounding variables did not alter the results.[73]

Hereditary Nonpolyposis Colon Carcinoma

At least five gene mutations have been identified in families with HNPCC. Women who inherit HNPCC susceptibility syndrome have a 60% chance of developing endometrial cancer as well as an 80% chance of developing colon cancer.[74] Microsatellite instability caused by mutations in DNA repair genes in HNPCC has increased interest in searching for additional mutations in microsatellite sequences that might be related to endometrial carcinoma.[75]

Oncogenes and Tumor Suppressor Genes

Poor survival has been correlated with overexpression of the HER-2/*neu* oncogene, which occurs in 10% of endometrial cancers. Mutations in the K-*ras* oncogene are present in 10% of American women and in 20% to 30% of Japanese women with endometrial carcinoma. Overexpression of p53 mutant protein resulting from mutation of the p53 tumor suppressor gene is present in 20% of women with endometrial adenocarcinomas.[75]

The two most common types of uterine cancer, endometrioid and serous, are significantly different in several molecular genetic alterations. Lax and associates[29] discovered significant differences between the two cancer types in K-*ras* mutations (15 of 58 endometrioid, 26%; 1 of 45 serous, 2%; $p < .001$) and in p53 mutations (7 of 42 endometrioid, 17%; 25 of 27 serous, 93%; $p < .001$). Microsatellite instability was also present in 16 of 57 endometrioid tumors (28%) and in none of the serous tumors ($p < .001$).

Microsatellite instability has been associated with favorable outcomes in endometrioid carcinomas. In a study of 131 endometrioid carcinomas, microsatellite instability was present in 29 (22%) of the tumors. There was no association between microsatellite instability and age, race, tumor grade or stage, or depth of myometrial invasion. Five-year survival was significantly improved in women with microsatellite instability (77% vs. 44%; $p = .03$) after controlling for confounding influences. Significant associations with *PTEN* mutation ($p = .002$) and lack of p53 overexpression ($p = .01$) were also found.[76]

A2 Allele of CYP17

Increases in endogenous steroid hormones have been linked to the presence of the A2 allele of CYP17. In a case-control study undertaken within the Nurses' Health Study (142 cases, 554 controls), however, women with the A2 allele did not have a significantly elevated level of any of the steroid fractions. Furthermore, they were at a decreased risk for endometrial carcinoma, and risk was lowest in those with the A2 allele on both chromosome pairs (A1/A2 genotype: OR 0.89, 95% CI 0.62-1.27; A2/A2 genotype: OR 0.43, 95% CI 0.23-0.80).[77]

PREVENTION AND EARLY DIAGNOSIS

There is no evidence that screening is beneficial to women at average risk for endometrial carcinoma with no identified risk factors. Further, the American Cancer Society (ACS) guidelines for endometrial carcinoma testing do not recommend screening for women at increased risk because of a history of unopposed estrogen therapy, late menopause, tamoxifen therapy, nulliparity, infertility or failure to ovulate, obesity, diabetes, or hypertension. Most endometrial carcinomas are diagnosed at an early stage because of abnormal uterine bleeding. For women at average or increased risk of endometrial carcinoma, patient education, especially in perimenopausal and postmenopausal women, should be aimed at early reporting of unexpected bleeding or spotting. Women at high risk who have HNPCC or are susceptible to developing HNPCC should be offered endometrial biopsy annually beginning at age 35, although there is insufficient information that endometrial cancers are detected at an early stage or that survival is improved with annual screening. The ACS guidelines also recommend that women with HNPCC who are undergoing surgery for colorectal cancer be counseled regarding elective prophylactic hysterectomy and oophorectomy at the same time.[78]

Abnormal Vaginal or Uterine Bleeding

Diagnosis of endometrial carcinoma depends on early differential assessment of abnormal vaginal bleeding, present in approximately 90% of women with cancer of the uterine corpus.[79] Women of all ages experience unusual vaginal bleeding, but the significance and likely causes vary with age. In premenopausal women, pregnancy-related disorders, infection, birth control methods, and dysfunctional uterine bleeding (DUB) associated with anovulation are likely causes. Abnormal vaginal bleeding near the time of the perimenopause is expected, but heavy abnormal bleeding requires evaluation. In postmenopausal women, endometrial carcinoma should be suspected. The possibility of malignancy is increased in all patients—regardless of age—who have a history of anovulation, who are obese, and who do not respond to initial medical management.[80] Histologic examination of the endometrium should be completed for patients regardless of age who report abnormal vaginal bleeding and have risk factors for endometrial carcinoma.[79,81]

Hyperplasia As a Predisposing Condition

The extent to which endometrial hyperplasia may be a precursor to endometrial carcinoma is related to classification of endometrial samples as simple or complex, with or without atypical histology (Box 10-2). Reports of how the risk of endometrial carcinoma relates to the various forms of hyperplasia vary widely among studies. Silverberg summarized four prospective studies in which the incidence of endometrial carcinoma was 0% to 10% for simple hyperplasia without atypia, 3% to 22% for complex hyperplasia without atypia, 7% to 8% for atypical simple hyperplasia, and 29% to 100% for atypical complex hyperplasia.[82]

A review of data from 136 patients with a diagnosis of endometrial hyperplasia who subsequently had a hysterectomy between 1970 and 1992 was undertaken by Hunter and associates.[83] No cases of endometrial carcinoma were identified among the 82 patients with simple or complex endometrial hyperplasia without atypia. Among the 54 patients with simple or complex hyperplasia with atypia, 19 (35%) exhibited endometrial carcinoma. The risk of endometrial carcinoma to patients with atypia was independent of other risk factors.

The timeline for hyperplasia to develop into carcinoma is unknown. Silverberg suggests that lesions found years after a diagnosis of atypical hyperplasia may represent carcinomas present that persisted rather than progressed and that hyperplasias thought to have progressed may actually be coexisting lesions in some cases.[82] At one institution the presence of coexisting endometrial carcinoma was evaluated in 45 patients who underwent hysterectomy for preoperatively diagnosed simple or complex endometrial hyperplasia with or without

BOX 10-2   **Classification of Endometrial Hyperplasia**

- Simple hyperplasia without atypia
- Complex hyperplasia without atypia
- Atypical simple hyperplasia
- Atypical complex hyperplasia

Source: Silverberg SG: Problems in the differential diagnosis of endometrial hyperplasia and carcinoma. *Mod Pathol* 2000;13:309-327.

atypia: 24 and 21 patients, respectively. Carcinoma was not found during surgery in any of the 21 patients without atypia. Half (12 of 24) of the patients with atypia had coexistent endometrial carcinoma; 9 of the carcinomas (37.5%) were staged at 1B or greater.[84] Regardless of whether endometrial hyperplasia progresses to endometrial carcinoma or coexists, there is a significant increased risk of endometrial carcinoma when atypia is present.

Treatment for Endometrial Hyperplasia with Atypia

Based on the risk of endometrial carcinoma in women with endometrial hyperplasia and atypia, hysterectomy is the treatment of choice in this group of women (Figure 10-2). In women who refuse hysterectomy or want to retain childbearing potential, progestins may be tried. Patient monitoring with endometrial biopsies every 3 months is recommended.[79]

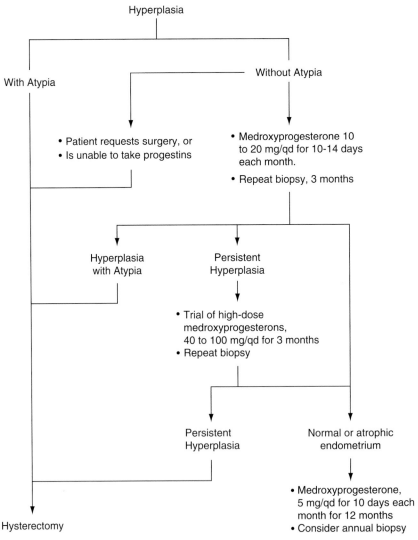

FIGURE 10-2
Algorithm for treatment of simple and complex hyperplasia with and without atypia. Adapted from Berek JS, Macker NF, eds. Practical gynecologic oncology. 2nd ed. Baltimore: Williams & Wilkins, 1994:285-326, with information from Karlsson B, Granberg S, Wikland M, et al. Transvaginal ultrasonography of the endometrium in women with postmenopausal bleeding: a Nordic multicenter study. *Am J Obstet Gynecol* 1995; 172:1433-1494.

Treatment for Endometrial Hyperplasia without Atypia

MPA has been shown to have an antiangiogenic effect on myometrium underlying complex endometrial hyperplasia.[85] MPA is the treatment of choice for patients without atypia unless they prefer hysterectomy or cannot take progestins (see Figure 10-2).[79] Patient monitoring should be undertaken for adverse effects of MPA on lipid profiles as well as possible increased insulin resistance, which leads to hyperglycemia.[86]

Use of Endometrial Biopsy

Endometrial assessment by means of biopsy or sampling of endometrial cells in the clinic or office is a minimally invasive alternative for dilatation and curettage (D&C) or hysteroscopy. Cervical stenosis, infrequently present in older postmenopausal women, may prevent adequate endometrial sampling. For the majority of women, the use of endometrial biopsy reduces risks associated with D&C and the cost of the diagnostic work-up without reducing accuracy.

Several flexible aspiration devices are available to the clinician, all with acceptable sensitivity and specificity. A metaanalysis of studies from 1966 to 1999 was undertaken to assess the accuracy of endometrial sampling devices in the detection of endometrial carcinoma and atypical hyperplasia. A total of 39 studies involving 7914 women were analyzed. In both premenopausal and postmenopausal women, the pipelle had the highest sensitivity. Detection rates of 91% in premenopausal and 99.6% in postmenopausal women were calculated from study findings. Specificity for all endometrial sampling devices was greater than 98%.[87] Transvaginal ultrasound, D&C, or hysteroscopy is recommended if bleeding persists after a negative biopsy.

Role of Hysteroscopy

Hysteroscopy permits direct inspection of the endometrium, biopsy of suspicious lesions, and removal of polyps and leiomyomas. The procedure is particularly useful when abnormal bleeding is not resolved and the endometrial biopsy sample is negative. The procedure has surgical risks similar to D&C.

There is evidence of the spread of cancer cells to the peritoneum because of irrigation under pressure during hysteroscopy in some but not all studies. To evaluate the viability of malignant cells transported in hysteroscopic fluid washing, transtubal fluid dissemination of cells was evaluated in 24 uteri removed from women with endometrial carcinoma. Transtubal fluid dissemination occurred in 20 of 24 (83%) uteri. Functionally viable tumor cells were found in 10 (42%) of the specimens cultured.[88]

A retrospective cohort analysis included 113 consecutive patients who had D&C with or without hysteroscopy. All had stage IA,B endometrial carcinoma treated between 1996 and 1997. Positive peritoneal cytology, obtained at staging laparotomy, was present in 10 (9%) of patients and was associated with a history of hysteroscopy ($p = .04$). Presence of peritoneal cytology was not associated with myometrial invasion, histologic subtype, grade, or time between D&C and surgery.[89]

Zerbe and associates[90] retrospectively reviewed charts of 222 patients with endometrial carcinoma. Among the patients, 64 had hysteroscopy with saline infusion, and 158 did not. After investigators adjusted for confounding variables, patients who had hysteroscopy were significantly more likely to have positive peritoneal cytology than those who did not have the procedure (OR 2.6, 95% CI 1.02-6.63, $p = .05$). Patients in each group were stratified according to low and high risk for positive peritoneal cytology. Significance of the effect of hysteroscopy persisted in the high-risk group (OR 3.46, 95% CI 1.3-9.12, $p = .01$). Evidence is sufficiently compelling for some clinicians to recommend reserving hysteroscopy for patients with negative endometrial samples.[90,91]

The Papanicolaou Test and Endometrial Carcinoma

The Papanicolaou (Pap) test, highly sensitive in identifying abnormal cells associated cervical cancer, is not a reliable predictor of endometrial carcinoma. It has been shown that the prevalence of normal endometrial cells in Pap smears of women with endometrial carcinoma or hyperplasia does not significantly differ from that in women without these conditions.[92] However, follow-up is mandated when endometrial cells are found on Pap tests in postmenopausal women who are not on hormone replacement therapy.[93]

Transvaginal Ultrasound

Transvaginal ultrasonography (TVUS) is particularly useful to determine the thickness of the endometrium or endometrial stripe. Early trials identified threshold values of 4 mm or indicated pathology.[94] More recently, threshold values of 5 mm or more are considered indicative of hyperplasia, carcinoma, polyps, or other abnormalities, whereas values below 5 mm are considered normal for women who are not on tamoxifen or are on ERT. For those who are taking tamoxifen or are on ERT, endometrial thickness is increased and a thickness of from 6 mm to 8 mm is considered normal, depending on the study.[95-97] The exact cause of thickening cannot be determined with TVUS, but the likelihood of serious problems can be ruled out with a 95% to 99% negative specificity.[98,99]

Evaluation of the significance of a thickened endometrial stripe was undertaken in 624 of 897 consecutive postmenopausal women evaluated for bleeding who had pelvic ultrasound and comprehensive evaluation of the uterus and adnexa between 1991 and 1995. In women with thickened endometrial stripe and symptoms, repeat endometrial sampling within 1 year doubled the identified additional cases of endometrial hyperplasia or carcinoma (from 9% to 18%). Among women with a thickened endometrial stripe who were asymptomatic, evaluation beyond initial endometrial biopsy did not reveal additional pathology.[97]

TVUS and endometrial biopsy together increase the chances of finding endometrial hyperplasia and carcinoma. Among 104 postmenopausal women with abnormal bleeding, the combination increased sensitivity to 94% and specificity to 96% (CI 91% to 99%). None of the women with endometrial hyperplasia or carcinoma were misdiagnosed.[100]

A recent review of evidence that compares TVUS and endometrial biopsy resulted in consensus agreement among clinicians that either method is safe and effective as a first diagnostic step. Both methods are identified as equally sensitive when abnormality is ascribed to TVUS values of 5 mm or greater and there is sufficient tissue obtained by endometrial biopsy. Decision on which modality to use depends on assessment of patient risk, nature of the practice, availability of high-quality sonography, and patient preference.[101] TVUS is very helpful in evaluating patients with cervical stenosis when endometrial biopsy cannot be performed.

Computed Tomography Scan and Magnetic Resonance Imaging

Routine preoperative computed tomography (CT) scanning is not indicated in endometrial carcinoma. CT scanning has been shown to be a poor predictor of nodal disease and does not tend to alter treatment. Furthermore, no difference in survival was found when CT scanning identified subclinical recurrence.[102]

Magnetic resonance imaging (MRI) has been shown to help distinguish between polyps and endometrial carcinomas based on morphologic features. Intratumoral cysts and a central fibrous core were more frequent in endometrial polyps. Myometrial invasion and necrosis were more common in carcinoma. Responses from three individuals who read the MRIs showed mean values for carcinoma of sensitivity 79%, specificity 89%, accuracy 86%, positive predictive value 82%, and negative predictive value 88%.[103]

TVUS was found to be almost as accurate as MRI in preoperatively assessing the depth of myometrial invasion when a diagnosis of endometrial carcinoma was made. Although MRI is the gold standard, TVUS may be used as an alternative to MRI in this instance.[94]

CA125

Findings related to the utility of CA125 as an adjunct to diagnosis and management of patients with cancer of the uterine corpus are mixed. Levels greater than 35 U/mL were present in 58% of patients with recurrent disease. High-risk patients, such as those with papillary serous histolopathology, were more likely to have elevated CA125 levels (8 of 9 patients with recurrence in this group). However, false elevations occurred in 13 patients, 12 of whom were receiving radiation therapy.[104] A study of 220 serum specimens from 15 patients with papillary serous carcinomas indicated that the five patients who died had clinical or radiographic evidence of tumor that CA125 failed to precede or predict.[105] The utility of CA125 as a diagnostic adjunct remains uncertain.

SPECIAL HISTOLOGIC TYPES

Uterine papillary serous and clear cell carcinomas have been shown to be associated with high relapse rate and poor survival. A study of 240 consecutive patients identified 216 with stage I or stage II disease. Extrauterine disease was present in 7 of the 12 patients with papillary serous or clear cell carcinoma, compared with 46 of 204 patients with endometrioid carcinoma ($p < .01$). Multivariate analysis confirmed that prognosis is related to cell type, grade, lymphovascular space invasion, and paraaortic node metastasis, which is more likely in these patients.[106] In a study of 574 women with clinical stage I and II cancers, 53 had papillary serous and 18 had clear cell carcinomas. The estimated 5-year survival for papillary serous and clear cell tumors with less than 2 mm myometrial invasion was 56%, compared with 93% for endometrioid carcinoma. Extrauterine metastases were present in 55% of patients with papillary serous and 45% of patients with clear cell carcinomas. Prognostic factors for survival included age, stage, and lymphovascular space invasion in this group of patients.[107,108]

Uterine Papillary Serous Carcinoma

Uterine papillary serous carcinoma is an uncommon and highly malignant variant of endometrial carcinoma with a high recurrence rate.[109] The most common type of endometrial carcinoma, endometrioid adenocarcinoma, seems to be related to endometrial hyperplasia and excess estrogen exposure. Serous carcinomas, however, seem to develop not from hyperplastic but from atrophic epithelium. In serous carcinomas malignant transformation of the endometrial surface epithelium occurs. These carcinomas are associated with p53 mutations and abnormal accumulation of p53 protein.[24]

There is also some evidence that women with papillary serous carcinoma are at increased risk for developing breast cancer. In a retrospective analysis of 592 patients with a diagnosis of cancer of the uterine corpus between 1983 and 1994, 536 had endometrioid,

23 had papillary serous, 10 had clear cell, one had mucinous, and one had squamous carcinomas. Twelve patients had a previous diagnosis of breast cancer. A concurrent or subsequent diagnosis of breast cancer occurred in 3.2% of patients with endometrioid carcinoma and 25% of patients with papillary serous carcinoma ($p < .001$).[110]

Clear Cell Carcinoma

Separate etiologic pathways are proposed for endometrioid and papillary serous carcinoma. The ability to explain pathogenesis of clear cell carcinoma within the dual approach was explored by Lax and associates.[111] Comparison of 21 clear cell, 30 serous, and 77 endometrioid carcinomas in relation to p53, Ki-67, and estrogen and progesterone receptor expression identified a distinctive immunoprofile for clear cell carcinoma. Immunonegativity for estrogen and progesterone receptors and a high Ki-67 proliferation index were similar to papillary serous carcinomas, but low immunoreactivity for p53 in clear cell carcinomas was a difference ($p < .05$). Unlike endometrioid carcinomas, clear cell is rarely associated with endometrial hyperplasia. Estrogen and progesterone receptor expression were significantly lower and Ki-67 proliferation index was significantly higher in clear cell compared with endometrioid cancers ($p < .05$). A subtype of clear cell carcinoma, clear cell with serous features, had a higher Ki-67 proliferation index than typical clear cell carcinoma. The conclusion is that clear cell carcinoma differs from both endometrioid and serous carcinomas, thus suggesting a different molecular pathway for this cancer.[111]

REFERENCES

1. Jemal A, Thomas A, Murray T, et al: Cancer statistics, 2002. *CA Cancer J Clin* 2002;52:23-47.
2. National Cancer Institute: *Endometrial cancer (PDQ): Prevention.* Washington, DC, National Cancer Institute, 2002.
3. Goff BA, Goodman A, Muntz HG, et al: Surgical stage IV endometrial carcinoma: a study of 47 cases. *Gynecol Oncol* 1994;52:237-240.
4. Ries LAG, Eisner MP, Kosary CL, et al: *SEER cancer statistics review, 1973-1998, National Cancer Institute.* Bethesda, MD, NCI, 2001.
5. Creasman W, Odicino F, Maisonneuve P, et al: *FIGO staging of gynecological cancer: carcinoma of the corpus uteri, vol 2002.* Milan, International Federation of Gynecology and Obstetrics, 1988.
6. Miller BA, Kolonel LN, Bernstein L, et al: *Racial/ethnic patterns of cancer in the United States 1988-1992,* NIH Pub No 96-4104. Bethesda, MD, National Cancer Institute, 1996.
7. Mundt AJ, Waggoner S, Yamada SD, et al: Age as a prognostic factor for recurrence in patients with endometrial carcinoma. *Gynecol Oncol* 2000;79:79-85.
8. National Cancer Institute: *Rates and trends for the top 15 cancer sites by sex and race/ethnicity for 1992-1998, SEER cancer incidence, 1992-1998, vol 2002.* Besthesda, MD, National Cancer Institute, 2001.
9. National Cancer Institute: *Rates and trends for the top 15 cancer sites by sex and race/ethnicity for 1992-1998, U.S. mortality, 1992-1998, vol 2002.* Besthesda, MD, National Cancer Institute, 2001.
10. Madison T, Schottenfeld D, Baker V: Cancer of the corpus uteri in white and black women in Michigan, 1985-1994: an analysis of trends in incidence and mortality and their relation to histologic subtype and stage. *Cancer* 1998;83:1546-1554.
11. Matthews RP, Hutchinson-Colas J, Maiman M, et al: Papillary serous and clear cell type lead to poor prognosis of endometrial carcinoma in black women. *Gynecol Oncol* 1997;65:206-212.
12. Plaxe SC, Saltzstein SL: Impact of ethnicity on the incidence of high-risk endometrial carcinoma. *Gynecol Oncol* 1997;65:8-12.
13. Clifford SL, Kaminetsky CP, Cirisano FD, et al: Racial disparity in overexpression of the p53 tumor suppressor gene in stage I endometrial cancer. *Am J Obstet Gynecol* 1997;176:S229-232.
14. Maxwell GL, Risinger JI, Hayes KA, et al: Racial disparity in the frequency of PTEN mutations, but not microsatellite instability, in advanced endometrial cancers. *Clin Cancer Res* 2000;6:2999-3005.
15. Colditz GA, Atwood KA, Emmons A, et al: Harvard report on cancer prevention, vol 4, Harvard Cancer Risk Index. *Cancer Causes Control* 2000;11:477-488.
16. Watson P, Vasen HF, Mecklin JP, et al: The risk of endometrial cancer in hereditary nonpolyposis colorectal cancer. *Am J Med* 1994;96:516-520.
17. Brinton LA, Berman ML, Mortel R, et al: Reproductive, menstrual, and medical risk factors for endometrial cancer: results from a case-control study. *Am J Obstet Gynecol* 1992;167:1317-1325.

18. McPherson CP, Sellers TA, Potter JD, et al: Reproductive factors and risk of endometrial cancer: the Iowa Women's Health Study. *Am J Epidemiol* 1996;143:1195-1202.
19. Albretsen G, Heuch I, Tretli S, et al: Is the risk of cancer of the corpus uteri reduced by a recent pregnancy?: a prospective study of 765,756 Norwegian women. *Int J Cancer* 1996;67:586-587.
20. Mogren I, Stenlund H, Hogberg U: Long-term impact of reproductive factors on the risk of cervical, endometrial, ovarian and breast cancer. *Acta Oncol* 2001;40:849-854.
21. Lochen ML, Lund E: Childbearing and mortality from cancer of the corpus uteri. *Acta Obstet Gynecol Scand* 1997;76:373-377.
22. Salvesen HB, Akslen LA, Albrektsen G, et al: Poorer survival of nulliparous women with endometrial carcinoma. *Cancer* 1998;82:1328-1333.
23. Hachisuga T, Fukuda K, Hirakawa T, et al: The effect of nulliparity on survival in endometrial cancer at different ages. *Gynecol Oncol* 2001;82:122-126.
24. Sherman ME: Theories of endometrial carcinogenesis: a multidisciplinary approach. *Mod Pathol* 2000;13:295-308.
25. Emons G, Fleckenstein G, Hinney B, et al: Hormonal interactions in endometrial cancer. *Endocr Relat Cancer* 2000;7:227-242.
26. Akhmedkhanov A, Zeleniuch-Jacquotte A, Toniolo P: Role of exogenous and endogenous hormones in endometrial cancer: review of the evidence and research perspectives. *Ann N Y Acad Sci* 2001;943:296-315.
27. Henderson BE, Feigelson HS: Hormonal carcinogenesis. *Carcinogenesis* 2000;21:427-433.
28. Westhoff C, Heller D, Drosinos S, et al: Risk factors for hyperplasia-associated versus atrophy-associated endometrial carcinoma. *Am J Obstet Gynecol* 2000;182:506-508.
29. Lax SF, Kendall B, Tashiro H, et al: The frequency of p53, K-ras mutations, and microsatellite instability differs in uterine endometrioid and serous carcinoma: evidence of distinct molecular genetic pathways. *Cancer* 2000;88:814-824.
30. Potischman N, Hoover RN, Brinton LA, et al: Case-control study of endogenous steroid hormones and endometrial cancer. *J Natl Cancer Inst* 1996;88:1127-1135.
31. Potischman N, Gail MH, Troisi R, et al: Measurement error does not explain the persistence of a body mass index association with endometrial cancer after adjustment for endogenous hormones. *Epidemiology* 1999;10:76-79.
32. Madigan MP, Troisi R, Potischman N, et al: Serum hormone levels in relation to reproductive and lifestyle factors in postmenopausal women (United States). *Cancer Causes Control* 1998;9:199-207.
33. Swanson CA, Potischman N, Wilbanks GD, et al: Relation of endometrial cancer risk to past and contemporary body size and body fat distribution. *Cancer Epidemiol Biomarkers Prev* 1993;2:321-327.

34. Folsom AR, Kaye SA, Potter JD, et al: Association of incident carcinoma of the endometrium with body weight and fat distribution in older women: early findings of the Iowa Women's Health Study. *Cancer Res* 1989;49:6828-6831.

35. Duska LR, Garrett A, Rueda BR, et al: Endometrial cancer in women 40 years old or younger. *Gynecol Oncol* 2001;83:388-393.

36. Troisi R, Potischman N, Hoover RN, et al: Insulin and endometrial cancer. *Am J Epidemiol* 1997; 146:476-482.

37. Kvale G, Heuch I, Ursin G: Reproductive factors and risk of cancer of the uterine corpus: a prospective study. *Cancer Res* 1988;48:6217-6221.

38. Kelsey JL, LiVolsi VA, Holford TR, et al: A case-control study of cancer of the endometrium. *Am J Epidemiol* 1982;116:333-342.

39. Pettersson B, Adami HO, Bergstrom R, et al: Menstruation span: a time-limited risk factor for endometrial carcinoma. *Acta Obstet Gynecol Scand* 1986;65:247-255.

40. Shoff SM, Newcomb PA: Diabetes, body size, and risk of endometrial cancer. *Am J Epidemiol* 1998; 148:234-240.

41. Grady D, Gebretsadik T, Kerlikowske K, et al: Hormone replacement therapy and endometrial cancer risk: a metaanalysis. *Obstet Gynecol* 1995; 85:304-313.

42. Effects of hormone replacement therapy on endometrial histology in postmenopausal women. The Postmenopausal Estrogen/Progestin Interventions (PEPI) Trial. The Writing Group for the PEPI Trial. *JAMA* 1996;275:370-375.

43. Woodruff JD, Pickar JH: Incidence of endometrial hyperplasia in postmenopausal women taking conjugated estrogens (Premarin) with medroxyprogesterone acetate or conjugated estrogens alone, the Menopause Study Group. *Am J Obstet Gynecol* 1994;170:1213-1223.

44. Pickar JH, Archer DF: Is bleeding a predictor of endometrial hyperplasia in postmenopausal women receiving hormone replacement therapy? Menopause Study Group (United States, Italy, Netherlands, Switzerland, Belgium, Germany, and Finland). *Am J Obstet Gynecol* 1997;177: 1178-1183.

45. Ziel HK, Finkle WD, Greenland S: Decline in incidence of endometrial cancer following increase in prescriptions for opposed conjugated estrogens in a prepaid health plan. *Gynecol Oncol* 1998;68:253-255.

46. Boroditsky RS. Balancing safety and efficacy focus on endometrial protection. *J Reprod Med* 2000;45:273-84.

47. Suriano KA, McHale M, McLaren CE, et al: Estrogen replacement therapy in endometrial cancer patients: a matched control study. *Obstet Gynecol* 2001;97:555-560.

48. Chapman JA, DiSaia PJ, Osann K, et al: Estrogen replacement in surgical stage I and II endometrial cancer survivors. *Am J Obstet Gynecol* 1996;175: 1195-1200.

49. DiSaia PJ: Hormone replacement therapy in the gynecologic and breast cancer patient. *Cancer Control J* 1996;3:101-106.

50. DiSaia PJ, Brewster WR: Hormone replacement therapy for survivors of breast and endometrial cancer. *Curr Oncol Rep* 2002;4:152-158.

51. Risks and benefits of estrogen plus progestin in healthy postmenopausal women. Principal results from Women's Health Initiative Randomized Controlled Trial Writing Group for the Women's Health Initiative Investigators. *JAMA* 2002; 288: 321-333.

52. Williams JK: Oral contraceptives and reproductive system cancer. Benefits and risks. *J Reprod Med* 1991;36:247-252.

53. Combination oral contraceptive use and the risk of endometrial cancer. The Cancer and Steroid Hormone Study of the Centers for Disease Control and the National Institute of Child Health and Human Development. *JAMA* 1987;257:796-800.

54. Vessey MP, Painter R: Endometrial and ovarian cancer and oral contraceptives: findings in a large cohort study. *Br J Cancer* 1995;71:1340-1342.

55. Stanford JL, Brinton LA, Berman ML, et al: Oral contraceptives and endometrial cancer: do other risk factors modify the association? *Int J Cancer* 1993;54:243-248.

56. Silfen SL, Ciaccia AV, Bryant HU: Selective estrogen receptor modulators: tissue selectivity and differential uterine effects. *Climacteric* 1999;2: 268-283.

57. Carlson RW: Scientific review of tamoxifen: overview from a medical oncologist. *Semin Oncol* 1997;24:S1-151-S1-7.

58. Assikis VJ, Jordan VC: Gynecologic effects of tamoxifen and the association with endometrial carcinoma. *Int J Gynaecol Obstet* 1995;49:241-257.

59. Barakat RR: Tamoxifen and endometrial cancer. *Cancer Control J* 1996;3:107-112.

60. Escobedo LG, Lee NC, Peterson HB, et al: Infertility-associated endometrial cancer risk may be limited to specific subgroups of infertile women. *Obstet Gynecol* 1991;77:124-128.

61. Solomon CG: The epidemiology of polycystic ovary syndrome: prevalence and associated disease risks. *Endocrinol Metab Clin North Am* 1999;28:247-263.

62. Lobo RA, Carmina E: The importance of diagnosing the polycystic ovary syndrome. *Ann Intern Med* 2000;132:989-993.

63. Hunter MH, Sterrett JJ: Polycystic ovary syndrome: it's not just infertility. *Am Fam Physician* 2000;62:1079-1088, 1090.

64. Gibson M: Reproductive health and polycystic ovary syndrome. *Am J Med* 1995;98:67S-75S.

65. Brinton LA, Barrett RJ, Berman ML, et al: Cigarette smoking and the risk of endometrial cancer. *Am J Epidemiol* 1993;137:281-291.

66. Newcomer LM, Newcomb PA, Trentham-Dietz A, et al: Hormonal risk factors for endometrial cancer: modification by cigarette smoking (United States). *Cancer Causes Control* 2001;12:829-835.

67. Daniell HW. More advanced-stage tumors among smokers with endometrial cancer. *Am J Clin Pathol* 1993;100:439-43.

68. Potischman N, Swanson CA, Brinton LA, et al: Dietary associations in a case-control study of endometrial cancer. *Cancer Causes Control* 1993;4: 239-250.

69. McCann SE, Freudenheim JL, Marshall JR, et al: Diet in the epidemiology of endometrial cancer in western New York (United States). *Cancer Causes Control* 2000;11:965-974.

70. Littman AJ, Beresford SA, White E: The association of dietary fat and plant foods with endometrial cancer (United States). *Cancer Causes Control* 2001;12:691-702.

71. Kasum CM, Nicodemus K, Harnack LJ, et al: Whole grain intake and incident endometrial cancer: the Iowa Women's Health Study. *Nutr Cancer* 2001;39:180-186.

72. Gruber SB, Thompson WD: A population-based study of endometrial cancer and familial risk in younger women, Cancer and Steroid Hormone Study Group. *Cancer Epidemiol Biomarkers Prev* 1996;5:411-417.

73. Olson JE, Sellers TA, Anderson KE, et al: Does a family history of cancer increase the risk for postmenopausal endometrial carcinoma?: a prospective cohort study and a nested case-control family study of older women. *Cancer* 1999;85:2444-2449.

74. Cedars-Sinai GenRISK Program: *Inherited endometrial cancer fact sheet*. Medical Genetics-Birth Defect Center, Cedars-Sinai Medical Center, 1999.

75. Berchuck A, Boyd J: Molecular basis of endometrial cancer. *Cancer* 1995;76:2034-2040.

76. Maxwell GL, Risinger JI, Alvarez AA, et al: Favorable survival associated with microsatellite instability in endometrioid endometrial cancers. *Obstet Gynecol* 2001;97:417-422.

77. Haiman CA, Hankinson SE, Colditz GA, et al: A polymorphism in CYP17 and endometrial cancer risk. *Cancer Res* 2001;61:3955-3960.

78. Smith RA, von Eschenbach AC, Wender R, et al: American Cancer Society guidelines for the early detection of cancer: update of early detection guidelines for prostate, colorectal, and endometrial cancers. Also: update 2001—testing for early lung cancer detection. *CA Cancer J Clin* 2001;51: 38-75; quiz 77-80.

79. Canavan TP, Doshi NR: Endometrial cancer. *Am Fam Physician* 1999;59:3069-3077.

80. Long CA: Evaluation of patients with abnormal uterine bleeding. *Am J Obstet Gynecol* 1996;175: 784-786.

81. Dunn TS, Stamm CA, Delorit M, et al: Clinical pathway for evaluating women with abnormal uterine bleeding. *J Reprod Med* 2001;46:831-834.

82. Silverberg SG: Problems in the differential diagnosis of endometrial hyperplasia and carcinoma. *Mod Pathol* 2000;13:309-327.

83. Hunter JE, Tritz DE, Howell MG, et al: The prognostic and therapeutic implications of cytologic atypia in patients with endometrial hyperplasia. *Gynecol Oncol* 1994;55:66-71.

84. Widra EA, Dunton CJ, McHugh M, et al: Endometrial hyperplasia and the risk of carcinoma. *Int J Gynecol Cancer* 1995;5:233-235.

85. Abulafia O, Triest WE, Adcock JT, et al: The effect of medroxyprogesterone acetate on angiogenesis in complex endometrial hyperplasia. *Gynecol Oncol* 1999;72:193-198.

86. Clarkson TB: Progestogens and cardiovascular disease: a critical review. *J Reprod Med* 1999;44: 180-184.

87. Dijkhuizen FP, Mol BW, Brolmann HA, et al: The accuracy of endometrial sampling in the diagnosis of patients with endometrial carcinoma and hyperplasia: a meta-analysis. *Cancer* 2000;89: 1765-1772.

88. Arikan G, Reich O, Weiss U, et al: Are endometrial carcinoma cells disseminated at hysteroscopy functionally viable? *Gynecol Oncol* 2001;83: 221-226.

89. Obermair A, Geramou M, Gucer F, et al: Does hysteroscopy facilitate tumor cell dissemination?: incidence of peritoneal cytology from patients with early stage endometrial carcinoma following dilatation and curettage (D&C) versus hysteroscopy and D & C. *Cancer* 2000;88:139-143.

90. Zerbe MJ, Zhang J, Bristow RE, et al: Retrograde seeding of malignant cells during hysteroscopy in presumed early endometrial cancer. *Gynecol Oncol* 2000;79:55-58.

91. Rose PG, Mendelsohn G, Kornbluth I: Hysteroscopic dissemination of endometrial carcinoma. *Gynecol Oncol* 1998;71:145-146.

92. Gomez-Fernandez CR, Ganjei-Azar P, Behshid K, et al: Normal endometrial cells in Papanicolaou smears: prevalence in women with and without endometrial disease. *Obstet Gynecol* 2000;96: 874-878.

93. National Cancer Institute: *Endometrial cancer (PDQ): Screening*. Washington, DC, National Cancer Institute, 2002.

94. Lerner JP, Timor-Tritsch IE, Monteagudo A: Use of transvaginal sonography in the evaluation of endometrial hyperplasia and carcinoma. *Obstet Gynecol Surv* 1996;51:718-725.

95. Valenzano M, Bertelli GF, Costantini S, et al: Transvaginal ultrasonography and hysterosonography to monitor endometrial effects in tamoxifentreated patients. *Eur J Gynaecol Oncol* 2001;22: 441-444.

96. Fong K, Kung R, Lytwyn A, et al: Endometrial evaluation with transvaginal US and hysterosonography in asymptomatic postmenopausal women with breast cancer receiving tamoxifen. *Radiology* 2001;220:765-773.

97. Brooks SE, Yeatts-Peterson M, Baker SP, et al: Thickened endometrial stripe and/or endometrial fluid as a marker of pathology: fact or fancy? *Gynecol Oncol* 1996;63:19-24.

98. Langer RD, Pierce JJ, O'Hanlan KA, et al: Transvaginal ultrasonography compared with

endometrial biopsy for the detection of endometrial disease. Postmenopausal Estrogen/Progestin Interventions Trial. *N Engl J Med* 1997;337: 1792-1798.

99. Briley M, Lindsell DR: The role of transvaginal ultrasound in the investigation of women with post-menopausal bleeding. *Clin Radiol* 1998;53: 502-505.

100. O'Connell LP, Fries MH, Zeringue E, et al: Triage of abnormal postmenopausal bleeding: a comparison of endometrial biopsy and transvaginal sonohysterography versus fractional curettage with hysteroscopy. *Am J Obstet Gynecol* 1998;178: 956-961.

101. Goldstein RB, Bree RL, Benson CB, et al: Evaluation of the woman with postmenopausal bleeding: Society of Radiologists in Ultrasound-Sponsored Consensus Conference statement. *J Ultrasound Med* 2001;20:1025-1036.

102. Connor JP, Andrews JI, Anderson B, et al: Computed tomography in endometrial carcinoma. *Obstet Gynecol* 2000;95:692-696.

103. Grasel RP, Outwater EK, Siegelman ES, et al: Endometrial polyps: MR imaging features and distinction from endometrial carcinoma. *Radiology* 2000;214:47-52.

104. Rose PG, Sommers RM, Reale FR, et al: Serial serum CA 125 measurements for evaluation of recurrence in patients with endometrial carcinoma. *Obstet Gynecol* 1994;84:12-16.

105. Price FV, Chambers SK, Carcangiu ML, et al: CA 125 may not reflect disease status in patients with uterine serous carcinoma. *Cancer* 1998;82:1720-1725.

106. Sakuragi N, Hareyama H, Todo Y, et al: Prognostic significance of serous and clear cell adenocarcinoma in surgically staged endometrial carcinoma. *Acta Obstet Gynecol Scand* 2000;79:311-316.

107. Cirisano FD Jr, Robboy SJ, Dodge RK, et al: The outcome of stage I-II clinically and surgically staged papillary serous and clear cell endometrial cancers when compared with endometrioid carcinoma. *Gynecol Oncol* 2000;77:55-65.

108. Cirisano FD Jr, Robboy SJ, Dodge RK, et al: Epidemiologic and surgicopathologic findings of papillary serous and clear cell endometrial cancers when compared to endometrioid carcinoma. *Gynecol Oncol* 1999;74:385-394.

109. Grice J, Ek M, Greer B, et al: Uterine papillary serous carcinoma: evaluation of long-term survival in surgically staged patients. *Gynecol Oncol* 1998;69:69-73.

110. Geisler JP, Sorosky JI, Duong HL, et al: Papillary serous carcinoma of the uterus: increased risk of subsequent or concurrent development of breast carcinoma. *Gynecol Oncol* 2001;83:501-503.

111. Lax SF, Pizer ES, Ronnett BM, et al: Clear cell carcinoma of the endometrium is characterized by a distinctive profile of p53, Ki-67, estrogen, and progesterone receptor expression. *Hum Pathol* 1998;29:551-558.

CHAPTER 11

Ethical and Legal Implications of Genetic Testing in Preventive Health

Michele A. Carter

INTRODUCTION

Predictive testing for genetic mutations that predispose individuals to cancer carries with it an enormous potential to enhance our understanding of human life and its cycles of growth, change, generation, decay, and death. As a tool of science, such testing promises to express this potential in ways that will revolutionize approaches to the discovery, treatment, and prevention of genetic diseases in human beings. Understanding the molecular basis for specific forms of cancer is an essential ingredient in the process of defining safe and efficacious prevention and treatment strategies. The public—and many researchers and clinicians as well—suggest that the widespread genetic testing capabilities now emerging from the completion of the Human Genome Project will usher in a new era of preventive medicine.[1] If so, traditional ways of categorizing preventive medicine will undergo new conceptualizations, thus deepening the ongoing debate about the meaning and scope of the field.

Preventive medicine historically is demarcated by three distinct but overlapping categories of health care services, each of which emphasizes a different set of priorities and values regarding health status. Primary prevention is concerned with generalized health promotion and specific protection against disease. It emphasizes the values of wellness and risk identification, and its interventions are applied to generally healthy individuals or groups. Traditional examples of primary prevention interventions include health education programs about accident and poisoning prevention, stress reduction, dietary modification, and immunizations. Secondary prevention emphasizes early detection and diagnosis of disease, prompt intervention, prevention of complications and disabilities, and health maintenance for individuals experiencing health problems. It includes screening surveys, self-monitoring procedures, and surveillance strategies. The predominant health-related value in secondary prevention is the assessment, understanding, and management of identified risks associated with the development of diseases, and the effective strategies to ward against their occurrence. Tertiary prevention is confined to the period of time after an illness begins, or when a defect or disability is fixed, stabilized, or rendered irreversible. The aim of tertiary prevention is to help individuals rehabilitate and to restore them to an optimal level of functioning within the constraint of the disability. Most physicians would agree that tertiary prevention has traditionally been the proper domain for the provision of medical services, principally because of the medical profession's acceptance of the biomedical model of disease and the profession's emphasis on treatment of the sick.

During recent decades, the boundaries between these levels of health care services have become increasingly vague, thus blurring the distinctions between preventive health and clinical care. Moreover, expansion of knowledge in genetic science is occurring at an unprecedented rate, and this knowledge is having an enormous impact on the medical community, health care consumers, and the health care system at large. Both the public and funding agencies continue to generate increased expectations that scientific discoveries should be rapidly translated into clinical applications that promise potential health benefits for individuals.

The ability to identify individuals who have inherited genetic susceptibilities for disease years before any symptoms develop is an extraordinary development. This not only challenges traditional frameworks for understanding disease prevention and health promotion but in a fundamental way shifts the practice of medicine from a biomedical model of disease to one that emphasizes genetically informed health care management. Widespread publicity in the lay and scientific media about inherited forms of cancer susceptibility syndromes has heightened interest in genetic screening technologies among healthy individuals, individuals at high risk for disease because of family history, public health administrators, and primary care health care providers. The isolation of several major tumor suppressor genes has made predictive genetic testing for cancer susceptibility a new reality. It also challenges conventional ideas about the meaning of "health," "risk," "disability," and "disease."[2] In the postgenomic age, these basic concepts are already taking on new meanings; this in turn has important implications for health care education, health policy, clinical care, and public health paradigms. This is especially true in the field of oncology, in which the pace of genetic knowledge of heritable forms of cancer is progressing at an astonishing rate. The isolation and identification of the BRCA1 and BRCA2 genes, whose mutations are believed to dispose those who possess them to breast or ovarian cancer, create new expectations regarding the power of genetic testing to predict, and perhaps forestall, the occurrence of disease. Clearly, discoveries of this magnitude are scientific milestones that open new avenues for the prevention and early detection of common disorders.

However, an increasing expansion of technological prowess in genetic sciences and health care is matched by a proliferation of ethically challenging issues regarding the responsible use of such technology in a society marked by a diversity of values. Many provocative questions about genetic technology can be raised, some that are broadly philosophical and others that are concrete and immediate. For instance, how can we justify informing a person that she will develop a lethal disease for which no cure or treatment exists? Does knowledge of one's future always confer a benefit, or might it be a harmful burden one need not assume? Should we permit individuals identified as carriers of catastrophic genetic disease to have children whose care will be a burden on society? Does our technical ability to detect disease in unborn humans fundamentally change the ends or goals of medicine? Finally, how can we translate the knowledge of molecular and biologic genetics gained in the research process into practical wisdom at the bedside, along with intervention aimed at improving the health and well-being of an individual patient?

As genetic knowledge expands and genetic services proliferate, these questions are likely to take on more urgency for the primary care practitioner. As genomic information increases, the range and frequency of genetic decisions will become so great that the typical referral to a clinical geneticist for each instance of decision making will become impossible, thus adding an entire new dimension to the primary care practitioner's ethical obligations regarding patient care. It is likely that in the next decade DNA testing for specific gene disorders and for multifactorial genetic predispositions will become commonplace, as will the development of individually tailored therapies to possibly correct, modify, or even replace poorly functioning genes. It is estimated that in the near future almost every known disease will have some aspect that is influenced by, if not directly caused by, mutations or polymorphisms in the genome of the patient. The genetic understanding of disease will allow more rapid and accurate diagnosis and risk assessment for a wide range of diseases as well as for less medically relevant traits.[3] These emerging transformations embody a critically important feature of the public's expectations regarding the promise of genetic medicine—that the new era of preventive medicine will revolutionize the practice of medicine and make possible the age-old ideal of perfect human health. These changes also reveal a fundamental tension between two human tendencies: the centuries-old belief that our lives are fated, currently reflected in debates regarding genetic determinism, and the more modern conviction that we should have control and mastery over what ails us.[4]

This chapter explores the ethical and legal dimensions of genetic testing in the context of preventing hereditary disease. The overall assumption is that genetic testing enhances the opportunity and rationale for increased surveillance and other prevention strategies but that it also carries the potential for harmful or unwanted consequences. The chapter is divided into three sections. The first describes issues related to the use and limitations of genetic testing for cancer susceptibility, using breast cancer as an illustration. The second section addresses the emerging ethical, legal, and social concerns associated with genetic testing. The third section provides an ethical framework for addressing these concerns in the clinical milieu.

THE USE AND LIMITATION OF GENETIC TESTS FOR HEREDITARY BREAST CANCER

Genetic tests involve the analysis, for various clinical purposes, of human DNA, RNA, chromosomes, proteins, and certain metabolites aimed at detecting heritable disease–related genotypes, mutations, phenotypes, or karyotypes. In the clinical context, "genetic testing" refers to the process of determining the genetic status of individuals who are already suspected to be at risk for a particular genetic condition or disorder on the basis of family history or clinical symptoms.[5] Some genetic tests are used to clarify a diagnosis and direct a physician toward appropriate treatments, whereas others identify individuals at high risk for conditions that may be preventable. Individuals already affected by cancer may seek genetic testing to define their personal cancer cause, clarify risk to offspring, ascertain appropriate surveillance strategies, or serve as an adjunct to the decision-making process in situations in which prophylactic surgery is being considered.[6] In some cases, genetic testing can dramatically improve an individual's health outcome or quality of life as in the case of aggressive monitoring for and removal of colon growths in those inheriting a gene for familial adenomatous polyposis.[7] In other cases, DNA-based testing confers intrinsic benefits such as increased knowledge about carrier status and therefore more informed decision making about work, family, reproductive, and retirement issues.

Gene tests for predisposition to a number of diseases are now available commercially to predict whether an individual will develop a disease or whether he or she is only at a higher risk of developing it. Gene testing for adult-onset disorders is usually targeted toward healthy individuals who are identified as being at high risk because of a strong family history for the disorder. However, predictive testing for disease susceptibility gives only a probability for developing the disorder; a positive finding of a disease-associated mutation does not mean that one will develop it. The probabilistic nature of susceptibility testing and the related difficulties associated with interpreting both positive and negative results in individual cases are a unique aspect of this technology. Obviously, an individual who receives a positive DNA result for the existence of a genetic mutation for which there is no effective treatment has a significant psychological burden to bear. Conversely, receiving a negative DNA result because of limitations of the test itself or the conditions under which it was conducted can create a false sense of well-being at a time when available interventions might reduce the risk of disease at a later time.

Although most cancers do have a hereditary component, it is important to ascertain those individuals who are at unusually high risk over a lifetime so that surveillance practices and risk management strategies can be employed.[8] Genetic knowledge is especially important for primary care practitioners because they will be called upon to identify those likely to benefit from genetic testing and to alert patients and families about issues associated with treatment, prevention, or reproductive options.[9] As genetic testing for cancer susceptibility becomes more common in clinical oncology practice, oncologists will face new challenges in identifying individuals for whom testing is appropriate, selecting optimal strategies to manage or reduce risks, and developing new treatment practices.

For instance, it has been estimated that approximately 10% to 15% of all breast cancer is familial in origin and that inherited alterations or mutations in the BRCA1 and BRCA2 genes are involved in about 30% to 70% of all inherited cases of breast cancer.[10] More specifically, a woman with certain known mutations in BRCA1 has a lifetime risk of 56% to 85% for developing breast cancer and an increased risk (63%) of developing ovarian cancer.[11] However, whether she actually develops breast or ovarian cancer is influenced by other genetic factors as well as by her hormonal and dietary status, and so the predictive power of susceptibility testing is limited. Clinicians must help patients understand that not all people with genetic alterations or mutations go on to develop the disorder for which they may be predisposed, and conversely that those individuals lacking a discernible genetic mutation will not necessarily spend their lives "disease-free."[2] In some cases, clinicians must be prepared to argue against the advisability of genetic testing, especially when no definitive treatment exists for what the tests reveal.[1] Because the majority of breast cancer cases are attributed to nonheritable factors, most women with a family history are not at sufficiently high risk to necessitate presymptomatic genetic testing, and the efficacy of genetic testing and screening as well as the meaning of the tests may be in doubt.[12] Increasingly, physicians will be called upon to manage the care of patients identified as being at an increased risk for inherited cancer even though definitive treatment or preventive measures have not been established.[13] However, several studies have documented many physicians' lack of preparation for discussing and communicating with patients about genetic testing.[9] Some surveys indicate that physicians who order commercial tests may misinterpret the results of the test,[14] lack knowledge about how best to communicate medical risk,[15] or fall prey to subtle versions of genetic determinism.[1] This has significant implications for clinical decision making, informed consent, counseling strategies, and patient satisfaction. As presymptomatic testing for cancer prediction and prevention continues to evolve into practice settings, patients and families should be aware of the limitations in the predictive value of available tests and seek appropriate referral to genetics professionals for individualized risk ascertainment and counseling.

Clearly, the availability of genetic testing for breast and ovarian cancer mutations intensifies the need to define the benefits and risks of early detection and preventive measures so that appropriate intervention methods can be designed. Currently there are no known methods for preventing breast or ovarian cancer that specifically pertain to women with mutated versions of these genes,[16] although clinical trials with tamoxifen and Raloxifene are under way. The options for managing cancer risk in individuals found to have a mutated gene currently include the following:

- Surveillance (clinical examination, mammography, pelvic ultrasound, and serum tumor marker testing)

- Prophylactic surgery (bilateral mastectomy or oophorectomy)
- Risk avoidance (reducing alcohol intake, increasing exercise, modifying diet)
- Chemoprevention (antiestrogens, dietary retinoids, vitamin E, and selenium)[17]

For many women the benefits of genetic testing for breast and ovarian cancer risk include the ability to obtain information relevant to medical, reproductive, and lifestyle decisions and to exercise their right to know whether they or their relatives have a greater than average chance of developing cancer. However, there are particular concerns associated with genetic testing for breast and ovarian cancer. First, no consensus has yet emerged on the optimal techniques and schedules for early detection procedures in this group.[18] Many screening intervention strategies are of unproved benefit and technically difficult to achieve. For instance, in evaluating whether genetic testing is a useful screening technology in the population as a whole, it is important to note that among women who develop breast cancer, only 5% to 10% are carriers of genetic mutations in BRCA1 and BRCA2. The baseline risk for an average woman in the United States without the genetic mutation is estimated to be 12.6%, or 1 in 8 women.[19] Guidelines adopted by the American Society of Human Genetics (ASHG) state that it is premature to offer population screening until the risks associated with specific BRCA1 mutations are determined and the best strategies for monitoring and prevention are accurately assessed. Specifically, the consensus of this professional society is that "until we know the probability that a particular mutation will occur in cancer, the efficacy and safety of follow-up interventions, and the reliability of the test, mass screening for BRCA1 mutations is not recommended."[20] Similarly, using criteria developed by the U.S. Preventive Services Task Force, the American Academy of Family Physicians endorses the following principles for its recommendations regarding population screening for genetic risk:

1. The population screened must have a significant burden of suffering.
2. There must be an asymptomatic period during which the disease can be detected in the clinical setting.
3. Screening must be accurate during the asymptomatic period.
4. The screening test must be acceptable to the patient.
5. Preventive intervention must be superior to conventional follow-up.[21]

Another issue has to do with the question of whether predictive testing for breast cancer should be offered to every patient. Some individuals may perceive the physician's offer to provide genetic testing to a specific patient as an endorsement of its efficacy, when in fact its clinical validity, analytical validity, and clinical utility have not been established.[22] Test validity incorporates the following three distinct parameters, all of which are based on probabilistic reasoning: sensitivity, the probability that a test will identify a mutation if one is present; specificity, the probability that the test results will be negative if an individual does not have a mutation; and positive predictive value, the probability that individuals who receive a positive test result will go on to develop the disease.

Until genetic testing of bodily material is performed under universal laboratory conditions, it is likely that the proficiency of a particular laboratory can influence the validity of a test. Although the American College of Medical Genetics has established standards for laboratory genetics services,[23] compliance is voluntary. In 1998, the Clinical Laboratory Improvement Amendments (CLIA) determined universal requirements for laboratory quality assurance, control, and proficiency that could be used in standardizing the way genetic testing is performed, even though no specific directives for genetic services are included in its requirements. Left hanging are the following insufficiencies:

- The clinical usefulness of genetic testing for predisposing cancer mutations is directly linked to available therapeutic options, but for the most part these options remain unproved.

- Information provided by genetic testing for hereditary predisposition to breast cancer is not matched by state-of-the art diagnostics and therapies. This is partially because current understanding of the molecular penetration of disease in known mutation carriers remains incomplete and because the clinical implications of carrier status are largely unknown.
- There is no established standard of care regarding the efficacy of prophylactic surgical procedures. Also, bilateral prophylactic mastectomy and oophorectomy remain controversial despite a few reports that in women with high risk family histories, prophylactic mastectomy significantly reduced the incidence of breast cancer.[24,25]
- A final consideration has to do with the costs associated with predictive testing, which can range from several hundred to several thousand dollars depending on how many family members are involved, with full gene sequencing estimated at $2400.[26] Insurance policies vary in their coverage of genetic testing.

On the other hand, from the perspective of primary or secondary prevention, identifying women at significantly increased risk of developing inherited forms of breast and ovarian cancers can be ethically justified once research establishes that more frequent mammograms or intensified screening and surveillance regimens allow for early diagnosis, diet modification, or avoidance of known carcinogens, thus preventing or delaying the onset of cancer.

Increasingly, many social scientists believe that nurses, family physicians, and other primary care practitioners will be the intermediaries between genetic technology and the patient. They will be expected to appraise critically the appropriate application and limitation of genetic tests to individual patients.[27] Clinicians must carefully weigh the concerns associated with genetic testing and then decide when to refer patients to appropriately trained specialists who will discuss the desirability, interpretation, and limitation of genetic tests in detail. Currently, offering or recommending predictive testing for heritable cancer to every patient does not fall within the accepted standard of care. Moreover, to date there is no reliable evidence that genetic testing for heritable cancer reduces morbidity or mortality.[28,29] Thus the recommendation of the American Society of Clinical Oncology (ASCO) stipulates the following:

> Cancer predisposition testing [should] be offered only when: 1) the person has a strong family history of cancer or very early age of onset of disease; 2) the test can be adequately interpreted; 3) the results will influence the medical management of the patient or family member.[30]

Primary care physicians will increasingly confront healthy individuals who request genetic testing, even when the results of those tests may reveal that they carry genes that may predispose them to serious medical problems. The risks associated with obtaining information about one's genetic inheritance are magnified when definitive treatment or preventive interventions are not yet available for the condition or disorder. In clinical care settings, health care providers must take into consideration how to help individuals who test positive to live with the prospect of unavoidable illness. Additionally, they must be aware that the manner in which a person's genetic information is treated can have a profound effect on the patient-provider relationship and the ethical value of trust inherent in it.[31] Moreover, they must provide accurate information regarding the implications of knowing one's genetic status, so that fears about insurability and employment can be properly addressed. In confronting decisions about the appropriate use of genetic testing for these individuals, clinicians take on three important obligations. First, they must keep themselves abreast of emerging scientific data regarding new surveillance and prevention interventions as well as developments in risk assessment and modification. Second, clinicians must communicate this information openly and honestly with patients and families so that these individuals can make authentic choices about health behaviors, lifestyle issues, procreation, parenting, and being categorized as "at risk," rather than healthy. Third, they must appreciate the emerging ethical, legal, and social implications of genetic testing for cancer susceptibility and learn how to navigate the ever-changing currents of the new genetic frontier.

ETHICAL, LEGAL, AND SOCIAL IMPLICATIONS OF GENETIC TESTING

The first decade of research into the ethical, legal, and social aspects of the Human Genome Project has produced a remarkable reservoir of knowledge and scholarship. As genetic scientists probe the depths of DNA and map the sequences of its predictable sites, ethicists, legal scholars, and social scientists are beginning to unravel the ethical and philosophical questions such discoveries imply. Their intellectual insights and theoretical perspectives are critical to the next phase of ethical, legal, and social implications of genetic testing (ELSI) research, which will likely address increasingly complex issues associated with the integration of molecular understandings of disease into patient-centered health plans and pharmacogenetics paradigms. As new developments in gene-based medicine continue to occur at an astonishing rate, old values we have come to take for granted assume new meaning in genetic discourse. For instance, the principle of individual liberty, arguably the most powerful of ethical ideals in American life and culture, is itself under the microscope. How can the value of individual autonomy and freedom of choice be sustained in the face of technology that detects disease mutations in the members of one's immediate or distant family? Alternatively, does the application of emerging knowledge about human genetics fundamentally threaten cherished beliefs about human dignity, the value of human diversity, the child's right to an open future, and the proper ends of medicine? Although many clinicians may find such questions too removed from the concerns of daily practice, they are a central component of the public debates about who should have access to and control of genetic information and material.

Genetic testing for cancer susceptibility reaches far beyond the technical domain of science and medicine. It is a tool of humanity, one that reveals information about individuals and their families and about the nature of their concerns regarding life, liberty, identity, and community. Genetic testing is a powerful tool not only because of the information it yields about disease markers but also because it reveals information about ourselves as unique individuals and about the families and social institutions in which we live. Genetic testing is a technology embedded within a unique cluster of cultural, political, social, economic, and moral contexts. The significance of genetic testing cannot be measured in purely objective terms because its meaning derives from the diversity of these perspectives and the different values ascribed to its worth. By itself, gene testing and other emerging genetic technologies are neither good nor bad. What confers moral legitimacy to them is the way in which they are employed in actual human situations. In a pluralistic society, each patient, family, or provider interprets the significance of genetic information in terms of his or her own set of personal values, experiences, and beliefs. Thus, in weighing the relative benefits and burdens associated with genetic testing, it is imperative that practitioners understand the humanistic context within which these technologies are applied.

Although genetic testing may be seen as a subset of medical testing in general, the following characteristics taken together suggest that it be given special consideration.[32]

1. Genetic information is familial, in that the information it generates about the individual has direct health implications for others who are genetically related.

2. Genetic information is laden with social and psychological meanings related to one's identity, in part due to the tendency to consider genes as deterministic of future health and behavior.

3. The predictive power of genetic information is limited to probabilistic inference, often with no independent means to confirm a diagnosis. Given the complex interactions of genes with environmental factors, predictions about whether disease will develop or how symptoms will manifest are often inexact.

4. The objective risks associated with genetic testing may not be readily understood because they are largely psychological rather than physical and vary among individuals and groups.

5. The clinical utility of genetic information may be limited because many late-onset genetic diseases are difficult to treat or prevent, thus challenging the assumption that knowledge of risk status would reduce morbidity and mortality.[33]

Given these concerns, it is easy to see why genetic testing for cancer susceptibility should be understood in a moral context as well as a medical or scientific one. A moral context requires consideration of the underlying values, rights, duties, and obligations that guide behavior and determine responsibility. The moral context for genetic testing has four principal areas of concern: informed consent, medical privacy, psychosocial risks, and the duty to warn.

Informed Consent

The doctrine of informed consent requires that any decisions regarding genetic testing be made as a collaborative effort between the patient and the health care provider. In genetic testing for cancer susceptibility, informed consent is understood to be giving permission for the creation of potentially meaningful information about an individual's risk for adverse consequences. This information may have a variety of clinical, psychological, social, and economic implications for the individual to whom it pertains. Additionally, it may have implications for members of that individual's family or for that individual's future offspring. The clinician must disclose information that a reasonable person would regard as germane to the decision to undergo genetic testing. This information includes assessments of risk: benefits, effectiveness, and available alternatives. It should also be communicated in a manner that is readily comprehended, while respecting the person's cultural, ethnic, and religious values. In the context of testing for BRCA1 and 2, the American Society of Clinical Oncology recommends that disclosure should include these elements:

(a) Information that the purpose of the test is to determine whether a mutation can be detected in a specific cancer susceptibility gene

(b) Current knowledge about the type and magnitude of health risks associated with a positive test and any risks that might remain even if a test is negative

(c) The possibility that no additional information will be obtained upon completion of the test

(d) Alternative options for ascertaining risk status, such as empirical risk tables

(e) Current knowledge about risks associated with passing a mutation on to children

(f) Accuracy of the test

(g) Any laboratory or counseling fees associated with the test

(h) The risks of psychological distress or family disruption if a mutation is found or not found

(i) The degree to which the confidentiality of results will be preserved as compared with the confidentiality of other medical tests

(j) Medical options and limited proof of effectiveness for surveillance and cancer prevention for those with a positive test as well as the accepted recommendations for
cancer screening even if the genetic testing is negative[30]

Informed consent should be viewed as a process of shared decision making that conjoins
the right of the person to make his or her own health care decisions based on personal and
cultural values along with the corresponding duty of the health care provider to promote the
patient's well-being. There is considerable debate surrounding the issue of a patient's ability
to make medical or surgical decisions about cancer treatments or to provide adequate
informed consent, especially given the anxiety and depression often observed in women
with early breast cancer.[34-38] However, in the United States the recognized ideal norm for
decision making about treatment intervention is the standard of shared decision making.
This standard refers to the assumption that well-informed patients and health care providers
each have value systems that affect decisions about treatment and prevention goals. These
differing value systems are believed to be expressions of different ways of ordering or ranking what one considers worth pursuing in life, whether this is in terms of one's health and
well-being, or other ideals such as happiness, justice, rationality, or liberty. This standard acknowledges that both patients and health care providers are agents of their own
values and beliefs regarding the meanings associated with life, death, health, disease, and
self-determination.

From an ethical and legal perspective, the standard of shared decision making is a nor-
mative ideal that informs the practice of clinical medicine. The model of shared decision
making is particularly relevant to the genetic context because it promotes respect for individual autonomy, self-determination, beneficence, and human dignity.

One of the primary ways to implement the standard of shared decision making in providing genetic services is by referral to a genetic counselor. The genetic counseling process is
fundamentally a method of communication aimed at helping individuals and families to
interpret and deal with information about a genetic disorder that has been diagnosed or is
suspected. Genetic counselors working in the field of oncology address the risks of having
an inherited form of cancer for an individual with either a personal or family history of a
particular condition. After ascertaining relevant medical facts and obtaining family history
information, genetic counselors present available options for managing risks associated with
a genetic condition. These may include prenatal testing, screening, or other preventive measures. A primary tenet of the Code of Ethics for National Society of Genetic Counselors
emphasizes the ethical value of individual autonomy and stipulates that genetic counselors
should strive to "respect their client's beliefs, cultural traditions, inclinations, circumstances,
and feelings."[39] Another tenet of genetic counseling is that information and available
options should be provided in a nondirective fashion, illuminating the necessary facts so
that their clients can make "informed independent decisions, free of coercion."[39] Although
some commentators challenge whether the norm of nondirectiveness is really feasible,[40]
morally neutral,[41] or accurate,[42] the principle of nondirectiveness is still stressed in genetic
testing.

Another important goal of genetic counseling is to assess the degree to which counselees comprehend risk information.[43] Interestingly, research studies investigating genetic
counseling demonstrate that most counselees have difficulty understanding probability
information.[44,45] Although genetic counseling often focuses on the family unit, studies show
that even when other family members do not participate in the testing themselves, they may
be profoundly affected by the genetic diagnosis of a family member.[46,47] Moreover, given the
information-rich nature of DNA analysis, genetic testing often exposes other family members

to psychological and social harms, frequently without their consent. This can challenge traditional professional obligations regarding confidentiality and the need to protect the individual's right to privacy. In addressing this point, the National Society of Genetic Counselors stipulates, "it is the right and responsibility of the individual to determine who shall have access to medical information, particularly results of testing for genetic conditions."[48] Furthermore, the personal and familial nature of genetic testing can challenge the autonomy-driven paradigms that have dominated the patient-provider relationship for several decades. Genetic counselors have special responsibilities to strengthen communication strategies as a means of resolving the familiar tensions often exacerbated by genetic information and the competing claims that individuals and their relatives make on behalf of it.[49]

Medical Privacy

Of all the types of personal information, medical data about one's state of health are considered among the most sensitive and deserving of protection. Keeping medical information confidential has been an ethical duty of physicians since the time of Hippocrates, in part because of the belief that doing so would increase patients' trust in their providers and improve their willingness to adhere to a treatment plan. While facilitating the exchange of highly personal health information continues to be a necessary component of a medically sound patient-provider relationship, there is a corresponding concern among patients and the public that such information could be used in unacceptable ways. Inappropriate disclosure of medical information can lead to personal embarrassment, increased vulnerability or exploitation, and loss of the patient's right to privacy. A number of states have sought to protect individuals by enacting legislation that restricts the use of genetic information by employers, insurance companies and others, but these efforts can be preempted by federal laws.[50] One of the federal protections against unwarranted disclosure of personal medical information is codified in the Privacy Act of 1974. This code asserts the right of an individual to discover what information is kept about him or her and to know how it is used. It gives the individual the right to correct or amend a record containing personal health information. In addition, it requires organizations that collect, maintain, use, and disclose personal data to take precautions to deter misuses of sensitive information.

Keeping individualized detailed genetic data private is one of the most talked-about concerns in genetic research and medicine. Recent reports suggest that individuals perceive the possibility of facing genetic discrimination in health care, employment, and insurance if they are identified as having a genetic condition or predisposition. For instance, a study published in *Science* reports that 15% of individuals at risk of developing a genetic condition said that they had been asked questions about heritable disease on their employment applications. Thirteen percent reported that they or another family member had been denied a job or fired because of information that a family member had a genetic condition.[51] To understand the context of these concerns, it is important to bear in mind two salient points. First, it is not abundantly clear what is meant by the term "genetic discrimination." One definition cited frequently throughout the literature suggests that genetic discrimination refers to "discrimination directed against an individual or against members of that individual's family solely because of real or perceived differences from the 'normal' genome of that individual."[52] Second, it must be noted that the current legal system for the regulation of patient information is inadequate. Although all states have laws that provide some form of protection of the privacy of medical records and the confidentiality of patient-provider discussions, there is little consistency in state law regarding genetic discrimination.[53] In 1996 Congress passed the Health Insurance Portability and Accountability Act (HIPAA), in part to modernize health privacy policy in the wake of extraordinary advances in electronic information technology. This legislation prohibits a health insurer from using genetic information to determine a person's eligibility for a group plan and assures people with medical conditions, including genetic predispositions, that they can obtain health insurance when they move from one job to the next. Thus, HIPAA is an important step forward in combating discrimination on the basis of health status, even though its provisions do not strongly protect genetic privacy outside the context of health insurance needs.[54]

Despite recent federal and state efforts banning "genetic discrimination," some commentators suggest that genetic privacy remains elusive and extremely difficult to ensure.[55] More comprehensive and meaningful legislation is needed to create uniform standards for the protection of patient privacy and the confidentiality of health information, while at the same time being flexible enough to encourage innovations in research, medical care, and community health practices. Safeguarding the individual's right of privacy is a fundamental ethical and legal imperative about which health care professionals should be appropriately trained and held accountable. On the other hand, we must acknowledge that personal medical information has a public and community purpose as well and could be an important benefit in such programs as health services research, epidemiologic surveillance, communicable disease control, quality assurance, clinical trials, and population-based research. In the future, it is likely that more prevention studies of health risks will be linking data sets on environmental exposures, behavioral risk factors, and the use of medical services and pharmaceuticals with other data sets involving genome information, thus increasing the challenge of protecting information of a personal and sensitive nature from unwarranted disclosure.

Psychosocial Risks

Genetic information is unique and more personal than medical information because it can predict an individual's likely medical future, divulge personal information about one's family members, and be used, as it sometimes has been, to stigmatize and victimize individuals.[56] Moreover, the act of labeling an individual with genetic variations as "diseased" has enormous personal, psychosocial, financial, and physical implications, even in the absence of disease symptoms. For instance, labeling someone as diseased may affect decisions about family planning, or it may result in unjust treatment by life, medical, and disability insurers, leading to significant distress. A review of the literature reveals that the most common psychological and social risks of genetic testing for hereditary disease include anxiety, cancer worry, guilt, social stigma, disfigurement, impaired self-esteem, and the fear of discrimination in insurance or employment. These potential risks must be explained to patients before any testing procedure because they are relevant to an individual's risk-benefit calculation and subsequent informed consent process. In addition to the emotional stigmatization of being labeled "at risk" or a "mutation carrier," learning one's genetic status can precipitate anger, perceived lack of control, negative body image, fear of disfigurement and dying, and a sense of isolation.[57] On the other hand, such labeling can be beneficial to some patients in that it helps to legitimize symptoms, clarify issues of personal responsibility, and improve one's motivation to access health care services.[2] Some studies indicate that identification of genetic disorders or carrier status can be a contributing factor in marital discord, divorce, or other family problems.[58] Clearly, inadvertent disclosure of genetic information may reveal painful facts about family relationships, such as the misattribution of parentage.[59] Clinicians must be sensitive to these potential consequences and know when to refer patients for appropriate psychological counseling if necessary.

Because gene testing reveals information not only about the individual but about his or her relatives as well, the results can challenge family and social dynamics. Although most genetic tests are undertaken to improve management and treatment options for patients, sometimes the disadvantages of knowing one's genetic status information outweigh the benefits. Given the traditional dictum of "First, do no harm," health care providers must weigh the relative merits of promoting individual autonomy against the harms that might result from unwarranted disclosure of test results to family members who may hold different value perspectives on this information. Moreover, although informed consent of the patient is a prerequisite to genetic testing, ethical dilemmas arise when the disclosure of genetic results is relevant to the health priorities and decisions of family members, even if they have not provided informed consent to be tested. Although there is a strong presumption in favor of the established norm to preserve the confidentiality of the patient's private medical information, the familial aspect of genetic risk information raises new and profound questions regarding the ethics of preserving confidentiality and preventing harm to others.

Duty to Warn

In the era of postgenomic medicine, new controversies are beginning to emerge about the responsibility of the clinician or researcher to share genetic information within families. This is a complex issue that requires sensitive balancing of the right of the individual to keep confidential any information disclosed within the doctor-patient relationship and that individual's ethical obligation to share information that could potentially benefit or forestall harm to his or her biologic relatives. Clinicians faced with the dilemma of whether to breach the prevailing standard of care with regard to patient confidentiality must weigh a number of critical factors, such as professional codes of ethics, current legislation regarding who has appropriate access to genetic information, evolving social standards regarding the prevention of high-risk activities associated with disease, and personal values regarding professional autonomy.

In its effort to provide guidance on this issue, the President's Commission for the Study of Ethical Problems in Medicine and Biomedical and Behavioral Research states that disclosure of a patient's confidential information is warranted only when these four conditions are met:

- Reasonable attempts to elicit voluntary disclosure are unsuccessful.
- There is a high probability of a very serious harm occurring if the information is withheld.
- There is reason to believe that disclosure of the information will prevent the harm.
- Appropriate precautions are taken to ensure that only information necessary for diagnosis and treatment of another identifiable person is disclosed.[60]

More recently, the Florida Supreme Court deliberated the case of a daughter whose mother was diagnosed as having medullary thyroid cancer, an autosomal dominant disorder. Three years later the daughter, Heidi Pate, was diagnosed with the same disease. The plaintiff Pate sued her mother's physicians and their employers for not warning her that she might be at risk of genetic transmission. Pate contended that if she had been told in 1987 of the genetic inheritance of the condition, she would have been tested for the disease, and would have taken preventive actions that would render her condition curable. In its ruling, the court upheld the state's law that protected the confidentiality of the patient's medical information, asserting that although the physician should have told the mother her condition was genetic, he had no legal duty to warn the daughter. In Pate *v.* Threlkel, the court held the following:

Our holding should not be read to require the physician to warn the patient's children of the disease. In most instances the physician is prohibited from disclosing the patient's medical condition to others except with the patient's permission. Moreover, the patient ordinarily can be expected to pass on the warning. To require the physician to seek out and warn various members of the patient's family would often be difficult or impractical and would place too heavy a burden upon the physician. Thus we emphasize that in any circumstances in which the physician has a duty to warn of a genetically transferable disease, that duty will be satisfied by warning the patient.[61]

One year later, the Superior Court of New Jersey took a different approach and denied that the physician's duty to warn is satisfied by informing the patient. In this case, over a period of years, a man received treatment for retroperitoneal cancer, ulcerative adenocarcinoma of the colon, and adenomatous polyps. He subsequently died at the age of 45, leaving a 10-year-old daughter, who 26 years later was diagnosed with primary carcinoma of the colon and multiple polyposis. In 1990, the daughter, Ms. Safer, sued the estate of her father's physician, Dr. Pack, alleging a violation of his duty to warn her of the hereditary risk to her health and thus denying her the benefits associated with early examination, monitoring, detection, and screening. Although the trial court held that a physician had no legal duty to warn a patient's child of a genetic risk, it dismissed the case on the grounds that there was no doctor-patient relationship between the father's doctor and the now adult child. The New Jersey Appeals Court, however, discerned no appreciable difference between this case and traditional "duty to warn" cases that involved communicable infection or threat of physical harm. It pointed out that in Safer the genetic risks are foreseeable and "the individual or group at risk is easily identified, and substantial future harm is easily identified or minimized by a timely and effective warning."[62] Thus the court held that a physician does have a duty to warn members of the immediate family of the patient known to be at risk of avoidable harm from a genetically transmissible condition, even though it failed to state just how the duty to warn might be discharged.

Although cases of this sort remain somewhat rare, they raise important questions about the appropriateness of informing a child of his or her genetic characteristics and whether there is a legal right to obtain confidential information about a genetically based medical condition even when no patient-physician relationship obtains. Among the issues to be considered are the accuracy of the genetic test, the specificity of the risk, the availability of treatment, whether disclosure actually prevents harm or induces more psychological distress, and the degree to which disclosure violates the rights of the patient whose confidentiality would otherwise be protected. At a minimum, these cases suggest that a health care provider has a duty to inform a patient about potential genetic risks to which the patient is susceptible but should disclose this information to at-risk relatives of the patient only where the potential harm is serious and treatment or prevention measures are available.

ETHICAL FRAMEWORK FOR GENETIC TESTING FOR HEREDITARY CANCER

As genetic technologies continue to be incorporated into clinical oncology practice, primary care providers will need to expand their knowledge of the ethical, professional, social, and legal issues associated with such advances. Because genetic testing and screening raise many complex issues about which there is only a wavering consensus, practitioners must work in collaboration with geneticists, genetic counselors, prenatal care providers, and other experts. These collaborations can be further guided by a framework of ethical commitments and recommendations that help resolve many of the value conflicts and ethical ambiguities associated with predictive testing for cancer susceptibility. Although ethical guidelines for genetic testing for hereditary cancer are similar to those that guide the practice of clinical medicine as a whole, two points deserve special attention. First, it is important to note that ethical and legal obligations with respect to genetic testing are evolving, shaped by existing scientific knowledge, social practices, and professional norms. As new data emerge regarding the risks and benefits of genetic testing, and new prevention, surveillance, and treatment interventions are developed, the duties and obligations of clinicians may change as well. Second, even though at present there is no established consensus or standard of care regarding the offering of genetic testing for cancer susceptibility, primary care providers play a key role in helping individuals understand and manage their risk, communicating with them about their concerns and when indicated, making appropriate recommendations for genetic testing.

From an ethical perspective, decisions about genetic testing should be guided by the ethical principles of respect for patient and family autonomy, a favorable risk-benefit analysis, and the just allocation of health care resources. Before undergoing genetic testing for cancer susceptibility, the patient should receive up-to-date and reliable information about how his or her risk status will be ascertained and communicated; who will have access to the genetic information revealed by the test; the availability of additional counseling, supportive, and educational services; and the degree to which rights to privacy and confidentiality will be maintained. This information should be provided in a way that shows respect for the individual's sense of vulnerability, cultural identity, and family dynamics. Genetic testing requires a meaningful and deliberate process of informed consent in which the clinician discloses all of these items:

1. Purposes and limitations of the testing procedure
2. Probabilistic nature of the genetic information and the risk estimates it yields
3. Information regarding access to and availability of alternatives to genetic testing
4. An assessment of the relative benefits and burdens associated with knowing one's genetic information
5. Notification of any legal or ethical requirements pertinent to the information obtained

Competent and well-informed patients and families should be free to make their own medical, lifestyle, and reproductive decisions based on the information generated through genetic testing. In addition, they should be free to exercise their "right not to know" unwanted details of their genetic inheritance, especially if there is no intervention or proven course of action that would benefit them.

The benefits of presymptomatic testing and intervention for cancer susceptibility must be weighed against potential harms such as anxiety, stigmatization, psychological distress, fear of employment or insurance discrimination—or both—and the burden of knowing one's carrier status in the absence of effective treatment. Because there are no definitive guidelines on genetic testing for hereditary cancer, the decision to undergo it largely rests with the patient and his or her physician. For this reason, it is imperative that physicians remain aware of the research developments in risk assessment, detection and surveillance, chemoprevention, prophylactic surgery, and quality-of-life measures. Physicians should provide open and honest discussions of the uncertainties associated with genetic testing and demonstrate vigilance with respect to the issues of trust inherent in the doctor-patient relationship. The relationship between the patient and the genetics professional provides the moral context within which the patient can express unique health-related values, needs, expectations, and hopes.[63] In addition, it provides a legal context within which the rights, duties, obligations, and judgments of the medical practitioners are ascertained and socially justified.

Finally, the current and future uses of genetic testing in the clinical context expand the debate about the role of social justice in the system of health care. Some bioethicists have warned that the genetic revolution will pose unprecedented challenges to equal opportunity, thus exacerbating social injustices against the poor and disadvantaged groups.[64] Current inequalities in access to health care seem likely to operate with respect to genetic testing and other genetic technologies.[65] Unless there are major changes in the health care system in this country, there will likely be a lack of equity in access to some genetic technologies, especially for individuals lacking health insurance. Ideally, any differences in access to or availability of genetic testing for cancer susceptibility should be ethically justified, and no individual at high risk for developing heritable cancer should be denied routine testing simply because of an inability to pay. In a just health care system, access to and availability of genetic testing for cancer susceptibility would be based on medical need and the promise of medical benefit. Although efforts to improve the effectiveness, safety, efficiency, and accuracy of predictive testing continue to advance, it is imperative that definitive criteria be established for its fair and equitable use. In addition, physicians, genetics professionals, and health policy analysts must develop ethically sound policies that prevent discrimination, stigmatization, exploitation, or disempowerment on the basis of genetic information. To the extent that genetic testing for cancer susceptibility can be proven to confer a favorable balance of realizable benefits over foreseeable harms for the well-informed and autonomous individuals consenting to it and it poses no inherent threat to the demands of distributive justice, such technologies are ethically justified.

REFERENCES

1. Bottles K: A revolution in genetics: changing medicine, changing lives. *Physician Exec* 2001;27:58-63.
2. Temple LKF, McLeod RS, Gallinger S, et al: Defining disease in the genomics era. *Science* 2001;293:807-808.
3. Leonard D: The future of molecular genetic testing. *Clin Chem* 1999;45:726-731.
4. Carson RA: The fate of the responsible self in a genetic age. In Carson RA, Rothstein MA, editors: *Behavioral genetics: the clash of culture and biology.* Baltimore, Johns Hopkins University Press, 1999.
5. Holtzman NA, Watson MS: *Promoting safe and effective genetic testing in the United States: Final report of the task force on genetic testing.* NIH-DOE Working Group on Ethical, Legal, and Social Implications of Human Genome Research, 1997.
6. Julian-Reynier C, Eisinger F, Chabal F, et al: Cancer genetic clinics: why do women who already have cancer attend? *Eur J Can* 1998;34:1549-1553.
7. Lynch HT, Watson P, Shaw TG, et al: Clinical impact of molecular genetic diagnosis, genetic counseling and management of hereditary cancer. *Cancer* 1999;86:2449-2463.
8. Ang P, Garber JE: Genetic susceptibility for breast cancer-risk assessment and counseling. *Semin Oncol* 2001;28:419-433.
9. Hofman KJ, Tambor ES, Chase GA, et al: Physicians' knowledge of genetics and genetic tests. *Acad Med* 1993;68:625-632.
10. Ford D, Easton DF, Stratton M: Genetic heterogeneity and penetrance analysis of the BRCA1 and BRCA2 genes in breast cancer families. *Am J Hum Genet* 1998;62:676-689.
11. Rosenthal TC, Puck SM: Screening for genetic risk of breast cancer. *Am Fam Physician* Jan 1, 1999; 59(1):99-106.
12. Gray J, Brain K, Norman P, et al: A model protocol evaluating the introduction of genetic assessment for women with a family history of breast cancer. *J Med Genet* 2000;37(3):192-196.
13. Worthen H: Inherited cancer and the primary care physician: barriers and strategies. *Cancer* 1999;86:1763-1768.
14. Giardiello FM, Brensinger JD, Peterson GM, et al: The use and interpretation of commercial APC gene testing for familial adenomatous polyposis. *N Engl J Med* 1997;336:823-827.
15. Bogardus ST Jr, Holmboe E, Jekel JF: Perils, pitfalls, and possibilities in talking about medical risk. *JAMA* 1999;281:1037-1041.
16. Haber D, Fearon E: The promise of cancer genetics. *Lancet* 1998;351:SII1-SII8.
17. The National Action Plan on Breast Cancer. *NAPBC fact sheet: genetic testing for breast cancer risk: it's your choice,* 1997 National Action Plan on Breast Cancer, U.S. Public Health Service's Office on Women's Health, U.S. Department of Health and Human Services, 200 Independence Avenue SW., Room 718F, Washington, DC 20201. *http://www.napbc.org*
18. Nayfield S: Ethical and scientific consideration for chemoprevention research in cohorts at genetic risk for breast cancer. *J Cell Biochem* 1996;63:123-130.
19. Peters JA: Familial cancer risk: II: breast cancer risk counseling and genetic susceptibility. *Journal of Oncology Management* 1994;14-22.
20. Statement of the American Society of Human Genetics (ASHG) on genetic testing for breast and ovarian cancer predisposition. *Am J Hum Genet* 1994;55:i-iv.
21. Puck SM: Screening for genetic risk of breast cancer. *Am Fam Physician* 1999; 59(1):99-104, 106. Review.
22. Holtzman NA: Primary care physicians as providers of frontline genetic services. *Fetal Diagn Ther* 1993;8:213-219.
23. American College of Medical Genetics: *Standards and guidelines: clinical laboratory genetics.* Bethesda, MD, American College of Medical Genetics, 1993.
24. Hartmann LC, Schaid DJ, Woods JE, et al: Efficacy of bilateral prophylactic mastectomy in women with a family history of breast cancer. *N Engl J Med* 1999;340:77-84.
25. Stephenson J: Study shows mastectomy prevents breast cancer in high-risk women. *JAMA* 1997;277:1421-1422.
26. Nelson NJ: Caution guides genetic testing for hereditary cancer genes. *J Natl Cancer Inst* 1996;88(2):70-72.
27. Whittaker LA: The implications of the human genome project for family practice. *J Fam Pract* 1992;35:294-301.
28. Burke W, Daly M, Garber J, et al: Recommendations for follow-up care of individuals with inherited predisposition to cancer: II: BRCA1 and BRCA2. Cancer Genetics Studies Consortium. *JAMA* 1997;277:997-1003.
29. Burke W, Petersen G, Lynch P, et al: Recommendations for follow-up care of individuals with inherited predisposition to cancer: I: hereditary nonpolyposis colon cancer. Cancer Genetics Studies Consortium. *JAMA* 1997;277:915-919.
30. American Society of Clinical Oncology. Statement of the American Society of Clinical Oncology: genetic testing for cancer susceptibility, adopted on February 20, 1996. *J Clin Oncol* 1996;14:1730-1736.
31. Carter MA: Patient-provider relationship in the context of genetic testing for hereditary cancers. *J Natl Cancer Inst Monographs* 1995;17:119-121.
32. Geller G, Botkin J, Green M: Genetic testing for susceptibility to adult-onset cancer: the process and content of informed consent. *JAMA* 1997;277:1467-1474.
33. American Academy of Pediatrics Committee on Bioethics: Ethical issues with genetic testing in pediatrics. *Pediatrics* 2001;107:1451-1454.
34. Lerman C, Schwartz M, Lin T, et al: The influence of psychological distress on use of genetic testing for cancer risk. *J Consult Clin Psychol* 1997;65:414-420.

35. Baum, A, Friedman A, Zakowski S: Stress and genetic testing for disease risk. *Health Psychol* 1997;16: 8-19.

36. Weber BL: Genetic testing for breast cancer. *Scientific American* 1996;Jan/Feb:12-21.

37. Williams CJ, editor: *Introducing new treatments for cancer, practical, ethical and legal problems.* London, John Wiley and Sons, 1992.

38. Maslin AM: A survey of the opinions on `informed consent' of women currently involved in clinical trials within a breast unit. *Eur J Can* 1994;3: 153-162.

39. National Society of Genetic Counselors (NSGC): Code of ethics. 1992. National Society of Genetic Counselors Executive Office, 233 Canterbury Dr., Wallingford, PA 19086-6617.

40. Johnson KA, Brensinger JD: Genetic counseling and testing: implications for clinical practice. *Clin Genet* 2000;35:615-626.

41. Caplan AL: Neutrality is not morality: the ethics of genetic counseling. In Bartels DM, LeRoy BS, Caplan AL, editors: *Prescribing our future: Ethical challenges in genetic counseling.* New York, Aldine de Gruyter, 1993.

42. van den Boer-van den Berg HMA, Maat-Kievit AA: The whole truth and nothing but the truth, but what is the truth? *J Med Genet* 2001;38: 39-42.

43. Sorenson JR, Swazey JP, Scotch NA, et al: Reproductive pasts, reproductive futures: genetic counseling and its effectiveness. *Birth Defects* 1981;17:1-192.

44. Wertz DC, Sorensen JR, Heeren TC: Client's interpretation of risks provided in genetic counseling. *Am J Hum Genet* 1996;39:253-264.

45. Chase GA, Faden RR, Holtzman NA, et al: Assessment of risk by pregnant women: implications for genetic counseling and education. *Soc Biolog* 1986;33:57-64.

46. Thompson RJ Jr, Gustafson KE, Hamlett KW, et al: Stress, coping, and family functioning in the psychological adjustment of mothers of children and adolescents with cystic fibrosis. *J Pediatr Psychol* 1992;17:573-585.

47. Thompson RJ Jr, Gill KM, Gustafson KE, et al: Stability and change in the psychological adjustment of mothers of children and adolescents with cystic fibrosis and sickle cell disease. *J Pediatr Psychol* 1994;19:171-188.

48. National Society of Genetic Counselors (NSGC): Position statements. 1991. National Society of Genetic Counselors Executive Office, 233 Canterbury Dr., Wallingford, PA 19086-6617.

49. Kelly PT: *Dealing with dilemma: a manual for genetic counselors.* New York, Springer-Verlag, 1977.

50. Bobinski MA: Genetic information, legal, ERISA preemption, and HIPAA protection. In Murray TH, Mehlman MJ: *Encyclopedia of ethical, legal, and policy issues in biotechnology.* New York, John Wiley & Sons, 2000.

51. Associated Press: President acts to bar genetic discrimination. *The New York Times* Feb 29, 2000: F7.

52. Billings PR, Kohn MA, de Curvas M, et al: Discrimination as a consequence of genetic testing. *Am J Hum Genet* 1992;50:476-482.

53. Carson WY: Legal issues associated with genetics. *Clin Genet* 2000;35:719-729.

54. Health Insurance Portability and Accountability Act, Pub. L. No. 104-191. (1996).

55. Rothstein MA: Genetic privacy and confidentiality: why they are so hard to protect *J Law Medicine and Ethics* 1998;26:198-204.

56. Annas GJ: Genetic prophecy and genetic privacy: can we prevent the dream from becoming a nightmare? *Am J Public Health* 1995;85:1196-1197.

57. Peters J: Breast cancer genetics: relevance to oncology genetics. *Cancer Control* 1995;195-208.

58. Suter SM: Whose genes are these anyway?: family conflict over access to genetic information. *Michigan Law Review* 1991;91:1854-1908.

59. Wertz DC: Ethical and legal implications of the new genetics: issues for discussion. *Soc Sci Med* 1992;35:495-499.

60. U.S. President's Commission for the Study of Ethical Problems in Medicine and Biomedical and Behavioral Research: *Screening and counseling for genetic conditions: a report on the ethical implications of genetic screening, counseling, and education programs.* Washington, DC, 1983.

61. Pate v. Threlkel, 661 So.2d 278 (Fla. 1995).

62. Safer v. Pack, 677 A.2d 1188 (N.J. Super. Ct. App. Div. 1996).

63. Carter MA: Ethical framework for care of the chronically ill. *Holistic Nurse Pract* 1993;8:67-77.

64. Murray TH: Introduction: the human genome project and access to health care. In Murray TH, Rothstein MA, Murray RF, editors: *The human genome project and the future of health care.* Indianapolis, Indiana University Press, 1996.

65. Murray TH: Genetics and the moral mission of health insurance. *Hastings Center Report* 1992;22: 12-17.

Complementary Therapies in Cancer Prevention

An Evidence-Based Analysis

Shiraz I. Mishra
Wadie I. Najim
Vivian Dickerson

Modalities and therapies currently called *complementary and alternative medicine (CAM)* have been in practice for centuries. Evidence of their existence can be traced back to Egyptian heliographs, Greek medical texts, and traditional folk practices. The World Health Organization (WHO) estimates that 65% to 80% of the world's population depends on these practices for their health care. During the last decade, interest in and study of CAM practices has gradually increased in the United States. Important factors contributing toward heightened interest include consumer-driven demand for and use of CAM modalities, increased media exposure, easy availability of therapies, and a trend toward a holistic approach to health care. U.S. national surveys indicate that more than 40% of the population has used CAM therapies and sought treatment from alternative medicine practitioners.[1]

Evidence supports use of CAM therapies by a significant proportion of cancer patients. A recent study indicated that between 7% and 64% of cancer patients used CAM therapies[2] and that nearly three fourths of patients have tried more than one therapy. Moreover, approximately 40% of cancer patients did not discuss CAM therapies with their physician.[3] Cancer patients who use CAM therapies are younger, have progressive cancer, and exhibit active coping behavior.[4] The more commonly used CAM modalities by cancer patients include dietary therapies, psychological therapies, prayer, exercise, and spiritual healing.[5] The majority of cancer patients learn about CAM therapies through family, friends, health food store advertisements, and personal research. A survey of health food stores in Hawaii identified 38 different health food products recommended for cancer, including shark cartilage, Essiac, and Maitake mushroom.[6]

Despite the popularity and use of CAM modalities, empirical evidence on their effectiveness for health promotion and treatment, including cancer prevention, is limited. This chapter provides some of the first evidence-based assessments of the use of CAM modalities such as micronutrients (i.e., vitamins, minerals), antioxidants, phytoestrogens, and green tea as chemopreventive agents against cancers of breast, lung, colon, skin, endometrium, and cervix. The efforts of those national institutions that are involved in CAM are described, review methodology is briefly summarized, and the potential anticarcinogenic mechanisms of action of the CAM therapies reviewed are discussed. Lastly, an in-depth analysis of various CAM therapies used as potential cancer chemopreventive agents is provided.

COMPLEMENTARY AND ALTERNATIVE MEDICINE

Over the years there have been several definitions, descriptions, and names given to CAM. In April 1995, a panel established by the former Office of Alternative Medicine (OAM) attempted to avoid confusion by defining CAM as a "broad domain of healing resources that encompasses all health systems, modalities, and practices and their accompanying theories and beliefs, other than those intrinsic to the politically dominant health system of a particular society or culture in a given historical period. CAM includes all such practices and ideas self-defined by their users as preventing or treating illness or promoting health and well-being. Boundaries within CAM and between CAM domains and the dominant health system are not sharp or fixed."[7]

In response to the overwhelming demand from consumers and health care practitioners, the National Institutes of Health established the Office of Alternative Medicine (OAM) in 1992-1993; this organization was later renamed the National Center for Complementary and Alternative Medicine (NCCAM). The OAM's mission was to develop a reliable database, foster research, and develop a clearinghouse for consumers. The NCCAM has accumulated a database with more than 180,000 references, sponsored several studies, and provided grants to establish 13 research centers. The NCCAM has identified more than 360 modalities as CAM. This list is far from exhaustive, and new therapies continue to be identified. By definition, CAM modalities vary by region and country. To help identify these modalities, the NCCAM (http://nccam.nih.gov/) has divided these modalities into five major domains (Table 12-1).

Cancer figures prominently among the priorities of the NCCAM. Three research centers are dedicated to studying the interface between CAM and cancer: the University of Texas, which is currently inactive; the Center for Cancer Complementary Medicine at Johns Hopkins University, which focuses on PC-SPES, soy phytoestrogens, tart cherry, and prayer; and the Specialized Center of Research in Hyperbaric Oxygen Therapy at the University of Pennsylvania, which focuses on angiogenesis, vascular integrity, and cell adhesion. In addition, current NCCAM-sponsored cancer-related studies include those that examine the use of green tea, black cohosh, soy supplements, shark cartilage, and distant healing. NCCAM has recently approved two new concepts for potential study: CAM for end-of-life care and phytoestrogens for breast cancer.

Table 12-1
Classification of Complementary and Alternative Therapies by the National Center for Complementary and Alternative Medicine

System	Modality
Alternative systems of medical practice	Traditional Oriental medicine; ayurveda; homeopathy; naturopathy; Native American practices; acupuncture; Tibetan medicine
Energy therapies	Biofield therapies (qi gong, reiki, etc.); electroacupuncture; magnetic (i.e., pulse fields, magnets, currents); electrostimulation and neuromagnetic devices
Biologic-based therapies	Herbs; nutritional supplements; special diets (i.e., Atkins, Ornish); macrobiotics; orthomolecular (i.e., megavitamins, minerals); biologic therapies (i.e., Laetrile, bee pollen)
Manipulative and body-based methods	Acupressure; chiropractic medicine; massage therapy; osteopathy; therapeutic touch
Mind-body interventions	Meditation; hypnosis; dance/music therapy; art therapy; prayer; mental healing

National Cancer Institute

In October 1998, the National Cancer Institute (NCI) established the Office of Cancer Complementary and Alternative Medicine (OCCAM) (*http://occam.nci.nih.gov*). The OCCAM is organized to support the development of high-quality CAM research. OCCAM does not directly fund research but develops an agenda for NCI-supported CAM cancer research and responds to the general public, health practitioner communities, and research communities on the role of CAM in cancer treatment. There are several NCI-sponsored trials currently under way. One trial at Columbia University examines the Gonzalez/Kelly regimen of proteolytic enzymes and intense nutritional support with the more conventional chemotherapy for pancreatic cancer. A multicenter U.S.-Canadian trial is assessing the effectiveness of shark cartilage versus conventional chemotherapy plus radiation for lung cancer. In addition, there are several studies where the relationship of diet to breast and prostate cancer is being analyzed.

Data from the NCI comprehensive cancer database, the Physician Data Query (PDQ), includes a summary of various CAM therapies. The NCI Cancer Information Services (CIS) interprets and explains research findings clearly and concisely. The publication "Questions and Answers About Complementary and Alternative Medicine in Cancer Treatment" is available on the CIS Web site: *http://cis.nci.nih.gov* or by calling 1-800-4CANCER. Appendix A lists additional CAM resources.

LITERATURE REVIEW METHODOLOGY

For this analysis, a systematic search of the Medline database (1966-2000) and pertinent literature identified in bibliographies of articles was conducted. The primary CAM modalities considered included micronutrients, vitamins, antioxidants, dietary supplements, minerals, Chinese herbs, herbs, Ayurveda, and alternative therapies used in the prevention of cancers of the breast, lung, colon, skin, endometrium, cervix, ovary, vulva, and vagina. Literature specific to diet (i.e., high- or low-fat diet, vegetables) was excluded because this information is reviewed in other chapters. Research was limited to human studies published in English. Randomized controlled trials, controlled trials, observational (case-control studies, and retrospective and prospective cohort studies) epidemiologic studies, systematic reviews, and metaanalysis were included. Few studies outside those centered on gynecologic organs focused solely on women. Hence some information presented in this chapter is gleaned from studies involving mixed genders or males only and so should be interpreted with some caution.

Despite an extensive literature search, study results are concentrated in a few areas. Current research focuses on chemopreventive CAM modalities for cancers of the breast, lung, colon, skin, endometrium, and cervix but not for cancers of the ovary, vulva, and vagina. Furthermore, the CAM therapies studied are primarily limited to vitamins, antioxidants, and occasionally minerals.

There are no published reports (based on human studies) that cover some CAM therapies, such as Maitake mushroom, kombucha tea, several types of herbs, and Chinese herbs that show some promise in experimental studies. The *Maitake mushroom* has been used in tonics, soups, teas or herbal formulas by Asian therapists to promote health. Experimental studies indicate that it has an immune-enhancing effect and inhibits the spread of tumors.[8] *Kombucha tea* is said to enhance and boost the immune system and to fight cancer in the early stages. However, there is no scientific evidence to support its use. In fact, after two reports of acidosis, the Food and Drug Administration (FDA) issued a cautionary warning.[9] Several *herbs* such as

Echinacea, cat's claw, amygdalin (Laetrile), Essiac, ginseng, HANSI, Hoxsey, mistletoe, sily-marin, turmeric, pycnogenols, shark cartilage, Coley's toxin, and immuno-augmentative ther-apy are marketed for their cancer-fighting and immune-enhancing abilities. Their use for can-cer prevention in humans remains scientifically unproved. Studies on *Chinese herbs* have focused mainly on their use as an adjuvant in the treatment of advanced cancer.

POTENTIAL ANTICARCINOGENIC ACTION OF CAM THERAPIES

In this section, the CAM therapies reviewed for their potential anticarcinogenic effects are briefly described. These therapies include vitamin A (i.e., retinol and its analogs, synthetic retinamides, carotenoids), vitamins C (ascorbic acid) and E (tocopherol), selenium, plant sterols, allium compounds and limonene, phytoestrogens, and green tea. Many of these agents are most active during early (premalignant) stages of carcinogenesis.[10]

Vitamin A, β-Carotene, Retinoids

Vitamin A includes two different families of dietary factors: a) retinyl esters, retinol, and reti-nal (preformed vitamin A); and b) β-carotene and other carotenoids (provitamin A), which serve as precursors to vitamin A.[11] The seven predominant carotenoids in humans are β-carotene, lycopene, lutein, α-carotene, α-cryptoxanthin, β-cryptoxanthin, and zeaxanthin. Retinamides are a new class of synthetic retinoids.[12]

The chemopreventive effects of vitamin A may result from antioxidant properties, inhi-bition of cell proliferation and differentiation, modulation of cytochrome P450 and immune function, inhibition of arachidonic acid metabolism and chromosome instability and damage, induction of gap junction communication, and apoptosis.[11-13] The chemopre-ventive effects of β-carotene may be independent of its provitamin A activity. N-(4-hydrox-yphenyl)retinamide (4-HPR) or fenretinide (a synthetic derivative of all-*trans*-retinoic acid), which has cell differentiation and cytostatic effects, may not mediate its effects via the retinoid receptors[14] but may selectively induce apoptosis rather than cell differentiation.

Vitamins C and E

Vitamin C (ascorbic acid) has broad biologic functions and plays an important role as an antioxidant and free radical scavenger.[15] Vitamin E, a major lipid-soluble antioxidant, includes two groups of compound—tocopherols and tocotrienols—that are present in vari-ous foods such as polyunsaturated vegetable oils, cereal seeds, and palm oil.

Selenium

Humans ingest organic forms of selenium especially as selenomethionine in cereals, grains, and vegetables. The anticarcinogenic effects of selenium are still unclear and may include its function as a cofactor for antioxidant enzymes (such as glutathione peroxidases), inducer of apoptosis, and as an inhibitor of cell growth and synthesis of proteins.[16]

Phytoestrogens

Phytoestrogens (isoflavonoids and lignans) form part of our diet as constituents of soybean products (mainly isoflavonoids including genistein and daidzein) and whole grain cereals, seeds, berries, and nuts (mainly lignans).[17] They may play a significant inhibitory role during the initiation and promotional phases of cancer development.[18] Ingested phytoestro-gens (isoflavonoids) are converted into hormone-like compounds, which exhibit mixed weak estrogen agonist or antagonist properties and antioxidative activity. Some of the other potential biologic cancer-protective effects of phytoestrogens, especially isoflavone genistein, include antioxidant activity, stimulation of the synthesis of sex hormone–binding globulin (SHBG), and inhibition of angiogenesis, tyrosine kinase, DNA repair enzymes, and signal transduction enzymes.[17,18]

Green Tea

Tea leaf (Camellia sinesis plant) extracts may have potential antimutagenic, antioxidant, and anticarcinogenic properties.[15] Extracts from dried tea leaves contain 25% to 40% of naturally occurring phenolic compounds (polyphenols), including flavonoids such as flavan-3-ols (i.e., flavanols including (+)-catechin and epigallocatechin 3-gallate [EGCG]), flavonol glycosides (quercetin and kaempferol), tannins, and phenolic acids.[15] In black tea, most of the catechins are oxidized to thearubigens and theaflavins. EGCG is the most prevalent catechin found in green tea. Green tea extract polyphenols have a number of biochemical immunomodulatory and antitumor actions and also inhibit platelet aggregation.[15]

Miscellaneous Therapies

The *shiitake mushroom* is regarded traditionally as anticarcinogenic, with studies focusing on lentinan (a polysaccharide component) as an adjuvant to chemotherapy.[19] *Garlic* is promoted for several medical problems, and experimental studies have indicated a potential anticancer effect.[20,21] *Olive oil*, because of its high content of vitamin E, squalene, and antioxidant, is believed to have anticarcinogenic activity.[22] *Monoterpenes*, found in many fruits, vegetables, and herbs, show anticarcinogenic effects in experimental studies,[23] although the exact mechanism is unclear. *Melatonin's* anticarcinogenic effects may be cause by its antioxidant activity, glutathione peroxidase stimulation, antiestrogenic activity, or the augmentation of the anticancer effects of interleukin-2. *Vitamin D*, through its hormonal form 1,25-dihydroxyvitamin D_3 $(1,25(OH)_2D_3)$ or calcitriol, regulates the growth and differentiation of a number of cancer cells, including breast cancer cells.[24] *Vitamin B_{12}* deficiency may induce carcinogenesis through an increase in the DNA strand break and an alteration of DNA methylation by the methyl folate trap.[25] *Folate* plays a key role in DNA synthesis, repair, and methylation, and folate deficiency in normal epithelial tissue may predispose it to carcinogenesis.[26]

BREAST CANCER

Several CAM therapies have been assessed for their breast cancer chemopreventive effects. The therapies to be reviewed include vitamins, selenium, phytoestrogens, green tea, and miscellaneous dietary constituents.

Vitamin A, β-Carotene, Retinoids

Interest in the breast cancer chemopreventive effects of vitamin A has focused on both synthetic vitamin analogs and natural compounds. The synthetic agents used in clinical trials include retinyl palmitate, 4-HPR, arotinoids, and etretinate. Most of the clinical studies involve the natural retinoids, retinol (vitamin A), tretinoin or all-*trans*-retinoic acid (t-RA), isotretinoin or 13-*cis*-retinoic acid (13-*cis*-RA), 9-*cis*-retinoic acid (9-*cis*-RA), and the retinoid-related molecule β-carotene, which is metabolized to retinol.

Synthetic Retinoid Fenretinide

Animal model studies indicate that retinoids such as fenretinide or 4-HPR show the most promise as chemopreventive agents.[23] Phase III clinical trials are currently under way to determine the effectiveness of fenretinide in cancer prevention. One trial evaluates the chemopreventive activity of a combination of tamoxifen and 4-HPR to prevent contralateral breast cancer among patients surgically treated for stage I-II breast cancer.[27] Another trial evaluates the effectiveness of 4-HPR in preventing contralateral primary tumors in women pretreated for breast cancer.[28,29] Preliminary results from this trial suggest that fenretinide treatment for 5 years did not have a significant effect on the incidence of contralateral or ipsilateral second breast malignancies,[30] although significant results were observed in the incidence of second breast malignancies based on menopausal status. The findings indicate that, compared with postmenopausal women, premenopausal women treated with fenretinide had a reduced incidence of contralateral breast cancer and ipsilateral breast cancer reappearance.[30]

Vitamin A or Precursors

The epidemiologic evidence for the breast cancer chemopreventive effects of vitamin A (or its precursors) is unclear. The vast majority of epidemiologic studies indicate that the risk of cancer in several target tissues is reduced in groups with a relatively high intake of carotenoids. However, in populations whose vitamin A status is not deficient, increases in vitamin A and carotene intake are not well correlated with increases in serum vitamin A.

In a recent review of the literature on dietary carotenoids and breast cancer risk, Cooper and associates[31] reiterated conclusions reached by Clavel-Chapelon and associates[32] that the majority of epidemiologic studies do not show statistically significant reductions in risk with β-carotene and that the evidence is conflicting. In the 10 case-control studies reviewed by Cooper and associates, six studies provided evidence for a protective effect of carotenoids (measured as dietary intake, serum levels, or adipose carotenoid levels) on breast cancer, and four studies showed no association. In addition, none of the three cohort studies reviewed by Cooper and associates provided evidence for an inverse association between breast cancer risk and carotenoid levels.

Metaanalyses of epidemiologic studies, however, provide conclusions different from those just presented. For instance, based on a metaanalysis of 11 studies, Gandini and associates[33] reported a significant protective effect for breast cancer resulting from a higher intake of β-carotene (relative risk [RR] of high consumption [7000 μg/day or more] compared with low consumption [1000 μg/day or less] = 0.82, 95% CI = 0.76-0.91). Similarly, Howe and associates,[34] based on a metaanalysis of 12 case-control studies of diet and breast cancer, reported some significant associations between intake of vitamin A and carotenoids and breast cancer risk, based on a metaanalysis of 12 case-control studies of diet and breast cancer. In the studies reviewed, vitamin A, β-carotene, and retinol intake were estimated from dietary history. There were statistically significant inverse associations between intake of vitamin A (RR 0.87, p = .04, comparing highest vs. lowest quintile of intake) and β-carotene (RR 0.85, p = .007, comparing highest vs. lowest quintile of intake) and breast cancer risk; however, the relationship between retinol intake and breast cancer risk was not significant. The inverse associations between breast cancer risk and intake of vitamin A and β-carotene were also significant among postmenopausal women, but the interactions between intake and menopausal status were not significant. Furthermore, when the effects of vitamin A and β-carotene on breast cancer risk were simultaneously compared, the effects were essentially significant for β-carotene.

Results from some studies not covered by the works of Gandini and associates, Howe and associates, and Cooper and associates also confirm the conflicting results. Jumaan and associates[35] reported that high consumption of β-carotene was associated with a lower risk of breast cancer. Furthermore, there was no evidence to suggest a critical time period when diets rich in β-carotene are more effective for cancer prevention. However, other studies reported no breast cancer chemopreventive association with serum β-carotene levels,[36] low carotene intake, low serum retinol levels,[37] carotenoids, and vitamin A.[38]

Vitamin C

Epidemiologic studies provide conflicting reports on the cancer preventive role of vitamin C. Gandini and associates,[33] based on a metaanalysis of eight studies, reported a significant protective effect for breast cancer because of higher intake of vitamin C (RR of high consumption [400 mg/day or more], compared with low consumption [50 mg/day or less] = 0.80, 95% CI = 0.68-0.95). Howe and associates,[34] based on a metaanalysis of 12 case-control studies on diet and breast cancer risk, reported a statistically significant inverse association between intake of vitamin C and breast cancer risk (RR 0.69, $p < .0001$, comparing highest vs. lowest quintile of intake). Vitamin C intake was estimated based on dietary history. Moreover, in multivariate models that included vitamin A, β-carotene, and vitamin C, the relative risk for breast cancer was only significant for vitamin C (RR 0.73, $p = .03$, comparing highest vs. lowest quintile of intake). Other epidemiologic studies, however, have found no inverse associations between breast cancer risk and higher intake of vitamin C from dietary sources[38-40] or supplements.[39] One study reported an increased breast cancer risk associated with higher levels of vitamin C supplemental intake.[41]

Vitamin E

A recent comprehensive review[42] of epidemiologic studies on the association between breast cancer risk and vitamin E intake provides mixed evidence. The review included seven retrospective case-control studies and three prospective studies, which assessed vitamin E intake based on either diet histories or food frequency questionnaires. In three of the seven case-control studies reviewed, there were statistically significant inverse associations between vitamin E intake (comparing highest quintile intake versus lowest quintile intake) and breast cancer risk. None of the prospective epidemiologic studies found an association between dietary vitamin E intake and breast cancer risk.

Epidemiologic studies that have examined the association between serum α-tocopherol levels and breast cancer also provide conflicting results. In three case-control studies reviewed by Kimmick and associates,[42] only one study reported increased odds of breast cancer risk with increasing levels of plasma vitamin E (comparing highest quintile versus lowest quintile of serum α-tocopherol levels), with the other two case-control studies reporting nonsignificant findings. Furthermore, only one of the five prospective studies reviewed by Kimmick and associates reported a significant inverse association between breast cancer risk and plasma levels of vitamin E. The other prospective studies had nonsignificant, mixed results on the relationship. Two studies not reviewed by Kimmick and associates suggest opposing effects of vitamin E on breast cancer risk. Negri and associates[40] reported a significant inverse association between vitamin E intake and breast cancer risk, whereas Potischman and associates[38] found no association between a reduction in risk of early-stage breast cancer and intake of dietary constituents such as vitamin E.

Vitamin D

Evidence from ecological studies indicates that breast cancer death rates in the United States are highest in regions (i.e., the northeast compared with Hawaii and the southwest) where ultraviolet B radiation levels and air pollution levels allow for decreased synthesis of vitamin D.[43] In addition, results from the National Health and Examination Survey (NHANES)

I Epidemiologic Follow-up Study (a national prospective cohort study) suggest a reduced breast cancer risk for women who lived in regions of high solar radiation and had moderate to considerable exposure to sunlight or had higher (≥200 IU versus <100 IU) dietary intake of vitamin D (relative risks ranged from 0.35 to 0.75).[44] The study had a small sample of breast cancer patients (n = 190) in a cohort of 5009 White women.

Vitamin B$_{12}$

Very little data exist on the association between vitamin B$_{12}$ and breast cancer risk. Evidence from a case-control study[45] suggests an increased breast cancer risk among postmenopausal women who had serum levels of vitamin B$_{12}$ in the lowest quintile, compared with women in the higher quintiles.

Folate

The little evidence on the association between folate levels and breast cancer risk is mixed. Evidence from a prospective cohort study (the Nurses' Health Study) among 88,818 women (3483 breast cancer cases) suggests that among women who consume at least 15 g/day of alcohol, a higher intake of folate (at least 600 μg/day) compared with lower intake (150-299 μg/day) was significantly associated with lower relative risk (RR 0.55, 95% CI 0.39-0.76) of breast cancer (p for trend = .001).[46] Furthermore, the study found no direct association between total folate intake and risk of breast cancer among the whole cohort or among premenopausal women but found a weak inverse association among postmenopausal women (p for trend = .02). A case-control study[38] found no association between a reduction in risk of early-stage breast cancer and folate intake.

Selenium

Epidemiologic studies provide conflicting results on the association between selenium levels and cancer incidence. Many case-control studies have reported no association between selenium levels and breast cancer incidence[47-49] or an increased site-specific risk for breast cancer.[50] Cohort studies on the relationship between selenium and breast cancer have not provided any significant positive results.[48,49,51-59]

Melatonin

Studies on melatonin in human breast cancer provide some promising results. For instance, lower levels of melatonin are reported in women with estrogen-receptor positive (ER-positive) breast tumor[60] and postmenopausal women with advanced breast cancer.[61]

Phytoestrogens

Both experimental[17,18] and observational studies (Table 12-2) provide some evidence for a cancer-protective role for phytoestrogens. Several studies[62-65] report a significantly decreased risk among premenopausal women for breast cancer associated with a high intake of soy products. One study[66] found no association between intake of soy foods and breast cancer risk. The study, however, reported a significant decrease in breast cancer associated with higher intake of foods rich in fiber. Fiber is an important source of lignans. There was no evidence for a significant protective effect of higher phytoestrogen intake on breast cancer risk among postmenopausal women.

There have been a few reports of negative effects of soy supplements. For instance, Petrakis and associates,[67] based on a pilot study on 24 women, reported that prolonged consumption (over 6 months) of soy protein isolate containing 38 mg of genistein had a

Table 12-2
Case-Control Studies on Soy Intake and Breast Cancer Risk

Study	Sample	Assessment	Main Outcome	Remarks
Lee et al[62]	200 cases and 420 controls aged 24 or older	Diet history	In premenopausal women, protective effect on breast cancer risk with higher intake of soy protein and soy products	No significant effects seen in postmenopausal women
Hirose et al[63]	1052 cases and 21,295 controls aged 20 or older	Diet history	In premenopausal women, protective effect on breast cancer risk with higher intake of bean curd	No significant effects seen in postmenopausal women
Yuan et al[66]	834 cases and 834 controls aged 20-69 years	Diet history	No significant effects of soy foods intake on breast cancer risk	
Wu et al[65]	597 cases and 966 controls aged 30-55 years	Diet history	In premenopausal women, protective effect on breast cancer risk with higher tofu intake	In postmenopausal women, a nonsignificant protective effect of higher intake of tofu was observed
Ingram et al[64]	144 cases and 144 controls aged 30-84 years	Diet history	Protective effect on breast cancer risk with an increased excretion of phytoestrogens (equol and enterolactone)	

stimulatory effect on the premenopausal female breast. The stimulatory effect included increases in breast fluid secretion, hyperplastic epithelial cells, and plasma estradiol levels.

Green Tea

A few studies have explored the cancer chemopreventive effects of tea (green or black). A prospective cohort study (without historical controls), among 8552 Japanese men and women aged 40 or older, reported that higher consumption of green tea (>9 cups/day) was associated with a significant slowdown in the increase of cancer incidence with age in females; a later onset of cancer; and a significant reduction of relative risk of cancer incidence among females (after adjusting for lifestyle factors).[68] Another prospective cohort study[69] reported that increased consumption (≥5 cups/day versus ≤4 cups/day) of green tea before clinical onset of breast cancer was significantly associated with improved prognosis of stage I and II breast cancer (i.e., decreased number of axillary lymph node metastasis with stage I and II breast cancer among premenopausal patients). The study also reported lower recurrence rate at follow-up among women who consumed greater quantities of green tea before the clinical onset of cancer. However, one prospective cohort study[70] among 3500 men and women followed over a period of 4.3 years reported no protective effect of black tea consumption on cancer risk, especially when the analyses controlled for potential confounders for the specific cancers.

Dietary Mixtures, Olive Oil, Monoterpenes

Humans studies have not corroborated the experimental findings[23] that dietary mixtures of plant origin such as cabbage, cauliflower, Brussels sprouts, broccoli, garlic, orange oil, seaweed, and rosemary extracts may inhibit the development of chemically induced breast cancer. A case-control study based on 469 breast cancer cases identified in the Netherlands Cohort Study and 1713 randomly selected female controls from the cohort reported that intake of onion, leeks, and garlic supplement was not associated with breast cancer risk. The relative risk (RR) for highest versus lowest intake categories were: 0.95, 95% CI 0.61-1.47 (for onion intake), 1.08, 95% CI 0.79-1.48 (for leeks), and 0.87, 95% CI 0.58-1.31 (for garlic supplement use).[71]

Epidemiologic studies have provided conflicting results of the cancer chemopreventive effects of olive oil. Some studies suggest that olive oil has an inverse association with breast cancer risk.[72-74] However, other studies have found no significant relationship between breast cancer risk and consumption of olive oil.[75] No clinical trials have examined the effects of olive oil as a cancer chemopreventive agent.

Monoterpenes' anticarcinogenic activity has been reported in chemically induced and spontaneous mammary tumors in animal models.[23] Human Phase I clinical trials are currently under way.[76]

Summary

Some CAM therapies such as vitamin A analogs, vitamin C, and phytoestrogens may have a chemopreventive effect on breast cancer risk. Vitamin E is unlikely to have a chemopreventive effect on breast cancer risk. Preliminary evidence of the effects of vitamin D, vitamin B_{12}, folate, melatonin, and dietary mixtures (including olive oil and monoterpenes) is intriguing. Dietary carotenoids (particularly β-carotene) may have a weak protective effect against breast cancer risk. However, it is unclear whether the breast cancer chemoprotective effect is due to a specific carotenoid or the effects of another agent found in carotenoid-rich food. Moreover, the inconsistent results on the association between dietary carotenoids (particularly β-carotene) and breast cancer risk may be due to limitations inherent in case-control studies (discussed elsewhere). However, the evidence for all the aforementioned studies is far from conclusive and warrants further investigation. Long-term prospective cohort studies and clinical trials to determine the link between these therapies and breast cancer risk are needed.

Evidence for a chemopreventive role for selenium and green tea is mixed. The conflicting findings about the association between selenium levels and cancer incidence may, in part, be due to limitations in the accurate assessment of selenium intake; measurements of biomarkers of exposure to selenium; lack of due consideration to confounders such as smoking and dietary factors; the biologic availability of selenium, which may be modified in the presence of trace elements; and the effect of preclinical disease on selenium levels.[16] For green tea, further research is needed to understand the biochemical and mechanistic effects of green tea constituents. In addition, there is a need to understand dose-response relationships, synergistic effects of green tea with other dietary constituents, length of consumption for protective effects, and differential effects between green and black tea consumption.

LUNG CANCER

A few CAM therapies have been examined for their chemopreventive role in lung cancer. These therapies include vitamins (A, C, E), minerals (i.e., selenium), melatonin, and dietary mixtures.

Vitamin A, β-Carotene, Retinoids

Initial animal and epidemiologic data suggested a protective effect of vitamin A and β-carotene on lung cancer.[77,78] Some of the earlier epidemiologic studies tried to distinguish the effect of vitamin A or carotenoids on lung cancer based on gender. Two studies found similar protective effects in both genders, [79,80] whereas other studies found a protective effect in men and an adverse effect in women.[81,82]

Several studies have evaluated the effects of β-carotene on lung cancer risk, with β-carotene levels estimated either through dietary intake of fruits and vegetables, serum or plasma β-carotene level, or use of supplements. Studies that estimated β-carotene levels based on the intake of vegetables and fruits have reported reduced lung cancer risk associated with higher intake of vegetables and fruits, an association that is stronger in case-control studies than in cohort studies.[83] Moreover, the association was stronger for vegetable and fruit intake than for β-carotene levels.

The inverse relationship between lung cancer risk and vegetable and fruit intake is not observed in studies that explored the effects of β-carotene on lung cancer risk. For instance, several prospective studies have reported nonsignificant associations between dietary β-carotene intake and lung cancer risk.[84-87] Furthermore, studies that reported lower prediagnostic plasma or serum β-carotene levels in subjects who subsequently developed lung cancer[87-90] are limited by potential confounding factors (i.e., single measurement of β-carotene level taken several years before the onset of cancer).

Multicenter double-blind controlled trials have also explored the possible role of β-carotene on lung cancer risk (Table 12-3). Two trials, the Alpha Tocopherol and Beta-Carotene Cancer Prevention study (ATBC) and the Beta-Carotene and Retinol Efficacy Trial (CARET), indicated a higher incidence of lung cancer among the group that received β-carotene supplementation.[91-93] The higher incidence of lung cancer was noted among current smokers, especially the heavy smokers (>20 cigarettes/day). In addition, above-average alcohol consumption was also noted to be a predisposing factor. The Physicians' Health Study (PHS)[94] did not report any association between β-carotene and lung cancer risk. The finding may be more a function of the low number of smokers (11%) in the trial.

The relationship between other carotenoids and lung cancer risk is unclear. Some studies suggest an inverse association between lung cancer and dietary intake of lutein and α-carotene. Prospective studies, however, report no association between lutein, α-carotene, and lycopene intake levels and lung cancer.[87,95]

Table 12-3
Results of Randomized Double-Blind Placebo Controlled Studies of β-Carotene Supplementation and Lung Cancer Risk

Study	Sample	Intervention	Main Outcome	Remarks
Albanes et al[91]	29,133 male smokers	a) α-tocophero 50 mg b) β-carotene 20 mg c) a + b d) placebo	Increased lung cancer risk in the group receiving β-carotene	Risk of lung cancer is greater in β-carotene group reporting above median alcohol use
Omenn et al[92,93]	18,314 men and women at high risk	a) β-carotene and retinol b) placebo	Increased lung cancer risk in the group receiving β-carotene	Risk increased among current smokers (≥ 20 cigarettes/day) and high alcohol users
Hennekens et al[94]	22,071 male physicians	a) β-carotene 50 mg b) placebo	No change in lung cancer risk	Relatively few smokers in the sample

Vitamin E

Evidence on the association between vitamin E (dietary intake of α-tocopherol) and lung cancer risk is inconsistent.[84-86] In addition, the ATBC trial[91] reported no protective effect against lung cancer among subjects who received α-tocopherol (50 mg/day). Furthermore, except for one study that reported an inverse association, most cohort studies have reported no association between lung cancer risk and serum concentration of α-tocopherol.[77]

Vitamin C

Limited data exists on the association between vitamin C and lung cancer risk. Among the prospective studies that have examined the effects of dietary vitamin C and lung cancer risk, some studies have reported no associations[80,87] whereas several more recent studies have indicated an inverse association.[84-86]

Selenium

Several epidemiologic and prospective randomized studies have evaluated the impact of selenium on the risk of lung cancer. Evidence from case-control studies (Table 12-4)[90,96-99] on the association between selenium levels and lung cancer risk are controversial, with some studies reporting an inverse relationship[55,96,97] and others reporting a direct relationship.[90,98] Findings from randomized studies (Table 12-5)[100,101] suggest a protective effect of selenium supplementation on lung cancer prevention.

Table 12-4
Results of Cohort Studies on the Relation between Selenium (Se) Levels and Lung Cancer Risk

Study	Sample	Assessment	Main Outcome	Remarks
Knekt et al[97]	95 cases and 190 controls	Serum Se level	Protective effect with higher serum level	Inverse association with current smokers but not among non-smokers
van den Brandt et al[96]	370 cases	Toenail Se level	Protective effect associated with higher level	Effect was not restricted to men Smoking was inversely related to toenail Se level
Menkes et al[90]	99 cases and 196 controls	Serum Se level	Positive association with lung cancer risk	
Nomura et al[99]	71 cases and controls	Serum Se level	No significant association with lung cancer risk	
Knekt et al[55]	189 cases and controls	Serum Se level	Protective effect on lung cancer risk among men	Slightly elevated risk in women and only at very low Se levels
Koo et al[98]	88 cases and 137 controls	Diet history	Direct relationship between Se intake and lung cancer risk	Results were more significant for fresh foods and adenocarcinoma or large cell cancer

Table 12-5
Results of Double-Blind Studies on the Relation between Selenium (Se) Supplementation and Lung Cancer Risk

Study	Design	Sample	Intervention	Main Outcome	Remarks
Yu et al[100]	CT	40 cases	300 μg Se	Increased glutathione peroxidase activity, and protected DNA repair capacity	
Clark et al[51]	CT	17 cases and 31 controls	200 μg Se (0.5 g brewer's yeast tablets)	Fewer lung cancers in the intervention group	A decrease in lung cancer mortality in the Se-supplemented group
Blot et al[101]	RCT	32 cases	50 μg Se (yeast) + β-carotene + α-tocopherol	Protective effect and reduced total mortality	

CT = clinical trial; RCT = randomized clinical trial.

Melatonin

The role of melatonin for the prevention of lung cancer is still to be determined. In one study, melatonin (10 mg/day) administered to patients with metastatic non–small cell lung cancer showed an increased 1-year survival and disease stabilization.[102,103]

Dietary Mixtures

The effects of diet on lung cancer are discussed in more detail elsewhere. We focus here on the effect of certain dietary foods considered as dietary supplements, such as onions, leeks, garlic, and tea (green and black). A cohort study found no evidence relating the consumption of onions, leeks, or garlic to the risk of lung cancer.[104] In addition, an observational study reported no protective effect of black tea consumption on lung cancer risk.[70]

Summary

The evidence reviewed earlier suggests that, except for selenium, most CAM therapies do not have a chemopreventive role for lung cancer. The evidence suggests that selenium may have a positive impact on lung cancer risk. However, despite these encouraging reports, questions regarding the use of selenium supplements still remain, especially in terms of the effective dose, the population it protects (smokers vs. nonsmokers, those with low levels vs. normal levels of selenium), and the length of time needed to achieve the protective effect. For vitamin A, the current evidence does not support a role for β-carotene alone in preventing lung cancer. In fact, β-carotene supplement seems to have an adverse effect, particularly among smokers and heavy alcohol users. The evidence suggests no association between vitamin E and lung cancer risk, and for vitamin C the result is mixed. Very few studies have been conducted to explore the of effects melatonin and dietary mixtures on lung cancer risk. Overall, there is a need for controlled randomized studies, especially to evaluate the effects of vitamin C, melatonin, dietary mixture, and green tea for lung cancer prevention.

COLON CANCER

CAM therapies studied as potential chemopreventive agents for colon cancer include vitamins, selenium, dietary mixtures (including garlic and fish oil), green tea, Panax ginseng, shiitake mushroom, and hydro-colon therapy. Diet, calcium, and vitamin D have also been studied extensively and are reviewed elsewhere.

Vitamins C, E, A, Carotenoids

Evidence from randomized controlled trials looking at associations between single or multiple vitamins and the treatment or prevention of colon cancer is mixed. One study that investigated at urinary excretion of N-nitroso compounds in 25 healthy women receiving vitamin C (250 mg or 1 g) or green tea (4 or 8 cups) found a protective effect of vitamin C and moderate amounts (4 cups/day) of green tea consumption.[105] Furthermore, results are encouraging for subjects with familial polyposis coli who use vitamin C. However, trials looking at the recurrence of adenomas conveyed mixed results. Vitamin A and E yielded mixed results for primary or secondary prevention of adenomas. One study showed an increased risk for bleeding adenomas in patients who received Vitamin E.[106] In addition, evidence from several trials suggests that high doses of vitamin A, C, E, and β-carotene supplementation do not reduce the risk of adenocarcinoma of the colon and rectum.[107] However, a WHO consensus statement on the role of nutrition in colorectal cancer, based on review of epidemiologic studies, indicated that low intake of certain vitamins may increase cancer risk (Table 12-6).[108-116]

Folate

Current evidence suggests that folate levels may influence colon cancer risk. For instance, evidence from case-control studies suggests that low folate intake is associated with higher risk

Table 12-6
Results from Randomized Controlled Trials on Vitamins and Colon Cancer Risk

Study	Sample	Intervention	Main Outcome
Bussey et al[108]	49 familial polyposis coli cases	vitamin C 3 g/day	Decreased polyp size
Moertel et al[109]	100 advanced colorectal cancer cases	vitamin C 10 g	No objective improvement
DeCosse et al[110]	58 familial polyposis coli cases	vitamin C 4 g + vitamin E 400 mg + grain fiber 22.5 g	Dietary grain fiber has a benefit on bowel neoplasm
Paganelli et al[111]	41 cases with history of adenoma	vitamin A 30,000 IU, vitamin C 1 g, vitamin E 70 mg	Decreased thymidine index
Roncucci et al[112]	209 cases with history of adenoma	vitamin A 30,000 IU, vitamin C 1 g, vitamin E 70 mg	Decreased recurrence of adenomas
Greenberg et al[113]	751 cases with history of adenoma	vitamin C 1 g, β-carotene 25 mg, vitamin E 400 mg	No reduction in adenoma risk
McKeown-Eyssen et al[114]	185 cases with history of adenoma	vitamin C 400 mg, vitamin E 400 mg	No significant effect
Malila et al[106]	146 male smokers	α-tocopherol 50 mg, β-carotene 20 mg	α-tocopherol increased risk and β-carotene had no effect
Cascinu et al[115]	Resected Duke stage B-C	vitamin A, C, and E	No reduction in cell kinetics of colon epithelium
Albanes et al[116]	135 male smokers	α-tocopherol 50 mg, β-carotene 20 mg	No beneficial effect of β-carotene and α-tocopherol on incidence

of colon cancer.[117,118] A similar association was observed between plasma folate levels and colon cancer risk in the Physicians' Health Study.[119] Furthermore, results from a prospective cohort study among 442 women recently diagnosed with colon cancer suggested that long-term use and higher total intake of folate (>400 µg/day) in a multivitamin may reduce the risk of colon cancer. [120] The association was stronger with supplemental folate than with dietary sources. A possible variable in interpreting this study is the potential role of other vitamins in the prevention of colon cancer.

Selenium

The evidence for an association between selenium levels and colorectal cancer is mixed. For instance, an Italian study reported low selenium levels associated with higher prevalence of cancer.[121] Another study reported an inverse association between toenail selenium (reflects long-term dietary selenium intake) and the risk of colon cancer for both genders, with the association persisting when women were analyzed as a separate group.[122] Other studies, however, have reported little or no association between serum selenium levels and colorectal cancer.[55,99] Moreover, a WHO consensus statement concluded that evidence was inconclusive for the use of minerals (selenium, zinc, molybdenum, and calcium) for the prevention or treatment of colon cancer.[107]

A randomized, double-blind placebo-controlled study examined whether selenium supplementation (200 µg as 0.5-g brewer's yeast tablet) can reduce risk of nonmelanoma skin cancer. The study reported no statistically significant differences in the occurrence of skin cancer between the two groups. However, the study reported that, compared with the placebo group, the treatment group had lower incidence of total cancer (39% lower) and of colorectal cancer (64% lower).[123]

Green Tea

Evidence for a chemoprotective role of green tea consumption on colon cancer is mixed. One observational study reported a protective effect of higher green tea (i.e, 10 cups of tea/day) on colon cancer risk.[68] However, a review of human studies on the role of green tea in cancer prevention reported mixed results for colon and rectal cancer (colon: inverse association in 3 of 5 studies, positive association in 1 of 5 studies; rectal: inverse association in 1 of 4 studies; positive association in 2 of 4 studies).[124]

Diet, Dietary Mixtures, Garlic, Fish Oil

There is clear evidence that diet plays a major role in the development of colon cancer. Studies indicate that vegetables, dietary fiber, and calcium may have a protective effect; however, a review of epidemiologic data remains controversial. Recent studies have looked at the Mediterranean diet (high in vegetables and fruits) as having a DNA adduct effect and possible role in cancer prevention. More detailed discussion of diet, calcium, and vitamin D is detailed elsewhere.

A large cohort study in the Netherlands failed to support an association between dietary use of onions, leeks, or garlic supplements and the incidence of male or female colorectal cancer.[125] The Iowa Women's Health Study, however, found that consumption of dietary garlic reduced the risk of colon cancer.[126] Metaanalyses of epidemiologic studies indicate that raw garlic might be associated with a protective effect against stomach and colorectal cancer; however, this may not hold true for garlic supplements.[127] Raw garlic's potential anticarcinogenic effect is affected by the method by which it is processed (i.e., length of heating, crushing).[128]

Animal studies suggest that ω-6 fatty acids induce colon cancer, whereas ω-3 fatty acids (eicosapentaenoic acid [EPA] and docosahexaenoic acid [DHA]) found in fish oils have an inhibitory effect.[129-132] Epidemiologic studies have confirmed a possible inhibitory effect of fish oil on the development of colon cancer.[133] In a double-blind clinical trial, 60 patients (34 men, 26 women) with a history of sporadic adenomatous colorectal polyps were randomly assigned to three different doses of fish oil and placebo for 30 days. Biopsy specimens of rectal epithelium were collected before and after the intervention to assess cell proliferation. Statistically significant inhibitory effect on rectal epithelial proliferation was found in subjects with elevated baseline values.[134] The onset of changes could be detected as early as 15 days after initiation of treatment and are maintained with long-term supplementation. In one study, ω-3 fatty acids in small doses (1.4 g EPA and 1.1 g DHA) seemed to improve rectal epithelial cell proliferation in subjects at high risk for colon cancer.

Panax Ginseng

Animal and observational studies of ginseng indicate a possible cancer prevention role. The effect is thought to be dose dependent.[135] In a case-control study, subjects who received Panax ginseng had lower (50% less) risk of developing cancer than the control group (odds ratio for colorectal cancer = 0.42).[136]

Shiitake Mushroom

There is scant information on the chemopreventive role of shiitake mushroom in colon cancer prevention. One randomized trial[137] of 166 subjects with gastric and colorectal cancer indicated a longer survival in subjects who received lentinan (a polysaccharide component in shiitake mushroom); the results, however, did not reach statistical significance.

Hydro-Colon Therapy (High Enema)

Hydro-colon therapy is commonly used for cleansing the colon and detoxifying the body with water or coffee. The therapy is often promoted for general health and prevention of disease. The FDA has not approved the colon irrigation machines for general use. There is no scientific evidence to support the use of hydro-colon therapy in the prevention or treatment of colon cancer.[138,139]

Summary

Evidence reviewed earlier suggests that folates may play a positive role in colon cancer chemoprevention. Evidence for the role of vitamins C, E, and A; carotenoids; and selenium is inconclusive. Preliminary evidence of the chemopreventive effects on colon cancer of garlic and fish oil is promising. Larger clinical trials are needed to examine the optimal dosage, onset of treatment, and clinical implications. In addition, there is inadequate research on the chemopreventive role of green tea, Panax ginseng, and shiitake mushroom. Lastly, there is no scientific evidence to support the use of hydro-colon therapy in the prevention or treatment of colon cancer.

SKIN CANCER

Several CAM therapies—including antioxidant vitamins, essential minerals, ayurvedic compounds, and mind-body interventions—have been studied as potential chemopreventive agents for skin cancer. Table 12-7 summarizes findings from randomized controlled trials and epidemiologic (case-control) studies.

Table 12-7
Findings from Randomized Controlled Trials and Epidemiologic Studies on Various CAM Modalities and Skin Cancer Risk

Study	Design	Sample	Intervention/Assessment	Main Outcome
Karagas et al[140]	CC	132 cases and 264 controls aged < 85 years	Serum levels of antioxidants	No significant associations of antioxidants
Green et al[141]	RCT	1383 patients in 4 treatment groups, aged 20-69 years	β-carotene (30 mg), sunscreen, placebo	Protective effect of sunscreen on occurrence of new NMSC
Moon et al[142]	RCT	2297 cases	Oral retinol (25,000 IU), placebo	Protective effect of oral retinol on occurrence of new NMSC, no effect on occurrence of new basal cell
Clark et al[51]	RCT	653 treated and 659 placebo patients aged 18-80 years	200 µg selenium (Se), placebo	No protective effect for basal or squamous cell cancer
Levine et al[143]	RCT	525 cases aged < 80 years	Retinol (25,000 IU), isotretinoin (5-10 mg), placebo	No protective effects of retinol or isotretinoin
Vinceti et al[147]	RC	63 cases of Reggio Emilia	Inorganic selenate	3.9-fold increased risk of melanoma in cases exposed to high Se levels
Reinhold et al[150]	RCC	101 cases and 80 controls aged 20-83 years	Serum Se levels	Stage dependent inverse correlation between serum Se levels and presence of melanoma

RCT = randomized controlled trial; CC = case-control; RCC retrospective case-control; RC = retrospective cohort; NMSC = non-melanoma skin cancer.

Nonmelanoma Squamous Cell Cancer
Vitamin A, β-Carotene, Retinoids

Both β-carotene and retinol have been studied in animal models and found to confer at least some protection against skin cancer. Epidemiologic data in both men and women found no association between prediagnostic serum levels of retinoids and the risk of subsequent primary or recurrent skin cancers.[140] A series of randomized placebo-controlled trials have been consistently unable to show a correlation between β-carotene supplementation and reduced skin cancer risk.[141] However, a single trial of more than 2000 patients did demonstrate a reduced risk of development of new nonmelanoma squamous cell cancers (NMSCs) in both low-risk (no previous skin cancers) and moderate-risk (at least two previous NMSCs) subjects given retinol supplementation for 5 years.[142] The designation of risk status is germane. Authors of a similar randomized study of high-risk patients (defined as patients with at least four previous NMSCs) demonstrated no protective effects of supplemental retinol or isotretinoin administration. End points included total new tumor number and time to first recurrence.[143]

Selenium

Early observational data from patients with basal or squamous cell skin cancers were conflicting. However, the trend toward significantly lower plasma selenium levels in cases than in controls led to a series of randomized controlled trials of selenium supplementation. These data consistently showed that supplementation had no effect on either incidence or recurrence of NMSCs. However, a secondary end point of reduced total cancer mortality was statistically significant, thus prompting the authors to suggest that further study is warranted.[51]

Malignant Melanoma
Vitamins A and E, β-Carotene, Retinoids
Studies that explored the use of antioxidant vitamins as chemopreventive agents for multiple melanoma prevention have provided mixed results. Observational and nested case-control studies of α-tocopherols, β-carotene, and retinols have been inconclusive in terms of diagnostic or prognostic significance, either due to marginally significant data or small study size.

Essential Minerals
Epidemiologic data show inverse, null, or direct correlations with melanoma risk and selenium levels. Some early studies demonstrated low serum selenium levels in melanoma patients, with levels inversely correlated to stage of disease, indicating a possible prognostic role.[144,145] Although two large selenium supplementation trials[51,146] showed selenium to be a likely chemopreventive agent against a variety of cancers, neither was specific for melanoma. In contrast, a long-term study of an Italian population, subject to increased selenium intake since 1984, revealed an unexpected 3.9-fold increase in melanoma in the exposed cohort.[147] Researchers have criticized this study because of its assumption that inorganic selenate is better absorbed and therefore more bioavailable than selenium supplements.[148,149] There are also questions of biologic plausibility because the findings are contrary to in vitro data on the effects of selenium on melanocytes as well as to two case-control studies.[51,150]

Studies of other minerals such as zinc, calcium, and magnesium on in vitro melanoma cells have produced conflicting data regarding differential effects. To date, no randomized controlled trials showing a protective effect of any of these minerals has been found. Iron and copper uptake in tissue culture has also been evaluated, but no prognostic significance has been revealed. Two studies in humans analyzed zinc serum levels have been attempted to identify an "early detection" marker. Unfortunately, the results were diametrically opposite, with one study finding hypozincemia[151] and the other finding increased serum levels[152] in melanoma patients.

Miscellaneous Therapies
There are a few promising developments in the field of prevention and early treatment of melanoma. A variety of ayurvedic compounds have demonstrated in vitro inhibition of growth of human melanoma cells.[153]

Research in the area of psychooncology (mind-body interventions) indicates the value of psychotherapeutic intervention on the activity of killer cells in patients with malignant melanoma.[154] Currently prevention appears to be of a secondary nature, with prolonged remission relative to controls. A role in primary prevention must be investigated.

Summary
Current prospective data is limited on the occurrence or recurrence risks of skin cancer with CAM therapies. New and carefully targeted research is necessary, particularly in high-risk populations. Only oral retinol has shown promise in randomized controlled trials, and evidence for essential minerals is mixed. The use of topical retinoic acid has been so widely documented and used that it can be removed from consideration as a "complementary"

modality. New therapies based on ayurvedic compounds, micronutrients, green tea extracts, and mind-body interventions are currently being tested. There is a need for appropriately powered randomized controlled trials to validate these epidemiologic findings.

ENDOMETRIAL CANCER

Obesity is known to be strongly associated with endometrial cancer risk. It is not surprising, therefore, that the effects of diet and exercise on endometrial cancer risk and prevention are the subjects of study in the CAM literature. To date there are relatively few published studies, and most of these are epidemiologic. Randomized placebo-controlled prospective trials have yet to be undertaken in any systematic way.

Vitamins A, C, E, β-Carotene, Retinoids

Studies to evaluate the role of dietary supplements on uterine cancer protection are limited (Table 12-8). In general, evaluation has included retinols (vitamin A), carotenoids (β-carotene), and antioxidants (vitamins C and E, and folate). Study designs included dietary questionnaires and, in some cases, serum levels. All were either cohort or case-control evaluations. Studies of β-carotene were conflicting, but most demonstrated some benefit or protection. Only Shu[155] and Heinonen[156] showed no reduction in relative risk. With only one exception,[157] vitamin C and vitamin E were not found to exert any effect in studies.[155,158] Neither data from animals nor the limited human data show a protective effect for folate.[158,159] Despite the theoretical foundation in animal and in vitro studies, neither retinol serum levels[156] nor intake[158] has shown a relationship to endometrial cancer prevention.

Physical Activity

Only three studies were identified that investigated physical activity and the risk of endometrial cancer.[160-162] With one exception,[160] no significant protective effect was noted when exercise was evaluated as a risk factor independent from body weight. Obviously, women who exercise more are less likely to be obese, and physical activity should be encouraged in women at risk.

Summary

Conclusions are difficult to draw regarding the effects of vitamins A, C, and E; β-carotene; retinoids; and physical activity on endometrial cancer because of the scarcity of data. An overall healthy lifestyle is to be encouraged and appears to have more to recommend it than

Table 12-8
Case-Control Studies on Dietary Supplements and Endometrial Cancer Risk

Study	Sample	Assessment	Main Outcome
Heinonen et al[156]	88 cases and 31 controls	Serum concentrations	No differences in levels of vitamins or carotene and risk
Levi et al[157]	274 cases and 572 controls	Micronutrient intake	Reduced risk with carotene and vitamin C intake (OR 0.5)
Shu et al[155]	268 cases and 268 controls	Micronutrient intake	No differences in risk with vitamin C or carotene intake
Negri et al[158]	368 cases and 713 controls	Micronutrient intake	Reduced risk for β-carotene (RR 0.6), folate (RR 0.7), vitamin E (RR 0.9)

OR = odds ratio; RR = relative risk.

the interventional strategies that have thus far been studied. There is a need for randomized prospective trials. Currently, the most promising nutraceutical for study appears to be β-carotene, and studies of β-carotene supplements and β-carotene available in the diet must be undertaken. Side effects of pharmaceutical doses would require further explanation as well.

CERVICAL CANCER

Numerous epidemiologic studies have explored the chemopreventive effects of micronutrients on cervical cancer risk. However, evaluation of the effects of nutrients on the natural progression of cervical neoplasia is complicated by its multifactorial etiology. Although many studies have failed to control for such factors as human papillomavirus (HPV) infection and smoking, a significant body of data has emerged regarding several nutrients. These include vitamin A (preformed vitamin A, vitamin A analogs, carotenoids), vitamins C and E, and folate. Data from the most seminal clinical trials and case-control studies are reflected in Table 12-9.[163-171]

Table 12-9
Micronutrients and Cervical Cancer Risk

Study	Design	Sample	Intervention/Assessment	Main Outcome
Wideroff et al[163]	CC	251 cases and 806 controls, mean age 33	Dietary assessment of vitamins A, C, E, folate, zinc, β-carotene	No associations noted between occurrence of precancerous lesion and micronutrient intake
Mackerras et al[164]	RCT	141 cases with mild atypia, aged >18 years	β-carotene (3 mg), vitamin C (500 mg), both, or placebo	No associations noted between treatment groups on regression of minor atypia
Butterworth et al[165]	C	47 cases with mild-moderate atypia, aged 16-28 years	Folic acid (10 mg) or placebo (ascorbic acid 10 mg)	Decreased biopsy scores in treatment group ($p < .05$)
Butterworth et al[166]	RCT	235 cases with mild-moderate atypia	Folic acid (10 mg) or placebo	No differences between treatment groups on regression of atypia
Childers et al[167]	RCT	331 cases with mild-moderate atypia, aged 15-59	Folic acid (5 mg) or placebo	No differences between treatment groups on regression of atypia
Manetta et al[168]	CT	25 patients with mild-moderate atypia	β-carotene (30 mg)	Positive correlation of treatment and serum levels and atypia
de Vet et al[169]	RCT	278 patients with dysplasia, aged 20-65	β-carotene (10 mg) or placebo	No treatment effect of β-carotene on regression of atypia
Romney et al[170]	RCT	69 patients with dysplasia, aged < 65 years	β-carotene (10 mg) or placebo	No treatment effect of β-carotene on regression of atypia
Meyskens et al[171]	RCT	301 patients with dysplasia	Topical all-*trans*-retinoic acid (1 mL of 0.372%) or placebo	Regression in treatment group for moderate dysplasia; no association in severe dysplasia

CC = case-control, RCT = randomized control trial, C = cohort, CT = controlled trial.

Vitamin A, β-Carotene, Retinoids

Epidemiologic studies have indicated conflicting degrees of association between dietary vitamin A and risk of cervical dysplasia, carcinoma in situ (CIS), or invasive cervical cancer. Early studies using dietary recall found an inverse correlation between dietary intake of retinol and risk of cervical disease.[172,173] Later investigators, in an attempt to evaluate the role of retinol in a more reproducible fashion, looked not only at dietary intake but also at serum levels. The results of these case-control studies were again conflicting.[174,175] In some cases, the dietary intake did not correlate with serum levels, which in turn did not correlate with tissue levels. A review of nutritional data and cervical neoplasia concluded that the majority of clinical and case-control studies showed no association of cervical neoplasia with either dietary vitamin A intake or serum retinol levels.[176] No subsequent study has established causality, and randomized prospective interventional trials are lacking. This is partially caused by high-dose retinol being contraindicated in women who might become pregnant. Investigators who have shown an association between low serum retinol and cervical neoplasia have been unable to determine whether the association indicates a true protective effect or altered metabolism secondary to the disease process itself.[177] It has been suggested that retinol may be required for adequate immunologic surveillance of HPV and may modify HPV-associated risk for cervical cancer.[178] Because of the recognized effects of vitamin A in cellular differentiation, these issues are still under investigation.

There has been considerable interest in the topical administration of retinoic acid, and a few trials using topical retinoic acid for patients with cervical neoplasia have been conducted. Pharmacokinetic evaluation demonstrates measurable tissue levels after topical administration, without detectable serum levels. A phase III interventional trial demonstrated statistically significant complete histologic regression of cervical intraepithelial neoplasia (CIN) II lesions over 26 months, after treatment at months one, three, and six.[171] HPV analysis was not done. No effect was noted on CIN III lesions. Subsequent studies have largely focused on retinoic acid in combination with other modalities in the treatment of advanced or recurrent cervical cancer.

The association between dietary deficiencies of β-carotene and the incidence of cervical neoplasias and cancers has been explored in numerous epidemiologic studies. The fact that smoking, a known risk for cervical neoplasia, reduces plasma levels of β-carotene in women older than 26 years of age lends credence to a causal relationship.[179] A phase II study confirmed that "a large percentage of patients with CIN I and II will respond clinically to PO β-carotene supplementation."[168] These data were not supported by the phase III randomized controlled trials of deVet and associates[169] and Romney and associates,[170] who found no effect of β-carotene on the regression percentages of cervical dysplasias. The latter findings were confirmed in another reported randomized placebo-controlled trial, in which markedly elevated serum levels of β-carotene in the supplemented arm showed no association with persistence of HPV infection or CIN.[180]

Vitamin C

Review of the literature that examines the relationship between fruit and vegetable intake and cervical cancer suggests a protective effect of vitamin C. The difficulty in extrapolating from this literature, however, stems from the fact that the protective effects of fruits and vegetables are multifactorial. Nonetheless, a significant protective effect for cervical cancers was shown in 11 of 13 epidemiologic studies reviewed.[181] End points included correlation of plasma ascorbic acid levels and dietary intake of vitamin C with progression or regression of cervical neoplasias. When specifically taking into account the presence or absence of HPV, however, Wideroff and associates[163] found no protective role for ascorbic acid in patients with low-grade squamous intraepithelial lesions. In the face of conflicting epidemiologic data, Mackerras and associates[164] undertook a randomized 2-year interventional trial to test whether high-dose ascorbic acid supplementation (500 mg) would retard the promotion or progression of precancers of the cervix. The results showed no statistically significant differences between those who were treated and those who were not, leading the authors to suggest that vitamin C in pharmacologic doses had no effect on the regression or progression of mild dysplasia of the cervix.

Vitamin E

Less attention has been paid to vitamin E, with the few studies that exist focusing on the α-tocopherols. An inverse correlation has been seen with serum vitamin E levels and higher grade premalignant cervical lesions.[182] Results from a case-control study indicated that low serum tocopherol levels represented a significantly increased risk for cervical cancer, even when the cancers in the first 2 years of follow-up were excluded.[183] The study used serum samples from a serum data bank and identified 23 cervical cancer patients 5 to 10 years after the original sample had been taken. The study had 44 age-matched controls. Adjustments were made for smoking, body mass index, and parity. The meaning of this association is, again, uncertain. The study populations have been small.

Folate

Interest in the role of folic acid deficiency stems from the early observations of megaloblastic cells in the epithelium of the uterine cervix.[184] Oral administration of folic acid induced methylation and reversed these megaloblastic changes in women taking oral contraceptives. The degree of hypomethylation of DNA in the cervix has been correlated with increased CIN severity.[185] Although early data appeared to support the hypothesis that folic acid administration inhibited the progression of CIN I and CIN II lesions,[165,186] the same authors later concluded that "folate deficiency may be involved as a co-carcinogen during the initiation of cervical dysplasia, but folic acid supplements do not alter the course of established disease."[186] A multiinstitutional, randomized placebo-controlled trial convincingly demonstrated that oral folic acid supplementation did not enhance regression of mild or moderate CIN; however, the authors raised the question of whether correction of folate deficiency before the initiation of the dysplastic process would be protective.[167]

It is postulated that low levels of folate, especially in an environment of low antioxidants, intensify cellular susceptibility to HPV infection and increase the risk of subsequent cellular transformation. Although this issue has not yet been answered directly, some newer epidemiologic data illustrate statistically lower levels of folic acid in women with CIN-HPV(+).[187] A recent nested case-control study, however, concluded that in the presence of viral DNA, folate is not a protective cofactor and that the association between low levels of serum folate and CIN-HPV+ may reflect little more than chance.[163]

Summary

Although there have been numerous studies evaluating the role of micronutrients in the prevention and treatment of cervical cancers, there are no current recommendations for specific dietary supplementation to prevent cervical cancer or other neoplasias. Currently, only topical retinoic acid shows any promise for the regression of cervical dysplasias. No randomized controlled trials support the use of β-carotene as a preventive agent. More worrisome is the fact that findings in the Romney study were consistent with a negative impact of β-carotene supplements on spontaneous healing and complete regression. In addition, no data support supplementation of vitamin C in patients with cervical disease or in healthy patients wishing to prevent precancerous lesions of the cervix. Furthermore, the evidence for use of folate in cervical cancer chemoprevention is inconsistent. Randomized placebo-controlled trials are needed as well as more site-specific evaluation of the presence and role of the micronutrient under investigation. The role of serum levels of micronutrients in the identification of high-risk patients is also being evaluated. Differentiating between serum levels of a specific nutrient as a causative or protective factor versus a marker for related compounds or processes will be essential. All future randomized controlled trials must continue for adequate periods of time and must control for all risk factors, including HPV infection. Given the invasive nature of current treatments for moderate and severe dysplasias and the disease burden of cervical cancer worldwide, it would be preferable if easily ingested or applied compounds were available to reverse the process.

CONCLUSION

The chemopreventive potential of various CAM therapies such as antioxidant vitamins, minerals, phytoestrogens, dietary mixtures, and green tea may show some promise. Vitamin A analogs appear to provide some benefit against cancers of the breast, skin, and cervix. In addition, there is some indication that selenium may reduce the risk of lung cancer, and vitamin C and phytoestrogens may positively affect breast cancer risk. Many other CAM therapies reviewed earlier such as vitamin D, folate, melatonin, dietary mixtures, fish oil, green tea, ginseng, mushroom, ayurvedic compounds, and mind-body interventions can have potential chemopreventive effects, but systematic evaluations of these therapies are lacking.

The evidence on the chemopreventive effectiveness of CAM therapies should be interpreted with some caution. With some exceptions, the majority of the review is based on observational epidemiologic (case-control or cohort) studies. Unlike clinical trials, observational studies are associative in nature and do not permit causal inference. Contradictory results between observational studies may be attributable to different study designs, accuracy of measurement of dietary intake, different follow-up times, differences between cases and controls, and selection biases introduced in the recruitment of cases and controls.

Observational studies examine the associations between intake of micronutrients or minerals either as part of a daily diet or in the form of supplements and cancer risk and are limited by problems of confounding. The confounding factor is diet. Diet and micronutrients in a diet are highly correlated with other nutrients of interest. The effects reported on individual micronutrients may be confounded by interactions between other micronutrients and yet undetermined factors.

Diet is typically measured through food frequency questionnaires or dietary histories. The measurement of diet is fraught with errors caused by recall bias, changes in diet because of disease, and disease-related differential metabolism. Diet may change because of risk profile. For instance, women with a family history of breast cancer may modify their dietary habits. In addition, people who consume high levels of vegetables and fruits are likely to be more health-conscious and would exercise other health-promoting practices that may not be measured. Recall bias is a problem in retrospective studies. Patients may be reluctant to recall dietary factors that may be implicated with their disease. The length of recall is also crucial, given that carcinogenesis is a long, slow process. Many previous observational studies of diet and disease did not assess the period and point of time of intake, and validation assessments of the primary predictors of interest were nonexistent. Future studies should determine period of intake of specific diet or nutrient before onset or diagnosis of disease because dietary patterns may change as a result of the disease.

There is an urgent need for well-designed randomized controlled trials, which systematically can address the chemopreventive potential of many of the CAM therapies. Moreover, these studies should address many clinical implications of the treatments including issues of dosage level, drug interactions, risk profile of patients, and optimal period to initiate chemoprevention therapy. Lastly, although some CAM therapies may show promise in experimental studies and epidemiologic observational studies, it may be premature to prescribe or encourage patients to consume products such as soy proteins, ginseng, green tea, and folates for their potential chemopreventive effects, given the absence of evidence from randomized controlled trials.

APPENDIX A
Books

American Cancer Society's Guide to complementary and alternative cancer methods. Atlanta, American Cancer Society, 2000.

Benson H, Stark M: *Timeless healing: the power and biology of belief.* New York, Scribner, 1996.

Blumenthal M, Busse WR, Goldberg, et al, editors: *The complete German Commission E monographs: therapeutic guide to herbal medicines.* American Botanical Council, 1998.

Boik J: *Cancer & natural medicine: a textbook of basic science and clinical research.* Princeton, MN, Oregon Medical Press, 1995.

Cohen MH: *Complementary and alternative medicine legal boundaries and regulatory perspectives.* Baltimore, The Johns Hopkins University Press, 1998.

DerMarederosian A, ed: *The review of natural products: facts and comparisons.* 111 West Port Plaza, # 300, St. Louis, MO 63146.

Fetrow CW, Avila JR: *Professional handbook of complementary & alternative medicine.* Springhouse, PA, Springhouse, 1999.

Fontanarosa P, ed: *Alternative medicine: an objective assessment.* Chicago, American Medical Association, 2000.

Foster S, Tyler VE: *Tyler's honest herbal: a sensible guide to the use of herbs and related remedies,* ed 4. New York, Hawthorn Herbal Press, 1999.

Gordon JS, Curtin S: *Comprehensive cancer care: integrating alternative, complementary, and conventional therapies.* Cambridge, MA, Perseus Publishing, 2000.

Jonas W, Levin J: *Essentials of complementary and alternative medicine.* Philadelphia, Lippincott Williams & Wilkins, 1999.

Packer L, Colman C: *The antioxidant miracle: your complete plan for total health and healing.* New York, John Wiley & Sons, 1999.

Spencer JW, Jacobs JJ: *Complementary/alternative medicine an evidence-based approach.* St Louis, Mosby, 1999.

Vincent C, Furham A: *Complementary medicine: a research perspective.* New York, Wiley, 1997.

Journals
Alternative Medicine Review

Alternative Medicine Alert (208) 263-1337
http://www.ahcpub.com

Alternative Therapies in Health and Medicine

InnoVision Communications LLC
169 Saxony Road, Suite 104
Encinitas, CA 92024
866-828-2962
http://www.alternative-therapies.com

Focus on Alternative and Complementary Therapies

An Evidence-Based Approach
Pharmaceutical Press
1 Lambeth High Street
London SE1 7JN
44(0)207-735-9141
http://www.ex.ac.uk/fact/

Herbalgram

American Botanical Council
6200 Manor Road
Austin, TX 78723
(512)926-4900
http://www.herbalgram.org

Journal of Ethnopharmacy

Elsevier Science Ireland, Ltd.
Madison Square Station, Box 882
New York, NY 10159
(212) 989-5800

Institutions
The Alternative Medicine Homage

http://www.pitt.edu/~cbw/altm.html

American Association of Naturopathic Physicians

3201 New Maxico Ave. NW, Suite 350
Washington, DC 20016
(866) 538-2267
http://www.naturopathic.org

American Association of Oriental Medicine

433 Front Street
Catasauqua, PA 18032
(800) 521-2262

American Botanical Council

6200 Manor Rd
Austin, TX 78723
(512) 926-4900
http://www.herbalgram.org

American Cancer Society

http://www.cancer.org

American Chiropractic Association

1701 Clarendon Boulevard
Arlington, VA 22209
(800) 986-4836
http://www.americhiro.org

American Holistic Health Association

PO Box 17400
Anaheim, CA 92817
(714) 779-6152
http://www.ahha.org

American Massage Therapy Association

820 Davis Street, Suite 100
Evanston, IL 60201
(847) 864-0123
http://www.amtamassage.org

Center for Mind/Body Medicine

5225 Connecticut Avenue, NE Suite 414
Washington, DC 20015
(202) 966-7338
http://www.cmbm.org

FDA, Center for Food Safety and Applied Nutrition

http://vm.cfsan.fda.gov/list.html

Federal Trade Commission

Room 130
600 Pennsylvania Avenue, NW
Washington, DC 20580
(877) 382-4357
http://www.ftc.gov/

Food and Drug Administration (FDA)

5800 Fishers Lane
Rockville, MD 20857
(888) INFO-FDA
http://www.fda.gov/

Health Oasis—Mayo Clinic

http://www.mayohealth.org

International Bibliographic Information on Dietary Supplements (IBIDS)

http://ods.od.nih.gov

National Center of Complementary and Alternative Medicine (NCCAM)

PO Box 8218
Silver Springs, MD 20907
(301) 495-4957
http://altmed.od.nih.gov

National Center of Homeopathy

801 North Fairfax Street, Suite 306
Alexandria, VA 22314
(877) 624-0613
http://www.homeopathic.org

Quackwatch

http://www.quackwatch.com

Tufts University Nutrition Navigator

http://www.navigator.tufts.edu

REFERENCES

1. Eisenberg DM, Davis RB, Ettner SL, et al: Trends in alternative medicine use in the United States, 1990-1997: results of a follow-up national survey. *JAMA* 1998;280:1569-1575.

2. Ernst E, Cassileth BR: The prevalence of complementary/alternative medicine in cancer: a systematic review. *Cancer* 1998;83:777-782.

3. Begbie SD, Kerestes ZL, Bell DR: Patterns of alternative medicine use by cancer patients. *Med J Aust* 1996;165:545-548.

4. Sollner W, Maislinger S, DeVries A, et al: Use of complementary and alternative medicine by cancer patients is not associated with perceived distress or poor compliance with standard treatment but with active coping behavior: a survey. *Cancer* 2000;89:873-880.

5. VandeCreek L, Rogers E, Lester J: Use of alternative therapies among breast cancer outpatients compared with the general population. *Altern Ther Health Med* 1999;5:71-76.

6. Gotay CC, Dumitriu D: Health food store recommendations for breast cancer patients. *Arch Fam Med* 2000;9:692-699.

7. Defining and describing complementary and alternative medicine: panel on definition and description, CAM Research Methodology Conference, April 1995. *Altern Ther Health Med* 1997 Mar;3(2):49-57.

8. Nanba H, Kubo K: Effect of Maitake D-fraction on cancer prevention. *Ann N Y Acad Sci* 1997;833:204-7.

9. Unexplained severe illness possibly associated with consumption of Kombucha tea—Iowa, 1995. From the Centers for Disease Control and Prevention. *JAMA* 1996;275:96-98.

10. Giacosa A, Filiberti R, Hill MJ, et al: Vitamins and cancer chemoprevention. *Eur J Cancer Prev* 1997;6(Suppl 1):S47-54.

11. Omenn GS: Chemoprevention of lung cancer: the rise and demise of beta-carotene. *Annu Rev Public Health* 1998;19:73-99.

12. Lippman SM, Kessler JF, Meyskens FL: Retinoids as preventive and therapeutic anticancer agents (part I). *Cancer Treat Rep* 1987;71:391-405.

13. Pryor WA, Stahl W, Rock CL: Beta carotene: from biochemistry to clinical trials. *Nutr Rev* 2000;58:39-53.

14. Kurie JM, Lippman SM, Hong WK: Potential of retinoids in cancer prevention. *Cancer Treat Rev* 1994;20:1-10.

15. Boik J: *Cancer & natural medicine: a textbook of basic science and clinical research.* Princeton, MN, Oregon Medical Press, 1995.

16. Vinceti M, Rovesti S, Bergomi M, et al: The epidemiology of selenium and human cancer. *Tumori* 2000;86:105-118.

17. Adlercreutz H, Mazur W: Phyto-oestrogens and Western diseases. *Ann Med* 1997;29:95-120.

18. Messina MJ, Persky V, Setchell KD, et al: Soy intake and cancer risk: a review of the in vitro and in vivo data. *Nutr Cancer* 1994;21:113-131.

19. Chihara G, Hamuro J, Maeda YY, et al: Antitumor and metastasis-inhibitory activities of lentinan as an immunomodulator: an overview. *Cancer Detect Prev Suppl* 1987;1:423-443.

20. Lin XY, Liu JZ, Milner JA: Dietary garlic suppresses DNA adducts caused by N-nitroso compounds. *Carcinogenesis* 1994;15:349-352.

21. Milner JA: Garlic: its anticarcinogenic and antitumorigenic properties. *Nutr Rev* 1996;54:S82-S86.

22. Newmark HL: Squalene, olive oil, and cancer risk: review and hypothesis. *Ann N Y Acad Sci* 1999;889:193-203.

23. el-Bayoumy K: Evaluation of chemopreventive agents against breast cancer and proposed strategies for future clinical intervention trials. *Carcinogenesis* 1994;15:2395-2420.

24. Christakos S: Vitamin D and breast cancer. *Adv Exp Med Biol* 1994;364:115-118.

25. Choi SW: Vitamin B12 deficiency: a new risk factor for breast cancer? *Nutr Rev* 1999;57:250-253.

26. Kim YI: Folate and cancer prevention: a new medical application of folate beyond hyperhomocysteinemia and neural tube defects. *Nutr Rev* 1999;57:314-321.

27. Decensi A, Formelli F, Torrisi R, et al: Breast cancer chemoprevention: studies with 4-HPR alone and in combination with tamoxifen using circulating growth factors as potential surrogate endpoints. *J Cell Biochem Suppl* 1993;17G:226-233.

28. Costa A, Formelli F, Chiesa F, et al: Prospects of chemoprevention of human cancers with the synthetic retinoid fenretinide. *Cancer Res* 1994;54:2032s-2037s.

29. Veronesi U, De Palo G, Costa A, et al: Chemoprevention of breast cancer with retinoids. *J Natl Cancer Inst Monogr* 1992;75:93-97.

30. Veronesi U, De Palo G, Marubini E, et al: Randomized trial of fenretinide to prevent second breast malignancy in women with early breast cancer. *J Natl Cancer Inst* 1999;91:1847-1856.

31. Cooper DA, Eldridge AL, Peters JC: Dietary carotenoids and certain cancers, heart disease, and age-related macular degeneration: a review of recent research. *Nutr Rev* 1999;57:201-214.

32. Clavel-Chapelon F, Niravong M, Joseph RR: Diet and breast cancer: review of the epidemiologic literature. *Cancer Detect Prev* 1997;21:426-440.

33. Gandini S, Merzenich H, Robertson C, et al: Meta-analysis of studies on breast cancer risk and diet: the role of fruit and vegetable consumption and the intake of associated micronutrients. *Eur J Cancer* 2000;36:636-646.

34. Howe GR, Hirohata T, Hislop TG, et al: Dietary factors and risk of breast cancer: combined analysis of 12 case-control studies. *J Natl Cancer Inst* 1990;82:561-569.

35. Jumaan AO, Holmberg L, Zack M, et al: Beta-carotene intake and risk of postmenopausal breast cancer. *Epidemiology* 1999;10:49-53.

36. Comstock GW, Helzlsouer KJ, Bush TL: Prediagnostic serum levels of carotenoids and vitamin E as related to subsequent cancer in

Washington County, Maryland. *Am J Clin Nutr* 1991;53:260S-264S.

37. Willett WC, Polk BF, Underwood BA, et al: Relation of serum vitamins A and E and carotenoids to the risk of cancer. *N Engl J Med* 1984;310:430-434.

38. Potischman N, Swanson CA, Coates RJ, et al: Intake of food groups and associated micronutrients in relation to risk of early-stage breast cancer. *Int J Cancer* 1999;82:315-321.

39. Hunter DJ, Manson JE, Colditz GA, et al: A prospective study of the intake of vitamins C, E, and A and the risk of breast cancer. *N Engl J Med* 1993;329:234-240.

40. Negri E, La Vecchia C, Franceschi S, et al: Intake of selected micronutrients and the risk of breast cancer. *Int J Cancer* 1996;65:140-144.

41. Rohan TE, Howe GR, Friedenreich CM, et al: Dietary fiber, vitamins A, C, and E, and risk of breast cancer: a cohort study. *Cancer Causes Control* 1993;4:29-37.

42. Kimmick GG, Bell RA, Bostick RM: Vitamin E and breast cancer: a review. *Nutr Cancer* 1997;27:109-117.

43. Lipkin M, Newmark HL: Vitamin D, calcium and prevention of breast cancer: a review. *J Am Coll Nutr* 1999;18:392S-397S.

44. John EM, Schwartz GG, Dreon DM, et al: Vitamin D and breast cancer risk: the NHANES I Epidemiologic follow-up study, 1971-1975 to 1992. National Health and Nutrition Examination Survey. *Cancer Epidemiol Biomarkers Prev* 1999;8:399-406.

45. Wu K, Helzlsouer KJ, Comstock GW, et al: A prospective study on folate, B12, and pyridoxal 5'-phosphate (B6) and breast cancer. *Cancer Epidemiol Biomarkers Prev* 1999;8:209-217.

46. Zhang S, Hunter DJ, Hankinson SE, et al: A prospective study of folate intake and the risk of breast cancer. *JAMA* 1999;281:1632-1637.

47. Basu TK, Hill GB, Ng D, et al: Serum vitamins A and E, beta-carotene, and selenium in patients with breast cancer. *J Am Coll Nutr* 1989;8:524-529.

48. Hunter DJ, Morris JS, Stampfer MJ, et al: A prospective study of selenium status and breast cancer risk. *JAMA* 1990;264:1128-1131.

49. van den Brandt PA, Goldbohm RA, van't Veer P, et al: Toenail selenium levels and the risk of breast cancer. *Am J Epidemiol* 1994;140:20-26.

50. Ewertz M, Gill C: Dietary factors and breast-cancer risk in Denmark. *Int J Cancer* 1990;46:779-784.

51. Clark LC, Combs GF, Turnbull BW, et al: Effects of selenium supplementation for cancer prevention in patients with carcinoma of the skin: a randomized controlled trial. Nutritional Prevention of Cancer Study Group. *JAMA* 1996;276:1957-1963.

52. Criqui MH, Bangdiwala S, Goodman DS, et al: Selenium, retinol, retinol-binding protein, and uric acid. Associations with cancer mortality in a population-based prospective case-control study. *Ann Epidemiol* 1991;1:385-393.

53. Dorgan JF, Sowell A, Swanson CA, et al: Relationships of serum carotenoids, retinol, alpha-tocopherol, and selenium with breast cancer risk: results from a prospective study in Columbia, Missouri (United States). *Cancer Causes Control* 1998;9:89-97.

54. Coates RJ, Weiss NS, Daling JR, et al: Serum levels of selenium and retinol and the subsequent risk of cancer. *Am J Epidemiol* 1988;128:515-523.

55. Knekt P, Aromaa A, Maatela J, et al: Serum selenium and subsequent risk of cancer among Finnish men and women. *J Natl Cancer Inst* 1990;82:864-868.

56. Overvad K, Gron P, Langhoff O, et al: Selenium in human mammary carcinogenesis: a case-referent study. *Eur J Cancer Prev* 1991;1:27-30.

57. van Noord PA, Collette HJ, Maas MJ, et al: Selenium levels in nails of premenopausal breast cancer patients assessed prediagnostically in a cohort-nested case-referent study among women screened in the DOM project. *Int J Epidemiol* 1987;16:318-322.

58. van Noord PA, Maas MJ, van der Tweel I, et al: Selenium and the risk of postmenopausal breast cancer in the DOM cohort. *Breast Cancer Res Treat* 1993;25:11-19.

59. Vinceti M, Rovesti S, Gabrielli C, et al: Cancer mortality in a residential cohort exposed to environmental selenium through drinking water. *J Clin Epidemiol* 1995;48:1091-1097.

60. Tamarkin L, Danforth D, Lichter A, et al: Decreased nocturnal plasma melatonin peak in patients with estrogen receptor positive breast cancer. *Science* 1982;216:1003-1005.

61. Bartsch C, Bartsch H, Jain AK, et al: Urinary melatonin levels in human breast cancer patients. *J Neural Transm* 1981;52:281-294.

62. Lee HP, Gourley L, Duffy SW, et al: Dietary effects on breast-cancer risk in Singapore. *Lancet* 1991;337:1197-1200.

63. Hirose K, Tajima K, Hamajima N, et al: A large-scale, hospital-based case-control study of risk factors of breast cancer according to menopausal status. *Jpn J Cancer Res* 1995;86:146-154.

64. Ingram D, Sanders K, Kolybaba M, et al: Case-control study of phyto-oestrogens and breast cancer. *Lancet* 1997;350:990-994.

65. Wu AH, Ziegler RG, Horn-Ross PL, et al: Tofu and risk of breast cancer in Asian-Americans. *Cancer Epidemiol Biomarkers Prev* 1996;5:901-906.

66. Yuan JM, Wang QS, Ross RK, et al: Diet and breast cancer in Shanghai and Tianjin, China. *Br J Cancer* 1995;71:1353-1358.

67. Petrakis NL, Barnes S, King EB, et al: Stimulatory influence of soy protein isolate on breast secretion in pre- and postmenopausal women. *Cancer Epidemiol Biomarkers Prev* 1996;5:785-794.

68. Imai K, Suga K, Nakachi K: Cancer-preventive effects of drinking green tea among a Japanese population. *Prev Med* 1997;26:769-775.

69. Nakachi K, Suemasu K, Suga K, et al: Influence of drinking green tea on breast cancer malignancy among Japanese patients. *Jpn J Cancer Res* 1998;89:254-261.

70. Goldbohm RA, Hertog MG, Brants HA, et al: Consumption of black tea and cancer risk: a prospective cohort study. *J Natl Cancer Inst* 1996;88:93-100.

71. Dorant E, van den Brandt PA, Goldbohm RA: Allium vegetable consumption, garlic supplement

intake, and female breast carcinoma incidence. *Breast Cancer Res Treat* 1995;33:163-170.

72. Martin-Moreno JM, Willett WC, Gorgojo L, et al: Dietary fat, olive oil intake, and breast cancer risk. *Int J Cancer* 1994;58:774-780.

73. la Vecchia C, Negri E, Franceschi S, et al: Olive oil, other dietary fats, and the risk of breast cancer (Italy). *Cancer Causes Control* 1995;6:545-550.

74. Trichopoulou A, Katsouyanni K, Stuver S, et al: Consumption of olive oil and specific food groups in relation to breast cancer risk in Greece. *J Natl Cancer Inst* 1995;87:110-116.

75. Toniolo P, Riboli E, Protta F, et al: Calorie-providing nutrients and risk of breast cancer. *J Natl Cancer Inst* 1989;81:278-286.

76. Gould MN: Cancer chemoprevention and therapy by monoterpenes. *Environ Health Perspect* 1997;105(Suppl 4):977-979.

77. Peto R, Doll R, Buckley JD, et al: Can dietary beta-carotene materially reduce human cancer rates? *Nature* 1981;290:201-208.

78. Ziegler RG, Mason TJ, Stemhagen A, et al: Carotenoid intake, vegetables, and the risk of lung cancer among white men in New Jersey. *Am J Epidemiol* 1986;123:1080-1093.

79. Hirayama T: Diet and cancer. *Nutr Cancer* 1979;1:67-81.

80. Kvale G, Bjelke E, Gart JJ: Dietary habits and lung cancer risk. *Int J Cancer* 1983;31:397-405.

81. Gregor SZDZA: Comparison of dietary histories in lung cancer cases and controls with special reference to vitamin A. *Nutr Cancer* 1980;2:93.

82. Hinds MW, Kolonel LN, Hankin JH, et al: Dietary vitamin A, carotene, vitamin C and risk of lung cancer in Hawaii. *Am J Epidemiol* 1984;119:227-237.

83. Koo LC: Diet and lung cancer 20+ years later: more questions than answers? *Int J Cancer* 1997;Suppl 10:22-29.

84. Bandera EV, Freudenheim JL, Marshall JR, et al: Diet and alcohol consumption and lung cancer risk in the New York State cohort (United States). *Cancer Causes Control* 1997;8:828-840.

85. Yong LC, Brown CC, Schatzkin A, et al: Intake of vitamins E, C, and A and risk of lung cancer: the NHANES I epidemiologic follow-up study, First National Health and Nutrition Examination Survey. *Am J Epidemiol* 1997;146:231-243.

86. Ocke MC, Bueno-de-Mesquita HB, Feskens EJ, et al: Repeated measurements of vegetables, fruits, beta-carotene, and vitamins C and E in relation to lung cancer, The Zutphen Study. *Am J Epidemiol* 1997;145:358-365.

87. Knekt P, Jarvinen R, Seppanen R, et al: Dietary antioxidants and the risk of lung cancer. *Am J Epidemiol* 1991;134:471-479.

88. Comstock GW, Alberg AJ, Huang HY, et al: The risk of developing lung cancer associated with antioxidants in the blood: ascorbic acid, carotenoids, alpha-tocopherol, selenium, and total peroxyl radical absorbing capacity. *Cancer Epidemiol Biomarkers Prev* 1997;6:907-916.

89. Stahelin HB, Gey KF, Eichholzer M, et al: Plasma antioxidant vitamins and subsequent cancer mortality in the 12-year follow-up of the prospective Basel Study. *Am J Epidemiol* 1991;133:766-775.

90. Menkes MS, Comstock GW, Vuilleumier JP, et al: Serum beta-carotene, vitamins A and E, selenium, and the risk of lung cancer. *N Engl J Med* 1986;315:1250-1254.

91. Albanes D, Heinonen OP, Taylor PR, et al: Alpha-tocopherol and beta-carotene supplements and lung cancer incidence in the alpha-tocopherol, beta-carotene cancer prevention study: effects of base-line characteristics and study compliance. *J Natl Cancer Inst* 1996;88:1560-1570.

92. Omenn GS, Goodman GE, Thornquist MD, et al: Risk factors for lung cancer and for intervention effects in CARET, the Beta-Carotene and Retinol Efficacy Trial. *J Natl Cancer Inst* 1996;88:1550-1559.

93. Omenn GS, Goodman GE, Thornquist MD, et al: Effects of a combination of beta carotene and vitamin A on lung cancer and cardiovascular disease. *N Engl J Med* 1996;334:1150-1155.

94. Hennekens CH, Buring JE, Manson JE, et al: Lack of effect of long-term supplementation with beta carotene on the incidence of malignant neoplasms and cardiovascular disease. *N Engl J Med* 1996;334:1145-1149.

95. Steinmetz KA, Potter JD, Folsom AR: Vegetables, fruit, and lung cancer in the Iowa Women's Health Study. *Cancer Res* 1993;53:536-543.

96. van den Brandt PA, Goldbohm RA, van 't Veer P, et al: A prospective cohort study on selenium status and the risk of lung cancer. *Cancer Res* 1993;53:4860-4865.

97. Knekt P, Marniemi J, Teppo L, et al: Is low selenium status a risk factor for lung cancer? *Am J Epidemiol* 1998;148:975-982.

98. Koo LC: Dietary habits and lung cancer risk among Chinese females in Hong Kong who never smoked. *Nutr Cancer* 1988;11:155-172.

99. Nomura A, Heilbrun LK, Morris JS, et al: Serum selenium and the risk of cancer, by specific sites: case-control analysis of prospective data. *J Natl Cancer Inst* 1987;79:103-108.

100. Yu SY, Mao BL, Xiao P, et al: Intervention trial with selenium for the prevention of lung cancer among tin miners in Yunnan, China: a pilot study. *Biol Trace Elem Res* 1990;24:105-108.

101. Blot WJ, Li JY, Taylor PR, et al: Nutrition intervention trials in Linxian, China: supplementation with specific vitamin/mineral combinations, cancer incidence, and disease-specific mortality in the general population. *J Natl Cancer Inst* 1993;85:1483-1492.

102. Lissoni P, Tisi E, Barni S, et al: Biological and clinical results of a neuroimmunotherapy with interleukin-2 and the pineal hormone melatonin as a first line treatment in advanced non-small cell lung cancer. *Br J Cancer* 1992;66:155-158.

103. Lissoni P, Barni S, Ardizzoia A, et al: Randomized study with the pineal hormone melatonin versus supportive care alone in advanced nonsmall cell lung cancer resistant to a first-line chemotherapy containing cisplatin. *Oncology* 1992;49:336-339.

104. Dorant E, van den Brandt PA, Goldbohm RA: A prospective cohort study on Allium vegetable consumption, garlic supplement use, and the risk of lung carcinoma in The Netherlands. *Cancer Res* 1994;54:6148-6153.

105. Vermeer IT, Moonen EJ, Dallinga JW, et al: Effect of ascorbic acid and green tea on endogenous formation of N-nitrosodimethylamine and N-nitrosopiperidine in humans. *Mutat Res* 1999; 428:353-361.

106. Malila N, Virtamo J, Virtanen M, et al: The effect of alpha-tocopherol and beta-carotene supplementation on colorectal adenomas in middle-aged male smokers. *Cancer Epidemiol Biomarkers Prev* 1999;8:489-493.

107. Scheppach W, Bingham S, Boutron-Ruault MC, et al: WHO consensus statement on the role of nutrition in colorectal cancer. *Eur J Cancer Prev* 1999;8:57-62.

108. Bussey HJ, DeCosse JJ, Deschner EE, et al: A randomized trial of ascorbic acid in polyposis coli. *Cancer* 1982;50:1434-1439.

109. Moertel CG, Fleming TR, Creagan ET, et al: High-dose vitamin C versus placebo in the treatment of patients with advanced cancer who have had no prior chemotherapy: a randomized double-blind comparison. *N Engl J Med* 1985;312:137-141.

110. DeCosse JJ, Miller HH, Lesser ML: Effect of wheat fiber and vitamins C and E on rectal polyps in patients with familial adenomatous polyposis. *J Natl Cancer Inst* 1989;81:1290-1297.

111. Paganelli GM, Biasco G, Brandi G, et al: Effect of vitamin A, C, and E supplementation on rectal cell proliferation in patients with colorectal adenomas. *J Natl Cancer Inst* 1992;84:47-51.

112. Roncucci L, Di Donato P, Carati L, et al: Antioxidant vitamins or lactulose for the prevention of the recurrence of colorectal adenomas, Colorectal Cancer Study Group of the University of Modena and the Health Care District 16. *Dis Colon Rectum* 1993;36:227-234.

113. Greenberg ER, Baron JA, Tosteson TD, et al: A clinical trial of antioxidant vitamins to prevent colorectal adenoma, Polyp Prevention Study Group. *N Engl J Med* 1994;331:141-147.

114. McKeown-Eyssen G, Holloway C, Jazmaji V, et al: A randomized trial of vitamins C and E in the prevention of recurrence of colorectal polyps. *Cancer Res* 1988;48:4701-4705.

115. Cascinu S, Ligi M, Del Ferro E, et al: Effects of calcium and vitamin supplementation on colon cell proliferation in colorectal cancer. *Cancer Invest* 2000;18:411-416.

116. Albanes D, Malila N, Taylor PR, et al: Effects of supplemental alpha-tocopherol and beta-carotene on colorectal cancer: results from a controlled trial (Finland). *Cancer Causes Control* 2000;11:197-205.

117. Freudenheim JL, Graham S, Marshall JR, et al: Folate intake and carcinogenesis of the colon and rectum. *Int J Epidemiol* 1991;20:368-374.

118. Meyer F, White E: Alcohol and nutrients in relation to colon cancer in middle-aged adults. *Am J Epidemiol* 1993;138:225-236.

119. Ma J, Stampfer MJ, Giovannucci E, et al: Methylenetetrahydrofolate reductase polymorphism, dietary interactions, and risk of colorectal cancer. *Cancer Res* 1997;57:1098-1102.

120. Giovannucci E, Stampfer MJ, Colditz GA, et al: Multivitamin use, folate, and colon cancer in women in the Nurses' Health Study. *Ann Intern Med* 1998;129:517-524.

121. Caroli S, Coni E, Alimonti A, et al: A pilot study on colon cancer occurrence as related to serum selenium levels. *Ann Ist Super Sanita* 1994;30: 243-247.

122. Ghadirian P, Maisonneuve P, Perret C, et al: A case-control study of toenail selenium and cancer of the breast, colon, and prostate. *Cancer Detect Prev* 2000;24:305-313.

123. Combs GF, Clark LC, Turnbull BW: Reduction of cancer risk with an oral supplement of selenium. *Biomed Environ Sci* 1997;10:227-234.

124. Bushman JL: Green tea and cancer in humans: a review of the literature. *Nutr Cancer* 1998;31: 151-159.

125. Dorant E, van den Brandt PA, Goldbohm RA: A prospective cohort study on the relationship between onion and leek consumption, garlic supplement use and the risk of colorectal carcinoma in The Netherlands. *Carcinogenesis* 1996;17: 477-484.

126. Steinmetz KA, Kushi LH, Bostick RM, et al: Vegetables, fruit, and colon cancer in the Iowa Women's Health Study. *Am J Epidemiol* 1994; 139:1-15.

127. Fleischauer AT, Poole C, Arab L: Garlic consumption and cancer prevention: meta-analyses of colorectal and stomach cancers. *Am J Clin Nutr* 2000; 72:1047-1052.

128. Song K, Milner JA: Heating garlic inhibits its ability to suppress 7, 12-dimethylbenz(a)anthracene-induced DNA adduct formation in rat mammary tissue. *J Nutr* 1999;129:657-661.

129. Reddy BS, Burill C, Rigotty J: Effect of diets high in omega-3 and omega-6 fatty acids on initiation and postinitiation stages of colon carcinogenesis. *Cancer Res* 1991;51:487-491.

130. Reddy BS, Maruyama H: Effect of dietary fish oil on azoxymethane-induced colon carcinogenesis in male F344 rats. *Cancer Res* 1986;46:3367-3370.

131. Reddy BS, Sugie S: Effect of different levels of omega-3 and omega-6 fatty acids on azoxymethane-induced colon carcinogenesis in F344 rats. *Cancer Res* 1988;48:6642-6647.

132. Sakaguchi M: Relationship of tissue and tumor fatty acids to dietary fat in experimental colorectal cancer. *Gut* 1989;30:A1449.

133. Willett WC, Stampfer MJ, Colditz GA, et al: Relation of meat, fat, and fiber intake to the risk

of colon cancer in a prospective study among women. *N Engl J Med* 1990;323:1664-1672.

134. Anti M, Armelao F, Marra G, et al: Effects of different doses of fish oil on rectal cell proliferation in patients with sporadic colonic adenomas. *Gastroenterology* 1994;107:1709-1718.

135. Yun TK, Choi SY: A case-control study of ginseng intake and cancer. *Int J Epidemiol* 1990;19: 871-876.

136. Yun TK, Choi SY: Preventive effect of ginseng intake against various human cancers: a case-control study on 1987 pairs. *Cancer Epidemiol Biomarkers Prev* 1995;4:401-408.

137. Wakui A, Kasai M, Konno K, et al: [Randomized study of lentinan on patients with advanced gastric and colorectal cancer, Tohoku Lentinan Study Group]. *Gan To Kagaku Ryoho* 1986;13:1050-1059.

138. Green S: A critique of the rationale for cancer treatment with coffee enemas and diet. *JAMA* 1992;268:3224-3227.

139. Brown BT: Treating cancer with coffee enemas and diet. *JAMA* 1993;269:1635-1636.

140. Karagas MR, Greenberg ER, Nierenberg D, et al: Risk of squamous cell carcinoma of the skin in relation to plasma selenium, alpha-tocopherol, beta-carotene, and retinol: a nested case-control study. *Cancer Epidemiol Biomarkers Prev* 1997;6: 25-29.

141. Green A, Williams G, Neale R, et al: Daily sunscreen application and betacarotene supplementation in prevention of basal-cell and squamous-cell carcinomas of the skin: a randomised controlled trial. *Lancet* 1999;354:723-729.

142. Moon TE, Levine N, Cartmel B, et al: Effect of retinol in preventing squamous cell skin cancer in moderate-risk subjects: a randomized, double-blind, controlled trial, Southwest Skin Cancer Prevention Study Group. *Cancer Epidemiol Biomarkers Prev* 1997;6:949-956.

143. Levine N, Moon TE, Cartmel B, et al: Trial of retinol and isotretinoin in skin cancer prevention: a randomized, double-blind, controlled trial. Southwest Skin Cancer Prevention Study Group. *Cancer Epidemiol Biomarkers Prev* 1997;6:957-961.

144. Clark LC: The epidemiology of selenium and cancer. *Fed Proc* 1985;44:2584-2589.

145. Willett WC, Polk BF, Morris JS, et al: Prediagnostic serum selenium and risk of cancer. *Lancet* 1983;2: 130-124.

146. Ip C: The chemopreventive role of selenium in carcinogenesis. *Adv Exp Med Biol* 1986;206: 431-447.

147. Vinceti M, Rothman KJ, Bergomi M, et al: Excess melanoma incidence in a cohort exposed to high levels of environmental selenium. *Cancer Epidemiol Biomarkers Prev* 1998;7:853-856.

148. Clark LC, Jacobs ET: Environmental selenium and cancer: risk or protection? *Cancer Epidemiol Biomarkers Prev* 1998;7:847-848; discussion 851-852.

149. Kristal AR, Moe G: False presumptions and continued surprises: how much do we really know about nutritional supplements and cancer risk? *Cancer Epidemiol Biomarkers Prev* 1998;7:849-850;discussion 851-852.

150. Reinhold U, Biltz H, Bayer W, et al: Serum selenium levels in patients with malignant melanoma. *Acta Derm Venereol* 1989;69:132-136.

151. Horcicko J, Pantucek M: Hypozincemia in patients with malignant melanoma. *Clin Chim Acta* 1983;130:279-282.

152. Ros-Bullon MR, Sanchez-Pedreno P, Martinez-Liarte JH: Serum zinc levels are increased in melanoma patients. *Melanoma Res* 1998;8: 273-277.

153. Prasad ML, Parry P, Chan C: Ayurvedic agents produce differential effects on murine and human melanoma cells in vitro. *Nutr Cancer* 1993;20: 79-86.

154. Greer S: Mind-body research in psychooncology. *Adv Mind Body Med* 1999;15:236-244.

155. Shu XO, Zheng W, Potischman N, et al: A population-based case-control study of dietary factors and endometrial cancer in Shanghai, People's Republic of China. *Am J Epidemiol* 1993;137: 155-165.

156. Heinonen PK, Kuoppala T, Koskinen T, et al: Serum vitamins A and E and carotene in patients with gynecologic cancer. *Arch Gynecol Obstet* 1987;241:151-156.

157. Levi F, Franceschi S, Negri E, et al: Dietary factors and the risk of endometrial cancer. *Cancer* 1993;71:3575-3581.

158. Negri E, La Vecchia C, Franceschi S, et al: Intake of selected micronutrients and the risk of endometrial carcinoma. *Cancer* 1996;77:917-923.

159. Jennings E: Folic acid as a cancer-preventing agent. *Med Hypotheses* 1995;45:297-303.

160. Levi F, La Vecchia C, Negri E, et al: Selected physical activities and the risk of endometrial cancer. *Br J Cancer* 1993;67:846-851.

161. Shu XO, Hatch MC, Zheng W, et al: Physical activity and risk of endometrial cancer. *Epidemiology* 1993;4:342-349.

162. Olson SH, Vena JE, Dorn JP, et al: Exercise, occupational activity, and risk of endometrial cancer. *Ann Epidemiol* 1997;7:46-53.

163. Wideroff L, Potischman N, Glass AG, et al: A nested case-control study of dietary factors and the risk of incident cytological abnormalities of the cervix. *Nutr Cancer* 1998;30:130-136.

164. Mackerras D, Irwig L, Simpson JM, et al: Randomized double-blind trial of beta-carotene and vitamin C in women with minor cervical abnormalities. *Br J Cancer* 1999;79: 1448-1453.

165. Butterworth CE, Hatch KD, Gore H, et al: Improvement in cervical dysplasia associated with folic acid therapy in users of oral contraceptives. *Am J Clin Nutr* 1982;35:73-82.

166. Butterworth CE, Hatch KD, Soong SJ, et al: Oral folic acid supplementation for cervical dysplasia: a clinical intervention trial. *Am J Obstet Gynecol* 1992;166:803-809.

167. Childers JM, Chu J, Voigt LF, et al: Chemoprevention of cervical cancer with folic acid: a phase III Southwest Oncology Group Intergroup study. *Cancer Epidemiol Biomarkers Prev* 1995;4: 155-159.

168. Manetta A, Schubbert T, Chapman J, et al: Beta-carotene treatment of cervical intraepithelial neoplasia: a phase II study. *Cancer Epidemiol Biomarkers Prev* 1996;5:929-932.

169. de Vet HC, Knipschild PG, Willebrand D, et al: The effect of beta-carotene on the regression and progression of cervical dysplasia: a clinical experiment. *J Clin Epidemiol* 1991;44:273-283.

170. Romney SL, Ho GY, Palan PR, et al: Effects of beta-carotene and other factors on outcome of cervical dysplasia and human papillomavirus infection. *Gynecol Oncol* 1997;65:483-492.

171. Meyskens FL, Surwit E, Moon TE, et al: Enhancement of regression of cervical intraepithelial neoplasia II (moderate dysplasia) with topically applied all-trans-retinoic acid: a randomized trial. *J Natl Cancer Inst* 1994;86: 539-543.

172. Romney SL, Palan PR, Duttagupta C, et al: Retinoids and the prevention of cervical dysplasias. *Am J Obstet Gynecol* 1981;141:890-894.

173. Wylie-Rosett JA, Romney SL, Slagle NS, et al: Influence of vitamin A on cervical dysplasia and carcinoma in situ. *Nutr Cancer* 1984;6:49-57.

174. Ramaswamy G, Krishnamoorthy L: Serum carotene, vitamin A, and vitamin C levels in breast cancer and cancer of the uterine cervix. *Nutr Cancer* 1996;25:173-177.

175. Harris RW, Forman D, Doll R, et al: Cancer of the cervix uteri and vitamin A. *Br J Cancer* 1986;53:653-659.

176. Potischman N, Brinton LA: Nutrition and cervical neoplasia. *Cancer Causes Control* 1996;7:113-126.

177. Nagata C, Shimizu H, Higashiiwai H, et al: Serum retinol level and risk of subsequent cervical cancer in cases with cervical dysplasia. *Cancer Invest* 1999;17:253-258.

178. Lehtinen M, Luostarinen T, Youngman LD, et al: Low levels of serum vitamins A and E in blood and subsequent risk for cervical cancer: interaction with HPV seropositivity. *Nutr Cancer* 1999;34:229-234.

179. Basu J, Palan PR, Vermund SH, et al: Plasma ascorbic acid and beta-carotene levels in women evaluated for HPV infection, smoking, and cervix dysplasia. *Cancer Detect Prev* 1991;15:165-170.

180. Palan PR, Chang CJ, Mikhail MS, et al: Plasma concentrations of micronutrients during a nine-month clinical trial of beta-carotene in women with precursor cervical cancer lesions. *Nutr Cancer* 1998;30:46-52.

181. Block G: Vitamin C and cancer prevention: the epidemiologic evidence. *Am J Clin Nutr* 1991;53: 270S-282S.

182. Potischman N: Nutritional epidemiology of cervical neoplasia. *J Nutr* 1993;123:424-429.

183. Knekt P: Serum vitamin E level and risk of female cancers. *Int J Epidemiol* 1988;17:281-286.

184. van Niekerk W: Cervical cytologic abnormalities caused by folic acid deficiency. *Acta Cytol* 1966;10: 67-73.

185. Whitehead N, Reyner F, Lindenbaum J: Megaloblastic changes in the cervical epithelium. Association with oral contraceptive therapy and reversal with folic acid. *JAMA* 1973;226:1421-1424.

186. Butterworth CE, Hatch KD, Macaluso M, et al: Folate deficiency and cervical dysplasia. *JAMA* 1992;267:528-533.

187. Kwasniewska A, Tukendorf A, Semczuk M: Folate deficiency and cervical intraepithelial neoplasia. *Eur J Gynaecol Oncol* 1997;18:526-530.

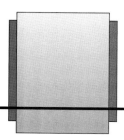

Index

A

A2 allele of CYP17, endometrial cancer and, 278
Aberrant crypt foci, 78
ACBE. *See* Air-contrast barium enema
Acetic acid application, vulvar intraepithelial neoplasia (VIN) and, 209, 213f, 223
ACF. *See* Human aberrant crypt foci
Actinic keratoses (AKs), 132f
 precancerous, 131
Adenocarcinomas, 16, 66
 cervical cancer and, 149
 extramammary Paget's disease (EMPD) of vulva and, 237
Adenomas. *See* Benign polyps
Adenomatous polyposis coli (APC), 88, 89
 diagram of, 91f
 mutation representation of, 92f
 ulcerative colitis (UC) and, 95
Adenomatous polyps
 color of, 87
 colorectal cancer (CRC) and, 81
 distribution of, 81
Adolescents
 cigarette advertising and, 31
 nicotine addiction and, 31, 34
 smoking cessation for, 34–35
 smoking incidence in, 32
 smoking prevalence in, 32–33, 32t, 33t
 smoking prevention for, 34
 smoking risk factors for, 33
 tobacco use and, 31–32
Advertising, smoking prevalence and, 12–13
Aerodigestive cancer, 15
African-American women, with breast cancer, 49
Agency for Healthcare Research and Quality (AHRQ), 23
AHRQ. *See* Agency for Healthcare Research and Quality
Air-contrast barium enema (ACBE), colorectal cancer (CRC) and, 100–101
AJCC. *See* American Joint Committee on Cancer
AKs. *See* Actinic keratoses
Alcohol abuse, smoking prevalence and, 18–19
Alcohol consumption
 breast cancer and, 54–55, 66
 hyperinsulinemia and, 54–55
Alpha-difluoromethylornithine (DFMO), cervical cancer and, 165

Alpha Tocopherol Beta Carotene (ATBC) study, 36
American Academy of Family Physicians, 293
American Cancer Society, 103, 122, 190, 278
 colorectal polyps/cancer screening guidelines of, 99t
American College of Medical Genetics, 293
American Joint Committee on Cancer (AJCC), 231
 Prognostic Factors Consensus Conference, 71–72
American Polyp Prevention Trial, 76
American Society of Clinical Oncology (ASCO), 294, 296
American Society of Human Genetics (ASHG), 293
Amygdalin, 309
Anastasiadis, P., 205
Andrieu. N., 51
Angiogenesis, 307
Anoscopy, vulvar intraepithelial neoplasia (VIN) and, 213
Anovulation, endometrial cancer and, 275
Antiviral agents, for vulvar intraepithelial neoplasia (VIN), 227, 228b
APC. *See* Adenomatous polyposis coli
Apoptosis, 152, 154
Arsenic
 Bowen's disease and, 129
 skin cancer and, 129
Asbestos, ovarian cancer and, 254
ASCO. *See* American Society of Clinical Oncology
ASCUS. *See* Atypical squamous cells of undetermined significance
ASHG. *See* American Society of Human Genetics
Ashkenazi Jews, breast cancer and, 58, 58t, 59
Aspirin, for colorectal chemoprevention, 107
Assiskis, V. J., 275
Asymptomatic status, cancer screening in, 2
ATBC study. *See* Alpha Tocopherol Beta Carotene
Atypical hyperplasia, 10
 breast cancer and, 53
Atypical squamous cells of undetermined significance (ASCUS), 167, 169, 173, 174, 175
Australian immigrants, colorectal cancer (CRC) and, 74–75
Australian Polyp Prevention Project, 76

B

Barium enema (BE), colorectal cancer (CRC) and, 100–101
Basal cell carcinoma (BCC), 122
    appearance of, 122–123, 123f
    incidence rates of, 122, 124
    location of, 122
    morpheaform of, 125f
    from occupational hazards, 128
Basset, A., 197
BCC. *See* Basal cell carcinoma
BE. *See* Barium enema
Behavioral Risk Factor Surveillance System, 104
Benign hyperplasias, 10
Benign polyps, colorectal cancer (CRC) and, 78
Bergen, S., 238
Berger, B. W., 218
Beta-carotene
    for breast cancer, 310, 311
    for cervical cancer, 326
    as complementary & alternative medicine (CAM), 309
    for endometrial cancer, 324
    for lung cancer, 315–316, 316t
    as retinoids, 36
    for skin cancer, 322–323
Bethesda system
    2001 cytology reporting system of, 170, 171b–172b
    of Papanicolaou (Pap) smear, 167–170
    strengths of, 167–170, 168b
Biomarkers, of lung cancer, 36. *See also* Molecular markers
Bjørge, T., 205
Black cohosh, 307
BMI. *See* Body mass index
Body mass index (BMI), 273, 277
    endometrial cancer and, 273
Bowen's disease, 200, 224
    arsenic and, 129
Brain, nicotine and, 20–21
BRCA1, 58, 59, 66, 253, 254, 296
    breast cancer and, 57, 57t
    genetic testing and, 292, 293
    molecular aspects of, 57t
    mutations of, 58t, 59, 60
    various ethnicities and, 58t
BRCA2, 58, 59, 66, 253, 254, 296
    breast cancer and, 57, 57t
    genetic testing and, 292, 293
    molecular aspects of, 57t
    mutations of, 58t, 59, 60
    various ethnicities and, 58t
Breast cancer, 15
    affected relatives with, 56, 56t
    African-American women with, 49
    age at first birth and, 50–51
    alcohol consumption and, 53, 54–55
    Ashkenazi Jews and, 58, 58t, 59
    atypical hyperplasia and, 53
    beta-carotene for, 310, 311
    BRCA1 and, 57, 57t

Breast cancer (*Continued*)
    BRCA2 and, 57, 57t
    breast-feeding and, 51
    breast/ovarian familial syndromes and, 56–57, 57t
    Cancer and Steroid Hormone (CASH) study on, 51
    chemoprevention and, 61, 62–63, 66
    complementary & alternative medicine (CAM) and, 310–315
    Cowden's syndrome and, 56, 57t
    dietary factors in, 50b, 54–55
    dietary fat and, 55
    early operable, 49
    endocrine factors in, 50b, 51–54
    endogenous hormones and, 51–52
    environmental risk factors of, 61–62
    estradiol and, 53
    exogenous hormones and, 52–54
    fenretinide and, 63
    fertility drugs and, 53–54, 66
    folate for, 313
    genetic/familial factors in, 50b, 56–61, 57t
    genetic testing for, 60, 292, 293
    green tea and, 314
    hormone replacement therapy and, 52–53
    incidence of, 48–50
        by ethnicity, 49
    individuals at risk of, 59
    ionizing radiation and, 61
    Li-Fraumeni syndrome and, 56, 57t
    lung cancer and, 14, 14t
    Lynch syndrome and, 56, 57t
    magnetic resonance imaging (MRI) and, 65
    mammography for, 63–64
    melatonin for, 313
    menarche/menstrual cycles and, 50
    monoterpenes and, 314–315
    Nurse's Health Study on, 52, 55
    obesity and, 53, 55, 66
    olive oil and, 314–315
    oral contraceptives and, 52
    organochlorines and, 61–62
    ovarian ablation and, 52
    ovarian cancer and, 57
    parity and, 51
    physical activity and, 55–56
    phytoestrogens for, 313–314
    prevention of, 48–66
    primary prevention of, 62
    proliferation lesions and, 53
    prophylactic mastectomy and, 62, 66
    raloxifene and, 63
    reproductive factors in, 50–54, 50b
    retinoids for, 63, 310
    risk by age, 49t
    risk factors of, 48–66, 50b
    screening for, 63–64, 66
    secondary prevention and, 63–65
    selenium for, 313
    soy intake and, 314t
    synthetic retinoid fenretinide for, 310–311

Breast cancer (*Continued*)
   tamoxifen and, 62–63
   testing for, 59–60
   vitamin A for, 310, 311
   vitamin B_{12} for, 313
   vitamin C for, 312
   vitamin D for, 312–313
   vitamin E for, 312
   White women with, 49
Breast Cancer Prevention Trial (BCPT), 62
Breast examination, 64–65
Breast-feeding, breast cancer and, 51
Breast/ovarian familial syndromes, breast cancer
   and, 56–57, 57t
Breslow, A., 231
Brinton, L. A., 151, 207
Burkitt, D. P., 76
Burkitt's lymphoma, 77
Buscema, J., 218, 219
Butler, L. M., 50

C
CA125, endometrial cancer and, 283
Calcium, as colorectal chemoprevention, 108–109
CAM. *See* Complementary and alternative medicine
Cancer
   detectable preclinical phase of, 10
   growth rapidity of, 10
   National Center for Complementary and
      Alternative Medicine (NCCAM) and, 307
   screening-detected outcomes of, 10
Cancer and Steroid Hormone (CASH) study, 275
   on breast cancer, 51
   on endometrial cancer, 276, 277
Cancer control phases, evaluation process for, 8
Cancer detection. *See* Cancer screening
Cancer Information Services (CIS), 308
Cancer intervention, cancer screening and, 9
Cancer mortality
   cancer screening and, 9
   from cervical cancer, 148
   from endometrial cancer, 267–270
   females rates of, 149f
   from lung cancer, 12, 36
   from melanoma, 137–138
   from nonmelanoma skin cancer (NMSC), 122
   rates of, 14t
Cancer prevention, 1–2
   of breast cancer, 48–66
   cancer screening and, 1–2, 9
   cervical cancer and, 160–179
   complementary & alternative medicine (CAM)
      and, 306–329
   of endometrial cancer, 278–283
   of melanoma, 143–144
   ovarian cancer of, 255
   of skin cancer, 131
   for vaginal cancer, 192
Cancer Registry, 122
Cancer screening
   abnormal results in, 2–3
   applicability of, 3

Cancer screening (*Continued*)
   asymptomatic status in, 2
   cancer intervention and, 9
   cancer prevention and, 1–2, 9
   for cervical cancer, 160–162
   community dissemination of, 9
   controversy over, 1
   cost-effectiveness of, 4
   costs of, 5b
   defined population for, 9
   definition of, 1
   demonstration/implementation programs and, 9
   diagnosis and, 2–3
   effectiveness of, 4
   efficacy of, 9
   for endometrial cancer, 278–279
   epidemiologic measurements and, 5–7
   evaluation process circumvention in, 9
   expected benefits of, 8
   familial adenomatous polyposis coli (FAP) and,
      91
   genetic markers and, 1
   goal of, 2
   governing principles of, 7–8, 7t
   for hamartomatous polyposis syndromes, 93
   lead-time bias in, 9, 10
   length bias in, 9, 10
   long-term measures of, 4
   methodological research in, 9
   molecular markers and, 1
   mortality reduction and, 9
   nationwide, 9
   normal results in, 2–3
   outcomes of, 4, 4b
   for ovarian cancer, 259, 261, 262, 262f
   overdiagnosis bias in, 9, 10–11
   pilot studies of, 9
   potential harm of, 8
   practitioner of, 2
   predictive value/cancer prevalence, 7t
   principles of, 1–11
   short-term measures of, 4
   for skin cancer, 133
   strategy/protocol for, 3
   survival times and, 9, 10
   target population of, 2, 3, 9
   test for, 2
   treatment and, 7
   types of, 1
   for vaginal cancer, 192
   validity measures of, 6t
Cancer screening strategy
   clinical acceptance for, 9
   community dissemination of, 9
   expense of, 9
   quality control process for, 9
Carbon dioxide laser vaporization therapy, for
      vulvar intraepithelial neoplasia (VIN),
      222–227, 227
Carcinoembryonic antigen (CEA), colorectal cancer
      (CRC) and, 72
Carcinogen metabolism, genetic factors in, 15

Carcinogenesis
    chemoprevention and, 35
    of colorectal cancer (CRC), 77, 78–79, 80f
Carcinogens
    polycyclic aromatic hydrocarbons (PAHs) as, 16
    in tobacco smoke, 16
Carcinoma, 10
CARET. *See* Carotene and Retinol Efficacy Trial
Carotene and Retinol Efficacy Trial (CARET), 36
Carotenoids, for colon cancer, 319
Carter, J., 208
CASH study. *See* Cancer and Steroid Hormone study
Cat's claw, 309
CCA. *See* Clear cell adenocarcinomas
CEA. *See* Carcinoembryonic antigen
Cell adhesion, 307
Center for Cancer Complementary Medicine, at
        Johns Hopkins University, 307
Centers for Disease Control, 51, 275
Cervical cancer
    adenocarcinomas and, 149
    alpha-difluoromethylornithine (DFMO) and,
        165
    beta-carotene for, 326
    chemoprevention for, 164–165
    complementary & alternative medicine (CAM)
        for, 325–329
    contraception and, 157–158
    dietary factors in, 158–159
    ethnicity groups and, 148, 149f
    folate for, 327
    folic acid and, 160
    herpes simplex virus (HSV) and, 155–156
    histologic types and, 148–150
    human immunodeficiency virus (HIV) and, 156
    human papillomavirus (HPV) and, 151–155,
        172–174
    incidence of, 148, 149f
    male sexual behavior and, 156–157
    micronutrients for, 325t
    mortality of, 148, 149f
    nomenclature of, 150t
    oral contraceptives and, 157–158
    Papanicolaou (Pap) smear and, 150, 161–163,
        165–170
    prevention and, 160–179
    prophylactic vaccines and, 163–164
    reproductive/sexual factors in, 151
    retinoids for, 164–165, 326
    risk factors for, 151–161, 157b
    screening for, 160–162
    sexual behavioral changes and, 160–162
    sexually transmitted diseases (STDs) and, 151
    squamous cell carcinoma (SCC) and, 149
    staging of, 148–150, 150t
    Surveillance Epidemiology and End Results
        (SEER) and, 158
    tobacco exposure and, 160–161
    vaginal cancer and, 190
    vitamin A for, 159, 326
    vitamin C for, 160, 326–327
    vitamin E for, 159, 327

Cervical intraepithelial neoplasia (CIN), 199
    cold knife cone biopsy for, 178
    cryotherapy for, 177
    laser vaporization for, 177–178
    loop electrosurgical excision for, 178
    management of, 177–179
    surgery for, 177
Chalmydia trachomatis, 207
Chemoprevention
    agents of, 106
    breast cancer and, 61, 62–63, 66
    carcinogenesis and, 35
    for cervical cancer, 164–165
    of colorectal cancer (CRC), 106–111
    epidermal growth factor receptor (EGFR) and, 36
    epidermal growth factor receptor (EGFR)
        inhibitors and, 38
    familial adenomatous polyposis coli (FAP) and,
        91
    of lung cancer, 35–38
    principles of, 35–36
    proliferation markers and, 106
    prostaglandin pathway inhibitors and, 37–38
    retinoid receptors RAR/RXR and, 36
    retinoids and, 36–37
    selenium and, 37
    targeted agents in, 37–38
Chemotherapy, colorectal cancer (CRC) for, 70–71
Chesterfield cigarettes, 13
Chie, W. C., 50
Chiechi, L. M., 53
Childhood sun overexposure, skin cancer and, 131
Chinese herbs, 309
Chippers, 19–20
Chlorofluorocarbons (CFCs), ozone layer and, 128
Chromosomal deletions, 78
Chung, A, F., 231
Cidofovir, for vulvar intraepithelial neoplasia
        (VIN), 230
Cigarette advertising, adolescents and, 31
Cigarette smoking. *See* Smoking
CIN. *See* Cervical intraepithelial neoplasia
Clarke, W. H. Jr., 231
Clear cell adenocarcinomas (CCA), vaginal cancer
        and, 191
Clear cell carcinoma, endometrial cancer and, 283,
        284
CLIA. *See* Clinical Laboratory Improvement
        Amendments
Clinical Laboratory Improvement Amendments
        (CLIA), 293
CO_2 laser vaporization, for vaginal intraepithelial
        neoplasia (VAIN), 193
Coley's toxin, 309
Collins, C. G., 212, 219
Colon cancer
    carotenoids for, 319
    complementary & alternative medicine (CAM)
        for, 318–321
    dietary mixtures for, 320–321
    fish oil for, 320–321
    folate for, 319–320

Colon cancer (*Continued*)
  garlic for, 320–321
  green tea for, 320
  hydro-colon therapy for, 321
  panax ginseng for, 321
  selenium for, 320
  shiitake mushroom for, 321
  vitamin A for, 319
  vitamin C for, 319
  vitamin E for, 319
  vitamins for, 319t
Colon/rectum, arterial blood supply of, 70f
Colonic epithelium, 78
Colonocytes, 78
Colonoscopy (CS), 104
  colorectal cancer (CRC) and, 97, 101–102
  hysterectomy and, 101
  ulcerative colitis (UC) and, 97
Colorectal adenocarcinomas, 84f, 85f
  histopathology spectrum of, 86f
  hyperplastic polyps (HPs) and, 85–88
  morphogenesis model of, 75f
  physical activity and, 76
  tobacco use and, 76
Colorectal adenomas, 80, 83f
Colorectal cancer (CRC), 69–110
  adenomatous polyps and, 81, 82
  air-contrast barium enema (ACBE) and, 100–101
  anatomy of, 69, 70f
  Australian immigrants and, 74–75
  barium enema (BE) and, 100–101
  benign polyps and, 78
  carcinoembryonic antigen (CEA) and, 72
  carcinogenesis of, 77, 78–79, 80f
  chemoprevention of, 106–111
  chemotherapy for, 70–71
  colonoscopy (CS) and, 97, 101–102
  curability of, 69
  diet and, 75–76
  dietary fat and, 75
  dietary fiber and, 76
  Dukes staging system for, 71
  environmental influence in, 74–75
  epidemiology of, 73, 74
  ethnicity/race incidence rates of, 73
  etiology of, 73
  familial adenomatous polyposis coli (FAP) and, 73, 74f
  familial causes of, 73, 74f
  fecal occult blood testing (FOBT) and, 98
  flexible sigmoidoscopy and, 98, 100
  gene-gene interactions and, 73
  genetic model of, 89f
  geographic differences and, 74–75
  hamartomatous polyposis syndromes and, 93
  hereditary, 88–95
  hereditary nonpolyposis colorectal cancer (HNPCC) and, 73, 74f, 93–95
  heterocyclic amines and, 76
  high temperature cooking and, 76
  histology of, 69–70, 71f
  human aberrant crypt foci (ACF), 80, 81, 81f, 82f

Colorectal cancer (CRC) (*Continued*)
  inflammatory bowel disease and, 95–97
  Japanese immigrants and, 74
  molecular genetics and, 77
  Nurses' Health Study of, 75, 76
  perineural invasion and, 72
  primary prevention of, 106–111
  prognostic factors for, 71–72
  proliferation zone of, 80
  radiation for, 71
  rare syndromes of, 74f
  recessive traits and, 73
  red meat and, 75–76
  screening and, 73, 103, 105–106
  sporadic, 74f, 78
  surgical resection for, 70–71
  Surveillance Epidemiology and End Results (SEER) and, 71
  survival rates for, 73
  susceptibility genes and, 75
  TNM staging system and, 71, 72t
  treatment cost-effectiveness and, 105–106
  treatment of, 70–71
  ulcerative colitis (UC) and, 95–97
  virtual colonoscopy (VCS) and, 102–103
Colorectal carcinogenesis, molecular genetics of, 88
Colorectal chemoprevention
  calcium as, 108–109
  difluoromethylornithine as, 109
  folate as, 109–110
  hormone replacement therapy as, 109–110
  nonsteroidal anti-inflammatory agents (NSAIDs) as, 107–108
  oltipraz as, 110
  urosidal as, 110
Colorectal crypt, proliferation zone of, 80, 80f
Colorectal polyps/cancer, early detection guidelines for, 99t
Colposcopy, cervical cancer and, 170, 172
Columbia University, 308
Community dissemination, cancer screening strategy and, 9
Complementary and alternative medicine (CAM), 306
  beta-carotene as, 309
  for breast cancer, 310–315
  cancer prevention and, 306–329
  for cervical cancer, 325–329
  classification of, 307, 307t
  for colon cancer, 318–321
  definition of, 306–307
  demand for, 307
  effectiveness of, 306
  for end-of-life care, 307
  for endometrial cancer, 324–325
  folate as, 310
  garlic as, 310
  green tea as, 310
  literature review methodology for, 308–309
  for lung cancer, 315–318
  melatonin as, 310
  monoterpenes as, 310

Complementary and alternative
   medicine (*Continued*)
   olive oil as, 310
   phytoestrogens as, 309–310
   potential anticarcinogenic action of, 309–310
   retinoids as, 309
   selenium as, 309
   shiitake mushroom as, 310
   for skin cancer, 321–324, 322t
   vitamin A, 309
   vitamin B$_{12}$ as, 310
   vitamin C as, 309
   vitamin D as, 310
   vitamin E as, 309
Computed tomography (CT)
   endometrial cancer and, 282–283
   lung cancer and, 38
   lung cancer screening and, 39–40
Conjugated equine estrogens, 275
Contraception, cervical cancer and, 157–158. *See
   also* Oral contraceptives
Cooking, high temperature
   colorectal cancer (CRC) and, 76
   lung cancer and, 17
Coronary heart disease, hormone replacement
   therapy and, 53
Counseling
   familial adenomatous polyposis coli (FAP) and,
     91
   genetic testing and, 91, 297–298, 299
   for hormone replacement therapy, 53
   tobacco use cessation and, 23
Cowden's syndrome, breast cancer and, 56, 57t
COX–2 inhibitors, prostaglandin pathway
   inhibitors and, 37–38
Cramer, D. W., 252
CRC. *See* Colorectal cancer
Cryosurgery
   for vulvar cervical intraepithelial neoplasia
     (CIN), 177, 228
   for vulvar intraepithelial neoplasia (VIN), 227,
     228b
CS. *See* Colonoscopy
CT scanning. *See* Computed tomographic
   scanning
CXR. *See* Traditional chest radiography
Cyclooxygenase inhibitors, prostaglandin pathway
   inhibitors and, 37
CYP1A1 genes, lung cancer and, 15
CYP1A2 genes, lung cancer and, 15
Cytochrome P450 activating enzymes, 15

D
D & C. *See* Dilatation & curettage
DCC genes. *See* Deleted in colorectal cancer genes
Deleted in colorectal cancer (DCC) genes, 88
Demonstration/implementation programs, cancer
   screening and, 9
Dermatology screening, for melanoma, 143
DES. *See* Diethylstilbestrol
DFMO. *See* Difluoromethylornithine
Diabetes, endometrial cancer and, 273

Dietary fat
   breast cancer and, 55
   colorectal cancer (CRC) and, 75
   endometrial cancer and, 277
Dietary mixtures
   for colon cancer, 320–321
   for lung cancer, 318
Dietary risk factors
   in breast cancer, 50b, 54–55
   cervical cancer in, 158–159
   colorectal cancer (CRC) and, 75–76
   endometrial cancer and, 276–277
   ovarian cancer and, 252, 254
   vulvar cancer and, 205
Dietary supplements, for endometrial cancer,
   324t
Diethylstilbestrol (DES), vaginal cancer and, 191,
   192
Differentiation markers, molecular risk assessment
   and, 230
Difluoromethylornithine (DFMO), as colorectal
   chemoprevention, 109
Dilatation & curettage (D & C), 281
Dinitrochlorobenzene (DNCB), for vulvar
   intraepithelial neoplasia (VIN), 227
DiSaia, P. J., 274
Distant healing, 307
DNA
   damage to, 77
   hereditary nonpolyposis colon cancer and
     (HNPCC), 93
   hypomethylation of, 88
   repair mechanisms of, 77
DNCB. *See* Dinitrochlorobenzene
Dolan, N. C., 132
Dopamine transmission, nicotine and, 15–6
Dose-response relationship, in tobacco use
   cessation, 23
Double-contrast barium enema (DCBE), 104
Dubrewilh, W., 233
Ductal carcinoma in situ (DCIS), 63, 66
Dukes staging system, for colorectal cancer (CRC),
   71
DUS. *See* Dysfunctional uterine bleeding
Duty to warn
   Florida Supreme Court ruling on, 300–301
   genetic testing and, 300–301
   Pate v. Threlkel case on, 300–301
   Superior Court of New Jersey on, 301
Dysfunctional uterine bleeding (DUS), endometrial
   cancer and, 279
Dysplastic epithelium, 78

E
Early detection. *See* Cancer screening
Early Lung Cancer Action Project (ELCAP), 40
Echinacea, 309
Education, smoking prevalence and, 18–19
EGFR. *See* Epidermal growth factor receptor
ELSI. *See* Ethical/legal/social implications
EMPD of vulva. *See* Extramammary Paget's disease
   of vulva

End-of-life care, complementary & alternative medicine (CAM) for, 307
Endocervical brush, for Papanicolaou (Pap) smear, 167f
Endocrine risk factors
    in breast cancer, 50b, 51–54
    for endometrial cancer, 272
Endocrinopathies, endometrial cancer and, 275
Endogenous hormones, breast cancer and, 51–52
Endometrial cancer, 282
    A2 allele of CYP17 and, 278
    abnormal vaginal bleeding and, 279
    anovulation and, 275
    beta-carotene for, 324
    biopsy for, 281
    body mass index (BMI) and, 273
    CA125 and, 283
    Cancer and Steroid Hormone (CASH) study and, 276
    Cancer and Steroid Hormone (CASH) study on, 277
    clear cell carcinoma and, 283, 284
    complementary & alternative medicine (CAM) for, 324–325
    computed tomography (CT) and, 282–283
    curability of, 267
    diabetes and, 273
    dietary fat and, 277
    dietary risks and, 276–277
    dietary supplements for, 324t
    dysfunctional uterine bleeding (DUS) and, 279
    early diagnosis and, 278–283
    endocrine risk for, 272
    endocrinopathies and, 275
    endometrial hyperplasia and, 279–280, 279b
    estrogen replacement therapy (ERT) and, 274
    ethnicity/race differences in, 269–270
    familial history and, 277
    genetic risks and, 277
    hereditary nonpolyposis colon cancer (HNPCC) gene and, 270, 277, 278, 279
    histopathologic types/grades, 268b
    hyperplasia and, 279
    hysteroscopy and, 281–282
    incidence of, 267–270, 269t
    Iowa Women's Health Study and, 270, 273
    lifestyle risks and, 276–277
    magnetic resonance imaging (MRI) and, 282–283
    menarche/menstrual cycles and, 273
    menstruation span and, 273
    mortality of, 267–270, 269t
    obesity and, 272–273
    oncogenes and, 278
    oral contraceptives and, 275
    Papanicolaou (Pap) test and, 282
    prevention of, 278–283
    raloxifene and, 275
    reproductive risks for, 270–272
    retinoids for, 324
    risk factors for, 270–278
    screening for, 278–279

Endometrial cancer (*Continued*)
    smoking and, 276
    staging for, 267, 269t
    Surveillance Epidemiology and End Results (SEER) and, 275
    survival rates of, 267, 268t, 271–272
    tamoxifen and, 62, 63, 275–276
    transvaginal ultrasound (TVUS) and, 282
    tumor suppressor genes and, 278
    uterine bleeding and, 279
    uterine papillary serous carcinoma and, 283–284
    vitamin A for, 324
    vitamin C for, 324
    vitamin E for, 324
Endometrial carcinoma. *See* Endometrial cancer
Endometrial hyperplasia
    endometrial cancer and, 279–280, 279b
    treatment for, 280, 280f, 281
Environmental risk factors
    of breast cancer, 61–62
    in ovarian cancer, 254–55
Environmental tobacco smoke (ETS), lung cancer and, 17
Epidemiologic studies
    cancer screening and, 5–7
    on lung cancer, 13
    negative predictive value of, 6
    positive/negative tests and, 5
    positive predictive value of, 6
    prevalence/incidence rates and, 5
    specificity of, 6
    on tobacco smoke, 13
Epidermal growth factor receptor (EGFR)
    chemoprevention and, 36, 38
    inhibitors of, 38
    overexpression of, 38
Epithelial dysplasia histopathology, of ulcerative colitis (UC), 96f
Epithelial ovarian cancer
    epidemiology of, 249–250
    oral contraceptives and, 275
ERT. *See* Estrogen replacement therapy
Erythroplasia of Queyrat, 200
Essential minerals, for skin cancer, 323
Essiac, 309
Estradiol, breast cancer and, 53
Estrogen, melanoma and, 141, 143
Estrogen replacement therapy (ERT), endometrial cancer and, 274
Ethical framework, for genetic testing, 301–303
Ethical/legal/social implications (ELSI), of genetic testing, 295–296
Ethnicity groups
    cervical cancer and, 148
    tobacco use and, 14
Etretinate, as retinoids, 36
ETS. *See* Environmental tobacco smoke
Evista. *See* Raloxifene
Exogenous hormones, breast cancer and, 52–54
Extramammary Paget's disease (EMPD) of vulva, 233–239
    adenocarcinomas and, 237

Extramammary Paget's disease (EMPD)
    of vulva (*Continued*)
    clinical appearance of, 236, 236f
    histology of, 237, 238
    incidence of, 235
    manifestations of, 235–236
    recurrence of, 239
    risk factors of, 236
    treatment for, 239

F
False-negative screening test, 3, 5, 8
False-positive screening test, 1, 3, 8
Familial adenomatous polyposis coli (FAP)
    chemoprevention and, 91
    colorectal cancer (CRC) and, 73, 74f, 88–91, 90f
    counseling and, 91
    gene testing for, 91
    proctolectomy and, 91
    screening and, 91
Familial history
    endometrial cancer and, 277
    melanoma and, 140–141
Familial retinoblastoma, 78
Family history, lung cancer and, 15
FAP. *See* Familial adenomatous polyposis coli
FDA. *See* Food and Drug Administration
Fecal occult blood testing (FOBT), colorectal cancer
    (CRC) and, 98
Fehr, M. K., 229
Fenretinide, breast cancer and, 63
Ferenczy, A., 224
Fertility drugs, breast cancer and, 53–54, 66
FIGO. *See* International Federation of Gynecology
    and Obstetrics
Fish oil, for colon cancer, 320–321
5-fluorouracil (5-FU)
    for vaginal intraepithelial neoplasia (VAIN), 193
    for vulvar intraepithelial neoplasia (VIN),
        227–228
Flexible sigmoidoscopy, colorectal cancer (CRC)
    and, 98, 100
Florida Supreme Court ruling, on duty to warn,
    300–301
FOBT. *See* Fecal occult blood testing
Folate
    for breast cancer, 313
    for cervical cancer, 327
    for colon cancer, 319–320
    as colorectal chemoprevention, 109–110
    as complementary & alternative medicine
        (CAM), 310
Folic acid, cervical cancer and, 160
Food and Drug Administration (FDA), 308
Forney, J. P., 219
Franklin, E. W., 206, 208
Fred Hutchinson Cancer Research Center, 204
Friedrich, E. G. Jr., 218, 219, 225

G
Gabrick, D. M., 52
Gadolinium injection, tumor enhancement and, 65

Gardiner, S. H., 219
Garlic
    for colon cancer, 320–321
    as complementary & alternative medicine
        (CAM), 310
Gender, lung cancer biology and, 16–17
Gene-gene interactions, colorectal cancer (CRC)
    and, 73
Gene mutation
    mammograms and, 65
    patient management of, 60–61
Genetic counselors, 298
Genetic discrimination, genetic testing and,
    298–299
Genetic/familial factors
    in breast cancer, 50b, 56–61, 57t
    in carcinogen metabolism, 15
    in lung cancer, 15–16
    ovarian cancer and, 252–254
    smoking behavior and, 15–16
Genetic polymorphisms
    tobacco addiction and, 14
    in tobacco carcinogen activating enzymes, 15
Genetic risks, endometrial cancer and, 277
Genetic testing
    benefits of, 289, 292–293
    BRCA1 and, 292, 293
    BRCA2 and, 292, 293
    for breast cancer, 60
    breast cancer and, 292, 293
    challenges of, 290
    clinical decisions from, 292–293
    clinical usefulness of, 293–294
    counseling and, 91, 297–298, 299
    duty to warn and, 300–301
    ethical framework for, 301–303
    ethical/legal/social implications (ELSI) of,
        289–303, 295–296
    for familial adenomatous polyposis coli (FAP), 91
    genetic discrimination and, 298–299
    Health Insurance Portability and Accountability
        Act (HIPAA) and, 298–299
    hereditary cancer and, 301–303
    informed consent and, 296–298
    insufficiencies of, 293–294
    limitations of, 291–295
    medical privacy and, 298–299
    ovarian cancer and, 292, 293
    President's Commission for Study of Ethical
        Problems in Medicine/Biomedical/Behavior
        Research and, 300
    Privacy Act of 1974 and, 298
    psychosocial risks of, 299–300
    risks of, 294
    shared decision making and, 297
    significance of, 295
    technological expansion in, 290
    uses of, 291–295
Genital tract infections, vulvar cancer and, 207
Genomic markers
    cancer screening and, 1
    molecular risk assessment and, 230

Germline mutations, in hereditary nonpolyposis colon cancer (HNPCC), 94
Gilda Radner Ovarian Detection Program, 258
Giles, G. G., 239
Ginseng, 309
Glands of Lieberkuhn, 69
Glutathione S-transferase (GST), detoxifying enzymes, 15
Glutathione S-transferase 1 (GSTM1)
    lung cancer and, 15
    skin cancer and, 131
Gorlin's syndrome, 131
Grant, P. T., 239
Green tea, 307
    breast cancer and, 314
    for colon cancer, 320
    as complementary & alternative medicine (CAM), 310
Grenz-ray therapy, skin cancer and, 129
Grossweiner, L. I., 229
GST. *See* Glutathione S-transferase
Gynecologic Oncology Group, 197, 254, 256

H
Hamartomatous polyposis syndromes, 93, 254
    colorectal cancer (CRC) and, 93
    screening for, 93
HANSI, 309
Hara, A. K., 103
Hard-core smokers, 20
Harvard Cancer Risk Index, for endometrial carcinoma, 270, 271t
Health behavior, transtheoretical model of, 162f
Health Insurance Portability and Accountability Act (HIPAA), genetic testing and, 298–299
Henson, D., 206
Herbst, Arthur, 191
Hereditary cancer, genetic testing and, 301–303
Hereditary colorectal cancer, 88–95
    familial adenomatous polyposis (FAP) coli and, 88–91, 90f
Hereditary flat adenoma syndrome, 91
Hereditary nonpolyposis colon cancer (HNPCC), 73, 74f, 93–95, 254. *See also* Lynch syndrome
    DNA repair and, 93
    endometrial cancer and, 270, 277, 278, 279
    germline mutations in, 94
    histology of, 93
    individuals with, 94
    screening for, 94–95
    survival rates of, 93
Herpes simplex virus (HSV)
    cervical cancer and, 155–156
    vulvar intraepithelial neoplasia (VIN) and, 204
Heterocyclic amines
    colorectal cancer (CRC) and, 76
    lung cancer and, 17
High enema. *See* Hydro-colon therapy
High grade squamous intraepithelial lesions (HSILs), 176
Hillemanns, P., 229
Hippocrates, 298

Histopathology spectrum, of colorectal adenocarcinomas, 86f
HIV. *See* Human immunodeficiency virus
HNPCC. *See* Hereditary nonpolyposis colon cancer
Holmes, M. D., 55
Hori, Y., 218
Hormone replacement therapy (HRT)
    breast cancer and, 52–53
    as colorectal chemoprevention, 109–110
    coronary heart disease and, 53
    counseling for, 53
    osteoporosis and, 53
Hoxsey, 309
HPs. *See* Hyperplastic polyps
HRT. *See* Hormone replacement therapy
HSV. *See* Herpes simplex virus
Human aberrant crypt foci (ACF), colorectal cancer (CRC) and, 80, 81, 81f, 82f
Human Ethical Committee at Karolinska Institute, 232
Human Genome Project, 295
Human immunodeficiency virus (HIV), 130
    cervical cancer and, 156
Human papillomavirus (HPV)
    cervical cancer and, 151–155, 172–174
    gene functions of, 152t
    genomic map of, 151, 151f
    p53 gene and, 155ff
    penile carcinoma and, 156
    prophylactic vaccines for, 163–164
    skin cancer and, 130
    squamous cell carcinoma (SCC) and, 130
    testing for, 172–174
    types of, 153t, 154t
    vaccine for, 192
    vaginal cancer and, 190, 192
    vaginal intraepithelial neoplasia (VAIN) and, 190
    vulvar cancer and, 197, 203–204, 220
Hydro-colon therapy, for colon cancer, 321
Hyperinsulinemia, alcohol consumption and, 54–55
Hyperplasias
    atypical, 10
    benign, 10
Hypomethylation of DNA, 88
Hysterectomy
    colonoscopy (CS) and, 101
    ovarian cancer and, 255
    vaginal cancer and, 191, 192
Hysteroscopy, endometrial cancer and, 281–282

I
Ileoanal anastomosis, ulcerative colitis (UC) and, 95
Ileostomy, ulcerative colitis (UC) and, 95
Immunohistochemical staining, 80
Immunosuppressive diseases, vulvar cancer and, 208
In vitro fertilization (IVF), 54
Industrial exposure, ovarian cancer and, 254
Inflammatory bowel disease, colorectal cancer (CRC) and, 95–97

Informed consent, genetic testing and, 296–298
Internal air pollution, lung cancer and, 17
International Federation of Gynecology and
        Obstetrics (FIGO), 150, 190, 201, 202, 267
International Society for the Study of Vulvar
        Diseases, 215
Interventions, for tobacco use cessation, 22–23
Ionizing radiation
    breast cancer and, 61
    skin cancer and, 129
Iowa Women's Health Study, endometrial cancer
        and, 270, 273, 277
Isotretinoin, as retinoids, 36
Italian Study Group on Vulvar Disease, 205
Iverson, T., 201
IVF. See In vitro fertilization

J

Japanese immigrants, colorectal cancer (CRC) and,
        74
Jernstrom, H. C. B., 59
Johns Hopkins Lung Project, lung cancer screening
        and, 39
Jones, R. W., 219
Jordan, V. C., 275

K

Kaplan, A. L., 225
Karagas, M. R., 129–130
Karlan, B. Y., 258
Kneale, B. L., 239
Knight, R. V. D., 224
Knudson's hypothesis, 78, 79f
Kombucha tea, 308
Kurjak, A., 260
Kurwa, H. A., 229

L

Lactose consumption, ovarian cancer and, 252
Laetrile, 309
Lagasse, L. D., 229
Lamina propria, 70
Laser vaporization, for cervical intraepithelial
        neoplasia (CIN), 177–178
LCIS. See Lobular carcinoma in situ
Lead-time bias, in cancer screening, 9, 10
LEEP. See Loop electrosurgical excision &
        fulguration procedure
Length bias, in cancer screening, 9, 10
Li-Fraumeni syndrome, breast cancer and, 56, 57t
Lipworth, L., 51
Lobraico, R. V., 229
Lobular carcinoma in situ (LCIS), 62
Loop electrosurgical excision & fulguration
        procedure (LEEP)
    for cervical intraepithelial neoplasia (CIN),
        178
    vulvar intraepithelial neoplasia (VIN) and, 224
Loss of heterozygosity (LOH), 78, 79f
Low-birth weight infants, tobacco use and, 30
Low-grade squamous intraepithelial lesions
        (LSILs), 155, 169, 173, 175–176

Low skin pigmentation, vulvar melanoma and,
        233
LPA. See Lysophosphatidic acid
LSILs. See Low-grade squamous intraepithelial
        lesions
Lucky Strikes cigarettes, 12–13
Lung cancer, 12–40
    anatomical distribution of, 16
    beta-carotene for, 315–316, 316t
    biology of, 16–17
    biomarkers of, 36
    breast cancer and, 14, 14t
    chemoprevention of, 35–38
    in Chinese women, 17
    complementary & alternative medicine (CAM)
        for, 315–318
    computed tomographic (CT) scanning and, 38
    cooking and, 17
    CYP1A1 genes and, 15
    CYP1A2 genes and, 15
    dietary mixtures for, 318
    environmental tobacco smoke (ETS) and, 17
    epidemiologic studies on, 13
    family history and, 15
    gender and, 16–17
    general incidence of, 12
    genetic factors in, 15–16
    GSTM1 genes and, 15
    heterocyclic amines and, 17
    host factors in, 15
    internal air pollution and, 17
    mainstream smoke and, 16
    melatonin for, 318
    men's incidenceof, 14
    mortality through, 36
    nonoccupational risks for, 17
    retinoids for, 315–316
    selenium for, 317, 317t, 318t
    sidestream smoke and, 17
    traditional chest radiography (CXR) and, 38
    vitamin A for, 315–316
    vitamin C for, 317
    vitamin E for, 317
    women 's risk factors in, 15–18
    women's incidence of, 13–14
        early diagnosis of, 38–40
        screening of, 38–40
    women's mortality through, 12, 13–14
Lung cancer risk
    molecular markers of, 40
    smoking cessation and, 38
Lung cancer screening
    computed tomographic (CT) scanning and,
        39–40
    Johns Hopkins Lung Project and, 39
    Mayo Lung Project and, 39
    Memorial Sloan Kettering Lung Project and, 39
    National Cancer Institute and, 39
    new imaging techniques in, 39–40
    overdiagnosis and, 39
    sputum cytology and, 39
    traditional chest radiography (CXR) and, 39

Lynch, Henry, 93
Lynch syndrome, 93
    breast cancer and, 56, 57t
Lysophosphatidic acid (LPA), ovarian cancer and,
    261

M
Macrophage colony-stimulating factor (MCS-F),
    ovarian cancer and, 261
Madeleine, M. M., 204
Magnetic resonance imaging (MRI)
    breast cancer and, 65
    endometrial cancer and, 282–283
    limitations of, 66
Mainstream smoke, lung cancer and, 16
Maitake mushroom, 308
Malignant melanoma, 230–233
    vulvar cancer and, 231
Malone, K. E., 59
Mammograms, 60, 63–64
    debate over, 64
    false-negative examinations of, 64
    false-positive examinations of, 64
    gene mutation and, 65
Mastectomy, prophylactic, 60, 61. See also Simple
    mastectomy
Mayo Lung Project, lung cancer screening and, 39
MCC genes. See Mutated in colorectal cancer genes
McLean, M. R., 219
MCS-F. See Macrophage colony-stimulating factor
Medical privacy, genetic testing and, 298–299
Medline database, 308
Medroxyprogesterone acetate (MPA), 274, 275
Melanocyte, basal skin layer and, 138f
Melanoma, 137–144. See also Skin cancer
    dermatology screening for, 143
    drawing of, 142f
    estrogen and, 141, 143
    etiology of, 138
    familial history and, 140–141
    incidence of, 137–138
    mortality of, 137–138
    nicotine and, 29–30
    nicotine replacement therapy (NRT) and, 25
    oral contraceptives and, 143
    pregnancy and, 141, 143
    presentation of, 137, 137f, 139f, 141f
    prevention of, 143–144
    risk factors for, 139–141
    self-examination for, 143
    smoking prevalence in, 29
    sun-senstive skin types and, 139
    sunscreens and, 143, 144
    tobacco use and, 29–31
    ultraviolet radiation (UVR) and, 139–140
Melatonin
    for breast cancer, 313
    as complementary & alternative medicine
        (CAM), 310
    for lung cancer, 318
Memorial Sloan Kettering Lung Project, lung cancer
    screening and, 39

Menarche/menstrual cycles
    breast cancer and, 50
    endometrial cancer and, 273
Menopause Study Group trial, 274
Menstruation span, endometrial cancer and, 273
Methodological research, in cancer screening, 9
Mezzetti, M., 55
Micronutrients, for cervical cancer, 325t
Microstaging systems, for vulvar melanoma,
    231–232, 232t
Minami, Y., 51
Minnesota Colon Cancer Control Study, 98
Mistletoe, 309
Mitchell, M. F., 178
Molecular genetics, colorectal carcinogenesis of, 88
Molecular markers. See also Biomarkers
    cancer screening and, 1
    of lung cancer risk, 40
Molecular risk assessment
    differentiation markers and, 230
    general genomic markers and, 230
    proliferation markers and, 230
    tumor markers and, 230
    of vulvar intraepithelial neoplasia (VIN), 230
Moller, R., 126
Monitoring the Future—the National Youth
    Tobacco Survey (MTF), 32
Monoterpenes
    breast cancer and, 314–315
    as complementary & alternative medicine
        (CAM), 310
Morgagni, John Baptist, 197
Mortality. See Cancer mortality
MPA. See Medroxyprogesterone acetate
MRI. See Magnetic resonance imaging
MTF. See Monitoring the Future—the National
    Youth Tobacco Survey
Mucosa, 69, 70, 71f
    hyperproliferation in, 80f
Mumps infection, ovarian cancer and, 254
Mundt, A. J., 267
Muscularis propria, 69, 71f
Mutated in colorectal cancer (MCC) genes, 88
Mutation carrier, 299

N
Narod, S. A., 256
NAT2 detoxifying enzymes, 15
National Cancer Institute, 39, 71, 73, 158, 204,
    206, 249, 267, 308
National Center for Complementary and
    Alternative Medicine (NCCAM), 307
National Health Interview Survey, tobacco use and,
    14, 18
National Household Survey on Drug Abuse, 14
National Institute on Drug Abuse (NIDA), 32
National Institutes of Health (NIH), 148, 274, 307
    Consensus Conference on cervical cancer, 148
National Society of Genetic Counselors, 298
National Youth Tobacco Survey (NYTS), 32
NCCAM. See National Center for Complementary
    and Alternative Medicine

Negative predictive value, of epidemiologic
  measurements, 6
Netherlands Cohort Study, 315
Newcomb, P. A., 51, 207, 208
Newmark, H. I., 108
Nicotine
  brain and, 20–21
  dopamine transmission and, 15–16
  pregnancy and, 29–30
  smoking behavior and, 15–16
Nicotine addiction, 19–20, 20–22
  adolescents and, 31, 34
  signs of, 21
  withdrawal from, 21
Nicotine replacement therapy (NRT), 23
  pregnancy and, 25
NIDA. *See* National Institute on Drug Abuse
NIH. *See* National Institutes of Health
Nitrosamines, as carcinogens, 16
NMSC. *See* Nonmelanoma skin cancer
Nonmelanoma skin cancer (NMSC), 122
  incidence rate of, 122
  mortality from, 122
  prevalence of, 122
Nonoccupational risks, lung cancer for, 17
Nonsteroidal anti-inflammatory drugs (NSAIDs)
  as colorectal chemoprevention, 107–108
  prostaglandin pathway inhibitors and, 37
NPCT. *See* Nutritional Prevention of Cancer Trial
NRT. *See* Nicotine replacement therapy
NSAIDs. *See* Nonsteroidal anti-inflammatory drugs
Nurses' Health Study
  on breast cancer, 52, 55, 56
  of colorectal cancer (CRC), 75, 76
Nutritional Prevention of Cancer Trial (NPCT),
  selenium and, 37
NYTS. *See* National Youth Tobacco Survey

O

OAM. *See* Office of Alternative Medicine
Obesity
  breast cancer and, 53, 55, 66
  endometrial cancer and, 272–273
  vulvar cancer and, 206
Occupational exposure, skin cancer and, 128
ODC. *See* Ornithine decarboxylase
Office of Alternative Medicine (OAM), 306, 307
Office of Cancer Complementary and Alternative
  Medicine (OCCAM), 308
Olive oil
  breast cancer and, 314–315
  as complementary & alternative medicine
    (CAM), 310
Olson, J. A., 66
Oltipraz, as colorectal chemoprevention, 110
Oncogenes, 77
  endometrial cancer and, 278
Oral contraceptives
  breast cancer and, 52
  cervical cancer and, 157–158
  endometrial cancer and, 275
  epithelial ovarian cancer and, 275

Oral contraceptives (*Continued*)
  melanoma and, 143
  ovarian cancer and, 255–256
  vaginal cancer and, 191
  vulvar cancer and, 207
Organochlorines, breast cancer and, 61–62
Ornithine decarboxylase (ODC), 109
Osteoporosis
  hormone replacement therapy and, 53
  raloxifene and, 63
Ovarian ablation, breast cancer and, 52
Ovarian cancer, 249–262. *See also* Epithelial
    ovarian carcinoma
  African-American women and, 249
  asbestos and, 254
  breast cancer and, 57
  dietary factors in, 252, 254
  early detection of, 259
  environmental factors in, 254–255
  genetic testing and, 252–254, 292, 293
  gynecologic surgery for, 255
  hormonal factors in, 251–252
  hysterectomy and, 255
  incidence of, 249–250
  industrial exposure and, 254
  lactose consumption and, 252
  lysophosphatidic acid (LPA) and, 261
  macrophage colony-stimulating factor (MCS-F)
    and, 261
  mumps infection and, 254
  oral contraceptives and, 255–256
  pelvic examination and, 259
  prevention of, 255
  prophylactic oophorectomy and, 256–258
  reproductive factors in, 251
  risk factors of, 250–251
  screening for, 259, 261, 262, 262f
  secondary prevention and, 259–262
  serum CA125 levels and, 260, 261
  staging of, 250, 250t
  surgery for, 255
  survival rates of, 249
  talc and, 254–255
  tobacco smoke and, 255
  ultrasound and, 259
Overdiagnosis bias
  in cancer screening, 9, 10–11
  lung cancer screening and, 39
Ovulation, 199
Oxford Family Planning Association contraceptive
    study, 275
Ozone layer
  chlorofluorocarbons (CFCs) and, 128
  skin cancer and, 127–128

P

p53 gene, 77, 88, 127, 152, 154, 270
Paget, Sir James, 233
Paget's disease, in vulva, 200–201
PAHs. *See* Polycyclic aromatic hydrocarbons
Palmer, J. R., 191
Panax ginseng, for colon cancer, 321

Papanicolaou, George, 165
Papanicolaou (Pap) test
    Bethesda system of, 167–170
    cervical cancer and, 150, 161–163, 165–170
    endocervical brush for, 167f
    endometrial cancer and, 282
    HIV-positive patient and, 176–177
    inaccuracies of, 166–170, 166b
    pregnant patient and, 179
    result classification of, 166b
    unsatisfactory smear of, 174, 174b
    for vaginal cancer, 192
    vulvar cancer and, 208
Parazzini, F., 205, 207
Parity, breast cancer and, 51
Pate v. Threlkel case, on duty to warn, 300–301
Pauerstein, C. J., 237
PC-SPES, 307
PCOS. See Polycystic ovary syndrome
Pearce, K. F., 192
Pelvic examination
    ovarian cancer and, 259
    vaginal cancer, 192
Penile carcinoma, human papillomavirus (HPV)
        and, 156
Perineural invasion, colorectal cancer (CRC) and,
        72
Peritoneal serous papillary carcinoma, prophylactic
        oophorectomy and, 258
Person-to-person intervention, in tobacco use
        cessation, 23, 24t, 25t
Peters, Ruth, 151
Peutz-Jeghers syndrome. See Hamartomatous
        polyposis syndromes
Pharmacologic therapies, for tobacco use cessation,
        24–25, 25t
Phoenix Colon Cancer Prevention Physicians'
        Network, 76
Photocarcinogenesis, ultraviolet radiation (UVR)
        and, 127
Photodynamic therapy, for vulvar intraepithelial
        neoplasia (VIN), 227, 229
Photoprotection. See Sunscreens
Physical activity, breast cancer and, 55–56
Physician Data Query (PDQ), 308
Physician intervention, for tobacco use cessation,
        26–27
Phytoestrogens
    for breast cancer, 313–314
    as complementary & alternative medicine
        (CAM), 309–310
Pike, Malcolm, 158
Placental complications, tobacco use and, 30
Polycyclic aromatic hydrocarbons (PAHs), as
        carcinogens, 16
Polycystic ovary syndrome (PCOS), 276
Population, of screening intervention, 9
Positive predictive value, of epidemiologic
        measurements, 6
Postmenopausal Estrogen/Progestin Interventions
        (PEPI) trial, 274
Potashnik, G., 53

Poverty, smoking prevalence and, 18–19
Prayer, 307
Prendiville, W., 178
President's Commission for Study of Ethical
        Problems in Medicine/Biomedical/Behavior
        Research, genetic testing and, 300
Prevention. See Cancer prevention; Primary
        prevention; Secondary prevention
Primary prevention, 289
    of breast cancer, 62
    of colorectal cancer (CRC), 106–111
    of skin cancer, 131–132
Privacy Act of 1974, genetic testing and, 298
Prochaska & DiClemente's Transtheoretical Model
        of Staged Change, tobacco use cessation and,
        26
Proctocolectomy
    familial adenomatous polyposis coli (FAP) and,
        91
    ulcerative colitis (UC) and, 95, 97
Proliferation lesions, breast cancer and, 53
Proliferation markers, chemoprevention and, 106
Proliferation zone, colorectal crypt of, 80, 80f
Prophylactic mastectomy
    breast cancer and, 62, 66
    simple mastectomy and, 62
    subcutaneous mastectomy and, 62
Prophylactic oophorectomy
    candidates for, 257
    indications for, 258
    ovarian cancer and, 256–258
    peritoneal serous papillary carcinoma and,
        258
    procedure for, 257
    risks of, 257
    unilateral, 257
Prophylactic vaccines
    cervical cancer and, 163–164
    for human papillomavirus (HPV), 163–164
Proposed screening strategy, evaluation of, 8–9
Prostaglandin pathway inhibitors
    chemoprevention and, 37–38
    COX-2 inhibitors and, 37–38
    cyclooxygenase inhibitors and, 37
    nonsteroidal anti-inflammatory drugs (NSAIDs)
        and, 37
Proto-oncogenes, 77
Pseudodisease. See Overdiagnosis bias
Psoralens phototherapy, skin cancer and, 129
Psychiatric disorders, smoking prevalence and,
        18–19
Psychosocial risks, of genetic testing, 299–300
PTEN tumor suppressor gene, 270
Pycnogenols, 309

R
Race, vulvar cancer and, 206
Radiation
    colorectal cancer (CRC) for, 71
    for vaginal intraepithelial neoplasia (VAIN),
        193–194
Ragnarsson-Olding, B. K., 232

Raloxifene
  breast cancer and, 63
  endometrial cancer and, 275
Ramani, M. L., 128
Ransohoff, D. F., 97
Rastkar, G., 203
Recessive traits, colorectal cancer (CRC) and, 73
Red meat, colorectal cancer (CRC) and, 75–76
Registry for Research on Hormonal Transplacental
    Carcinogenesis, 191
Relatives, affected, with breast cancer, 56, 56t
Reproductive cancers, pathogenesis of, 199, 200t
Reproductive history, vulvar cancer and, 207
Reproductive outcomes, tobacco use and, 29
Reproductive risk factors
  in breast cancer, 50–54, 50b
  in cervical cancer, 151
  for endometrial cancer, 270–272
  in ovarian cancer, 251
Retinoid receptors RAR/RXR, chemoprevention
    and, 36
Retinoids
  beta-carotene as, 36
  for breast cancer, 63, 310
  for cervical cancer, 164–165, 326
  chemoprevention and, 36–37
  as complementary & alternative medicine
      (CAM), 309
  for endometrial cancer, 324
  etretinate as, 36
  isotretinoin as, 36
  for lung cancer, 315–316
  retinol as, 36
  retinyl palmitate as, 36
  for skin cancer, 322–323
Retinol, 36
Retinyl acetate gel, for vulvar intraepithelial
    neoplasia (VIN), 227, 229
Retinyl palmitate, retinoids as, 36
Rex, D. K., 101
Ricci, E., 54
Richart, R. M., 199
Risk factors
  of breast cancer, 48–66, 50b
  for endometrial cancer, 270–278
  of extramammary Paget's disease (EMPD) of
      vulva, 236
  in lung cancer, 15–18
  for melanoma, 139–141
  of ovarian cancer, 250–251
  for skin cancer, 126–131
  for vaginal cancer, 190–191
  of vulvar cancer, 203–205
Rockhill, B., 56
Rodriquez, G. C., 256
Roswell Park Memorial Institute, 253
Rutledge F. D., 206, 208, 225

S
Safe sun guidelines, skin cancer and, 136b
Sappey, Philibert Constant, 197
SCC. *See* Squamous cell carcinoma

Science, 298
Screened individuals, 2
Scrotal malignancy, squamous cell carcinoma
    (SCC) and, 128
Seats & Causes of Diseases Investigated by Anatomy
    (Morgagni), 197
Secondary prevention, 289
  breast cancer and, 63–65
  ovarian cancer and, 259–262
  of skin cancer, 135
Secondary primary tumor (SPT), 36, 37
SEER. *See* Surveillance Epidemiology and End
    Results
Selby, J. V., 98
Selective estrogen receptor modulators (SERMS),
    275
Selenium
  for breast cancer, 313
  chemoprevention and, 37
  for colon cancer, 320
  as complementary & alternative medicine
      (CAM), 309
  for lung cancer, 317, 317t, 318t
  Nutritional Prevention of Cancer Trial (NPCT)
      and, 37
  for skin cancer, 322–323
Self-examination, for melanoma, 143
Serosa, 69, 70, 71f
Serum CA125 levels, ovarian cancer and, 260, 261
Sexual behavior
  cervical cancer and, 160–162
  vulvar cancer and, 207
Sexual risk factors, in cervical cancer, 151
Shapiro, S., 52
Shared decision making, genetic testing and, 297
Shark cartilage, 307, 309
Shiitake mushroom
  for colon cancer, 321
  as complementary & alternative medicine
      (CAM), 310
Sidestream smoke, lung cancer and, 17
SIDS. *See* Sudden infant death syndrome
Silverberg, S. G., 279
Silymarin, 309
Simple mastectomy, prophylactic mastectomy and,
    62
Simplex carcinoma in situ, 200
Sinclair, M., 225
Sirovich, B. E., 64
Skin cancer, 122–179. *See also* Melanoma
  arsenic and, 129
  beta-carotene for, 322–323
  chemoprevention of, 136
  childhood sun overexposure and, 131
  complementary & alternative medicine (CAM)
      for, 321–324, 322t
  essential minerals for, 323
  genetic/familial risk of, 130–131
  glutathione S-transferase 1 (GSTM1)
      and, 131
  Grenz-ray therapy and, 129
  high-risk individuals for, 135

Skin cancer (*Continued*)
  human papillomavirus (HPV) infection and, 130
  inducing agents of, 127t
  ionizing radiation and, 129
  management for patients with history of, 135
  occupational exposure and, 128
  ozone layer and, 127–128
  patient resources on, 144b
  premalignant lesion identification of, 132–133
  primary prevention of, 131–132
  psoralens phototherapy and, 129
  retinoids for, 322–323
  risk factors for, 126–131
  safe sun guidelines and, 136b
  screening for, 133
  secondary prevention of, 135
  selenium for, 322–323
  skin type and, 128
  smoking and, 129–130
  statistics on, 123t
  sunscreen use and, 131
  sunscreens, 133–135
  tanning history and, 128
  tar and, 129
  ultraviolet A phototherapy and, 129
  ultraviolet radiation (UVR) and, 126–127
  vitamin A for, 322, 323
  vitamin E for, 323
Skin phototypes
  skin cancer and, 128
  sun reactive, 133t
Skinner, M. S., 218
Skinning vulvectomy, 225, 226f, 227f, 228f
Smith, Harriet, 158
Smoking. *See also* Tobacco
  endometrial cancer and, 276
  skin cancer and, 129–130
  vulvar cancer and, 207
Smoking behavior
  genetics and, 15–16
  nicotine and, 15–16
Smoking cessation
  for adolescents, 34–35
  lung cancer risk and, 38
Smoking incidence, in adolescents, 32
Smoking interventions, 23
Smoking prevalence
  in adolescents, 32–33, 32t, 33t
  alcohol abuse and, 18–19
  education and, 18–19
  gender gap in, 13
  image advertising and, 12–13
  poverty and, 18–19
  pregnancy in, 29
  psychiatric disorders and, 18–19
  substance abuse and, 18–19
  in women, 12–13, 18–19
  from World War II, 13
Smoking prevention, for adolescents, 34
Smoking risk factors, for adolescents, 33
Socioeconomic factors, of vulvar cancer, 206–207

Soy
  breast cancer and, 314t
  phytoestrogens of, 307
  supplements of, 307
Specialized Center of Research in Hyperbaric Oxygen Therapy, at University of Pennsylvania, 307
SPF values, of sunscreens, 133
Spicer, Darcy, 158
Sporadic neoplasia, 90f
SPT. *See* Secondary primary tumor
Sputum cytology, lung cancer screening and, 39
Squamous cell carcinoma (SCC), 16, 122, 125f
  appearance of, 124
  cervical cancer and, 149
  human papillomavirus (HPV) infection and, 130
  incidence of, 124
  of lower lip, 126f
  metastatic risk of, 126
  scrotal malignancy and, 128
  vaginal cancer and, 190
  of vulva, 219f, 220f
  vulvar cancer and, 198f
  vulvar histologic section of, 199f
Standard chest radiography. *See* Traditional chest radiography (CXR)
Stern, R. S., 129
Subcutaneous mastectomy, prophylactic mastectomy and, 62
Submucosa, 69, 70, 71f
Substance abuse, smoking prevalence and, 18–19
Sudden infant death syndrome (SIDS), tobacco use and, 30–31
Sun-senstive skin types, melanoma and, 139
Sunscreens
  attenuation principles of, 133
  melanoma and, 143, 144
  skin cancer and, 131, 133–135
  SPF values of, 133, 134t
  UVB/UVA absorbing, 134t
Superior Court of New Jersey, on duty to warn, 301
Surgeon General's Report on Women and Smoking, 31
Surgery
  for cervical intraepithelial neoplasia (CIN), 177
  for colorectal cancer (CRC), 70–71
  for ovarian cancer, 255
  for vaginal intraepithelial neoplasia (VAIN), 193
  on vulvar cancer, 197
  for vulvar intraepithelial neoplasia (VIN), 222
Surveillance Epidemiology and End Results (SEER), 201, 206
  cervical cancer and, 158
  colorectal cancer (CRC) and, 71
  endometrial cancer and, 275
  endometrial cancer survival rates and, 267, 268t
  ovarian cancer and, 249
Survival rates
  cancer screening and, 9, 10
  of endometrial cancer, 267, 268t, 271–272
  of ovarian cancer, 249
  of vulvar cancer, 202–203, 203f

Susceptibility genes, colorectal cancer (CRC) and, 75

Susceptibility genes. *See* Recessive traits

Swedish National Cancer Registry, 232

Swedish National Data Inspection Authority, 232

Synthetic retinoid fenretinide, for breast cancer, 310–311

T

Talc, ovarian cancer and, 254–255

Tamoxifen, 66
    breast cancer and, 62–63
    endometrial cancer and, 62, 63, 275–276

Tanning history, skin cancer and, 128

Tar, skin cancer and, 129

Target population, of cancer screening, 2, 3, 9

Tarone, R., 206

Tart cherry, 307

Taussig, Frederick J., 197

Teens. *See* Adolescents

Tertiary prevention, 289

Thin Prep (TP) test, 169

Thune, I., 55

Tilanus-Linthorst, M. M. A., 65

TNM classification scheme. *See* Tumor-node-metastasis classification scheme

TNM staging system, for colorectal cancer (CRC), 71, 72t

Tobacco addiction, genetic polymorphisms and, 14

Tobacco cessation, 22–29
    AHRQ guidelines for, 23
    counseling and, 23
    dose-response relationship in, 23
    interventions for, 22–23
    person-to-person intervention in, 23, 24t, 25t
    pharmacologic therapies for, 24–25, 25t
    physician intervention for, 26–27
    Prochaska& DiClemente's Transtheoretical Model of Staged Change, 26
    relapse reasons in, 28
    success predictors for, 27–28
    weight gain and, 28

Tobacco exposure, cervical cancer and, 160–161

Tobacco smoke. *See also* Smoking
    carcinogens in, 16
    epidemiologic studies on, 13
    ovarian cancer and, 255

Tobacco use, 18–19
    adolescents and, 31–32
    cessation techniques and, 22–23
    colorectal adenocarcinomas and, 76
    by ethnic groups, 14
    hard-core smokers and, 20
    low-birth weight infants and, 30
    placental complications and, 30
    pregnancy and, 29–31
    quitting smoking and, 20
    reproductive outcomes and, 29
    smoking rates and, 20
    sudden infant death syndrome (SIDS) and, 30–31

Toronto Polyp Prevention Trial, 76

TP test. *See* Thin Prep test

Traditional chest radiography (CXR)
    lung cancer and, 38
    lung cancer screening and, 39

Transvaginal ultrasound (TVUS), endometrial cancer and, 282

Treating Tobacco Use and Dependence Clinical Practice Guideline, 23

Treponema pallidum, 207

True-negative screening test, 5, 8

True-positive screening test, 8

Tumor enhancement, gadolinium injection and, 65

Tumor markers, molecular risk assessment and, 230

Tumor-node-metastasis (TNM) classification scheme, for vulvar melanoma, 231

Tumor suppressor genes, 77, 78, 88, 278

Tumor thickness, of vulvar melanoma, 231

Turmeric, 309

TVUS. *See* Transvaginal ultrasound

U

U. S. Surgeon General's report, on smoking, 13

UC. *See* Ulcerative colitis

Ulcerative colitis (UC), 90f
    adenomatous polyposis coli (APC) and, 95
    APC gene mutation and, 95
    colonoscopy (CS) and, 97
    colorectal cancer (CRC) and, 95–97
    epithelial dysplasia histopathology of, 96f
    ileoanal anastomosis and, 95
    ileostomy and, 95
    proctocolectomy and, 95

Ultrasound
    ovarian cancer and, 259
    techniques of, 260, 260t

Ultraviolet radiation (UVR)
    melanoma and, 139–140
    photocarcinogenesis and, 127
    skin cancer and, 126–127

University of Texas, 307

Urosidal, as colorectal chemoprevention, 110

U.S. Public Health Service, 23

Uterine bleeding, endometrial cancer and, 279

Uterine corpus cancer. *See* Endometrial cancer

Uterine papillary serous carcinoma, endometrial cancer and, 283–284

UVR. *See* Ultraviolet radiation

V

Vaccine, for human papillomavirus (HPV), 192

Vaginal bleeding, abnormal, endometrial cancer and, 279

Vaginal cancer, 190–194
    cervical cancer and, 190
    chronic pessary trauma and, 191
    clear cell adenocarcinomas (CCA) and, 191
    diethylstilbestrol (DES) and, 191, 192
    etiology of, 190–191
    histological types of, 190
    human papillomavirus (HPV) and, 190, 192
    hysterectomy and, 191, 192

Vaginal cancer (*Continued*)
  incidence of, 190
  oral contraceptives and, 191
  Papanicolaou (Pap) test for, 192
  pelvic exams and, 192
  prevention for, 192
  risk factors for, 190–191
  screening for, 192
  squamous cell carcinoma (SCC) and, 190
  staging of, 190, 191t
  vaginal intraepithelial neoplasia (VAIN) and, 190
Vaginal intraepithelial neoplasia (VAIN)
  CO_2 laser vaporization for, 193
  5-fluorouracil (5-FU) for, 193
  human papillomavirus (HPV) and, 190
  management of, 193–194
  radiation for, 193–194
  surgery for, 193
  treatment for, 193–194, 194t
  vaginal cancer and, 190
VAIN. *See* Vaginal intraepithelial neoplasia
Vascular integrity, 307
Venn, A., 54
VIN. *See* Vulvar intraepithelial neoplasia
Virginia Slims cigarettes, 13, 32
Virtual colonoscopy (VCS)
  colorectal cancer (CRC) and, 102–103
  sensitivity of, 102–103
Vitamin A. *See also* Retinol
  for breast cancer, 310, 311
  for cervical cancer, 159, 326
  for colon cancer, 319
  as complementary & alternative medicine
      (CAM), 309
  for endometrial cancer, 324
  for lung cancer, 315–316
  for skin cancer, 322, 323
Vitamin B_{12}
  for breast cancer, 313
  as complementary & alternative medicine
      (CAM), 310
Vitamin C
  for breast cancer, 312
  for cervical cancer, 160, 326–327
  for colon cancer, 319
  as complementary & alternative medicine
      (CAM), 309
  for endometrial cancer, 324
  for lung cancer, 317
Vitamin D
  for breast cancer, 312–313
  as complementary & alternative medicine
      (CAM), 310
Vitamin E
  for breast cancer, 312
  for cervical cancer, 159, 327
  for colon cancer, 319
  as complementary & alternative medicine
      (CAM), 309
  for endometrial cancer, 324
  for lung cancer, 317
  for skin cancer, 323

Vitamins, for colon cancer, 319t
Vulva
  anatomy of, 198f
  biopsy of, 214, 214f
  lymphatics of, 197
  squamous cell carcinoma (SCC) of, 220f
Vulvar cancer, 197–239. *See also* Vulvar
      intraepithelial neoplasia (VIN)
  dietary risk factors and, 205
  early diagnosis/detection of, 200, 209
  etiology of, 197
  genital tract infections and, 207
  geographic distribution of, 205
  human papillomavirus (HPV) and, 197,
      203–204, 220
  immunosuppressive diseases and, 208
  malignant melanoma and, 231
  obesity and, 206
  oral contraceptives and, 207
  Papanicolaou testing frequency and, 208
  pathogenesis of, 199, 200t
  race and, 206
  reproductive history and, 207
  risk factors of, 203–205
  sexual behavior and, 207
  smoking and, 207
  socioeconomic factors, 206–207
  squamous cell carcinoma (SCC) and, 198f
  staging of, 201–202
  studies on, 221t, 222t
  superficially invasive, 218f
  surgery on, 197
  survival rates of, 202–203, 203f
  symptoms of, 209
Vulvar carcinoma in situ (CIS), 209, 210, 211, 213,
      215, 217
Vulvar cervical intraepithelial neoplasia (CIN)
  cryosurgery for, 228
  treatment of, 222–230
Vulvar intraepithelial neoplasia (VIN), 199, 204
  acetic acid application and, 209, 213f, 223
  anoscopy and, 213
  antiviral agents for, 227, 228b
  biopsy of, 214, 214f
  carbon dioxide laser vaporization therapy for,
      222–227, 227
  cidofovir for, 230
  clinical examination of, 209, 211–212
  clinical presentation of, 209–214, 210f, 211f, 212f
  cryosurgery for, 227, 228b
  dinitrochlorobenzene (DNCB) for, 227
  5-fluorouracil (5-FU) for, 227–228
  functional morbidities of, 227
  herpes simplex virus (HSV) and, 204
  histology of, 214–217, 215f, 216f, 217f
  invasive cancer incidence and, 201
  loop electrosurgical excision & fulguration
      procedure (LEEP) and, 224
  management algorithm for, 224, 225f
  molecular risk assessment of, 230
  multifocal nature of, 209–213
  natural history of, 217–222

Vulvar intraepithelial neoplasia (VIN) (*Continued*)
  nonsurgical approaches to, 227, 228b
  photodynamic therapy for, 227, 229
  postoperative care and, 224
  retinyl acetate gel for, 227, 229
  surgical procedure for, 222, 225, 226f, 227, 227f
  symptoms of, 209
  terminology of, 200
  treatment of, 222–230
  vulvar biopsy and, 214, 214f
  vulvectomy for, 224
Vulvar melanoma, 234f
  low skin pigmentation and, 233
  microstaging systems for, 231–232, 232t
  pathogenesis of, 233
  preexisting nevus and, 233
  presenting symptoms of, 233
  quality of life and, 233
  superficial spreading melanoma and, 231
  tumor-node-metastasis (TNM) classification
      scheme for, 231
  tumor thickness of, 231

Vulvectomy, 197
  risks of, 224
  skinning, 225, 226f, 227f, 228f
  for vulvar intraepithelial neoplasia (VIN), 224

W

Wagner, J. L., 101
Weight gain, tobacco use cessation and, 28
Weitraub, I., 229
Western New York Diet Study, 277
White women, with breast cancer, 49
WHO. *See* World Health Organization
Winawer, S. J., 100
Women's Health Initiative, 274
Women's mortality, from lung cancer, 12
Woodruff, J. D., 219, 225, 234, 237
World Health Organization (WHO), 252, 306

Z

Zerbe, M. J., 281
Ziegler, A., 127
Zur Hausen, H., 151